Library of Congress Cataloging-in-Publication Data

Griffin, John C., author.
 [Client-centered exercise prescription]
 Client-centered exercise prescription with web resource / John C. Griffin. -- Third edition.
    p. ; cm.
 Preceded by Client-centered exercise prescription / John C. Griffin. 2nd ed. c2006.
 Includes bibliographical references and index.
 ISBN 978-1-4504-5332-5
 I. Title.
 [DNLM: 1. Exercise. 2. Exercise Movement Techniques. 3. Exercise Therapy. 4. Patient-Centered Care. 5. Physical
Fitness--physiology. QT 255]
 RM725
 613.7'1--dc23
                            2014013410

ISBN: 978-1-4504-5332-5 (print)

The web addresses cited in this text were current as of October 2014, unless otherwise noted.

Acquisitions Editor: Diana Vincer; **Developmental Editor:** Judy Park; **Managing Editor:** Derek Campbell; **Assistant
Editor:** Tyler Wolpert; **Copyeditor:** Joyce Sexton; **Proofreader:** Anne Rumery; **Indexer:** Sharon Duffy; **Permissions
Manager:** Dalene Reeder; **Graphic Designer:** Dawn Sills; **Cover Designer:** Keith Blomberg; **Photograph (cover):** ©
Human Kinetics; **Photographs (interior):** © Human Kinetics, unless otherwise noted; **Photo Asset Manager:** Laura
Fitch; **Visual Production Assistant:** Joyce Brumfield; **Photo Production Manager:** Jason Allen; **Art Manager:** Kelly
Hendren; **Associate Art Manager:** Alan L. Wilborn; **Illustrations:** © Human Kinetics, unless otherwise noted;
Printer: Sheridan Books

Printed in the United States of America   10 9 8 7 6 5 4 3 2 1

The paper in this book is certified under a sustainable forestry program.

Human Kinetics
Website: www.HumanKinetics.com

United States: Human Kinetics
P.O. Box 5076
Champaign, IL 61825-5076
800-747-4457
e-mail: humank@hkusa.com

Canada: Human Kinetics
475 Devonshire Road Unit 100
Windsor, ON N8Y 2L5
800-465-7301 (in Canada only)
e-mail: info@hkcanada.com

Europe: Human Kinetics
107 Bradford Road
Stanningley
Leeds LS28 6AT, United Kingdom
+44 (0) 113 255 5665
e-mail: hk@hkeurope.com

Australia: Human Kinetics
57A Price Avenue
Lower Mitcham, South Australia 5062
08 8372 0999
e-mail: info@hkaustralia.com

New Zealand: Human Kinetics
P.O. Box 80
Torrens Park, South Australia 5062
0800 222 062
e-mail: info@hknewzealand.com

E5946

To my wife, who is my journey to now,
along an active road, ever mindful of our joy

Mary

To my son, who carves a path of adventure from the shifting sands
of life and leaves those close to him feeling cared for

Jay

To my daughter, whose body is her temple,
whose soul is her goodness, and whose spirit is her passion

Laura

To my parents, who shared with unconditional love the values most
sought in life: compassion, respect, responsibility, and fairness

Gord and Ruth

Contents

Form Finder

(continued)

(continued)

Preface

The third edition of *Client-Centered Exercise Prescription* substantially expands prescription theory and applications and is easy to use as a resource or as a primary course textbook. This edition maintains the previous edition's emphasis on the individual client and broadens the usual scope of books on this subject from exercise prescription alone to activity counseling, design modification, exercise demonstration, functionally integrated exercise, injury prevention, and follow-up monitoring for a variety of clients. Central to the book are seven models that present the skills involved in counseling, prescription, and working with clients. Each model serves as a template that provides a menu of options for each decision in the prescription process. The theory and application required for making informed, client-centered decisions are provided following each model. These models cover the client-centered approach to

- activity counseling,
- musculoskeletal exercise design,
- exercise demonstration,
- cardiovascular exercise prescription,
- resistance training prescription,
- muscle balance and flexibility prescription, and
- weight management prescription.

Included in the third edition are simple design tools (worksheets) to facilitate the flow from the prescription models to the prescription cards. In effect, the worksheets provide a transition for the trainer to easily move from the specific questions in the model to the applied prescription on the card.

What Does "Client Centered" Mean?

Like the first two editions, the third recognizes that exercise prescription is about helping people adopt, enjoy, and maintain an active lifestyle. How well we help our clients do this is the true measure of our success. Having knowledge of exercise sciences, having technical skills, and having a fit body do not guarantee success in one-on-one training. Thus, this text continues to feature an unusually personalized approach for anyone who prescribes exercise: It takes clients off the assembly line and establishes them as the center of decision making. You will discover that counseling is a central concern of this book. I do not intend to suggest that the personal fitness trainer should be a psychological therapist. I use the term to refer simply to the art of listening intently to client feedback and modifying the program appropriately. It is not a simple art, but it is essential to develop if one is to be the best trainer possible. This art is also achievable, and this text makes clear in many ways and on many levels how this type of activity counseling can be learned.

As shown in figure 1, the prescription process is a journey taken by the personal fitness trainer and client along a road leading to a uniquely tailored and progressive program of activity. Each stage of the journey has its own set of client-centered outcomes. This book will guide you, as an exercise specialist or personal trainer, in what questions to ask, what interventions to use, and what decisions to make along the way. The text challenges you to provide far more than a list of exercises. It will guide you through the stages of training, each characterized by "counseling"— that is, carefully listening to client feedback and modifying the path as necessary in response.

Parts I and II of the book follow from foundations to applications of exercise prescription. The process begins with an inquiry from someone who needs help. Every time we take on a client, we encounter a new set of circumstances, a new personality, a new history, and a new journey. The first challenge is to get a clear picture of the client's history, needs, and hopes for achievement. This picture will develop, and perhaps change, as our relationship progresses. Determining the client's level of commitment to change will help you know how to help him move to the next level. The counseling must challenge the client to create clear priorities for measurable and progressive objectives. More detailed information is gathered through the selective assessment of physical fitness. Without some physiological parameters to set prescription factors or monitor progress, we can use only broad guidelines that are not specific to our client's needs.

Next in the design process we select appropriate exercises, from a wide menu of choices, according to how they fit our client's goals. We can prescribe exercise programs to produce three potential outcomes: increased general fitness, performance improvements, or health enhancement. A variety of training methods allow us to match specific benefits to specific clients. The client's own preferences and availability of equipment will also influence our prescription. The details of the personalized exercise prescription are based on two main criteria: the physiological rationale and the needs of the client.

As to the client, she needs to see the exercises demonstrated and then try them with some expert feedback. The exercise may need to be modified or the dosage reset. The follow-up program demonstration, along with the type of monitoring designed into the program, can strongly affect the client's motivation and self-esteem and ultimately determine the client's adherence to the program.

Who Should Read This Book?

In recent years, a number of factors have encouraged a shift toward more client-centered exercise prescription. First, understanding of the effects of physical activity on human health and aging has advanced and has increased the knowledge and skill base for exercise specialists, which has increased the demand for competent practitioners. Second, fitness consumers want specific results, more choices, and guidance about where and how to exercise; they also want service along with prescriptions. Third, personal fitness trainers are increasing in number and are establishing new employment opportunities in private, clinical, and community sectors.

As one of these professionals—perhaps you are a clinical kinesiologist, a personal trainer, a strength training coach, or a fitness specialist in a private or community setting or retirement facility—you no doubt recognize the scarcity of available resources. This text is written for you. Physical therapists, athletic trainers, chiropractors, professors, activationists (gerontology), and physical educators will also benefit from it. This text draws on applied exercise physiology, the art of counseling, and personal experience to provide skills that will help you prescribe and administer safe, effective, and enjoyable activities for your clients. Practical examples, applied models, and background scientific knowledge make the text well suited for undergraduate health and fitness courses such as those in physical activity, health, biophysical sciences, or theory of conditioning and training methods. The text may also be used in conjunction with a traditional exercise physiology or exercise science course. It provides

- a bridge between industry practices and recent literature;
- a reliable method of matching client priorities with appropriate prescription factors; and
- specific examples, models, and case studies that demonstrate the skills of prescription.

A critical career step for many fitness employees and exercise science students is a personal training certification. *Client-Centered Exercise Prescription, Third Edition,* is a primary resource for candidates preparing for the Canadian Society for Exercise Physiology's Certified Personal Trainer (CSEP-CPT) certification practical and written examinations. It provides comprehensive treatment of the theory and applications covering more than 90% of the competencies needed for the CSEP-CPT and spans most of the requirements of other American and Canadian personal training certifications. The text will help you develop your confidence with the application of the knowledge and skills and contribute to your success on the certification exams.

Of particular note are several learning aids that you will find throughout the text. At the start of each chapter the expected competencies are listed. Greater emphasis is placed on sequenced learning, starting from a prescription model and proceeding to a case sample that includes detailed design justifications from a physiological and client-centered perspective. This progression highlights matching client priorities with appropriate prescription applications. Many chapters contain highlight boxes, which are summaries of the scientific basis of the applied material. The text also contains many forms and charts that you will find useful to copy and have at hand for

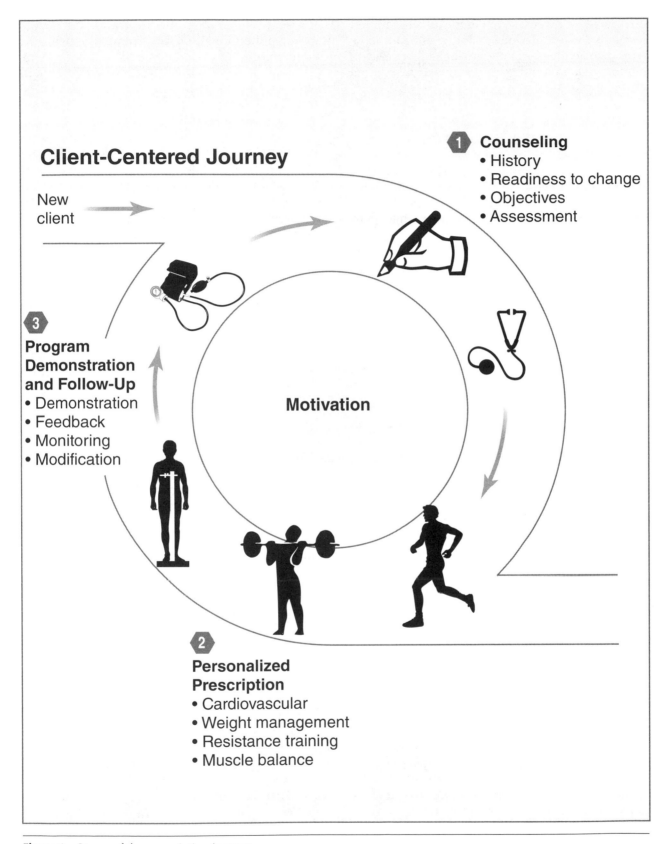

Client-Centered Journey

New client

1 Counseling
- History
- Readiness to change
- Objectives
- Assessment

3

Program Demonstration and Follow-Up
- Demonstration
- Feedback
- Monitoring
- Modification

Motivation

2

Personalized Prescription
- Cardiovascular
- Weight management
- Resistance training
- Muscle balance

Figure 1   Stages of the prescription journey.

direct use; an extensive list of recent and applied research in the references; and exercise photos with instructions formatted to make them easy to photocopy and hand out to clients as take-home visual and textual aids.

Online Resource

A web resource, available at www.HumanKinetics. com/ClientCenteredExercisePrescription3E, provides the forms found in this book in an easy-to-print format. They are organized by chapter to assist you with locating the forms that you need for each stage of working with your client. The forms in this book have been carefully prepared to help you gather the key information you need to help your clients succeed in reaching their fitness goals.

What Is New in the Third Edition?

This third edition of *Client-Centered Exercise Prescription* expands the scope and facilitates the application of new and established knowledge of effective training and client motivation. It continues with the practical client-centered approach through simulated initial client interview, teaching cues for demonstration, a sample of the first two sessions, more counseling dialogue, a team approach to scope of practice, and personality and learning style integration. It also continues with a practical skill approach using effective tools for personal fitness trainers. The number of reproducible forms has doubled to over 40, and this toolbox of forms is now included in a web resource. Included are simpler design tools (worksheets) to facilitate the flow from the prescription models to the prescription cards. The expanded and more detailed table of contents and index and new chapter summaries make it easy to find what you are looking for. The text includes five new case studies and other case study additions or updates; many new special elements, exercises, and graphs; and an updated reference list.

In terms of content, this edition has continued to focus on practical and reliable field tests, introducing Cook's Functional Movement Screen, Rikli and Jones' Senior Fitness Test, and the older adult Functional Mobility Screening Tool. Within

the scope of practice of the trainer, it covers more applied nutrition, for example, nutritional concerns for active clients and the recent U.S. and Canadian guidelines. It discusses new small equipment for cardiovascular and resistance training and offers more on exercise modification and progressions with a unique biomechanics approach to principles of modifications and functional progressions. Chapter 8 on functionally integrated exercise recognizes that we need to treat the human body as a highly integrated structure instead of a series of independent parts. Functionally integrated exercise is presented as an approach that will improve any performance, reduce the risk of overuse injuries, address muscle imbalances, and allow trainers to be more creative in their exercise design. Updates on injury prevention and recovery include information on delayed-onset muscle soreness, neuromuscular progression, tennis elbow, core stability, safety and referrals, and many new exercises.

Perhaps the most notable scope expansion is the addition of three new chapters on the older client in part III: "Exercise Prescription for Injuries and Older Adults." This retains the valuable resource on exercise prescription for clients recovering from or having a history of orthopedic injury but contains many new exercise designs for stretching and strengthening. However, talk to anyone over 50 and you will hear laments about how long it takes to recover from an injury. The first of the new chapters (chapter 12) addresses this and other exercise considerations for musculoskeletal conditions. Chapter 13 is a comprehensive discussion of successful aging, physiological changes, and the effects of specific exercise or activity prescriptions for the wide range of clients in this demographic. The final chapter focuses on functional mobility and aging, identifying causes, providing screening tools, and applying functional exercise design principles.

Client-Centered Exercise Prescription, Third Edition, is a front-line resource that will help you focus on the individual in creating your initial prescriptions and in following up with service excellence. Whether used for learning the essentials of exercise prescription and personal training or preparing for a certification examination, *Client-Centered Exercise Prescription, Third Edition,* is a valuable reference.

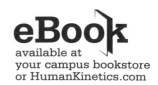

eBook available at your campus bookstore or HumanKinetics.com

Acknowledgments

My personal gratification from the work on this text was much greater with the involvement of my family and friends. Mary, my talented wife, was not only my artistic advisor but always a voice for relevance.

I am very happy to have maintained the wonderful images of my daughter, Laura; my sister, Gail Collins; and my good friend, John Villiers while capturing new images from an outstanding Human Kinetics team during my visit to Champaign.

I would also like to acknowledge my students over the years at George Brown College and in particular those who modeled for the book. It was the need for such a text that first emerged from the Fitness Program, and it was the students, my colleagues, and clients at the college that fueled many of the practical anecdotes.

Finally, my experiences with Human Kinetics during all editions have been a delightful learning environment thanks to an outstanding, dedicated, and caring team of professionals.

Introduction

The best salespeople tell us that the first step in making a sale is to find out what consumers need or perceive themselves as needing. Similarly, a big part of what we do is to help clients "buy in" to their exercise. If we act merely as experts, our success will be limited. Preaching the merits of fitness can create a frenzy of activity in our clients that can die out just as quickly as it began. Our first job is not to preach—it is to listen. We must hear what the people we are serving say to us. Our clients need our attention and our guidance, especially at the beginning of their commitment.

Several years ago, I invited a colleague to present a guest lecture on counseling skills for exercise prescription to my students at George Brown College. After I introduced her, she said, "For the next 15 minutes, I am your client." This was followed by a very long and awkward silence. Finally, a student said, "But we don't know anything about you." Of course, that was the whole point! Very quickly the floodgate of questions opened, and the students and the guest were well on their way.

Clients constitute the starting point of the prescription and training process. Rather than trying too early to design a solution, we must help our clients empower themselves by working with them to identify and develop their underused potential. Program designs are not ends in themselves. Our role is to formulate the right questions and choices and to provide the pros and cons from the clients' perspective and help them develop the skills to become independent exercisers. We cannot help anyone we do not understand. So we must listen before we talk, keep listening, and remember that the journey to helping clients has many options for rerouting and that the map is in our clients' hands.

All too often in our exercise prescription, we limit ourselves by selecting or designing exercises that only suit the equipment we have in the facility or that follow traditional fitness components (e.g., strength or aerobics) rather than real client concerns. By taking a client-centered approach, we partner with our clients during the counseling stage to collect information or assess their personal interests and needs. In this way, we are better able to effectively and precisely prescribe exercise that addresses the complex issues that each client presents, such as fatigue, aches, tightness, joint pain, lack of energy, and body image.

Each client represents a new journey. Even if the choices are similar, the perspective of each client is different. This difference creates the challenge and the joy of exercise prescription and exercise-centered health care. It calls for us to become skilled not only in the science but also in the art of exercise prescription, and it is the reason why we all must be client centered.

PART I

Foundations of Client-Centered Exercise Prescription

Many new clients start out with the best of intentions but quickly find that change is difficult. They find reasons to avoid their daily workout or their session at the gym. They may want to exercise more or lose weight, but when the day is full and stressful, it is hard to tie up the laces and head out. So people get discouraged and perhaps, as in the past, feel as though they tried and failed again. Although they believe they want to change their lifestyle to include more activity, somehow the shift doesn't happen.

The problem is that these clients have not even reached the point of being ready to adopt regular exercise. Activity and exercise are vague terms to them. Their idea of what is involved and even what they really want to achieve may not be well formed in their minds and is far from concrete. For these clients, before you can even consider designing an exercise prescription, you must change how they think about exercise. Your focus should be not only on fitness improvement (such as weight loss or improved strength) but also on a heightened awareness of personal fitness benefits and their own confidence that they can succeed. For example, discussing how far or how fast a client walks should emphasize the encouraging point that walking provides stress relief and higher energy levels; when walking is a regular habit, positive health benefits will accrue.

But success with such clients is more than a matter of enthusiasm and pep talks. To motivate them you must, in the first stage of your journey, create a rapport through which your clients learn to trust you and develop confidence in your competence. Such rapport will free clients to discuss frankly both their present situation and their vision of the future. It will also allow you to help them clarify their experiences so they can better understand themselves.

The techniques you use for discovery and self-exploration will vary with the client's personality, but they will always include effective questioning and probing to determine the client's needs, wants, and lifestyle. The areas in which a need and a want coincide and lifestyle is compatible are the areas with the greatest potential for success. Understanding your client's history through intelligent and empathetic listening will enable you to set priorities and formulate an effective motivational strategy.

In the first stage of the journey, we encounter a new set of circumstances, a new personality, a new history, and perhaps a new set of obstacles. To motivate our clients, we can use the change process strategies, presented in chapter 2, that are appropriate at each stage of change. This will help clients recognize the personal relevance of the message and understand how it fits with their personal needs. The counseling must challenge the client to create clear priorities for measurable and progressive objectives. More detailed information is gathered through the selective assessment of physical fitness, allowing us to set prescription factors specific to our client's needs. Basic prescription principles including specificity, individuality, and progression will help you design balanced, safe programs that are modified to suit your client.

In preparation for personalized exercise prescription, we must be able to analyze various exercises, sport skills, and work tasks. Chapter 5 outlines a process for anatomical analysis of exercise that allows us to select or modify the exercise by recognizing the joint movements, muscles used, and types of contraction. Applying other prescription principles can optimize exercise benefits for our clients and at the same time attend to their limitations through alterations of the exercise. A final safety check can identify high risk in the design and later in the execution. The person-to-person demonstration of an exercise combines our counseling skills and technical knowledge, allowing us to teach and modify each movement. Features included in the text like an initial client interview, case studies, and a sample of the first two sessions with a client help to bridge the gap between theory and the real skills and the confidence you will need to be client centered in your training.

This is the foundation of client-centered exercise prescription, and part I will give you the tools to build it.

Activity Counseling Model

Chapter Competencies

After completing this chapter, you will be able to demonstrate the following competencies:

1. Apply the three steps of the Activity Counseling Model.
2. Apply strategies, skills, and tools to establish rapport with your client.
3. Apply strategies, skills, and tools to gather client information.

4. Apply strategies, skills, and tools to work effectively with the stages of change.
5. Apply effective questioning and the Activity Counseling Model to establish measurable objectives in a client interview.

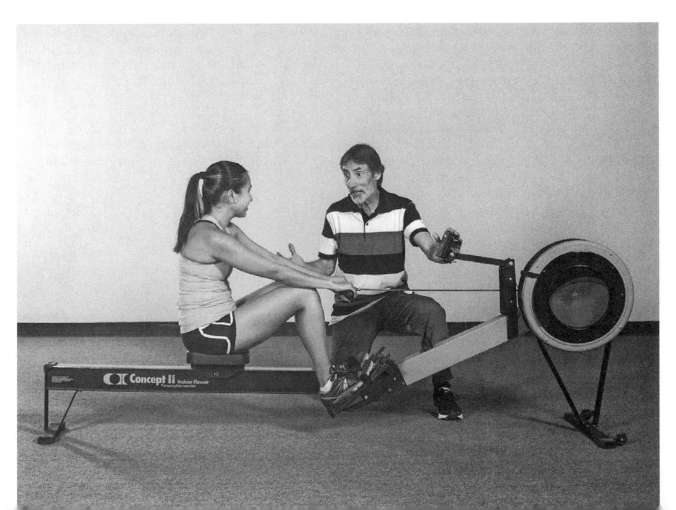

It was my first year teaching at the college. I had completed my graduate work, was running a fitness consulting business, and was up for any challenge when it came to designing conditioning programs. The word traveled quickly around the college that we were setting up a new employee fitness program, and before the doors were open I had received many calls, one from a staff member in the admissions office. Suzanne was in her mid-40s and wanted some help but was too self-conscious to go to the fitness center. With a naive desire to help, I jumped into the case. I explained that we started with a series of assessments and that then I would interpret the data and design a home program for her. The home program sounded fine, but Suzanne didn't want anything to do with the assessment. Although preprogram assessment was a standard approach I had always used with my practice and was the procedure that I was teaching my students, I told Suzanne that I would still design a program. During our first meeting, she seemed as cautious as I was impetuous. The meeting was brief, but I came out with the impression that she wanted something that was short, was easy to do at home, and would help her lose weight and tone her upper body. Armed with this I worked that night on what I thought was an effective program that combined skipping with a series of biomechanically modified exercises designed to tone her body. She was apprehensive about using any equipment, so I designed several creative movements lifting soup cans to strengthen her arms. The next day, I went to her area at lunch to demonstrate the exercises. She was unable to participate, but I enthusiastically went through each exercise for her. Her response seemed ho-hum, but I had classes and just left the program card with her. About 2 weeks later I ran into Suzanne coming in to work and asked her how the program was going. She discreetly pulled me over and explained that she had incontinence after giving birth to three children and that jumping up and down was not something she could do. As for the soup can lifts, they were hurting her shoulder. After two sessions she stopped doing the program. Even more disheartening were her comments that nothing seemed to work for her, and, despite my offer, she did not want a new program. I knew that I had failed Suzanne and vowed from that point to serve my clients more than simply design programs.

Recently, we were having an open house for an expansion of our employee fitness center and one of my staff introduced me to Marg, a woman from our college's human resources department who had called earlier for a private meeting. She had told my colleague that she was hypertensive and overweight and had been sedentary since her college days, 20 years earlier. I was concerned that she did not want to come to the center, but I wanted to support any desire to become more active. We talked about her past experiences that she saw as failed opportunities. As we continued, several doors opened as she shared her feelings about gyms, embarrassments, and more recent health concerns. I knew it was important to gain her trust and reinforce the benefits of following through on these early intentions. Marg's last medical exam had given her a bit of a scare, and she was looking for the connection between exercise and her high blood pressure. Despite some progress, she was still not comfortable exercising in the center with students and other fit staff. I walked away from that first meeting with a sense that we had connected and that Marg had a renewed hope of reaching her goals. Subsequent meetings over the next few weeks were shorter, but each seemed to bring us closer to determining what Marg wanted to do and getting a commitment from her. Our program was planning its annual hike, and I invited Marg to come along. It was a comfortable setting; she now knew some of our staff, and I assured her that there were routes for all levels. She accepted the invitation and walked with one of our senior students. By the end of the day, Marg had linked up with her new friend as her personal trainer! Marg hired our student (graduate) over the summer and now is being trained by a new student through regular attendance in the fitness center.

What made the difference between Marg's success and the failure to affect Suzanne's health and quality of life? The two women had similar histories, health problems, and anxiety about public exercise. In both cases a sincere effort was made to help. Why did Marg eventually take responsibility for her health and become an enthusiastic convert to fitness? The difference was in the focus, which was always on Marg's well-being. With Suzanne, I had been preoccupied with assessment, prescription, and getting on with the exercise regimen before establishing a commitment. There was little rapport, critical pieces of information were not gathered, her activity intentions were not clear, and my prescription did not meet her needs.

Client-Centered Approach

This book is about taking the "client-centered" approach. This approach involves more than having the knowledge and skills of an assessor or program designer. In fact, it involves more than caring and wanting to help. But if you can use these characteristics as part of a client-centered approach, then you will be able to experience constant and rewarding success. We are always challenged to find ways to help our clients whether they are young athletes, professional people, community members, or older adults. Fitness programming often feels like an endless pursuit of the newest techniques and latest equipment. However, with the client-centered approach, your success will come from integrating the mosaic of applied experiences in this text with the unique physical, emotional, and social needs of each client. This book will allow you to put together the client-centered models and skill sets needed to help your clients achieve personal satisfaction and success.

Counseling skills are essential for anyone with aspirations to clinical practice. Learning how to talk to your client and what to talk about is one of the most difficult skills to acquire for a personal fitness trainer. Your job as an "activity counselor" is to help clients take charge of their own exercise regimens. You help them pursue their own objectives, whether these are an active lifestyle, recovery from injuries, or better athletic performance. By careful listening and empathetic conversation, you encourage your clients to tell their stories. Effective questioning helps you gather sufficient information and assemble a history for each client. The value of the final prescription depends on how well you empower clients to plan personal strategies to set priorities for their actions—priorities that will satisfy their needs and wants within the limitations of their lifestyle. This kind of structured activity counseling can make a difference. A recent Canadian study has shown that the addition of a physical activity counselor to the primary health care team providing six patient-centered counseling sessions over 3 months produced significantly higher levels of physical activity (Fortier et al. 2011). Others have found that those receiving exercise counseling were more likely to report positive behavioral changes and increases in exercise duration (Duffy and Schnirring 2000). The benefits of counseling interventions have been well documented in the health care field (Sotile 1996). Several similar counseling models are based on fundamental problem solving (Wheeler 2000). For more than a decade, the Canadian physical activity, fitness, and lifestyle approach (Canadian Society for Exercise Physiology [CSEP] 2003) has been used to train thousands of fitness consultants using a multiple-step counseling strategy. The Activity Counseling Model is designed to prepare activity specialists or personal trainers to counsel their client toward goals and strategies of increased personal physical activity.

The Activity Counseling Model is based on three steps:

1. Create a **rapport** that allows openness to new information through effective conversation.

2. **Gather information** through effective questioning to identify your client profile and determine the client's degree of commitment to change.

3. Use **strategies for behavioral change** that are designed to increase your client's perceptions of personal control through effective strategic planning.

The Activity Counseling Model retains the rapport-building and information-gathering steps from earlier similar models (CSEP 2003; Wheeler 2000) but expands on the skills and tools for each step. The stages and strategies for change become a focal point for the client's behavioral change (Prochaska et al. 1992). Physical assessment and activity planning steps, although part of the strategy that is built from the counseling, are not core elements in the process of behavioral change. Thirty years of clinical, consulting, and teaching experience have led me to the undeniable conclusion that this three-step Activity Counseling Model is simple to use, natural in its progression, and effective in providing a framework for activity counselors.

Personal characteristics and attitudes or beliefs about fitness and lifestyle are the basis for the counseling style that naturally evolves. By recognizing different counseling styles, you can respond more appropriately to different clients in different situations. A skilled personal fitness trainer will be able to use the appropriate counseling style depending on the client, his needs, and the situation. In one-on-one counseling, a personal fitness trainer or lifestyle coach will often need to switch hats several times within a single session. The highlight box "Counseling Styles" defines some of the more commonly used counseling styles. In table 1.1, consider the following four types of clients you may encounter and the counseling style(s) that would be most effective.

Table 1.1 Clients and Counseling Styles

Type of client		Counseling style
Unable and insecure	Reluctant and somewhat unwilling; no previous knowledge or experience; may have been told to attend.	Activity counselor provides specific instructions (e.g., what, how, when, where). Follow-up is important. [Primary style: Director]
Unable but confident	Client lacks experience and knowledge but is willing; may have never exercised before; has a goal in mind.	Activity counselor provides support and encouragement and two-way communication; explains why, helps in decisions and goal setting, and helps the client "buy-in" to the new behavior. [Mixture of styles: Counselor, Educator, Preacher]
Able but insecure	Client has experience or knowledge but is not confident to stay with it; may have relapsed.	Activity counselor facilitates decisions, shares ideas, and listens in a nondirecting, supportive way. [Primary style: Counseling, with possible times for soft Preaching]
Able and confident	Client has abundance of experience, knowledge, and integration skills; has high desire to achieve; is dedicated and willing to take responsibility.	Activity counselor takes a low-profile, delegating stance. May identify problems but leave the responsibility of action to the client. [Lesser role needed; use an emergent style, i.e., the style most appropriate for that moment]

Counseling Styles

- **Preacher.** The preacher often delivers minilectures on healthy behaviors, describing to the client what she should be doing. A judgmental lecture will ruin the establishment of any rapport, but the endorsement of positive choices and practical advice may be an effective way to respond to a client's question. This style may infuse energy into the session and reinforce some behaviors.

- **Director.** The director gives instructions or specific prescriptive guidance. The design and demonstration of the exercise prescription are an appropriate use of this style. This style does not exclude slipping into the counseling role to get a client's input. Directors should be aware that clients need to explore and dialogue about personal lifestyle preferences.

- **Educator.** An educator provides relevant information about health and fitness to facilitate decisions about behavioral change. Some clients feel reassured when information comes from an expert. At times, an educator may provide written material; keep the information short and readable and make sure your client is interested in receiving it.

- **Counselor.** A counselor uses a collaborative problem-solving approach to help clients make informed decisions. This will be the style of choice most often throughout counseling. As new issues and interests evolve during training, this is also an effective style to implement action plans and change strategies. Counselors still need structure and direction to the process but the focus is on the needs of the client.

Within the Activity Counseling Model, you may be more likely to use the counselor style to establish strategies for change (step 3, table 1.2); however, gathering information (step 2) may be more efficiently done as a director. It is important to engage in interactive rather than didactic communication. To be most effective, you will have to empower your clients to take control of the process, to learn for themselves, and to engage actively in the activity counseling.

In addition to the style of counseling employed, the nature of the communication needs to be applied with some informed flexibility. Establishing rapport (step 1) involves the creation of a real and sustained relationship with your client. The counseling skills and tools needed for this are fundamental to all healthy relationships, and the nature of the communication is best described as conversational. For step 2 (gathering information), the counseling skills and tools are most effectively

Table 1.2   Activity Counseling Model, Skills, and Tools

Counseling steps	Counseling skills and tools
Step 1: Establish rapport • Create a friendly welcome: Be receptive and responsive • Discuss the counseling process and the reason for attending • Ensure you have received your client's messages	Conversational: • Nonverbal skills • Active listening skills • Supportive communication
Step 2: Gather information • Examine past, present, and future • Identify needs, wants, and lifestyle • Determine your client's stage of change	Questioning: • Form 1.1 FANTASTIC Lifestyle Checklist • Form 1.2 Inventory of Lifestyle and Activity Preferences • Form 1.3 Gathering Information Interview Worksheet • Form 1.4 Activity Preferences Questionnaire • Form 1.5 Focus on Lifestyle • Form 1.6 Stages of Change Questionnaire
Step 3: Establish strategies for change • Select strategies that match your client's stage of change • Maximize benefits from the client's perspective • Set priorities for change • When goal setting, use measurable objectives	Strategic planning: • Summarizing and clarification • Form 1.7 Decision Balance Summary • Form 1.8 Objective-Setting Worksheet • Strategies for Change Process (table 2.1)

delivered when the nature of the communication is questioning. By the time we reach step 3 (establishing strategies for change), the method of applying the tools and the nature of the communication are strategic planning.

The counseling steps shown in table 1.2 provide a framework that will enable you to change your clients' activity behaviors. As you develop the skills and use the tools listed in the table and taught in this chapter, you will receive the direction and confidence you need to achieve each step and develop productive relationships with your clients.

Step 1: Establish Rapport

In this chapter, we will use the following scenario to work through the steps of the Activity Counseling Model demonstrating the skills and tools that you would use.

Carol, a 42-year-old female client (CL), has come to you, the fitness professional (FP), to start an exercise program. She has not been successful in sticking with a program in the past. The client is concerned about her weight and has some back stiffness. Her doctor has encouraged her to be more active and presented no restrictions to increased activity. Carol works 9 to 5 in a human resources department and has a husband and two children, ages 10 and 12.

At various points in this discussion, dialogues between the fitness professional (FP) and Carol

(CL) illustrate material that has just been presented. Although these dialogues are abbreviated compared with an actual dialogue, they still demonstrate how you might apply the preceding material in a real-life setting.

Counseling is a client-centered process that leads to new behaviors. Building on a foundation of caring, rapport, and comfort, we help clients commit to changing their habits. We keep our clients at the center of this process by listening more than we talk and by encouraging them to learn from their own experiences. Counseling is an opportunity to help clients develop more options—to lead clients to open new doors, throw off chains, and stretch!

Our first objective is to put our client at ease and develop a comfortable working relationship.

Rapport and Trust

Recently I accompanied a friend to an initial therapy session. The therapist began by saying that she wanted to start by building trust. On the drive home my friend said, "Did she think that I would fully trust her after one meeting?" This led me to think about my own expectations when counseling. My goal is to establish an affinity or rapport with my client. At times, this is a challenge that demands attentive behavior and a listening style that respects his feelings and clarifies his message; empathy and support must always be provided.

In establishing this rapport, be receptive and responsive while outlining the counseling process and discussing the reasons for attending. Before moving to step 2 (gathering information), we should confirm what we have heard and ensure that we have received the messages sent by our client.

Create a Friendly Welcome: Be Receptive and Responsive

For your client to make a lifestyle change, she must first examine her existing lifestyle for areas of desired change. She is most likely to do so when she feels comfortable with you. Establish rapport from the onset by being open, receptive, and responsive. Be aware of your impact on your client at all times. Sheer enthusiasm may show your level of dedication, but if your client is quiet and easily intimidated, your enthusiasm can create more harm than good. Something as comfortable to you as your place of work may be threatening to your client.

- **Prepare the environment.** Try to have people fill out most forms before they arrive. Showing new clients around your facility may help them relax, increase their comfort zone, and take the counseling out of the traditional office setting. Your clients will be poorly focused if their basic needs for comfort are not met. When you are ready to sit down together, be sure you have good lighting, appropriate temperature, good air flow, and comfortable chairs (avoid a desk). As appropriate, familiarize clients with various facilities, equipment, washrooms, and club procedures. A friendly welcome is essential. When you first meet, avoid pressure of any kind and start a short chat (conversation) about an area of mutual interest (e.g., home, work, children, sports). As part of being receptive and responsive, you must show that you care and be aware of body language.

- **Show that you care.** Accepting your clients as they are makes it easier for them to accept themselves and therefore to change. Being sensitive to their concerns and demonstrating sincere interest will build trust. Your clients will be able to tell whether you care about making a difference. Desmond Tutu once said, "A person is a person because he recognizes other persons." Listening well shows that you care, which is one of the most important elements in establishing rapport, building a relationship, and maintaining continued trust.

- **Be aware of body language.** Body language or nonverbal skills involve your own "attending" behavior and your ability to perceive your client's nonverbal messages. Effective attending does two things: It tells clients that you are with them, and it puts you in a position to listen. Posture and gestures may be starting points that show you are interested. Egan (1990) suggested a series of nonverbal skills that are summarized by the acronym SOLER:

S: Face the client **squarely**. You may be at a slight angle—what is important is the quality of the attention. Remember, a **smile** can go a long way!

O: Adopt an **open** posture. Avoid crossed arms or legs, as they are seen as defensive postures.

L: At times **lean** toward the client. Leaning forward shows involvement, whereas leaning backward may be interpreted as a lack of interest.

E: Maintain good **eye contact**. The level of reluctance or comfort may be revealed by the consistency of eye contact.

R: Be **relaxed**. Your being natural helps put the client at ease.

These are only guidelines, because your clients differ individually and culturally. Reading your client's nonverbal communication can increase rapport and improve the effects of your listening. Watch the whole body, not just the face and eyes. Hand gestures, body movement, the use of touch, and the way the person occupies space can be very expressive. For example, recently I had a daughter-and-mother session using an exercise ball. As I was demonstrating I noticed that the mother was very tactile, sitting and moving on the ball and experimenting with different shifts in body position. The daughter was slow to even sit on the ball, and she kept her hands crossed on her thighs. I discovered after the session that the training was definitely the mother's idea and that building rapport with the daughter would be somewhat more difficult.

Observe shifts in your client's body posture, facial expressions, vocal tone, or rate of speech, particularly in response to your questions. Are the verbal and nonverbal messages telling you the same thing (Jones 1991)? A client may say that she understands how to start the treadmill, but squinting, perplexed looks, and cocked head provide another message when she is standing on the treadmill. Of course, you must check the accuracy of your interpretation with the client and avoid jumping to conclusions. Also be aware that just as you are watching your client's nonverbal cues, she will be watching yours. Finally, there does seem to be consistent research indicating that women are better than men at accurately reading body language.

Discuss the Counseling Process and the Reason for Attending

Clients want to know what they are "letting themselves in for." When they can see the complete picture, it helps them focus and pace themselves. Outline what will be done and why. Organize your message into successive steps with particular emphasis on the essential aspects. Briefly describe options and choices clients will have throughout the program. Show them a copy of a sample questionnaire, assessment form, or prescription. Allow enough time for questions. Try to link the answers to clients' particular situations and don't move on until you are sure they are satisfied with the explanation. Avoid rushing through this stage.

In the first few minutes, avoid discussing health and fitness concerns in any detail. Once you have explained the counseling process, ask clients why they are there and what they hope to change. Some clients may elaborate and possibly continue to talk about physical problems or other barriers. When clients speak about themselves to you, they start a process of commitment to you and are more inclined to trust you.

Without sounding boastful, explain your qualifications and experience. Not only does this establish your own credibility, it also provides your clients with confidence and shows them what expertise there is to draw on. For example: "You mentioned some previous back stiffness. . . . I had an opportunity to be part of the Healthy Back program staff at the YMCA while finishing my kinesiology degree. . . . I'm looking forward to helping you with that problem."

Ensure You Have Received Your Client's Messages

The field of health and fitness is rich in interpersonal communications, yet most of us have never received formal training on how to be effective listeners. A great listener makes people feel as if they are the only thing that matters to the other person at the moment. Listening is the process of receiving verbal and nonverbal messages, analyzing them for meaning, understanding them, and responding to the sender (Kolovou 2011). Figure 1.1 shows a graphic of a communication loop from the listener's perspective. The speaker, the client in this model, has his own filter and noise; however, our challenge as personal trainers is that elusive skill of active listening.

Good listening takes a lot of work and requires a constant awareness of the elements of "listener-centered communications" within the process of activity counseling. Effective listening responses such as paraphrasing, clarifying, and matching the speaker's emotion can improve your

---

The Initial Client Interview

If the first thing you do is probe with reams of paperwork or prod and induce fatigue from testing or exercise, clients who are not totally committed may leave with less resolve to change than when they entered. Take sufficient time to establish your clients' commitment, question them carefully, and focus on their areas of concern. And most of all, listen carefully.

The interview process is a comfortable way to begin gathering information and establishing a relationship. Be organized and efficient with your questions, perhaps following a pattern with your interview as shown in table 1.3. With effective rapport and organization in the initial counseling interview, clients should reveal their fitness goals and areas of greatest concern. This interview gives them a forum to discuss expectations and speak further about themselves. By asking appropriate and probing questions, you will be able to select strategies that match the client's stage of change and refine his goals as measurable objectives. Information you gather from this conversation will help you determine not only where potential weaknesses may exist but also what assessments should be done to help you determine where the training program should begin.

Table 1.3   The Initial Client Interview

Counseling area	Counseling outcome	Sample questions and statements
Greeting, broad goals	• Create a friendly welcome: Be receptive and responsive. • Discuss the counseling process and the reason for attending. • Leave the impression that you are working on things together.	• Today we will just get to know each other a little better and explore your goals and how I can help you be successful. • People get involved in activity for many different reasons. What are your main priorities? • We'll work together to help you reach those goals.

Past, present, future	• Describe past, present, and future activities and goals, whether they be recreational, occupational, or training. Whenever clients mention any type of activity, be it recreational, household chore, fitness training, or active social, always ask about the FIT—how frequently, how intensely, and for how long (time).
	• For example, walking is a common activity for many middle-aged adults; be sure to probe for detail.
		• What activities in your past would you like to try again?
		• What are you currently doing for activity?
		  • F:
		  • I:
		  • T:
		  • T:
		• How often do you walk? When was the last time you went for a walk? For how long do you walk? Is it a brisk walk or a stroll? Do you walk your dog? Describe the nature of those walks.

Needs, wants, lifestyle	• Identify needs, wants, and lifestyle. • Start with lifestyle including inquiries about employment, daily routines (time), transportation, and so on. • Find out where clients are working and living and about their family situation. • Review the questions on form 1.4, Activity Preferences Questionnaire, and select the ones you think will be most relevant for your client. Try to determine if her preferences and expectations coincide with her needs (perceived or real).	• Tell me about a typical week in your life. • Is any part of your work physical? • How do you spend your time away from work? • When are the most convenient times to exercise? • What specific things do you do for the upkeep of your home inside and out? • Do you belong to any clubs or cultural groups, and are there activities associated with them?
Barriers, injuries, motivation	• Good problem-solving skills are helpful to overcome barriers, but take sufficient time to listen empathetically to your client. • Most clients have a history of injuries. A good health and lifestyle questionnaire can gather considerable information in this area. • Perhaps the most important factor in motivation is the client's own belief that she is capable of committing to her goals.	• Let's just chat about potential barriers and how we might deal with them. • I will be part of your support, but do you have someone else who can be supportive of your efforts, perhaps even a training partner? • Have you had any recent injuries? • Did you undergo any rehabilitation? • Do you experience any pain during the activity? • How long does it take for the pain to subside? Is your doctor aware of this pain, and has the doctor ever restricted your activity because of the pain? • Do you believe that this is important in your life?

quality of overall listening and make the client feel appreciated. Good communication is represented by the need to send messages clearly and the need to receive—hear—them just as clearly. Asking good questions is useless if you are not actively listening. The following skills will make you a more effective listener.

Focus on Feelings

Repeat or reflect a client's feelings. Match her depth of meaning, whether light or serious. Give clues that you are trying to be empathetic. For example, a client recovering from a motor vehicle accident or a work-related injury may harbor pent-up feelings that emerge during her exercise

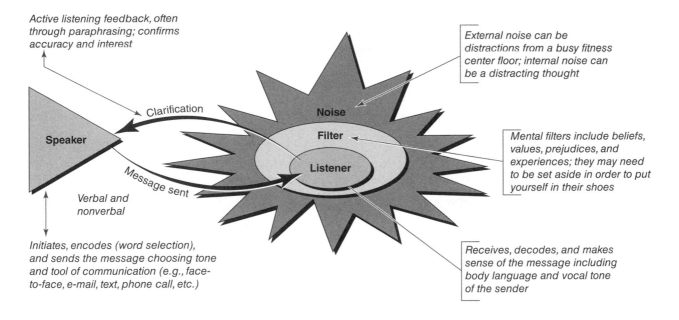

Figure 1.1   Listener-centered communications.

rehabilitation. You might say, "The time it has taken to recover from your injury must be hard for you." You should not assume that you know accurately how a client feels, of course, but you should acknowledge feelings and communicate empathy. Verifying feelings and not assuming immediately that you understand can build trust and reduce negative feelings. Avoid the temptation to give an "autobiographical response," an interjection that this has happened to you too.

Remember that the relationship with your client is not all about facts and science but includes elements of a social relationship (albeit professional) and is as much about feelings as about facts. As such, important conversations with your clients may be focused on feelings, and their motivation will come from how they feel about an issue, not the facts of the issue. Feelings are the brain's descriptive statistics: They are the summary of previous experiences along with thoughts and abstractions. This makes them valuable to the client and an important force in any conversation.

Check for Clarity or Accuracy

Clarifying, or paraphrasing, is an attempt to verify your understanding of what your client is saying. "It sounds like you are concerned with . . ." and "I'm a little unsure about . . ." are useful phrases for clarifying. Restate the client's basic ideas, emphasizing the facts. Although restatement is a check for factual content, it also can encourage the client to continue with her thoughts. For example, you might say, "Uh-huh, so it sounds like

it's hard to find time with your new schedule. Is that right?" A check like this is also valuable as a method of summarizing major ideas and feelings at the end of a session. It pulls important ideas and facts together and may offer a springboard for further discussion. Try to be brief and use your own words: "Let's see now, I think I heard you saying that . . ." Paraphrasing keeps things on track in two different ways: It requires that you listen very carefully to what is being said and, by restating things in your own words, requires that you think about and try to understand what was said.

Clarification involves exploring your clients' feelings as well as behaviors. By clarifying emotions, you help clients understand their emotions. You need to catch the meaning of a message without interpreting or analyzing the meaning. The following two responses illustrate this difference:

CL: The XYZ Club said they would do a fitness assessment and design a personalized program for me. They took a few measurements and gave me the same program card as everyone.

FP response 1: Do you feel cheated and angry that they have not provided the services they promised?

FP response 2: So you think you were ripped off for your money and feel embarrassed that you were taken in by the club.

Response 1 reflects what the client said and asks for clarification of the client's feelings. By clarifying the client's feelings, you have begun to establish empathy and are in a better position to understand what the client wants. Response 2 may be true, but it is not what the client said and may not be an accurate interpretation of how she feels. It is critical that the client feel understood, not analyzed.

Supportive Communication

Supportive communication preserves the trust and positive relationship between you and your client during discussion of any issue. It is a two-way process that allows you to empathize with your client and appreciate her uniqueness. Supportive communication avoids top-down conversation and rigid predetermined personal agendas. This aspect of active listening is far more than robotic head bobbing and deadpan "yeahs" and "uh-huhs." It involves selecting the appropriate response once you figure out the purpose of the conversation.

For example, if you need more information about your client's back stiffness, use a "probing" response. "Does your back stiffness affect daily activities or give you any problems when you sleep?" If the client describes a continual ache in her low back while at work, show empathy without deflecting the conversation to you. "When the ache is unrelenting, it sounds like it can affect your whole day." Advising your client is a good coaching technique, but avoid giving advice as a first response. For example, if the client asks what equipment is best for burning calories, ask at least one more question before advising.

Sometimes clients come to you because there is a discrepancy between what they want to be and what they are. Their goals may not be realistic or attainable. In that case, do not condemn or suggest by words or body language that the client is unrealistic. Instead, listen carefully to your client, recognizing that a helping role is necessary. Never judge the merits of what your clients say in terms of good or bad, right or wrong, relevant or irrelevant. The following exchange took place between one of my student trainers and a member of our employee fitness program:

Member: Well, the knee is still a little sore. The exercises are good, but I played hockey with my children over the weekend and it flared up again.

Student: That's the problem, isn't it? Why don't you stick to your program and forget the hockey?

This might well be sound counsel, but the student responded in his "advice-giving mode," with little empathy and no acknowledgment of the person's feelings. A better approach for the student would have been this:

Student: Do you think there is a way we can modify your play to avoid the flare-up, or is rest the best at this stage? I am pleased to hear that the exercises are good. Keep it up!

Accepting your clients as they are makes it easier for them to accept themselves and therefore to change. Being sensitive to their concerns will build trust and show genuine interest. Listening well shows that you care.

Now that you have learned important ways of establishing rapport, and mistakes to avoid, look at this opening conversation between Carol (CL) and her personal fitness trainer. Note how the fitness professional (FP) communicates being receptive, responsive, and caring and how she is nonjudgmental, encouraging, and informative about how they will work on Carol's issues together.

FP: Hi, Carol. It's nice to meet you. How are you this morning?

CL: Well, pretty good. . . . I'm here to give it another try.

FP: The fact that you are here is a great start. And don't worry that you have to "get up and do" right now. Today we will just get to know each other a little better and explore how I can help you be successful this time around.

CL: Will I have to be tested today?

FP: Not at all! Let's just chat about your goals, any changes you may want to make, and any concerns that you have.

CL: You may have your hands full. . . . I haven't done very well in the past.

FP: Don't worry about that. We'll take another look at why those changes that you want to make are important and we'll work together to help you reach those goals. What is it that has you so concerned that you aren't going to stick with the program we develop together?

CL: I work with people all day and by 5 o'clock it's all I can do to get home, make dinner, and have a little time with my family.

FP: That really does sound full. It may be all the more reason to keep you healthy! And I'm sure that we can find some great benefits for you personally as well.

CL: That sounds good.

FP: I understand you have two children . . . so do I. What types of activities do you do as a family?

Step 2: Gather Information

In this age of information, we have made great gains in storing and retrieving data, but little advance in our skills or techniques for effectively gathering client information. What do we ask about and in what order? How do we deal with barriers or lifestyle issues as they arise? We need some refined questioning skills that are suited to the learning and personality styles of our clients. We also need tools to collect and prioritize needs and preferences and to understand our clients' lifestyles well enough to anticipate areas of integration.

The initial consultation with a client is one of the most challenging aspects of personal training. The purpose of this counseling step is to gather information about the client that will help you design a safe and appropriate exercise program and motivation strategy (see table 1.2). Getting clients to talk about themselves is one thing; asking the right questions is another.

The type and timing of questions can make or break a counseling session. Listen carefully to your client's issues and gather additional information about her wants, needs, and lifestyle. The clearer the profile we have of our client, the better the information and support we can provide.

Questionnaires, inventories, and checklists can increase the efficiency of counseling. They may be filled out in advance, allowing time during the counseling to discuss and clarify the most relevant information. See forms 1.1 (Fantastic Lifestyle Checklist) and 1.2 (Inventory of Lifestyle and Activity Preferences) at the end of this chapter for sample questionnaires. Develop the techniques of questioning detailed next.

- **Open or broad question strategy.** Start questions with a broad framework, narrowing to specifics later. For example, "Where do you see your fitness and health needs in the next few years?" Open-ended questions are used to gather information and are increasingly effective as your client feels more comfortable with you. Use them to learn how your client thinks about something. For example, "I'd like to hear more about your past experience with health clubs," or "How did you come to be involved in old-timers baseball?"

- **Closed or narrow question strategy.** After obtaining general information, use a series of narrow questions to focus the client's attention on a specific topic. Closed-ended questions provide detailed information, verify accuracy, and clarify understanding. They may help the client recall facts or choose options from a list. For example, "You mentioned that you wanted to start weight training—would you prefer free weights, machines, or calisthenics?" Closed-ended questions are also effective in getting agreement or commitment. For example, "How many days per week do you think you can devote to this part of your prescription?" Be careful, however, not to overuse narrow questions, lest the conversation become too centered on your concerns rather than on the client and her concerns.

- **Probing strategies.** Probing techniques help your clients think more deeply about the issues. When initial responses to questions are superficial, use probing questions to prompt clients to provide more information, meaning, critical awareness, or reflective thinking. Listen carefully, then proceed from "where the client is." Acknowledge previous responses before presenting the next probe. There are several types of probes. Clarification probes ask for more information or meaning: "Can you give me an example of . . . ?" "What do you mean by muscle tone?" Probes for critical awareness analyze, justify, or evaluate a response. They usually deal with values and attitudes: "Why do you think that is the best way to get in shape?" "How does the old diet compare with the new one?" The intention of perception probes is to anticipate a cause and effect or probable consequences: "If you sprinted without warming up, what do you think would happen?" "How do you think you would feel if . . . ?" Often the discussion needs to shift back to the main issue by the use of refocusing probes: "How does that relate to your fitness goals?" "That's right, and how can that time be managed to allow . . . ?"

- **Softening a question.** Questions can be threatening. Use of a lead-in statement can soften the impact of an open-ended question, particularly if clients are being asked about their values or lifestyles. For example, "There has been a lot written recently about the effects of smoking—how do you feel about your own smoking habits?" or "Many people have trouble starting an exercise program—what would help motivate you?" Note that the softening statements that introduce the questions are in the third person.

Where do you start? You are usually faced with a limited period of time and a daunting task of finding out "all about" your client! Counseling skills and tools like effective probing techniques and interview questionnaires can be very effective. However, some structure to the collection of information can reduce your anxiety about the session, save time, and provide more complete information. There are two effective methods: (1) past, present, future, and (2) needs, wants, lifestyle. Either method of approaching information gathering can stand alone, but merging the two methods is the most comprehensive and client-centered approach.

Examine Your Client's Past, Present, and Future

Begin by asking your client about **past** exercise and activity. The objective here is to understand your client's interests, physical aptitude, and skills. For example, if your client tells you that she has felt awkward exercising and has never done anything except walking and some cycling, this might indicate that the prescription should begin at a basic level. With little sport background, she may have issues with coordination and dynamic balance. Further questioning may reveal that she has avoided some physical activities because she was embarrassed by her body. Try to glean information about her feelings during discussions about past activities. It would not be surprising if this bias continued to the present.

Questions about what your client is doing at **present** will provide information about the quantity, intensity, and type of exercise you should prescribe. For example, the client may state that she is involved regularly with various types of exercises but still has a high body fat level. You need to know if she is exercising adequately to create a negative caloric balance and lose weight. Appropriate questions can help you determine how and where to start the exercise prescription.

A **future**-oriented line of questioning may reveal specific information about the direction that the program should take. What does your client want to get out of his program, and how much time and effort can he put into the program? Notice what makes your client's eyes light up; this will help you design the motivation strategy.

Identify Your Client's Needs, Wants, and Lifestyle

Needs are not the same as wants (Trottier 1988). **Needs** originate in human biology and in the human social condition. In the case of our clients, needs are basic requirements related to an injury, a specific weakness in a fitness component, a health risk factor, or some other personal situation such as participation in a sport or a problem with motivation. **Wants** are desires to meet these needs in specific ways or perceptions of value for things that may not be related to needs at all. Wants often determine our clients' choices about how to address their needs; wants, of course, are

influenced by social forces. **Lifestyle** includes time, facilities, partners, travel, and employment. The areas of overlap—where a need and a want coincide and the lifestyle is compatible—intuitively are the areas of the greatest potential for success. It is on these overlapping areas that we should focus.

Figure 1.2 depicts the client history as a Venn diagram showing the overlap of three primary areas of that history: needs, wants, and lifestyle. Form 1.3 is a useful worksheet to gather such information during the interview.

Types of Needs

Client needs may be related to medical, high-risk, educational, or motivational factors; needs also can be defined by results of fitness assessments, by lack of self-esteem, or by special designs necessitated by physical limitations.

- **Medical needs.** A questionnaire can identify medical issues and help determine if you need clearance from a health care specialist. Gather information on past medical history, present symptoms, medications, and existing medically prescribed limitations to exercise. Clients may be quite general in their comments ("I'd like to feel more healthy or have more energy"), or they may be specific ("My doctor says I have to lower my blood pressure and reduce my cholesterol"). If clients believe that exercise will produce the desired health effects and they are willing to

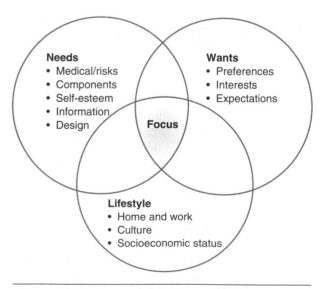

Figure 1.2   The areas with the greatest potential for success are where needs and wants coincide with a compatible lifestyle.

commit to realistic goals, these health needs will be effective motivators.

- **High-risk needs.** Always determine coronary heart disease risk factors such as smoking, high blood pressure, obesity, inactivity, and poor diet. Age, previous injuries, or low back pain may present special limitations. Risk factors can be identified with specific screening tools such as PAR-Q+ and RISK-I, with follow-up clearance from a physician obtained with the use of e-PARmed-X+ (see chapter 4).

- **Educational or informational needs.** Whether a client actually changes his lifestyle often depends on well-timed sharing of information. This need for information may emerge from a conversation. For example, a client tells you that he joined a health club, tries different pieces of equipment each time he goes, and is disappointed that he hasn't seen results after five visits over the last 3 weeks. This client may need information about what he can realistically expect from exercise. In addition, literature is readily available concerning exercise and chronic conditions, and a compendium of medications is a valuable resource. Referrals to clinics specializing in hyperlipidemia, hypertension, or obesity can provide credible supplements to exercise guidance. If you do not have appropriate information for a particular condition or situation, know when and where to refer your client. For example, if your client has significant pain with any exercise, he should discontinue and seek advice from a health care practitioner.

- **Special motivational needs.** Depending on their reasons for participation and their stage of change, clients may have specific motivational needs. Your strategies can include self-testing, logging, supervision, and support systems. I recently had a client who returned to exercise after almost 15 years. At that earlier time he had religiously followed the Cooper aerobics point-based exercise system and wanted to use it again with the new equipment in our facility. Using the physiological value of an "aerobic point," I prescribed a program of cardiovascular cross-training that allowed him to continue using a system of motivation with which he was comfortable.

- **Fitness needs.** A fitness assessment can indicate your client's fitness component needs. However, if you first determine the client's priorities—before doing the fitness assessment—you will be able to select only those test items that relate to those priorities. The prescription model is flexible, allowing you to loop back and verify needs through selective assessment. No matter when it is done, fitness assessment is a vital source of information for both writing the prescription and monitoring progress.

- **Self-esteem needs.** Good self-esteem can help people adopt more healthful lifestyles. Physical self-esteem may include how a client feels about his appearance, his perception of personal skill levels, or his realistic expectations of an ideal self (CSEP 2003). Counseling should encourage the continuation of healthy habits and develop an awareness of the value of changing high-risk behaviors. This assistance will improve overall self-esteem. Avoid setting standards for clients that are not realistic or are judgmental, such as looking like someone with an ideal body build. Self-esteem traps like these can prevent clients from enjoying the intrinsic aspects of activity. Motivation to continue physical activity usually comes from the sheer pleasure of the experience. But positive feelings about oneself as an active, fit person can also be powerful motivators.

- **Special design needs.** Special design needs may include the need for specific equipment (e.g., special shoes or orthotics needed for running), a focus on a specific sport or skill for training (e.g., energy systems and anatomical demands), or limitations of the venue or facility (e.g., lack of resistance equipment in a home program, requiring biweekly visits to the Y).

Focusing on Wants

Wants relate to clients' preferences. Wants may include what your clients enjoy, their special interests, or their expectations or aspirations. Marketing trends and other societal influences shape your clients' wants, which in turn will affect the way you address their needs.

To focus on your clients' wants, you need to examine their activity preferences, interests, and expectations. Form 1.4, Activity Preferences Questionnaire, will assist with this important function. Use it as a guide and ensure that your questioning is client centered, allowing liberty to expand on important areas that emerge in the dialogue.

You may want to present clients with a list of possible activities and ask them to check which ones they most enjoy. They may also enjoy a particular method of training, type of equipment, training partner, or location. Clients may also have special interests and be attracted to something old or new, a specific challenge, or background information on their interest.

The desire for a more muscular body or one with less fat brings huge numbers of people to fitness clubs and exercise specialists. But be careful not to encourage the pursuit of the fashion industry ideal. The desire to change body image and appearance can be positive, but you must exploit that desire responsibly by helping your client establish realistic goals.

In the following dialogue, the client revealed her fitness goals and areas of greatest concern. The dialogue gave the client a forum to discuss expectations and speak further about herself. By asking some probing questions, the fitness professional was able to discover more detail for the eventual prescription and some underlying motivations. Finally, the rapport from step 1 was further reinforced.

FP: Now that we have had a chance to chat about your past activities and the things that you are doing right now, tell me, Carol, exactly what you want to get out of your program. Do you have any specific expectations?

CL: Well, I want to lose some weight, tone up, and just have a little more energy. But somewhere in the future I would like to be able to run a long distance, maybe a marathon, with my son—he's really interested in running.

FP: That's really exciting! Let's talk about the marathon in just a moment, but first, are there any areas of your body that you want to tone up?

CL: Certainly my trunk and thighs are my problem areas for flabby muscles and fat. My back is often tight too, probably because of work.

FP: Are your thighs and back weak or do they tire easily, or do you believe the muscles are not toned?

CL: It is partially an appearance thing but I think my back could benefit from some stronger stomach muscles. What do you think?

FP: That's pretty perceptive. Your trunk should benefit from strengthening and building some muscular endurance in your abdominal muscles but we'll also plan some stretching for your back for some relief.

CL: Good.

FP: I see that you have written on the Inventory of Lifestyle and Activity Preferences that you want a structured plan that you can do on your own.

CL: Yes, that may be best with my schedule.

FP: Carol, you also mentioned that you would like to get a treadmill to make things a little more convenient.

CL: Will the treadmill help me tone up and reduce my weight?

FP: Certainly in combination with your exercises and meal plan you will notice a difference. Walking on the treadmill will be a good calorie burner. It will also address a couple of your other goals by helping condition your legs and being a first step toward running with your son.

CL: This is exactly what I am looking for. I'm looking forward to getting started.

FP: That's great, Carol. I'm excited too!

Lifestyle Considerations

Good tools and some skillful questioning can help at the early stages of an action plan. If your client's prescription comprises activities she has chosen and considers important to meeting her

---

Conversations During Personal Training Sessions

Asking questions during a personal training session can be challenging. Try to keep questions brief. Often a client will bring up a problem or issue during the workout. In this case, your questions and dialogue should follow a process similar to the Activity Counseling Model but should be suited to an intermittent format flowing between or during exercises.

- Focus on the client's issue, listen carefully to what he has to say, and encourage him to elaborate on details that will help you later. Gather specific information on barriers to change and what he has tried or might try to alleviate the problem.

- Determine his thoughts on how important the issue is and what would be different in his life and workout if it were resolved.

- Work with your client to establish what needs to happen, determine who or what can help him, and start to formulate an action plan.

For example, during a warm-up stretch, a client mentions to her trainer that she has booked a massage. Seeing an opportunity to probe further, her trainer asks what motivated that decision. The client talks a little more about the stiffness she often has in her back. Still gathering information, the trainer asks if the stiffness is the result of an injury or a chronic problem. At this point, the trainer is starting to process the information. Depending on the answers, she may refer her client, perform a postural assessment, or introduce a stress reduction technique. This illustrates that the more you know about your client, the better able you are to support her.

lifestyle needs, her chances of long-term compliance will be significantly improved. Form 1.2, Inventory of Lifestyle and Activity Preferences, helps people identify their three most important lifestyle needs from a list of 35 suggestions. It is an excellent counseling tool to help your clients identify activities that will satisfy these three needs. When Carol came to her trainer, she wasn't sure what activities would be best for her. They talked about barriers in the past and what the future might look like. Together they filled out the inventory and identified three lifestyle needs: to have a structured activity, to improve her health, and to be time efficient.

You may get ample information about your client's lifestyle wants and needs if you start with an open-ended question such as "Tell me about your favorite activities." But many people need a bit of help to recall even what is important to them. So unless you are completely convinced that your client has "revealed all," you can use forms 1.4, Activity Preferences Questionnaire, and 1.5, Focus on Lifestyle, at the end of the chapter to check and gather additional information about your client's wants, needs, and lifestyle.

Determine Your Client's Stage of Change

Early discussions should clarify what clients hope to gain or learn and why they are there. Determining their level of commitment to change will help you move them to the next level of readiness to change. One effective way to work with a client's readiness to change is to think in terms of the five "stages of change" postulated by Prochaska and colleagues (1992) in their Transtheoretical Model.

Emerson once said, "One who lacks the courage to start is already finished." This is a motivational quote and an apparent truism but falls short of explaining human behavior. People start things when they are ready to start. Our role is to recognize how close they are to initiating a change in behavior. Once we determine their stage of readiness, we can provide the appropriate type of counseling support.

The stages of change describe the motivational readiness of clients. Chapter 2 provides specific motivational strategies for each stage. These stages are as follows:

1. **Precontemplation**—Not intending to make changes
2. **Contemplation**—Considering a change
3. **Preparation**—Making small changes or ready to change in the near future
4. **Action**—Actively engaging in the new behavior
5. **Maintenance**—Sticking with the behavior change

Table 1.4 lists some characteristics of the different stages of change. Watch your clients for these characteristics to help you determine their stages

Table 1.4   Stages of Change and Characteristics

Stage	Characteristics
Precontemplation	• Has no intention to change • Has low awareness • Never considered it • Believes that cons outweigh pros
Contemplation	• Intends to change in next 6 months • May be ambivalent • May have low self-confidence
Preparation	• Intends to take action in next 30 days • Is making some small changes • May have tried in past year
Action	• Has changed behavior in last 6 months • Has a high risk of relapse • Needs support—challenging time mentally • Is changing beliefs and attitudes
Maintenance	• Continues program 6 months or more • Has high confidence • Has learned strategies to deal with lapses to prevent relapse • May not get further support

Reprinted by permission from the Canadian Society for Exercise Physiology 2003.

of change. Just as with any New Year's resolution, your client's degree of commitment can fluctuate and she may fall back to a preparation rather than an action stage. The Canadian Society for Exercise Physiology (2003) has developed the Stages of Change Questionnaire, designed to establish the stage of motivational readiness of clients (see form 1.6). The questionnaire identifies five stages of change corresponding to the number of the statement selected. Even when using the Stages of Change Questionnaire, you can't always be sure that your client's self-reported level is correct. You may also be misled by the apparent determination of her speech. Sometimes planning specific time slots and discussing what must change to open up slots can avert this problem. Regular contact in the early stages seems to be the best method of maintaining adherence and helping clients move through their stages of change.

Precontemplation Stage

A client comment at the precontemplation stage may be "Exercise may be fine for young people, but I'm too old to start." Your strategy here should be to increase his awareness of the importance of appropriate exercise at any age. Here is a typical conversation between a precontemplative client (CL) and a fitness professional (FP):

FP: I'm really happy to meet you, and I'm sure that I can help you achieve the goals that brought you here.

CL: Frankly, I'm only here because my wife made me come. I figure we can talk for a bit and then I can get out of here and back to my armchair.

FP: Oh. Well, OK. Then I guess we'd better have that conversation! So, were you active when you were younger?

CL: Oh, yes. I was always involved in sports and activities in the neighborhood.

FP: Why were you so active at that time?

CL: Well, it was fun and the better shape I was in, the more competitive I was in sports.

FP: That's great! Sounds like being active suited your goals at that time. For that matter, having fun at any age is a worthwhile goal.

CL: Yes, but I can't still do those activities, and why would I want to?

FP: Good question. You certainly aren't training for the Olympics, but the training effects from even light exercise at your age can be very substantial. Your interests have changed, but activity can help you reach new goals.

CL: Yeah, sure. Can it help my tired feet or give me more energy?

FP: It can do that, and the experience you've gained since your youth can help you shape your activity to get what you want from it. Let me tell you a bit about what it can do. . . .

Contemplation Stage

Once some awareness of the problem arises, the client enters a period characterized by ambivalence. The contemplator both considers change and rejects it. To move to the preparation stage, clients must be able to begin seeing themselves in the future as persons who behave differently than they do at present.

The most common excuse of contemplative clients is "I know I should exercise, but I just don't have time." Help the client examine things that will keep her motivated; discuss what might make it hard for her to stick with exercise. Your goal is for her to decide for herself that the gains outweigh the losses. Here is another typical conversation between such a client and her personal fitness trainer:

CL: I just never seem to have enough time to take up a regular fitness program.

FP: I'm amazed at how much you accomplish in a day. You are very organized.

CL: Sometimes I feel like too many things are pulling in too many directions.

FP: You seem to enjoy much of what you do.

CL: Yes, I just need more hours in the day and more energy to last.

FP: Well, I can't change the hours in a day, but with your skill for time management, I think we could come up with a strategy for rejuvenation. You already have your priorities well established—a convenient activity break can actually help you meet your commitments.

CL: You've got my ear and 20 minutes of my time. . . .

Preparation Stage

You might say that a client entering this stage has become motivated. He has found those personal thoughts that will activate him, that will overcome his ambivalent feelings and his doubts that he can, in fact, succeed. The preparation stage may include two different types of clients: those who are making their first serious attempt to incorporate enough regular physical activity in their lives to improve their health, and those who have tried before and failed:

• "I play baseball once a week but I think I'll start doing more," may be a comment from a client in the preparation stage who is trying "serious exercise" for the first time. Now you must seek a commitment. Booking an assessment at this stage may still be too threatening: Rather, schedule a consultation to find out what the client really wants to achieve, and establish short-term goals like learning a baseball warm-up routine or getting a few stretches for an old groin pull. A check-off log incorporated into the prescription reinforces every positive action taken in the early activity stages.

• Another client at this stage may be like our 42-year-old mother of two from our counseling scenario. She appears to have made an initial commitment although she has had some unsuccessful attempts in the past. Probe for the true measure of success she expects from her efforts, because any changes she may have attempted in the past probably have not met these criteria. Provide opportunities for her to believe in her ability to make change. Frequent contacts and simple encouragement in the first 30 days are extremely important. Keep your own journal of contacts and comments you have with all your clients. Your care and attention will impress them when you can recall earlier conversations.

Action Stage

The client in the action stage may be a new club member who says, "I started 6 weeks ago at three to four times a week but I'm not working out as often now. Perhaps I need a personal trainer?" This client has made some very positive actions and needs to hear praise.

Maintenance Stage

For many maintenance clients, regular exercise is a self-reinforcing, positive behavior. If they stop for too long, they do not feel well and are almost impelled to take up their activity again. Once at the maintenance stage, your clients must work to prevent relapse and to consolidate their gains—especially if they are involved in rehabilitation (Sotile 1996). Remind these clients of their prior state of health, and encourage activities that might help their transition from clinical exercise to active lifestyle: Increase their awareness of an exercise technique, for example, or of a method for self-monitoring.

Step 3: Establish Strategies for Change

Clients are often at different points in their desire to commit, which often changes with the introduction of a new activity or component of fitness. Many longtime athletes have a difficult time adopting regular exercise routines. Similarly, avid runners who know that they should be doing some upper body resistance work are struggling on either side of the preparation stage even though they have been maintenance runners for years. In such cases, you must use counseling skills and tools that will help your clients either adopt or maintain their new behavior.

We must help our clients establish which of their concerns should be dealt with first. To set those priorities, begin with your client's concerns, not your strengths. Although health issues need attention, unless you choose manageable problems that can show improvement, you may be setting your client up for failure. Once you have established priorities, help your client translate these into action and provide visualization of a future outcome (see table 1.2). This should be a fun process that moves your client from theory to reality. Skills and tools for establishing strategies for change include how to write a good objective and the effective use of a self-contract, self-talk, self-efficacy, and the Relapse Planner (chapter 2, form 2.2). Some of the skills and tools to establish change are mentioned in this chapter only because they are all motivational tools for promoting or restoring commitment—and that is a subject that needs an entire chapter to itself (chapter 2).

Select Strategies That Match Your Client's Stage of Change

Once you know your client's stage of change, you can choose strategies that are effective for that specific stage. Becoming client centered requires that you match your frame of reference to that of your client. We will discuss in detail how to do this in chapter 2. For the present, simply consider the following examples, which will give you an idea of what it means to match your client's stage of change.

• **Precontemplation.** Consider one of my clients, Gerry, who was rehabilitating from a motor vehicle accident and had not previously been active. He had never considered what regular exercise would be like and had taken no voluntary steps toward doing it—the "cons" to regular exercise outweighed the "pros" in his mind. If I had simply assigned him an exercise prescription, I would have set him up for failure. Recognizing that he was at a precontemplation or contemplation stage, I knew that he had not yet made a commitment to take action. I knew that no matter how appropriate a plan is, if it is presented at the wrong time, it won't be heard. If I moved too quickly or sent Gerry off on his own, a trust relationship might never develop. I wanted to be there at the right time, so I made sure that I was predictably reliable for every session. I worked at helping him over his negative perceptions, always looking to highlight his personal benefits. I knew my goal was about creating positive feelings about his sessions as much as it was about continued rehabilitation. Providing positive feedback merely for his attendance at the sessions and giving encouragement for reaching even a small goal showed Gerry that his behavior was worthwhile and acceptable. Then one day a gear mechanism on one of the pieces of equipment was malfunctioning and he saw me struggling with it. Without hesitation, Gerry fixed it in no time. Praise soon came from other patrons and staff. This small equipment repair episode gave him a feeling of empowerment based on his knowledge of mechanics. This positive experience played a pivotal role confirming in Gerry's mind the relationship between his rehab effort and feeling better. Gerry still comes in once a month or on call to do my fitness equipment maintenance, and we always have a workout together.

• **Preparation.** Another client was considering an increase in her physical activity but seemed to be putting it off because of a lack of self-confidence. If I had presented her with a program featuring a wide variety of activities and detailed self-monitoring, I probably would have scared her off. She was at the preparation stage: Small changes were within her abilities, but large, complex changes would have set her back. Working together, we established a step-by-step plan that helped build her confidence.

• **Action or maintenance.** Josie felt great about one of her newer clients, Tony. Tony had been working hard under Josie's direction and was starting to meet many of his short-term goals. Josie looked forward to working with Tony but knew he could easily do the workouts on his own and should move into a maintenance stage.

Josie: Tony, I wanted to take a few minutes today and review your progress.

Tony: Yeah, it's great! I feel like a new man.

Josie: Tony, you certainly know what you are doing with each workout and I'm sure you can handle working out on your own from this point on. Congratulations.

Tony pulled back awkwardly, apparently not as pleased with the graduation.

Tony: Well . . . you know I really like working out with you . . .

Josie: I like training with you, too, but I thought you wanted to eventually be independent.

Tony: I did say that, Josie, but I've made such good progress with you, I'm not sure if I can do that on my own.

Josie realized that the transition was moving too rapidly for Tony and that she may have left him with the feeling that she did not want to continue on with him.

Josie: Tony, why don't we work toward that goal a little more slowly? Why don't we work out together twice a month and see how that goes?

Tony: I'll still have a chance to touch base with you but I think that might just work. Thanks for the confidence, Josie.

Find out what your clients know, think, and feel about physical activity before actively engaging them in exercise. The more information you discover about your clients, the better able you are to determine the right combination of strategies for them. You can help your clients move from one stage to another most effectively if you understand what stages they are in and devise your strategies with them accordingly.

You must define the important issues for your client and her intentions to change. You can help identify her willingness to commit to these priorities by using summarizing and clarifying techniques. In the following dialogue between Carol and her trainer, notice how the fitness professional uses the summarizing technique to recognize Carol's frustration and even despair about her condition and her past experiences—and then introduces hope into the situation with his response. In our scenario, the client, Carol, has described to the fitness professional a number of unsuccessful attempts at regular exercise. At this point, she is quite pessimistic.

FP: Let's take a look at what we have so far. After almost 20 years of serving the public first, your body and health are feeling the toll. Your experiences in school with physical education and sports were not positive and at times embarrassing. In the last 3 years, you have joined two different health clubs that appeared to welcome you initially, but there was little follow-up assistance. You want to look and feel better, but you appear to have little support.

CL: (Pauses.) Not a rosy picture, but that about sums it up. Maybe I wasn't thinking straight for a while, but until lately, I haven't wanted to stop and look at my situation. Maybe the time has come for a serious change. I do feel anxious that I need to turn things around.

FP: One way of doing that is to take a look at what you have accomplished and enjoyed in the last few years. Let's work together on a general vision of where you would like to be, and we can build on these things as we create some short-term objectives.

You can see that the trainer not only used summarizing to state the facts but also suggested an approach to turn things around one step at a time. This helped refocus the client's feelings.

The first challenge, then, is to get your clients to clarify the issues before them; the second is to move them toward committing to appropriate plans of action. The process of clarification can help them determine what needs to be changed and get ready to move forward. Here is another sample dialogue in which the exercise professional uses clarification to set the stage for commitment. In our scenario, the client, Carol, talks to her personal fitness trainer about her difficulties with her weight.

CL: My problem is that I am overweight. I just don't like how I look.

FP: How does this make you feel?

CL: I'm frustrated with myself and embarrassed. . . . It just makes me so angry because I do more to watch my weight than a lot of my skinny friends!

FP: Carol, you sound disappointed by the results of your efforts to lose weight.

CL: Yeah . . . but I don't know what to do about it.

FP: The causes of overweight are different for different people. Could you tell me why you think you have put on the weight?

CL: Well, I don't think I eat that badly, but I've never been very active. So I think maybe my avoidance of exercise is the main reason.

FP: So you're suspecting lack of exercise as a major culprit in your gaining weight, but you also know that regular exercise causes you some difficulty. Any examples of an attempt that has gone astray?

CL: Yes, I bought an exercise bike last year and used it regularly for 3 weeks, but after about 6 weeks it was out in the garage. I got bored easily, and the seat was very uncomfortable.

FP: You want to do something about your weight, but stationary cycling didn't keep your interest. The club has spin classes during the winter or you could cycle outdoors when the weather is good. Would either of those work, since they'd probably solve the boredom problem?

CL: I don't think so. I think I'd rather give my seat a bit of a rest!

FP: OK, then. Besides biking, what sort of other exercise choices do we have?

CL: Well, I don't like sports and jogging seems difficult right now, but I like to walk if the scenery is pleasant or I'm with a friend. I'm pretty much a homebody in the winter except to walk the dog, but I like to garden in the nicer weather. I have been thinking about buying an exercise video.

FP: Carol, those are great ideas! We've come a long way. That is a good list that we can work from. Which do you think are the most likely choices from that list that you can see yourself doing on a regular basis?

Notice how the personal fitness trainer established early trust by avoiding judgment and premature advice. The trainer's reflective listening, probing, and clarifying helped the client get a clearer picture of the problem. The trainer then moved into the analysis step of decision making. We leave the pair as they are about to select the best combination of options (priorities) and the most effective strategy for achieving those priorities. Chapter 2 expands on techniques for motivating clients to act.

Maximize Benefits From the Client's Perspective

Value is determined by your clients, not by you. Value is the consumers' estimate of the service's capacity to satisfy their needs and wants. Most exercise specialists know well the positive effects of exercise. But clients select their program priorities based on the benefits they see from their own perspective ("What does it do for me?" [Weylman

Counseling a Client to Develop Options

Don, an automotive worker and avid lacrosse coach, suffered a heart attack during a father–son game. At first, he was devastated, feeling that his identity and role in life had been taken away. Feelings of "Why me?" progressed to frustration and helplessness. Medical and corporate counseling helped Don readjust to a modified work environment; however, his doctors set lacrosse out of bounds. Then a lacrosse friend of Don's (a certified personal trainer) provided some "counseling" advice. He had Don take a closer look at different roles he could take on with the team. He helped Don discover that his years of experience were invaluable as a strategist and advisor and that being on the floor was not the only option for a coach. His friend also showed Don how to build his cardiovascular stamina and monitor his exertion levels and symptoms. Today, Don is co-coaching and providing a service to the team that goes beyond what he provided before the heart attack.

1995]). The challenge is knowing how to describe effects of exercise in a way that will clearly demonstrate how those effects will fill the clients' needs and wants while not introducing negative factors into their lives (such as interfering with family life or being terribly inconvenient). Three steps that will increase your chances of doing this are to identify options, rank the options, and lead the client to commitment.

Identify Options

A client wants to develop a flatter stomach and increased muscular support for a low back problem, all in a home program (lifestyle). After brainstorming with the client, you present her with the following prescription choices:

- Perform sit-ups.
- Reduce body weight and body fat.
- Stretch muscles that pull the back into lordosis.
- Join an aerobics or aquafit class specializing in abdominal work.
- Use a video that teaches abdominal exercises or prevention of low back problems.
- Perform a variety of abdominal strengthening exercises.
- Practice sitting abdominal exercises at her work desk or standing exercises at the bus stop.
- Do a short routine before bed each night.

Rank the Options

The next step is to weigh or rank the options. You can eliminate some options immediately because they are impractical or do not meet criteria required by the client. Your client may discard the aquafit class suggestion, for example, because it cannot be done at home. Working with your client, rank the rest of the options according to interest, time, and availability, which are the features of any given option. One way to help rank the options is to list the personal benefits of any given feature. Try using a simple chart (see table 1.5) to describe the benefits of any given feature.

Some approaches to counseling may work better for some clients than others. Form 1.7, Decision Balance Summary (CSEP 2003), is a tool to help clients weigh the pros and cons of changing their activity behavior. The client who is analytical and technical should respond very well to this approach. It allows clients to consider the potential benefits and costs not only for themselves but also for family and others around them. Decisions will be realistic and informed after clients weigh the gains and losses anticipated from physical activity.

Figure 1.3 is an example of how you might fill out the Decision Balance Summary as you and Carol, the client in our scenario, discuss the pros and cons and weigh the importance of the gains over the losses of her becoming active.

Lead the Client to Commitment

Finally, help your client commit to an action based on the analysis—select the highest priority, the best combination of options, and the most effective strategy for your client. For example, the client described here may choose to work out at home with a prescription that includes stretching the back muscles, performing a variety of abdominal strengthening exercises, and doing some aerobic work to burn calories. You can also provide a list of appropriate home videos to provide variety in the workouts.

Set Priorities for Change

Strategies for change are not simply a list of recommendations. The strategies are the final product of a progressive narrowing exercise. After pertinent

Table 1.5   Describing the Benefits of a Prescription Feature

Feature	Benefits
The prescription is designed to suit the space and equipment within your home.	• Suits your busy schedule • Saves time, because you don't have to wait for equipment or commute • Is less expensive in the long run • Will produce desired results • Provides a personalized approach • Allows you to circuit train
The prescription includes using exercise videos for education and leadership.	• Requires less reading or attending special classes on back care • Helps you understand your body and how to move it correctly • Can be performed any time • Is less expensive after several uses • Provides motivation through music and visuals

information has been gathered and the stage of commitment established, you help your client set his priorities. Then looking to the future, you and your client envision goals. With further focus and specific measurability, the exercise culminates in working objectives tailored to your client.

Your client has come for guidance and consultation. She has expectations but wants you to help develop a plan that will produce results. What is most important? What should you tackle first? What will make a difference in her life? Our clients usually have several concerns, and we must help them establish which is to be dealt with first. You must use all the listening and questioning

skills discussed earlier if you are to understand your clients' true priorities and discern what action should be taken first.

The following three principles can serve as guidelines to help you set those priorities: Begin with client concerns, choose manageable issues that can show improvement, and highlight the client's health concerns.

1. **Begin with client concerns.** Do not confuse what is important to you with what is important to your clients. Not everyone places the same priority on fitness that you do, and you cannot expect all of your clients to immediately buy in

Gains from physical activity (to self, family, and others)	Losses from physical activity (to self, family, and others)
• I may finally lose those extra pounds that I put on after my last child. • My energy levels should increase. • I will be a less stressed, happier person for my family.	• I may miss transporting my kids to some of their events. • My husband may have to prepare dinner if I work out after work.
Strategies (to maximize gains)	**Strategies (to minimize losses)**
• Although some of your gains will be physical and some psychological, it looks like both are dependent on being regular. • Keep a calendar posted at home with the dates and times of anticipated workouts clearly marked. • Don't be hard on yourself if you miss some!	• Take your husband out for dinner this week and talk to him about how important this is to you and that you recognize and appreciate his extended role. • Your family is obviously an important part of any change that you make and maintain. Perhaps you can organize something the whole family can do together on weekends like hiking, biking, or skating. • We will avoid back fatigue in every workout.

Figure 1.3   Carol and her trainer weigh the pros and cons of becoming more active.

Cautionary Note

At this crucial point of commitment and implementation, a host of things can happen to challenge this rational process. Many clients demonstrate ambivalence by stating that they can see why they should exercise but the costs of making that change are a significant deterrent (Prochaska 1994). You can work positively with this ambivalence if you guard against these potential pitfalls:

- Skipping or ignoring the analysis stage and moving quickly to a decision.

- Allowing the client to fall into "defensive avoidance" (Egan 1990), that is, rationalizing a delay in choice or commitment: "Yeah, that sounds good but I'll have to wait until this busy time at work is over."

- Letting the client seize on a comfortable short-term option. For example, "OK, that first step was new walking shoes. . . . I can do that at the end of the month when I get paid. I love to shop!"

- Suggesting a course of action more because it is highly recommended or popular than because it is suitable for the client.

- Pushing before the client is ready to change a lifestyle habit.

- Allowing the client to translate the decision into action half-heartedly. For example, "I'll probably get started sometime next week."

to your enthusiasm for exercise. Begin with the concerns (needs, wants, or lifestyle issues) that the client sees as important. You may believe that her focus should be broadened, but beginning at this point will send an important message: "Your interests matter to me." For example, a sedentary client with elevated blood lipids wants to start a weight training program to tone up. You soon see that she is more interested in her appearance than in the health issue. So for the present, you address the client's chief concern: With appropriate prescription precautions and monitoring, she begins light weight training. Later you will look for opportunities to address the lipid problem. Or if an overweight office worker comes to you with hypertension, stress, and muscular tension, you may discover as you gather information that you need to address his work environment before becoming too specific with an exercise prescription.

2. **Choose manageable issues that can show improvement.** Although you neither can nor should try to force your clients to adopt your views about what their priorities should be, it is your job to show your clients the benefits of certain choices. If clients are skeptical or fearful, give them information and encouragement to see the issues in focused, realistic, and concrete ways.

If you help them picture the benefits of relatively undemanding strategies and imagine what things would be like if they were to use those strategies, such clients will often adjust their priorities. If you can help a hesitant client buy in to a simple prescription, the reinforcement he experiences may empower him to attack more difficult tasks. Clear and measurable results that show up early in the training can magnify commitment. Intervention and monitoring provide feedback and help the client to focus on his gains. This can sometimes be more difficult for clients who have multiple tasks in their lives or for those who may be overwhelmed with new or busy challenges. The story of Jay, a teenage athlete suffering from tiredness, reflects one of these situations.

3. **Highlight the client's health concerns.** Consider seriously any health issues the client wants to change. Determine the client's primary goal: general fitness, performance-related fitness (e.g., for athletic competition), or health-related fitness (chapter 3). If he is open to modifying his behavior in any health-related area, cautiously seize the opportunity. He may expect immediate and tangible results, however, so educate him while still sympathizing with his impatience. Careful screening will reveal any cardiovascular or metabolic problems the client may have. If

Prioritizing for a Young Athlete

Jay, a young athlete, was brought to me by his parents. He was part of an active family with a very full agenda. I had worked with Jay's hockey team the previous year, and his parents knew that I worked one-on-one with many young athletes. Jay enjoyed sports, but his parents had noticed some fatigue and anxiety about meeting all his obligations, including doing homework and spending time with friends. They asked if I would try to help improve his energy level and what they called a waning attitude.

My first conversation with Jay was about how he managed all the demands on his time. I identified the areas where he was doing well and also those that showed a lack of self-discipline. Jay wanted to please everyone: his parents, teachers, and coaches. As the demands increased, he found himself overwhelmed and feeling as though he was not meeting anyone's expectations. I explained that it is hard to set things aside temporarily to allow focus on an immediate concern, yet that skill is the cornerstone of setting priorities. He agreed to try.

Jay and I pulled out a large calendar and listed all the things he had to do for the next 2 months. Then we went back over each one and tried to give it a priority rating of 1, 2, or 3. This was not easy, because Jay initially saw everything as a priority 1! We made sure to include all the 1s and managed to drop a few of the 3s. Jay maintained the monthly calendar and continued not only to list all his sport activities and school assignments but also to schedule blocks of free time that he could spend with his friends. He enjoyed checking off accomplishments and seeing progress.

I gave Jay's parents a list of symptoms of overtraining that they were to be watchful for. They also agreed to assist Jay during the busy times to focus on the higher-priority activities and to celebrate any and all accomplishments. Jay decided to play hockey for a less demanding team, which provided not only more time but a psychological break. He continues to use his calendar to record important dates and assignments, and the last time I called, he was out with his friends.

Alternatives: High-Intensity Interval Training

DeBusk and colleagues (1990) examined an alternative to the traditional prescription. They showed that three 10 min jogging workouts a day, 5 days a week for 8 weeks at moderate intensity, increased $\dot{V}O_2max$ by 8% in healthy middle-aged men. Another group who performed a standard 30 min jogging workout increased their $\dot{V}O_2max$ by 14%. This shows that more vigorous exercise is not necessary for initial conditioning in more sedentary clients.

Another recent alternative is high-intensity interval training, commonly referred to as HIIT, for well-conditioned, younger clients. It can give a natural boost to human growth hormone (HGH) production—which is essential for optimal health, strength, and vigor—and has been shown to significantly improve insulin sensitivity, boost fat loss, and increase muscle growth. While there are a large number of variations, the HIIT routine can involve going all out for 30 s and then resting for 90 s between sprints for 8 repetitions. The total workout is about 20 minutes two or three times a week.

necessary, work closely with other health care practitioners and consider other lifestyle issues (e.g., diet, reducing stress, eliminating smoking) along with the exercise prescription. Many clients with fitness or performance goals have a limiting musculoskeletal problem. Determine the stage of the injury, its seriousness, and the original or ongoing cause. Address this hurdle first or at least in parallel with other prescriptions. Chapter 11, "Exercise Prescription for Specific Injuries," is a valuable resource for such clients.

Use Measurable Objectives

Goals are broad, general (usually long-term) statements that describe overall intentions. They translate priorities into action and specify a future outcome. Working with your clients to write their goals down, you clarify your own thinking and make sure that you are using the same vocabulary as your clients. The act of writing down goals sometimes triggers a design idea that opens up new ways of approaching a problem.

The vagueness of many goals makes them easy to ignore. "I'm going to become more active this year" is a common New Year's resolution, yet it rarely leads to action. People need specificity. Ask the question, "What will you be doing or what will be different when you make the change?" The answer may be "I'm going to spend 3 days a week in an exercise class at my health club and ride my bike to work each day." Notice how specific this statement is. It describes a pattern of behavior that will be put in place, not a vague concept of greater activity.

A goal is a clear, broad statement of intention. It is a start to making a behavioral change. Write each client priority as a goal statement that includes an action verb. Then, try this simple checklist to judge the quality of each of your client's goals:

- Is it a broad statement based on a single priority?
- Does it describe the client's intentions?
- Is it easy to understand?
- Is it good for the client's overall health?

A goal is often defined by a series of objectives that break the strategies down into a number of distinct and sometimes progressive steps. Here are some sample goals and objectives:

Goal: To learn more about my personal diet.
Objectives:

1. To attend a weekly seminar this semester and keep a binder of all the course notes.
2. To have my diet analyzed before and after the course and calculate the improvements.

Goal: To improve my ability to work with free weights.
Objectives:

1. To attend a second program demonstration session next week with my exercise specialist to get personal feedback.
2. To ask my friend, who has more experience, to be a training partner 1 day per week.
3. To keep a training log that records my performance and my subjective feelings of improvement.

Recently, I had a client whose history, assessment results, and priorities centered around her cardiovascular improvement. Her goal was "to feel less tired and to last longer when doing aerobic activities." Her objectives were

1. to complete 10 walk–jog sessions within 3 weeks at her training heart rate,

2. to increase the length of each session (duration) by 10% each week, and

3. to monitor her feelings of fatigue at the end of each aerobic session and at the end of each day with an overall outcome of increased energy by the end of 3 weeks.

Note that each objective proposes clearly defined steps and describes the desired outcome of the goal more precisely. Objectives are action oriented. They tell how well and under what conditions the outcome should be performed. Working in small, measurable chunks gives people frequent successes in the journey to their goal, empowering them and feeding their enthusiasm and persistence in reaching the long-term goal.

A simple technique used to create and evaluate objectives is the SMART system (CSEP 2003). In this system, exercise objectives have five characteristics: specific, measurable, attainable, realistic, and timed. Francis (1990) recommended that the term **attainable** be replaced with the term **action oriented** because **attainable** and **realistic** are so similar as to be redundant and because **action oriented** is an important characteristic of an effective objective. Thus, we have the modified SMART system to include objectives that are

- specific,
- measurable,
- action oriented,
- realistic, and
- timed.

Setting objectives can take as little as 10 min and can improve your client's awareness of her "future vision." Use SMART to help clients develop objectives that have some probability of success. For one client, this may mean focusing on being clear and specific. You may help another client devise a way to measure improvement and another to develop realistic time frames. Most clients need some help with at least one of the five criteria. SMART not only helps to devise objectives but also provides a menu for intervention.

Form 1.8, Objective-Setting Worksheet, is designed to guide the process of setting objectives following the SMART criteria.

Specific

Objectives should be clear and specific enough to drive action. Effective use of questioning, probing, and paraphrasing can help your client articulate the level of specificity he needs in order to act. If a client whose objective is to get in shape does not state for what reason or in what component areas, she makes it impossible for you to prescribe an exercise program—let alone be client centered. By contrast, the objective of "running 40 min nonstop" is a specific and measurable outcome.

Measurable

For most clients, being able to measure progress is an important incentive. Moreover, if the objective is not specifically measurable, how will the client know when it is accomplished? Always have your clients ask themselves, "What will I be doing or what will be different when I make the change?" You can gauge progress on some objectives through measuring and others by rating or clearly describing the desired outcome.

You can easily measure changes in cardiovascular fitness, body composition, strength and endurance, flexibility, posture and muscle balance, and performance-related fitness. Conducting fitness assessments and providing periodic evaluations are two important motivational strategies known to improve exercise compliance (Francis 1990).

It is difficult to objectively quantify a goal such as "To feel better about exercising." One suggestion is to construct a rating scale from 1 to 10, with 1 representing the poorest and 10 the best (Clark and Clark 1993). The client estimates where on the scale he thinks he is at a given time and logs any trends.

Another method is to describe, in advance, what is meant or implied by the objective. For example, your client who wants to feel better about exercise might verify this accomplishment if he looked forward to each workout, saw activity as a break in the day, enjoyed the social aspect of the activity, and felt much more relaxed and energized after exercise. If you can't quantify, measure, rate, or otherwise describe an objective, then you should forget it, because your client will never be able to attain it!

Along with measurable, and keeping with the alliteration, the objective should be "meaningful." Of course, this is meaningful to the client, providing importance and personal reward at some level.

Here is another sample dialogue in which the exercise professional continues to focus and provide specific measurability, which culminates in working objectives tailored to Carol, the client.

FP: Now that we have had a chance to chat about your past activities and the things that you might like to do, tell me, Carol, exactly what do you think your weekly commitment could be?

CL: Well, until the weather gets a bit warmer and I can work in the garden, I know that I could walk the dog every day.

FP: Great start, and it fits into your daily pattern of activities. How fast does the dog go and how long are the usual walks?

CL: She tugs me along as fast as I can go with very few stops! I usually do kind of a double loop that takes about 20 min and sometimes on the weekends I'll go down to the creek for 30 to 40 min but it is a bit slower.

FP: Carol, can you see yourself doing a brisk 20 to 25 min walk with the dog Monday through Friday and two extended 30 to 40 min hikes down to the creek each week?

CL: Oh yeah. My husband will appreciate me taking over that chore and I think that I will enjoy getting outside. Is that in addition to my program?

FP: Actually, that will be a big part of your aerobic exercise prescription and a significant objective in itself. I'm glad it sounds realistic.

Action Oriented

The cornerstone of an effective objective is the specific activity or exercises that will accomplish the objective. It is not a detailed prescription, but the client must be able to visualize what she will be doing. "I want to start doing some exercise" is a nonspecific activity, whereas "Within 6 months, I will be running 3 miles in less than 30 minutes at least four times a week" is a specific outcome that your client can visualize. To check your objectives, look for the verbs; they are the action words and should reflect the activity needed to accomplish the outcome.

Realistic

Many people quit exercising because they are disillusioned when their program fails to accomplish the anticipated results. The exercise objective might have been unrealistic to begin with. An objective is realistic if

- the resources necessary for its accomplishment are available (exercise noncompliance is often related to inconvenience of location or inaccessibility of equipment),
- it is under the client's control (her genetic background may never allow her to look like a thin fashion model), and
- it has a high priority for the client (it is something your client wants to do because it will satisfy her most important needs in a way that accommodates her lifestyle) (Egan 1990).

An objective is most realistic when these three elements coincide. Objectives are unrealistic if they are set too high, but they are inadequate if

---

Evaluating Objectives

Your client's goal is to improve cardiovascular fitness. Use the SMART criteria as a checklist to evaluate the following objectives.

1. To walk briskly in the evenings for 40 min, 4 days per week.
2. To monitor weekly my walking time and heart rate over a measured distance and to have my cardiovascular (CV) fitness remeasured at 3 and 6 months—targeting a 10% increase every 3 months.

Objective 1:

S ___ Walk for CV fitness improvement

M ___ 40 min, 4 days/week

A ___ To walk briskly

R ___ Accomplishment has been demonstrated repeatedly in research and in personal experience; time commitment and resources such as walking shoes must be confirmed.

T ___ Ten percent improvement every 3 months for one-half year

Objective 2:

S ___ Monitor the walk for CV fitness improvement

M ___ Monitor heart rate over a measured distance and CV reassessments

A ___ Monitor duration and intensity (heart rate)

R ___ A 10% increase every 3 months is valid for the prescription.

T ___ Weekly monitorings are short-term checks, and the 3- and 6-month reassessments are longer-term benchmarks.

they are set too low. They must be relevant to the goal, painting a manageable picture of what success looks like while challenging the client.

Timed

A timed objective provides a powerful motivation for following an exercise program. To set realistic target dates, consider each objective from a time perspective. An objective can be long-term (months) or short-term (perhaps within a day). Losing 25 lb (11 kg) in 4 months may be realistic, but a short-term objective of losing 1.5 lb (0.7 kg) per week may seem more manageable. Short-term objectives, successfully completed early in your client's program, can start a cycle of challenge and achievement that enhances his self-confidence.

Summary

The Activity Counseling Model involves three steps: rapport, information, and strategies for change. In this model, the primary objective when counseling about activity is to create a rapport that allows openness to the gathering of information. Only then can you determine your client's degree of commitment to change and help her set action-oriented objectives that will enable her to visualize where she wants to be.

Your first objective is to put your client at ease and develop a comfortable working relationship. In establishing this rapport, be receptive and responsive while outlining the counseling process and discussing the reasons for attending. Rapport demands attentive behavior and a listening style that clarifies your client's message.

There are two effective methods to gather client information: (a) past, present, future and (b) needs, wants, lifestyle. Either method of approaching information gathering can stand alone, but a combination of the two methods will be most comprehensive and client centered. The type and timing of questions can make or break a counseling session. The clearer the profile of your client, the better the information and support you can provide.

One effective way to work with a client's readiness to change is to think in terms of the five stages of change. Once you know your client's stage of change, you can choose strategies that are effective for that specific stage, which you will read about in chapter 2. Begin with your client's concerns to set priorities; then set goals to translate the priorities and provide a visualization of a future outcome. Objectives take a goal and make it "SMART." They describe a pattern of behavior that will be put in place that is specific, measurable, action oriented, realistic, and timed. This culminates in working objectives tailored to your client.

FORM 1.1   FANTASTIC Lifestyle Checklist

Instructions: Unless otherwise specified, place an 'X' beside the box that best describes your behavior or situation in the past month. Explanations of questions and scoring are provided on the third page.

Family Friends	I have someone to talk to about things that are important to me	almost never		seldom		some of the time		fairly often		almost always	
	I give and receive affection	almost never		seldom		some of the time		fairly often		almost always	
Activity	I am vigorously active for at least 30 min per day (e.g., running, cycling, etc.)	less than once a week		1-2 times/ week		3 times/week		4 times/ week		5 or more times/ week	
	I am moderately active (gardening, climbing stairs, walking, house-work)	less than once a week		1-2 times/ week		3 times/week		4 times/ week		5 or more times/ week	
Nutrition	I eat a balanced diet (see explana-tion, third page)	almost never		seldom		some of the time		fairly often		almost always	
	I often eat excess: (1) sugar, or (2) salt, or (3) animal fats, or (4) junk foods	four of these		three of these		two of these		one of these		none of these	
	I am within _____ kg of my healthy weight	not within 8 kg (20 lb)		8 kg (20 lb)		6 kg (15 lb)		4 kg (10 lb)		2 kg (5 lb)	
Tobacco Toxics	I smoke tobacco	more than 10 times/week		1-10 times/ week		none in the past 6 months		none in the past year		none in the past 5 years	
	I use drugs such as marijuana, cocaine	sometimes								never	
	I overuse pre-scribed drugs or over the counter drugs	almost daily		fairly often		only occasion-ally		almost never		never	
	I drink caffeine-containing coffee, tea, or cola	more than 10 times/week		7-10/day		3-6/day		1-2/day		never	

(continued)

(continued)

		more than 20 drinks		13-20 drinks		11-12 drinks		8-10 drinks		0-7 drinks	
Alcohol	My average alcohol intake per week is _____ (see explanation, third page)	more than 20 drinks		13-20 drinks		11-12 drinks		8-10 drinks		0-7 drinks	
	I drink more than four drinks on occasion	almost daily		fairly often		only occasion-ally		almost never		never	
	I drive after drink-ing	sometimes								never	
Sleep Seatbelts Stress Safe sex	I sleep well and feel rested	almost never		seldom		some of the time		fairly often		almost always	
	I use seatbelts	never		seldom		some of the time		most of the time		always	
	I am able to cope with the stresses in my life	almost never		seldom		some of the time		fairly often		almost always	
	I relax and enjoy leisure time	almost never		seldom		some of the time		fairly often		almost always	
	I practice safe sex (see explanation, third page)	almost never		seldom		some of the time		fairly often		always	
Type of behavior	I seem to be in a hurry	almost always		fairly often		some of the time		seldom		almost never	
	I feel angry or hostile	almost always		fairly often		some of the time		seldom		almost never	
Insight	I am a positive or optimistic thinker	almost never		seldom		some of the time		fairly often		almost always	
	I feel tense or uptight	almost always		fairly often		some of the time		seldom		almost never	
	I feel sad or depressed	almost always		fairly often		some of the time		seldom		almost never	
Career	I am satisfied with my job or role	almost never		seldom		some of the time		fairly often		almost always	

Step 1   Total the Xs in each column   → ☐ ☐ ☐ ☐ ☐

Step 2   Multiply the totals by the numbers indicated (write answers in box below)   → 0   ×1   ×2   ×3   ×4

Step 3   Add your scores across bottom for your grand total   → ☐ ☐ ☐ ☐ ☐

A Balanced Diet

According to Canada's Food Guide to Healthy Eating (for people four years and over):
Different People Need Different Amounts of Food

The amount of food you need every day from the four food groups and other foods depends on your age, body size, activity level, whether you are male or female, and if you are pregnant or breast feeding. That's why the Food Guide gives a lower and higher number of servings for each food group. For example, young children can choose the lower number of servings, while male teenagers can select the higher number. Most other people can choose servings somewhere in between.

Grain products	Vegetables and fruit	Milk products	Meat and alternatives	Other foods
Choose whole-grain and enriched products more often.	Choose dark green and orange vegetables more often.	Choose lower fat milk products more often	Choose leaner meats, poultry and fish, as well as dried peas, beans, and lentils more often.	Taste and enjoyment can also come from other foods and beverages that are not part of the 4 food groups. Some of these are higher in fat or calories, so use these foods in moderation.
Recommended number of servings per day:				
5-12	5-10	Children 4-9 yrs: 2-3 Youth 10-16 yrs: 3-4 Adults: 2-4 Pregnant and breast-feeding women: 3-4	2-3	

Alcohol Intake

1 drink equals:

		Canadian	Metric	U.S.
1 bottle of beer	5% alcohol	12 oz.	340.8 ml	10 oz.
1 glass of wine	12% alcohol	5 oz.	142 ml	4.5 oz.
1 shot of spirits	40% alcohol	1.5 oz.	42.6 ml	1.25 oz.

Safe Sex

Refers to the use of methods of preventing infection or conception.

What does the score mean?				
85-100 Excellent	70-84 Very good	55-69 Good	35-54 Fair	0-34 Needs improvement

Note: A low total score does not mean that you have failed. There is always the chance to change your lifestyle—starting now. Look at the areas where you scored a 0 or 1 and decide which areas you want to work on first.

Tips

1. Don't try to change all the areas at once. This will be too overwhelming for you.
2. Writing down your proposed changes and your overall goal will help you to succeed.
3. Make changes in small steps toward the overall goal.
4. Enlist the help of a friend to make similar changes or to support you in your attempts.
5. Congratulate yourself for achieving each step. Give yourself appropriate rewards.
6. Ask your physical activity professional, family physician, nurse, or health department for more information on any of these areas.

From J.C. Griffin, 2015, *Client-centered exercise prescription,* 3rd ed. (Champaign, IL: Human Kinetics). Adapted with permission from the Fantastic Lifestyle Assessments © 1995, Dr. Douglas Wilson, Department of Family Medicine, McMaster University, Hamilton, Ontario, Canada L8N 3Z5.

FORM 1.2   Inventory of Lifestyle and Activity Preferences

I feel it is important to me to

___ like the people I'm with.

___ be in a group.

___ be independent.

___ get to know other people well.

___ meet many new people.

___ be a leader.

___ feel confident.

___ learn something.

___ be in pleasant, attractive surroundings.

___ be alone.

___ have a structured activity.

___ be able to do things at the last minute.

___ follow rules.

___ be praised.

___ have fun and enjoy myself.

___ release frustration.

___ release energy.

___ have common interests with other people.

___ improve my health.

___ be able to contribute something to a group.

___ have other people like me.

___ be physically active.

___ use my imagination.

___ create something.

___ find the activity challenging.

___ feel safe and secure.

___ try something new and different.

___ be myself.

___ use my talents.

___ improve myself and my skills.

___ accomplish something.

___ relax.

___ spend time with my family.

___ take a risk.

___ enjoy the outdoors.

Once you have checked the lifestyle needs that are important to you, list the three most important and identify which activities would most probably satisfy these needs.

Lifestyle needs	Activity preferences
1.	
2.	
3.	

FORM 1.3   Gathering Information Interview Worksheet

Trainer's name: _____

Client's name: _____

```
            _____         _____
          /             \     /             \
         /               \   /               \
        /                 \ /                 \
       /     Needs         X      Wants        \
      |               ___/   \___               |
       \             /  Focus    \             /
        \           /             \           /
         \         |               |         /
          \        |               |        /
           _____\             /_____/
                    |             |
                    |  Lifestyle  |
                     \           /
                      _____/
```

Injuries or health issues: _____

_____

_____

Current activities—FITT: _____

_____

_____

Preferred activities: _____

_____

_____

Commitment (stage of change): _____

Summary of top two objectives:

   1. _____

   2. _____

From J.C. Griffin, 2015, *Client-centered exercise prescription,* 3rd ed. (Champaign, IL: Human Kinetics).

FORM 1.4   Activity Preferences Questionnaire

Activity Reference

What type of training activity (e.g., jog, cycle, hike, ski) do you prefer? _____

What method of training (e.g., interval or continuous) do you prefer? _____

Do you prefer group or personal training? _____

Do you enjoy competitive or noncompetitive activities? _____

What type of location do you prefer? _____

What is your favorite type of equipment? _____

What aspects of a past prescription did you enjoy? _____

Is there anything in your type or level of current activity that you want to maintain? _____

Special Interests

Do you have any current or past skills that you want to pursue? _____

Do you want more information or resources on particular activities, health, or lifestyle topics? ____

_____

Do you definitely want to avoid anything? _____

Are you interested in accomplishing something specific or being challenged? _____

Are you looking for something new or some variety in your prescription? _____

Expectations

Do you have any objectives that are particularly important? _____

How will we know when you have reached your objective (be specific about measurable areas of improvement)? _____

Are there major behaviors that you wish to change (e.g., eating habits)? _____

Do you have expectations for changes in a medical condition? _____

Do you have any performance or sport-specific expectations? _____

Do you want to know your status or improvement with respect to population standards or in comparison with your own previous efforts? _____

Can you set priorities for your expectations? _____

From J.C. Griffin, 2015, *Client-centered exercise prescription*, 3rd ed. (Champaign, IL: Human Kinetics).

FORM 1.5   Focus on Lifestyle

One way of increasing activity is by altering daily routines to encourage more exercise. Ask your client questions that will indicate which of the following aspects of her lifestyle you can target to provide the best prescription. Use the following list to record appropriate notes and check off the ones you can target for modification.

___ Current work routine

___ Current leisure routine

___ Most convenient times

From J.C. Griffin, 2015, *Client-centered exercise prescription,* 3rd ed. (Champaign, IL: Human Kinetics).

FORM 1.6   Stages of Change Questionnaire

Physical activity can include such activities as walking, cycling, swimming, climbing stairs, dancing, active gardening, walking to work, aerobics, and sports. Regular physical activity is 30 min of moderate activity accumulated over the day, almost every day, or vigorous activity done at least three times per week for 20 min each time.

Here are a number of statements describing various levels of physical activity. Please select the one that most closely describes your own level:

(Please pick one.)

I am not physically active and I do not plan on becoming so.   1

I have been thinking about becoming physically active, but I haven't done   2
anything about it yet.

I am physically active once in a while, but not regularly.   3

I have become involved in regular physical activity within the past 6 months.   4

I participate in regular physical activity and have done so for more than 6 months.   5

(Answer if not currently active.)
I was physically active in the past, but not now.   Yes   No

FORM 1.7 Decision Balance Summary

Gains from physical activity (to self, family, and others)	Losses from physical activity (to self, family, and others)

Strategies (to maximize gains)	Strategies (to minimize losses)

From J.C. Griffin, 2015, *Client-centered exercise prescription,* 3rd ed. (Champaign, IL: Human Kinetics). Source: *Canadian Physical Activity, Fitness & Lifestyle Approach: CSEP-Health & Fitness Program's Appraisal and Counselling Strategy,* 3rd edition, © 2003. Reprinted with permission from the Canadian Society for Exercise Physiology.

FORM 1.8   Objective-Setting Worksheet

Goal (broad statement of intention):

_____

_____

Objective 1 (activity and outcome):

_____

_____

Check each SMART criterion that is fulfilled by the objective.

❏ Specific

❏ Measured

❏ Action oriented

❏ Realistic

❏ Timed

Objective 2 (activity and outcome):

_____

_____

Check each SMART criterion that is fulfilled by the objective.

❏ Specific

❏ Measured

❏ Action oriented

❏ Realistic

❏ Timed

Objective 3 (activity and outcome):

_____

_____

Check each SMART criterion that is fulfilled by the objective.

❏ Specific

❏ Measured

❏ Action oriented

❏ Realistic

❏ Timed

From J.C. Griffin, 2015, *Client-centered exercise prescription*, 3rd ed. (Champaign, IL: Human Kinetics).

FORM 1.9 Activity Counseling Model Checklist

Step 1: Establish rapport	Action checklist
Create a friendly welcome: Be receptive and responsive	❏ Friendly environment ❏ Caring demonstrated ❏ Clients talking about themselves
Discuss the counseling process and the reason for attending	❏ Clients share why they are there and what they hope to change
Ensure you have received your client's messages	❏ Clear messages sent ❏ Effective listening (paraphrasing)

Step 2: Gather information	Action checklist
Examine past, present, and future	❏ Discuss activity patterns ❏ Establish why client likes (dislikes) current activity . . . window to motivation
Identify needs, wants, and lifestyle	❏ Wants: activity preferences, special interests, or expectations identified ❏ Needs: injury, fitness component, health risk factors, special design, education, or motivational support identified ❏ Lifestyle: time, facilities, partners, travel, employment, and so on ❏ "Routines," for example, work, activity, sleep, eating, family identified ❏ Effective questioning
Determine your client's stage of change	❏ Stage of change (commitment) identified

Step 3: Establish strategies for change	Action checklist
Select strategies that match your client's stage of change	❏ Stage of change strategy identified (including major barriers)
Maximize benefits from the client's perspective	❏ Options identified (pros and cons) ❏ Check back with client regarding priorities
When goal setting, use measurable objectives	❏ Goals identified and refined as measurable objectives ❏ Discussion regarding follow-up applications: assessment, general action plan, prescription, and so on

From J.C. Griffin, 2015, *Client-centered exercise prescription*, 3rd ed. (Champaign, IL: Human Kinetics).

Client-Centered Motivational Strategies

Chapter Competencies

After completing this chapter, you will be able to demonstrate the following competencies:

1. Apply motivational strategies to help clients through various stages of exercise adoption.

2. Use the change process strategies that are appropriate at each stage of change.

3. Provide client support based on client profiling (learning styles and personality styles).

4. Describe the role and provide examples of extrinsic motivation and apply motivational techniques that will reinforce intrinsic change to healthy behaviors.

5. Apply motivational strategies to help clients commit to their objectives.

6. Suggest some client-centered approaches to coping with barriers and solving problems that will increase exercise adherence.

7. Apply appropriate client-centered motivating tactics learned in case study scenarios.

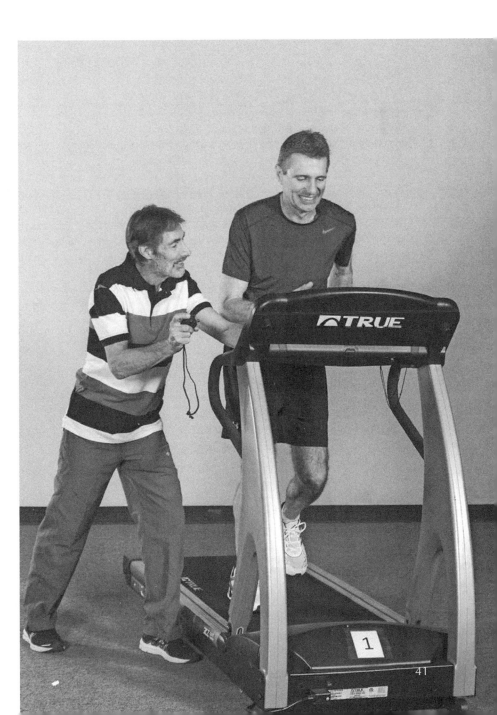

If the key factors in helping people to become regular exercisers were *what* to do in exercise and *how* to do it, we would be far more successful. But it is clear that the *motivation to make changes* and *how to go about mobilizing motivation* are the central factors in helping people to make health-promoting personal behavioral changes. Each stage of change is different and each client unique, which creates the challenge of selecting a motivation strategy and support tools to help each individual when early enthusiasm wanes. We can cajole, encourage, or threaten, but in the long run clients become active only because they think it is good for them. They will stick with an activity because they enjoy it and believe they are achieving something. The heart of effective motivation is learning what drives a particular client at a particular time. In this chapter we explore in detail how to work with clients to keep them motivated, following their priorities and objectives within the context of their lifestyles.

The counseling skills and tools outlined in the previous chapter include a number of strategic plans to help clients through various stages of exercise adoption. Each of these should be used appropriately as your client's stage of change varies. Strategies to facilitate personal behavioral change can be initiated in the counseling session. There are tools that can help support the various stages of change such as setting objectives, self-contract, self-talk, encouraging self-efficacy, and using form 2.2, the Relapse Planner. Listen carefully to your client's issues, because a tool may not work with one client but will with the next.

Stages of Change

Living in the developed world discourages physical activity, leading many people to exert as little physical effort as possible. Drive; don't walk or bike or run. Buy a robotic vacuum cleaner; don't push the old-fashioned kind. Watch basketball on television; don't play the game yourself. And on and on. Many people are aware that they should be physically active but have never been able to overcome their inertia.

The Transtheoretical Model (TTM) describes changes in behavior, such as regular exercise, as occurring through a series of five stages. The TTM also describes a number of "processes of change" (e.g., consciousness raising, enlisting social support, using stimulus control techniques) that are matched to these stages. The TTM also recognizes the roles of *decisional balance* (weighing pros and

cons of changing behavior) and *self-efficacy* (confidence in one's ability to engage in or continue behavioral change in specific high-risk situations) on behavior (Gabriele et al. 2011).

Table 2.1 lists the change processes (third column) that are most likely to increase motivation at each stage of change; specific strategies to encourage the appropriate change process are listed in the next column. (Refer to definitions of change process [Prochaska 1992] for 6 of the 10 processes if you are unsure what the listed change processes mean.) For example, if you have a precontemplative client, raise her consciousness of the importance of activity for her health. As this precontemplative person becomes aware of the message about activity and health, she moves to a level of comprehension where she recognizes and understands the problem. By informing her, conversing with her, and emphasizing the specific benefits she could experience from activity, you are likely to move her to the next level: contemplating the idea of becoming active. The Alberta Centre for Active Living (2011a) surveyed the predictors of physical activity and found that if Albertans had moderate or high "intention" to participate in regular physical activity (i.e., preparation stage), they were four to six times more likely to be sufficiently active compared to those with low intention. By declaring an intention, a client demonstrates a change process called self-liberation, which is the belief that one has the power to change ones' own life.

Look through the skills and tools presented in chapter 1 and identify which can be used to implement each strategy. For example, you can

- inform the client by using the assessment tools and discussing with her the results and their implications,
- facilitate dialogue by using a tool like form 1.7, Decision Balance Summary (chapter 1), and
- use active listening skills combined with questioning skills to help her understand the specific benefits she can experience.

Relapse is almost inevitable, and you should be prepared for it. You must help the client resume the process of change through simple, short-term objectives, because his confidence will be bolstered by the success that comes with small changes. Match his current stage (he will have regressed!) with a stage in table 2.1; think about the change processes that are necessary to move him forward again, and use the strategies associated with those change

Table 2.1   Strategies for Change Process

Stage	Client behavior	Change process strategy	Counseling and motivating strategies
Precontemplative	• Is somewhat aware of the message	• Consciousness raising	• Increase awareness of importance. • Start a dialogue. • Increase "pros" for activity.
Contemplative	• Is aware of and interested in the message • Recognizes the problem	• Consciousness raising • Contingency management	• Increase intention to action by addressing ambivalence, highlighting personal benefits, and building self-confidence. • Create an understanding and acceptance.
Preparation	• Identifies a course of action • Is ready to take action	• Consciousness raising • Contingency management • Self-liberation	• Help client plan (e.g., set date, location). • Focus on the "pros." • Strengthen self-confidence. • Provide helpful resources (knowledge and skills).
Action	• Makes a decision to implement a course of action • Tries the activity • Makes short-term adoption	• Contingency management • Self-liberation • Helping relationships	• Teach client how to deal with lapses. • Promote social support. • Deal with lapses; reevaluate next action step. • Provide encouragement.
Maintenance	• Makes long-term commitment • Achieves permanent lifestyle change	• Helping relationships • Counterconditioning • Stimulus control	• Refine and add variety to program. • Prepare in case of relapse. • Provide support in maintaining behavior to prevent relapse.

processes. To help lessen the chances of relapse, don't let new enthusiasts skip a stage, lest they miss a mechanism of support and be less successful in the long run. Success requires stage-to-stage transitions. The challenge is to match your strategy with natural progression through the stages of change.

By understanding your client's stage of change, the change process appropriate to that stage, and the strategies that will facilitate change, you will help your client recognize the importance of fitness and how it meets her personal needs. This recognition is the beginning of motivation.

Client Profiling

Unlocking the mysteries of how people think and learn will also help you be more effective with your clients. The clearer the "profile" you have of your client, the better the information and support you can provide at the most appropriate times. Two areas of profiling that present opportunities for better understanding of what is needed to change behavior are preferred learning style and personality style.

Preferred Learning Style

By keeping in mind the preferred learning style of your client, you can decide the best method to demonstrate an exercise, teach a monitoring technique, explain test results, introduce a new piece of equipment, and much more. If you select an approach that does not match the learning style of your client, you run the risk of moving at the wrong pace, providing too little or too much information, and generally not making a useful connection with your client regardless of earlier rapport. See "How Does Your Client Learn?" for one good way to understand your client's learning

Psychological Change Process Terminology

- **Consciousness raising** happens when the unconscious becomes conscious. Individuals become aware of new alternatives, and there is increased information about self and health. Consciousness raising may be brought about by changes in environment (e.g., a new bike path or employee fitness center) or a change in a stage of life. It usually requires education and feedback. Other techniques using this process may include watching an instructional program, visiting a physiotherapist, taking a class, or listening to others who are well informed.

- **Contingency management** is a self-evaluation that involves reinforcement made contingent on behavior. It depends on the individual's value of the particular consequence. We can help the client assess the impact of current or future behaviors. For example, by questioning, we may find that clients believe that if they were to take a yoga class, they would be less stressed and more productive. Other techniques using this process may include visualizing oneself overcoming a problem (e.g., binge eating), listing advantages and disadvantages (e.g., of regular exercise), or taking a fitness test to determine health status needs.

- **Self-liberation** is the belief that one has the power to change one's own life, which is based on the sense of self-efficacy. If my client believes that she can strengthen her ankle after injury, her thoughts and actions will increase her commitment to change. Other techniques using this process may include drawing from previous personal successes or purchasing jeans that are a size too small, then starting a daily walking routine.

- **Helping relationships** are provided by caring, understanding, and committed trainers, especially in the areas of acquiring skill and achieving self-efficacy. From the client's perspective, this process involves accepting support and trusting others. Other techniques using this process may include associating with people who have the same exercise goals as yourself or joining a well-led community program designed to deal with your problem (e.g., eating disorder).

- **Counterconditioning** is a strategy that involves changing one's response to particular stimuli. The objective is to counteract old habits and to reinforce new habits. For example, you can help your client change his thinking so that the break between classes that used to trigger a trip to the cafeteria becomes instead a signal for a walk to the local park. Other techniques using this process may include reading a book during TV commercials rather than snacking, or stretching with your towel after a shower.

- **Stimulus control** involves changing one's environment to minimize negative stimuli. This involves recognizing, controlling, or avoiding anti-exercise stimuli; an example is to avoid turning on the television until one has worked out (Brooks 2000). Other techniques using this process may include avoiding having junk food in the house, avoiding relationships that lead to problem behaviors, using posted notes to remind yourself about healthy habits, or simply spending more time in the park.

style. Once you have determined that, here are ways you can match each style:

- **Applying the information to individual situations:** "Up until now, to gauge how hard you were working, I would palpate your heart rate. By wearing this heart rate monitor, you can have that information whenever you want. Even during the hard interval training, you could use that information to judge your recovery."

- **Learning by observation:** "The watch that I have on is a new heart rate monitor that we can use. By presetting these controls, we can set the target zone. I'll show you, when I go below that zone . . . that is the sound of the buzzer that prompts me to speed up."

- **Learning by knowing the theory:** "This heart rate monitor displays the updated average of the last five beats. It's good during exercise but for a person like you with such a low casual heart rate, it may be misleading at rest or light exercise. Why don't we keep a chart comparing the monitor and palpation in different situations?"

- **Learning by doing:** "Check out this new heart rate monitor. Try it for a few workouts and let me know what you think and how it works for you."

Often, as we move from one client to the next, we catch ourselves explaining, demonstrating, or counseling using the same methods and style that we used for the earlier clients. It is natural to fall back to the comfort level of our own preferred style. Catching yourself is a great start; it means

How Does Your Client Learn?

Here is an exercise you can do with your client to determine his learning style:
"The new computer you ordered has just arrived. After you take it out of the box, what do you do?"

- Rely on past experience with a similar computer.
- Call my friend over to get some instruction and a good start on what I should be doing.
- Read the manual carefully and figure out the problems that emerge.
- Set it up, plug it in, and start playing.

If the client elects to rely on past experience, he prefers to learn by applying the information to individual situations. If he calls his friend, he prefers to learn by observation. If he reads the manual carefully, he likes to learn by knowing the theory. And if he just sets up the computer and starts playing, he prefers learning by doing.

your intention is to be truly client centered. If you sense that your client is having difficulty following something or is showing signs of frustration, think about your client's preferred learning style and try to match it.

Fitness professionals have a real challenge guiding clients who are exposed to a barrage of new gimmicks, gadgets, apparel, gym settings, and the latest industry offerings. Many new clients are intimidated and believe that they cannot perform the exercises that other clients can. From their past experiences, clients developed preconceived images of what they believe they can achieve. When the trainer nurtures self-confidence, the client's rate of learning and success will grow. We have an amazing opportunity to not only teach new skills but also to improve our client's confidence to overcome barriers.

Success with motivating and teaching your clients involves using their learning style and your skills to build their confidence. We must help our clients develop the confidence to act by tapping into opportunities such as these:

- Base delivery of the information on clients' preferred learning styles.
- Draw on information from the initial counseling or testing.
- Discover exactly what your client may be concerned about (i.e., source of anxiety).
- Determine level of comfort and understanding.
- Identify tasks that can be performed to facilitate success.
- Concentrate on teaching mastery of the task but at their preferred learning rate.

- Give clients permission to be themselves; show pleasure in what they are doing; provide protection from negative forces (e.g., negative self-talk, interruptions, intimidating atmosphere).
- Provide feedback to the client that is specific, positive, and helpful (provides success).
- Obtain feedback from client (specific probing).
- Modify design if necessary; make sure the client accepts the exercise.
- Observe body language, question the client effectively, provide clarifications, and encourage two-way feedback.

Personality Style

Identifying a client's personality style can help you understand how she sees and reacts to things. If you effectively adapt to her style, it will make her feel more comfortable and trusting. This will go a long way toward helping reach her objectives. Being client centered involves adapting to others' needs. In a counseling setting, use your listening skills (step 1, Activity Counseling Model) to determine the client's predominant personality style.

Of course, most people combine their styles somewhat, but the value of this profiling is that it will help you choose a strategy that will be effective with each client (Prukop 1997). Table 2.2 presents motivational strategies for three common personality styles.

Even with effective client profiling, recognition of learning styles, knowing how and where to build confidence, and recognizing personality characteristics, there are still some difficult client–trainer match-ups. With the growing middle-aged

Table 2.2 Personality Styles and Treatment Strategies

Personality style	Client characteristics	Motivational strategy
Technical	• Systematic • Analytic • Questioning • Organized • Reflective • Theoretical	• Explain pros and cons of choices. • Be accurate. • Allow time—moderate pace. • Provide tangible evidence (educate). • Follow up.
Sociable	• Friendly • Attentive • Supportive • Amiable • Relationship oriented • Demonstrative	• Address the whole person. • Maintain relaxed and moderate pace. • Be a partner in the change. • Be a good listener. • Make eye contact. • Invite feedback.
Assertive	• Leader • Controlling • Pragmatic • May be competitive • May be energetic • Opinionated	• Be stimulating. • Increase pace, once successful. • Be businesslike. • May need to limit options but incorporate input. • Find the client's dreams or hidden agenda.

and older demographics, many young personal trainers will be challenged to relate to their clients. In any successful relationship, both parties play a role in relating effectively to one another. Nationally recognized certifications coupled with formal postsecondary education is a good start, but look for courses or workshops in gerontology or physical changes with aging. Provide your client with specific examples of how you stay current about exercise and aging issues. Before getting too far into the initial session, ask your clients about any injuries and areas of pain and what they have done about them. And finally, build trust. Be attentive and listen to what your client has to say. You don't have to be the same age to enjoy each other's personality enough to spend a few hours a week together. Work at making your client a good match for you.

Goal Setting

Training your mind is just as important as the physical aspects of conditioning, and doing so begins with goal setting. It is often helpful with new clients to ask them to tell you in detail about their goals. When they verbalize or write down their goals, they are forced to consider them carefully. This is important because knowing their goals is what motivates them as they pursue their achievement.

Helping clients develop goals can have a number of advantages (Egan 1990):

- It can focus attention. Clients with clear goals are less likely to engage in aimless behavior, such as walking down a row of weight machines wondering which one to try.
- Setting goals mobilizes energy and effort. It is not just a mental exercise but often arouses in clients a need to act.
- Setting goals seems to increase persistence. Clients with clear goals work harder and don't give up as easily.
- Setting goals motivates clients to search for strategies to accomplish them.

Kyllo and Landers (1995) performed a meta-analysis involving 36 studies on goal setting in sport and exercise. They found that moderately difficult goals led to greater improvement than goals that were too easy or too difficult. These authors reported that critical variables for success included

- specifying goals,
- setting both long- and short-term goals,
- allowing individuals to participate in setting their own goals, and
- making goals public.

Types of Goals

Goal setting can enhance performance, but it needs to be implemented properly to maximize its benefits. Implementation begins with the realization that there are different types of goals:

- **Outcome goals** focus on final results. For some clients, the result may involve weight or size. With athletes, it may be the outcome of a competitive event such as winning a game or beating an opponent on the squash ladder.

- **Performance goals** focus on improving a personal best and are usually independent of others' performance. Examples include reducing your time to complete a circuit, improving a one-repetition maximum (1RM) lift, or bettering your 10K time. Performance goals should be broken down into smaller units, each still measurable but short enough to provide regular positive reinforcement.

- **Process goals** focus on behaviors during training or competition. This may include a client's form or technique during a series of lifts or stretches, or the maintenance of core stability throughout an abdominal workout. Completing a behavior (e.g., an exercise session) means immediate success. Process goals can focus on positive intrinsic experiences with movement and exercise. They can be very effective especially when it is difficult to see regular measurable performance-type improvements (e.g., changes in weight or fitness).

Process goals improve performance more quickly than do longer-term performance goals and are associated with lower anxiety, greater self-confidence, and improved concentration (Tod and McGuigan 2001).

To help your clients get started on their goals, consider the 5 W's of a physical activity plan (Alberta Centre for Active Living 2011b):

What	What type of physical activity(ies) do you want to do?	Nordic walking
Why	Why is this physical activity important to you?	Help control my weight; more energy
Where	Where would you do the activity(ies)?	On the park path near my home
When	When can you be active?	After work every day for 30 min
Who	Who can you be active with?	With my husband

Using Extrinsic Motivators

Many clients start exercise expecting rewards or outcomes such as weight loss, disease reduction, performance, or other health outcomes. If these changes do not happen quickly (and they generally do not), these clients may become discouraged or quit because their expectations are not being met. To prevent this from happening, you must become skilled at using extrinsic and intrinsic motivators. Extrinsic motivators are not essentially part of the goal: for example, the chance to win a monetary award by completing a fitness program at work. Intrinsic motivators are an essential outcome of something valued for its own sake: for example, exercising because you love how it increases your energy. Most clients must be kept motivated extrinsically long enough to experience the positive effects of activity that will give them the intrinsic motivation critical in maintaining long-term exercise (Kimiecik 1998).

Extrinsic motivators are great to get people going. But the rewards and recognitions you use must be psychologically satisfying to your client. At my college, we have tried gift certificates, free personal training sessions, and even money. However, by asking clients directly, we found that they preferred either a recognition T-shirt that they would proudly wear in the center or their name up on the display. The concept that behavior rewarded is repeated appears to be true only if the extrinsic incentive is client focused. Another example: We get a much more positive reaction to sending a card on the client's birthday than to sending a thank-you e-mail that is perceived as standard issue; both take the same effort and expense. Responsiveness to your client's needs means customizing the services and motivation you provide whenever possible. The better hotels and restaurants are masters at customized motivation. They will greet you by name, find your favorite table, or mention something thoughtful from the last visit. Each is an extrinsic motivator, but because it is client centered it shapes our behavior and we return our patronage.

Clients who expect quick results (usually people just entering the action stage of change) are often so disappointed that they quit. Extrinsic motivators are crucial for these people. I have found that some of the extrinsic motivators in the following list can be effective:

- **Motivation through a phone call.** Call your client periodically. If he knows you will be calling, he may work out just so he can honestly tell you he did it.

- **Motivation through variety.** Get involved with clients to refine or add variety to their programs.

- **Motivation through music.** Find out what music your client likes and use it. This may help to prolong his energy during a cardiovascular workout.

- **Motivation through change.** Organize a novelty activity, perhaps with a new social group.

- **Motivation through a partner.** Pair your client with a partner. If the partner is reliable, the ongoing commitment is very helpful. People are more likely to exercise if they know someone is waiting for them.

- **Motivation through the dog.** A greater proportion of those who regularly walked their dogs were more likely to meet the recommendations of 150 min of physical activity per week. Dogs serve as a motivational support for their owners' walking practices through fair and foul weather (Temple et al. 2011).

Developing Intrinsic Motivators

There is clearly a role for well-designed extrinsic motivators, but unless clients develop some intrinsic motivators, they're not likely to continue regular activity. People simply never reach the maintenance stage without intrinsic motivators. Wheeler (2000) reminded us that change must occur within the person (intrinsic change). To support this process with our clients, we must constantly reinforce facts and ways of thinking to ensure the following:

1. They are aware of the reasons and need for making changes.

2. They perceive the meaning and importance of the change.

3. They see that benefits for the change outweigh the costs.

4. They feel confident in their abilities to maintain new behaviors.

5. They have realistic outcome expectations and revisit them often.

6. They recognize that change takes time and effort.

These are elements that you must help clients grasp and remember if they are to achieve intrinsic motivation. The process is often an accumulation of experiences that come as the client stays with the program for a significant period of time—experiences that will tend to create intrinsic motiva-

tion. We can facilitate and support this process within our clients based on principles such as those just listed. Let's take a look at some motivational techniques and how they can reinforce intrinsic change.

- **Motivation through monitoring.** Dr. Daniel Pink, who spoke about the science of motivation at the 2011 International Health, Racquet and Sportsclub Association convention, says, "If you can show somebody that they are making progress, then there is nothing more [influential] you can do to motivate them" (Williams 2011). There is no better immediate and ongoing method of showing the benefits of a training program than well-designed monitoring of progressive improvement. Some clients will want to see concrete changes attributable to their fitness programs. For example, your client may want to see if his heart rate is decreasing with the same amount of work over a period of 2 months. Visually recording or plotting items that are monitored clearly shows clients the benefits of their efforts.

- **Motivation through increased knowledge.** Knowing good reasons for exercise and for correct diet may encourage your client to make additional changes in his lifestyle. In addition, some of your clients will be very interested in the technical side of the exercise process. Once I recognize that a client has a specific interest, I often bring in a related article or brochure and discuss how it pertains to his situation.

- **Motivation through retesting.** If your client knows you will be retesting him in 3 weeks, this may encourage him to continue faithfully with the program. To move this from extrinsic to intrinsic, provide some guidance as to what is realistic; the test results can provide your client with confidence in his ability to reach outcome expectations.

- **Motivation through goal and program modification.** Set a time to update goals and reinforce the goals already achieved. Intrinsic rewards come from reaching goals and setting down more challenging prescriptions.

- **Motivation through supervision.** Through personal contact, a personal trainer or staff supervising within a facility can increase awareness and importance of regular activity. Your support can help build confidence and prevent relapse.

To reach the maintenance stage, most clients need to adopt the mind-set of an intrinsic exerciser. The transformation from an extrinsic to an intrinsic exerciser is dependent on this change in mind-set from a product-based motivation such as weight loss to a process-based motivation such as enjoyment. Most clients do not permanently change their exercise behavior based on extrinsic or long-term outcomes. Clients may start an exercise program in this manner, but as personal trainers and lifestyle coaches we need to shift the focus toward the process of developing positive, intrinsic experiences with movement and exercise. There needs to be an emotional feedback more immediate to the activity experience that becomes the driving force behind why they are active and what makes them feel good about what they are doing. Intrinsic motivation focuses on doing a behavior for its own sake, and this process gives clients empowerment. To move toward the intrinsic side of the motivation continuum, we need to be present in the situation and help the client become more mindful during her physical activity experience. The desire to exercise for its own sake results from frequently experiencing being immersed totally in the activity without self-consciousness (Kimiecik 1998). The important thing is to enjoy the activity for its own sake and to know that what matters is not the result, but the control and close attention you have to the activity at hand. The focus is on the doing, not the results.

There are a number of strategies that may help. Start by actively involving your client in setting process-oriented goals that will help make the psychological connection between extrinsic goals, for which they have to do activity for some future reward, to intrinsic process goals that focus on their feelings during exercise. Personally, parts of my goal setting are to focus my attention on the task at hand. For example, some days my goal is to run more slowly and focus on nature around me; other days I run with my friends, and the goal is to be social and enjoy the contact with those I care about; other times I will spend most of the run listening to my breathing and sensing the pressure changes on the soles of my feet. It is so important for your clients to find an activity that they really like and to understand where they get their enjoyment from it. Another effective strategy is to show "progress on the process," such as highlighting the ease with which they are doing things that were once a struggle. You can also help your client focus on process by asking for feedback after exercise, such as "How did your body feel during the activity today?" "How was your energy level?" When I ask regularly active people why they exercise, they almost always mention their positive, intrinsic experiences with the exercise behavior itself: "I

Effective Motivation

Recently at a workout session, I got talking to a woman in her early 30s who was a referee for roller derby. She mentioned that she was following an app program on her iPhone called Fitocracy. According to the website, the program provides motivation: "Motivation: Activities earn you points. Points lead to level ups. Earn badges for significant achievements. The community will reward your hard work with props. Groups are small communities where you can talk about the things that really matter to you." She said: "I know that it is all external motivation but when I have trouble getting myself back on track, I will use the app." Many of your clients will fluctuate between sufficient levels of intrinsic motivation and lapses at other times when some extrinsic technique may be the right cue at the right time.

If "willpower" is defined as *the conscious mental ability to follow through on plans to make change and to maintain the change once it is made,* it is clear how important this is for behavioral change. Effective motivation almost always comes from within. You can guide your clients through the process of internal motivation mobilization and goal setting leading to self-discovery and action, provide positive reinforcement, highlight good role models, and offer technical assistance—but that's all. You cannot motivate other people for lifestyle behavioral change. You can only help clients locate their own motivation and mobilize it within themselves by taking control of the process.

enjoy it"; "I like the feelings I get when I exercise." They are intrinsic exercisers.

Motivation and Commitment

You can expect resistance from your clients when they need to make decisions and when they need to move from discussion to action. Making decisions and moving into action involve a commitment of the client's physical and psychological resources. This involves both the initial commitment to exercise objectives and an ongoing commitment to the full strategy. The client should attempt to make steady progress toward the objectives; however, after a lapse, the client must get back on track and move forward.

Several factors that we can control can help our clients commit to, then follow through on, their objectives:

• **Ownership.** Make sure the objectives are the client's, not yours. Jogging is still one of the most popular suggestions for a start-up activity. However, it also has the highest attrition rate—particularly when it was someone else's choice. If you work through form 1.4 (Activity Preferences Questionnaire) and form 1.5 (Focus on Lifestyle) with your client and pay close attention to the results, you will be able to offer activity options that came from the client, not you.

• **Options.** Provide a choice of activities that can produce similar training results. The Energy Deficit Point System (chapter 9) groups activities with similar caloric costs. These activities are virtually interchangeable in an exercise prescription.

• **Reinforcement.** Encourage any action taken toward the client's objective. Teach clients how to monitor themselves (chapter 6), because this will show them their progress and help build self-confidence. Even during an exercise demonstration, recognize the things your client is doing well.

• **Regularity.** Begin by focusing first on the habit of regular exercise by building the time for exercise into the lifestyle schedule. Before your client can succeed in committing to any given activity, he needs to convince himself that he can do it on a regular basis.

• **Appeal.** Look for ways to increase the appeal of the exercise program or to change the source of interest. A training partner, new exercises, a change of equipment, even a change of workout time can make the workout more pleasant.

• **Obstacle management.** Help clients see how to manage disincentives. One of the appeals of personal trainers is the expectation that they will help to remove obstacles or at least work around them. If your client tells you that he can't get started on his weight reduction program until work slows down, tell him that every calorie counts and help him find some active living habits like taking the stairs.

• **Challenge.** Help clients set objectives that are not just substantive but challenging. Small, measurable victories toward an objective can feed the drive to achieve. One of my clients was getting bored with the small gains in weight he was lifting, so I set up a recording chart that summed every pound he lifted. The totals accumulated quickly and soon he was lifting "tons."

• **Contracts.** Use contracts to help clients commit themselves to their choices. Form 2.1 will help guide your clients through a self-contracting process of commitment to their exercise objectives (Canadian Society for Exercise Physiology [CSEP] 2003).

Perhaps the most important factor in commitment, however, is the client's own belief that she is capable of committing to her goals and objectives, following through on that commitment, and reaching her goals. Two excellent strategies for helping a client embrace this belief are encouraging self-talk and promoting self-efficacy.

Encouraging Self-Talk

Any time you think about something, you are talking to yourself. Negative self-talk, such as making excuses for skipping exercise, is counterproductive. Positive self-talk can be used to focus attention, build confidence, modify poor habits, and increase energy. Your client may engage in negative thinking that interferes with his intentions to work out. When you sense that this is the case or when your client appears keen but repeatedly cancels, he may benefit from a technique to change his thoughts, called cognitive restructuring (Brehm 2003). Cognitive restructuring involves thinking about a situation in a new way and serves as a vehicle for making perceptions and beliefs conscious, which is the key to gaining cognitive control.

Clients may have trouble sticking to an exercise program because of misconceptions that underlie their negative thoughts. Some may believe that exercise is a waste of time and that other things take precedence. This may be a subconscious belief that it is selfish to take care of yourself. Help these clients see that their health is a priority and that exercise is a good use of time. Teach them to talk back to this negative self-talk: "What can be more important than my health, and without good health how can I take care of my family?"

Other clients may avoid exercise because they feel too tired or believe that an exercise program adds to their stress. They may feel emotionally tired, and we need to help them discover how exercise can make them feel energized or revitalized. Help them construct reinforcing self-talk like "I'll need the energy from this workout to get through that presentation this afternoon." Once underlying beliefs are clarified, clients can use a rehearsed positive self-talk to counter negative thoughts. With practice, we can help our clients develop more positive ways of thinking that will support regular activity.

We can use this technique in a number of ways. Many of our clients have developed unsafe movement habits by the time they reach us. Self-talk can help them overcome the habit if you teach them to interject a mental reminder at a well-chosen time in the execution of the exercise. Sometimes all it takes is a single word like "squeeze" or "breathe" or a short phrase like "pinch those scapulae together" or "hold the core" to cue the movement behavior. Clients can create their own positive statement to repeat to themselves while engaged in their activity of choice. I have a hill on my running route, and when I am near the top, my self-talk mantra is "Keep moving those feet!"

My editor provided a wonderful personal account of how this technique worked for her. "I used the self-talk strategy about 5 years ago. I talked to myself out loud primarily while walking to and from the bus—very early in the morning and then evening, so not many people were around to wonder about this woman talking constantly to herself! The topic of my self-talk was how great it was to have better eating habits. I would list all the new habits I wanted to have but would talk as if I already had them. I'd rhapsodize about how great it was not to be enslaved to food, how much more pleasant my encounters with food were, how empowering it was to eat slowly and savor small amounts of the food I loved instead of pigging out and then feeling fat and disgusted with myself. I didn't 'diet' at all. I simply found that after a few weeks of doing this, my habits began to change to be consistent with my self-talk. I lost 20 pounds in the first year and have lost 15 more since then. I don't believe I would have been successful had I not, in the first few months, held these extensive 'conversations' with myself. Hearing the statements repeatedly out loud helped me remember, when tempted by an unhealthy eating choice, to challenge the poor eating habits that were so ingrained in my head. If I find myself slipping, I use the strategy again until I get back on track."

Negative self-talk is as destructive as positive self-talk is helpful. Thus, you must learn the technique of **reframing** to help clients avoid negative self-talk that can sabotage their motivation. For instance, reframe guilt about time away from the office as an earned time-out and an investment in future energy. Encourage your client to regard that minor muscle soreness as the stage before the important rebuilding phase. After a shortened

Positive Self-Talk

Positive self-talk can be a powerful tool for your clients who are trying to change their eating habits. Encourage them to talk positively to themselves about how they eat—they can even do this out loud whenever they use a mirror—provided there are no bystanders!

workout, remind your client that the smallest good deed is better than the grandest intention.

Promoting Self-Efficacy

Dishman (1990) referred to an individual's self-efficacy as an ability to match behavior to behavior intentions in the face of competing external pressures. Self-efficacy is extremely important in the early stages of exercise adoption and critical in its role of confronting barriers. Self-efficacy is one of the strongest predictors of exercise behavior. Our role as an expert and our knowledge of fitness and training may undermine our client's sense of self-efficacy. For example, while 10 min of daily walking is below the recommended physical activity guidelines, accomplishing this initial goal improves the client's health and, importantly, raises her confidence to achieve further behavioral changes. When our clients take responsibility for their health behaviors and begin to achieve small goals, they gain the confidence to become an authority over their own health.

We must help our clients develop the confidence to act by tapping into these opportunities to facilitate self-efficacy. Six principal sources of self-efficacy have been identified (Ball 2001). Here they are, along with examples of how you can provide them to your clients:

1. **Performance accomplishment:** Look for opportunities to identify training successes to raise the level of self-efficacy. Help clients see themselves as a person who is physically active.

2. **Vicarious experience:** Use techniques such as exercise demonstrations and your own personal example to help clients learn new skills.

3. **Verbal persuasion:** Use encouragement and verbal cueing to keep clients positive and focused.

4. **Imaging experiences:** Use imagery to build confidence. For example, during balance or proprioceptive tasks, ask your client to close his eyes and visualize full stability and flawless execution.

5. **Physiological states:** Some clients may associate an elevated heart rate with anxiety and perceived incompetence. Try to reframe it as a sign of readiness for performance.

6. **Emotional states:** Depression and low self-efficacy may accompany a client with an injury. Have her picture full function and then show some progress; she will feel more energized about rehabilitation and may experience enhanced self-efficacy.

Clients may be anxious based on their past exercise history, your judgment of their abilities, or not being able to perform to their own standards. From experience, clients have developed preconceived images of what they believe they can achieve. Discovering exactly what your client may be concerned about will help establish a framework of goals wherein any anxieties are confronted and hopefully overcome. A client's belief in her ability begins when we demonstrate or teach the exercises and have the client attempt them. Try these three suggestions when doing an exercise demonstration:

1. The key to improving self-efficacy beliefs lies in designing tasks or exercises that can be performed to facilitate success.
2. Repeat the "client trial" phase of the demonstration a number of times, providing clear and concise feedback specific to the physical action.
3. Encourage positive imagery. For example, "During this lifting action, feel your core activating early. When you do that, you know that you are protecting your back."

Planning for Relapse

A *lapse* is merely a temporary stoppage of exercise, followed by a quick return. A *relapse* is abandonment of activity to the extent that positive outcomes disappear (Jonas and Phillips 2009). To reverse relapse requires first figuring

Relapse Risk Situations and Strategies

Here are some examples of typical high-risk situations and some approaches that have worked in dealing with them:

High-Risk Situation
People at work ask me to go for drinks after work, which is my usual workout time.

Suggested Solutions
- Tell everyone my regular workout schedule so they'll consider it when they're choosing a time to go out.
- Join them later.
- Schedule a makeup time every week to cope with any unplanned changes.
- Restrict how many times a week I go out for drinks after work; if I do want to go out, schedule alternative workout times a couple of times a week.

High-Risk Situation
I'm afraid to walk after work when it gets dark and rainy in the winter.

Suggested Solutions
- Ask my friend to join me.
- Use the community "safe walk" program.
- Walk at lunch or only when it is daylight.

High-Risk Situation
I can't jog or even walk briskly when my shin splints return.

Suggested Solutions
- Get fitted for orthotics.
- Start cross-training or rest at the first signs of discomfort.
- Ask my trainer to prescribe some supplemental exercises to help prevent the onset of shin splints.

out what happened, why the relapse occurred. Then, it requires going back to the planning, recommencing the change process and remobilizing motivation.

As noted earlier, relapse is almost inevitable, and you should be prepared for it. Simply understanding how common it is to lapse from an exercise program will help your client to get back on track when this occurs. Help your clients recall the core motivators for becoming physically active. Remind them that regular exercise is healthier than no extra physical activity at all. Other building blocks along the way may be revisited, for example reconnecting with the support structure or reviewing the strategies to overcome obstacles.

By working through form 2.2, Relapse Planner, with your client in the early stages of his program, you may be able to minimize serious relapse. When small lapses occur, remind your client of the strategies you have already used. If new challenges arise, discuss them and add them, along with tactics for countering them, to Relapse Planner. And if a major relapse occurs, use Relapse Planner to motivate the client to address the problem.

Be sure that the client always has a copy of the most recent version of the planner, and encourage him to review it periodically. Always be positive and encouraging as you try to help your client overcome the tendency to drop out. Use statements like the following to help clients deal positively and effectively with relapse: "I know you may feel discouraged, but it's normal for everyone to experience these setbacks. If we keep working together, we'll find that key or strategies that will work for you. So don't give up!"

Lifestyle Coaching

Despite all your efforts to help your clients overcome relapse (or inertia at the beginning of your work together), some of them may still have problems organizing their lives to support a more holistic, balanced lifestyle. For these clients, consider suggesting that they add lifestyle coaching to their repertoire of relapse-fighting tools. Lifestyle coaching is a collaborative effort in which clients present a situation and then work with a coach to set goals, explore possibilities, remove barriers, and create an action plan that suits the client's needs and values. The coach's job focuses on providing support to enhance the skills, resources, and creativity that the client already has (Cantwell 2003). Lifestyle coaching provides the framework to help clients work through their own personal barriers to living a healthy lifestyle. A well-trained coach helps people figure out where they are today and where they want to be in the future and helps them navigate the gap.

If your client is considering using a coach, give her the following tips:

- Select a coach very carefully, because the relationship between you and your coach is critical.
- Although the Internet is a good way to initially check for rates and any niche market specialists, rely on word of mouth from a reliable reference.
- Check credentials and experience.
- Ask a prospective coach to give you a complimentary first session, which provides a great opportunity to judge the fit before you commit.

What clients do outside of their personal training sessions has an impact on the results they are able to achieve from their training. In many ways, the roles of a personal trainer and lifestyle coach are similar. Both these professionals help design pathways to success. The lifestyle coach offers a more holistic health service and assistance with a more balanced lifestyle. Lifestyle coaching, when done well, is a natural fit for personal trainers whose goal is to help others lead a healthy lifestyle.

An excellent example of a lifestyle coaching tool is form 1.1, Fantastic Lifestyle Checklist. This checklist (see chapter 1) allows clients to understand the effects of various habits and attitudes on their health (Wilson and Ciliska 1984). Most lifestyle behaviors can be modified, including activity, nutrition, tobacco or alcohol use, sleep, stress, and personality. The scoring system provides a straightforward interpretation of health benefits associated with behavior change. The structure of the checklist makes it easy to discuss results with clients. The checklist directs clients to their lifestyle areas that need attention and provides tips to help people make the appropriate changes.

Motivation and Adherence

Forty to sixty-five percent of new clients will drop their exercise regimens within three to six months' time. This despite virtually every member acknowledging the positive effects regular activity will have on their lives—both physically and mentally. A puzzling paradox. (Annesi 2000, p. 7)

Annesi's observation is both powerful and discouraging, and it highlights how crucial it is that we learn how to motivate clients. The good news is that working with personal trainers can increase exercise adherence by 40% over 24 weeks (Pronk et al. 1994).

Barriers to Adherence

It has probably happened to many of your clients. Despite best intentions, their new fitness plans began to fade after a few months. Their Pilates instructor moved, their bike broke down, or they had an injury and they never started up again. We need to understand barriers to exercise and strategies that will enable our clients to overcome these barriers. Barriers can be internal or external.

External barriers are the product of our environment and lifestyle. Circumstances such as socioeconomic status, educational background, age, cultural or ethnic factors, and home or work environment are external barriers that may make it difficult to adopt a healthy lifestyle. Check your client's personal external barriers:

- No convenient facilities
- Financial limitations
- Significant work demands
- Significant family demands
- No support from family or friends
- Inclement weather
- Injury or medical problems
- Lack of free time
- Lack of interesting programs
- Lack of child care
- Lack of transportation

We need a plan that anticipates the barriers ahead and creates an effective defense. Encourage your client to ask himself some introspective questions, outlined in form 2.3, Beat-the-Barriers Plan. The answers to these questions will be his personal "beat-the-barriers" plan.

Internal barriers are personal thoughts, perceptions, and feelings about exercise and ourselves that may prevent us from being active. Despite a desire to become fit, those starting a program may be deterred by intimidation, physique anxiety, or lack of self-esteem and self-efficacy. Clients attempting to maintain an exercise routine face other barriers to exercise maintenance: lofty goals, perceived lack of time, and boredom (Kimiecik 2000). You need to help clients recognize and deal with whatever interior barriers they may have. Table 2.3 describes how the barriers manifest themselves in the client's behavior and some strategies for overcoming the barriers.

Elements of a healthy lifestyle include a positive attitude toward self and others and a love of life. If these positive attitudes are missing, the client faces serious internal barriers. You must develop a sense of empathy and good problem-solving skills to find practical ways to help clients overcome both internal and external barriers so they can change their lifestyles. Consider this sample dialogue for dealing with barriers:

Convenience Brings Compliance

Marie almost never used her previous club membership because of its inconvenience. In her new place of employment, she learns of a small fitness center in the company. She wants to "tone up" and lose some weight, but the center at her job has only resistance machines and one bike, and cycling holds limited attraction for her. She has slightly elevated blood lipids and some motivational needs. Where do her needs, wants, and lifestyle overlap?

The obvious part of convenience is proximity; that is, the fitness center is right there. We often do not pick up on things that could be convenient in our lives. Marie knows the center has potential, but at first glance it is obvious how the equipment will suit her needs. This client will benefit from a special program design. If the machines using large body parts are set up in a circuit with low resistance and high reps (see chapter 9 description of circuit training) and every other station is designed as an aerobic calisthenic, the training results should include weight loss, increased muscular endurance, and reduced blood lipids (Goldfine et al. 1991).

It became the challenge of the health and fitness professional to overcome barriers, design a plan, and shape the environment to satisfy the client. Working out at her place of employment will ensure better compliance. A "workout buddy" would provide additional support. Marie's needs, wants, and lifestyle may change, but for the time being she feels good about her start in the corporate fitness center.

Table 2.3 Internal Barriers and Coping Strategies

Internal barriers	Strategies for overcoming barriers
Intimidation and embarrassment are frequently quoted as reasons for not joining health clubs, especially for those who are overweight or out of shape.	• Adopt a one-on-one approach for personal training. • Start with a lifestyle approach to behavioral change. • Discuss exercise barriers, goal setting, and other client concerns.
Physique anxiety is a concern about visibility and judgment of one's body.	• Avoid the use of mirrors. • Be sensitive in how you dress and speak to anxious clients. • Focus on their positive physical points.
Self-esteem is how positive a client feels about herself. Self-efficacy refers to a client's belief in her ability to complete a goal.	• Choose a level at which the client can be successful. • Take time to teach and demonstrate carefully. • Provide personal attention and sincere positive feedback, encouragement, and follow-up (e.g., e-mail can be an effective follow-up).
Outcome objectives get clients started but are too long-term to maintain motivation. Clients need to shift their focus to the process of daily activity.	• Set short-term goals for each exercise session (e.g., maintain excellent form in last 2 reps of each set). • Monitor regularly, and assign subsequent progressive increases (e.g., increase resistance by 10% when reps have gone from 8 to 12).
Perceived lack of time is most often mentioned as the major barrier. We must help clients see exercise as a higher priority for their allocation of time.	• Work with clients to set priorities. • Examine the inactive parts of your client's day to see if an activity can be substituted or integrated (e.g., walking instead of driving). • Schedule your exercise; make it at a regular time. • Be prepared. For tomorrow's workout, pack your exercise clothes the night before. • Combine activity and socializing—meet for a walk rather than for coffee.
Boredom is common with activities that are continuous and repetitive. We must incorporate variety and change.	• Try different equipment; TheraBands and Swiss balls are cheap alternatives. • Use digital displays and personal progress reports to keep interest high.

FP: Carol, tell me about the difficulties you have had sticking to an activity regimen.

CL: Well, the goal usually looks good at the start. I say that I want to lose a certain amount of weight and they tell me how long and how often I need to exercise.

FP: Why do you think that approach doesn't work for you?

CL: It's not so much that it is hard work. It is just so long before I see any improvements.

FP: Absolutely. We all need some regular feedback and encouragement. Without losing sight of those long-term goals months away, let's work out some short-term goals for each week.

CL: I won't be able to lose much weight in a week.

FP: That will come if you keep yourself motivated with other benchmarks, like monitoring the number of steps you take with a pedometer.

CL: Can I count the steps that I put in at work?

FP: Exactly. That's the idea. Something that keeps you engaged in activity even when you don't think that you have the time!

"Motivation is a mental process that connects a thought or feeling with an action" (Jonas and Phillips 2009). "Getting motivated" is not a question of developing or importing the mind-state. Rather, it is a matter of activating a presently dormant process, of mobilizing it, and of removing barriers to its expression. Our task is to help the client locate these barriers and then help her to mobilize the mental process needed to remove them.

Improving Adherence With Effective Problem Solving

The process of problem solving calls for brainstorming to modify the original exercise prescription, adjusting expectations, and looking for opportunities to learn and grow despite the hindrance. Through the problem-solving process, clients understand that impediments invariably arise and that being flexible enables them to experiment with new strategies that may present other opportunities.

We assume that our clients have good intentions to start or maintain an exercise program. There will be times, however, when they discontinue the program for various reasons. They may have long periods of time when other priorities preclude regular physical activity, leading to feel-

ings of guilt and a drop in self-esteem. Emphasize to these clients that they are not failures, and help them seize this opportunity to refocus on some start-up strategies. The Relapse Planner (form 2.2) is useful for those who have discontinued their regular activity (CSEP 2003). Table 2.4 suggests some client-centered approaches to solving problems and increasing adherence.

Table 2.4 Effective Problem Solving to Improve Adherence

Client information	Problem-solving strategies
Overweight clients may have to struggle more and may have unrealistic expectations about what can be accomplished.	• Be honest and help clients form realistic goals. • Provide monitoring techniques that clearly show their progress. • Avoid positive feedback that is undeserved, but look for opportunities for recognition of progress. • Use social support systems such as "buddies" or a personal trainer if good rapport is present.
Clients need to be aware of the benefits and costs of their fitness program.	• Help your clients list the benefits they hope to experience and also the inconveniences and difficulties they may encounter. • Discuss how they will deal with these.
Smokers have difficulty sticking with exercise.	• Give permission to feel winded and less energized after exercise. • Avoid making smoking a big issue, but have literature available.
A client's personality problems or mood may affect attendance.	• Don't assume that you are responsible for how your clients feel or for the fact that they often miss sessions because of mood disturbances.
Improvement of health is often given as a reason for initiating exercise.	• Point out the specific health benefits that may be expected from their type of prescription. • Use screening tools (e.g., PAR-Q or FANTASTIC Lifestyle Checklist) to assure clients that they are ready for exercise and increase their health-related awareness.
There are large differences in goals and activity for specific ages and sexes. In one study, competition was seen as a benefit for young men and health for young women, whereas health was seen as a barrier for older men and women (De Bourdeauhuij and Sallis 2002).	• Emphasize to seniors that improved health should reduce that barrier. • Use careful monitoring and appropriate prescription to keep activities manageable and safe.
Satisfaction with you as an exercise specialist is an important issue for many clients.	• Seek your clients' input on many aspects of goal setting, techniques of training, variations in routines, and satisfaction. • Give your clients feedback about their progress and solicit their feedback about your abilities as a trainer. • Provide support and be available; show you care.
Clients often have trouble getting past common road blocks.	Consider the following responses, as suggested by Patrick and colleagues (1994): • If time is the barrier: "We're aiming for three 30-minute sessions each week. Do you watch a lot of TV? If so, maybe cut out three TV shows a week?" • If enjoyment is a problem: "Don't exercise. Start a hobby or an enjoyable activity that gets you moving." • If exercise is boring: "Listening to music during your activity keeps your mind occupied. Walking, biking, or running can take you past lots of interesting scenery."

When clients are not compliant with your exercise prescriptions, review their situation and behavior over the previous weeks in a nonthreatening manner. Listen carefully to what they tell you and try a rational problem-solving approach to get them back on track as soon as possible, perhaps coming up with a new routine that works with their new situation. Here is a process with some questions to ask:

Question

Does the program still seem like it is meeting your needs?

Process

- Establish whether the client clearly understands the link between your prescription and her goals.

- Have her priorities changed?

Question

Is the prescription appropriate or are you having any problems with the exercises?

Process

Establish if the program is appropriate for her levels of fitness.

Question

Are external barriers getting in the way of regular activity?

Process

- For example, establish if the program's time frame is realistic.
- Has there been a change in the client's work or home life?

Convincing the Unconvinced

I recall a client, Geneviève, who worked outside the home and had two children, ages 6 and 8. She had a low estimation of her physical capabilities and had even expressed doubts about her need to exercise. She exercised with me two times a week for 3 weeks but did not work out at all during the fourth week. Her reason was that she had deadlines at work. In an emotional confessional she gave me the following reasons for stopping her exercise program:

1. I want to exercise, but by the time 5:00 comes around, I am not able to leave. I have too many things left to do.
2. I don't have the time. I have too many other responsibilities: I work, I have to do grocery shopping, pick up the kids, take them to lessons, help with their homework, cook dinner, make lunches. . . . Get the picture?
3. It will take too long to make a dent in my weight gain. I am so heavy, why even bother?

Of the reasons Geneviève gave, what do you think is the main issue and how would you address it?

Geneviève was overwhelmed. Exercise seemed like just one more thing to fit into a busy day. Our six sessions were prescheduled and prepaid, and that, along with the motivation of having a training partner (me), was enough to get her started. But once those sessions were over, her enthusiasm fizzled. She thought that the prescription was meeting her fitness needs and was at the appropriate level, but there were too many barriers in the way of making it a regular habit. I sensed that we needed to change the way Geneviève thought about her activity. She was more concerned about providing justification to me than she was about her own well-being. She had to reconnect with her original reasons for starting and the meaning and importance of making the change.

We spent a fair amount of time talking about the demands of her work and home life . . . and they were significant. We talked about some of the ways that she might get back on track and how the fitness benefits could outweigh the costs of committed time. But the real breakthrough came when we talked about her children. She truly wanted to be fit enough to be an active mom, but sheer "kid maintenance" was leaving her drained. So I said, "Why not take a break for 30 minutes every day with no kids, no work . . . time just for you to enjoy some activity!" Her eyes widened! "Think of it as an active mini-vacation. Line up your favorite music, forget about the task of weight loss, and just enjoy the time to yourself. Your relaxation and confidence will increase if you accept that change is a process, and although it takes time, there is every reason to enjoy the process." Geneviève's energy level increased over the weeks and although some of it was attributable to the physiological improvements, the commitment was caused by her frame of mind, realistic expectations, and refocus on a new reinforcement.

Question

What alternatives can get you back on track?

Process

Musing on the issues identified, brainstorm some possibilities.

Question

Considering the pros and cons of each alternative, what do you think is your best choice?

Process

Help your client examine the choices, consequences, and personal benefits.

Question

What do you think will help you stick with this program?

Process

Establish a follow-up that is consistent with your client's preferred reinforcement system and establish strategies for commitment.

Case Studies

In the three case studies that follow, consider how you would apply appropriate client-centered motivating tactics. It may be helpful to think of yourself in three distinct roles—as a leader, as a designer, and as an educator. **Leadership** involves the way in which you approach and support your client. **Design** includes developing creative programs, devising incentives, and meeting goals. **Education** relates to how you provide information in a client-centered way, how you engender feedback, and how you create autonomy in your client.

Case Study 1: Initial Leadership With a New Client

Dan was a young, single social worker who had just joined a local club. Andrea worked at the club as a personal trainer and met Dan for the first time during his appointment for an assessment. Andrea learned quickly that Dan lacked experience and knowledge and had never regularly exercised. Dan was willing but apprehensive and somewhat uncomfortable.

Counseling and Assessment

The assessment was a good time to build rapport and gather more information.

A: I know this is your first time in a fitness center, Dan. It must feel strange with the new equipment and activity. I'll guide you through all of this, and we'll have a chance to talk about each stage of the assessment and program. I really can appreciate how hard it is to make the changes in your lifestyle that you'd like to make.

D: Yeah, I have a lot going on right now. I was thinking of applying for the police force but I am not sure that I can pass the physical testing.

A: I'm familiar with the screening tests; perhaps we can integrate some of those elements into your assessment?

D: That'd be great! I know I need to step up my fitness, and that will give me an idea about when I'll sign up for the testing.

Andrea's feedback during and after the assessment was both specific and encouraging.

A: Dan, you have excellent flexibility in most of your joints, and adequate strength as a good base upon which to work.

D: I didn't realize that these tests provided that much detail.

A: Yes, in fact, your aerobic capacity places you in an above-average category. You scored better than 75% of other men your age.

D: Well that's something! But I'm not about to run a marathon tomorrow.

A: Maybe not, but we'll set some progressive goals that will prepare you for the police aerobic run.

Dan had remarked on the professional quality of the test result information. Andrea was pleased at how the test results led to discussion about goals and possible outcomes. In addition to his exercise prescription, Dan was keen to get a better idea if he was capable of passing the police physical.

D: About these goals: I am not sure if I am capable of reaching the police standard.

A: Well, the good news is that you'll set your own objectives. I'll help you make them measurable, but the commitment will be to yourself.

D: I want to be able to finish all the items on that entrance test.

A: That's both realistic and challenging. It will help us plan your exercise prescription, and if we monitor your perceived exertion during the training, we can keep track of your progress.

Keys to Getting Started

Andrea provided support and encouragement and two-way communication. She explained why, helped in decisions and goal setting, and helped Dan "buy in" to the new behavior. Because Dan was unfamiliar with the equipment, Andrea scheduled her time to be with him for his entire workouts during the first week. This gave her time to improve Dan's technical skills and to share many personal anecdotes about her own training. At the end of the week, Andrea presented Dan with a club T-shirt and her phone number and e-mail address in case of problems.

Andrea used the counselor style to establish strategies for change; however, she was a director while gathering information. It is important to engage in interactive rather than didactic communication. She empowered Dan to take control of the process, to start to learn for himself, and to engage actively in the activity counseling. Andrea assisted Dan to move from a preparation stage of change to an action stage by helping Dan plan, focusing on the "pros," instilling self-confidence, and providing helpful resources such as the police assessment protocol.

Questions

- How did feedback in the early encounters affect Dan's motivation?
- How did Andrea's support of Dan change the focus of his goal?
- How did the modifications and additions to the assessment protocol assist in consciousness raising or contingency management (processes in stages of change)?

Case Study 2:
Motivating an Intermittent Exerciser

Jane, a single mother of two, had a busy schedule that found her on and off exercise for many years. The community fitness center had asked Tony, a personal fitness trainer, to work with her because both still played some competitive baseball. Jane was just returning to the center after her second child and wanted to get in shape before the baseball season. Tony realized that Jane's yo-yo pattern occurred when exercise was crowded out by her work schedule, home duties, or vacations. She also admitted that her exercise routine would take a downward spiral when she couldn't see any results, it wasn't fun, or it was boring.

Tony helped Jane become active through targeted counseling based on their conversations: He enabled her to identify and deal with the guilt she felt about taking time for herself; showed her how to build exercise into her busy routine through active living; and introduced her to new and interesting exercise activities.

Counseling and Assessment

"I know at times you don't see the type of progress you'd like, but you are very effective when you do work out more regularly. Everyone I work with goes through short relapses for various reasons. I appreciate that it's hard to make an ongoing commitment. I've struggled with this myself. We can take a look at your overall approach to an exercise habit."

Jane always believed that she was taking time from someone or something else when she exercised. Tony started their second meeting by discussing these feelings. He wanted to help Jane realize that slippage in attendance did not imply failure and that the time

spent exercising would more than pay back benefits and quality of time to job and family.

"Jane, I've noticed how concerned you are about your family and about the time you spend away from them. I admire your devotion and care. They are rare qualities. Your support and encouragement are important. In working with many single parents, I've found it important to remember that the better care you take of yourself—physically and emotionally—the better you can care for the people you love."

Tony tried to convey that there needs to be emotional feedback from Jane's activity experience that becomes the driving force behind why she is active and what makes her feel good about what she is doing. This intrinsic motivation focuses on doing a behavior for its own sake, and this process gives clients empowerment. To move toward the intrinsic side of the motivation continuum, Tony tried to encourage Jane to be present in the situation and become more mindful during her physical activity experience.

He worked with Jane on some positive self-talk. They developed some questions that highlighted the benefits of regular workouts. Whenever Jane started to feel guilty about taking time to exercise, she reviewed these questions in her mind:

- "How does exercise make me feel later in the day?"
- "How do I feel after completing a workout that I originally had planned to skip?"
- "What are some of the positive feelings I get with a good workout?"

Dealing With Time Commitments

Tony's second approach tackled the problem of not enough time. He introduced Jane to the concept of **active living,** whereby, during hectic weeks, she could substitute walking to work, taking the stairs, and doing manual chores for her formal workout. Since Jane's exercise pattern was usually irregular (fewer than six workouts per month), Tony discussed the benefits of adding only a few more sessions per month and slightly increasing the intensity of her workouts.

Knowing that injury can be a major reason for dropping out, Tony adjusted her previous prescription and introduced some interesting cross-training variety in her new program. Subsequent progressions were regular and became more specific to baseball. Jane thought she now had the right attitude and approach to maintain a more regular, healthy, and balanced lifestyle.

Questions

- What leadership qualities did Tony demonstrate that were well suited to helping Jane?

- Select one feature of Tony's exercise prescription and explain why it was appropriate for Jane.
- How did Tony influence Jane's attitude toward regular exercise?

Case Study 3: Motivating an Impatient Client

It occurs more often than you may think. You are scheduled to meet a client for the first time and within a few minutes you realize that his expectations are to get moving as soon as possible. The client may not say "Let's get moving," but you read this in his nonverbal communication. This does not mean that you should discard the Activity Counseling Model or that you necessarily have a problem. This situation becomes a problem only if you don't recognize and adapt to it. You should begin by being supportive, empathetic, and appreciative of the uniqueness of your client.

Counseling and Information Gathering

Kaveh spent a long time deciding to begin an exercise program, and now wanted to get started right away. This required that his trainer, Luke, reduce the initial time with the interview and exploration. After some essential counseling, he quickly engaged Kaveh in activity and integrated more information gathering and selected counseling strategies as the sessions progressed.

Clients "on the go" are often systematic, analytic, organized, pragmatic, energetic, and a leader in their own domains. Luke recognized that, and aimed for a treatment strategy that was businesslike, fast-paced, and included Kaveh's input. As an activity counselor, he took a low profile and a delegating stance. He identified problems but left the responsibility of action to the client. Luke and Kaveh worked together to come up with a few prioritized objectives and then broke the goals down into a number of distinct and sometimes progressive steps.

Luke: We've done the health history questionnaire and I think we can safely move on.

Kaveh: Good. I'm anxious to get out on the floor. I'd like to do some free weights and the treadmill.

Luke: I'm sure we can accommodate that request.

Kaveh: Will we get at it today?

Luke: What we can do today is get acquainted with some of the equipment and find out what level would be best for you to start at. Let's focus for a minute on your specific goals.

Kaveh: I want to get back into running and build some muscle.

Luke: You mentioned the charity 10K run in 4 months' time. We can set up a training schedule for that. Did you have a more specific objective for the weights? Why was this an area of concern?

Kaveh: The running schedule sounds doable. As for the muscle work, I want to strengthen my abs. They are starting to look and feel flabby, and if I can make some improvements, I'll feel a lot better about my fitness and appearance.

Luke: OK. If you are interested in trying some new techniques, I can show you a short ab routine on the Theraball.

Kaveh: Hey, that sounds like more fun than sit-ups.

Luke: Yes, but it is still a challenge. Next session I'll have some of these things documented on your program card, but right now let's move to the floor and we'll get started.

Safe and Snappy Prescription Guidelines

Luke ensured that all screening and health forms were completed (see chapter 4). He used the warm-up as an opportunity to see how Kaveh reacted to light aerobic loads, as well as basic body mechanics and confidence. He monitored intensity and form, continuously looking for any signs of distress, discomfort, or imbalance. He also kept the exertion levels moderate, below the level that he anticipated prescribing in the future.

With safety well established, he turned his focus to Kaveh's enjoyment of the workout and designed a program that was dynamic and continuous, mixing an ample share of new and interesting exercises. Luke kept them simple, allowing for minimum teaching and maximum use, with a brisk pace and an organized series of exercises to hold Kaveh's interest. Luke also used continuous verbal encouragement and positive feedback to keep the pace of the session high. He also reinforced Kaveh's objectives and any emotional connection made earlier (e.g., "This should make those morning bicycle rides a little easier!").

Luke checked with Kaveh during the cool-down as to how the workout felt physically and from an enjoyment perspective. Important information gathering took place during the partner-assisted stretching.

Monitoring on the Go

Luke used passive, active, and interactive monitoring tools as he worked with Kaveh. Passive monitoring involved watching, observing, and tracking the safety and form of his exercise techniques. Active monitoring involved taking heart rate, monitoring perceived exertion, adjusting workloads, resisting or assisting partner exercises, and checking angles and alignments. Interactive monitoring requires a close and continuous communication with your client. Luke found that nonverbal cues were as effective as spoken ones.

By creating standardized segments of his prescription, monitoring was an effective alternative to formal assessment. The information derived from monitoring provides personalized feedback and a basis for making changes or progressions in the program. Finally, the support, interest, and motivation provided by the monitoring are well suited to our systematic, pragmatic, "on the go" client.

In fact, it is common that after clients begin activity, they experience an increase in interest and a greater recognition of the benefits and enjoyment. Once Kaveh was "hooked," he was much more responsive to new information and suggestions.

Questions

- Are there any safety issues that have been compromised by moving at this pace?
- During the dialogue, did it appear that Kaveh was motivated? Extrinsically or intrinsically? How could you help him increase the awareness of his intrinsic changes?
- How does careful and selective monitoring allow the trainer to effectively deal with the impatient client?

Summary

The concepts behind the *motivation to make changes* and *how to go about mobilizing it* are the central factors in helping people to make health-promoting personal behavioral changes. By understanding your client's stage of change, knowing the change process appropriate to that stage, and choosing strategies that will facilitate the change process, you will help your client recognize the relevance of the message for herself and understand how it fits with her personal needs.

Unlocking the mysteries of how people think and learn will also help you be more effective with your clients. Knowing your client's preferred learning style and personality style are two areas of profiling that present opportunities for better understanding of what is needed to change behavior.

There is clearly a role for well-designed extrinsic motivators, but unless clients develop some intrinsic motivators, they're not likely to continue regular activity. Intrinsic motivation focuses on doing a behavior for its own sake, and this process gives clients empowerment. They will stick with an activity because they enjoy it and believe they are achieving something.

Several factors can help our clients commit to, then follow through on, their objectives: ownership, options, reinforcement, appeal, obstacle management, challenge, and contracts. Perhaps the most important factor in commitment, however, is the client's own belief that she is capable of committing to her objectives, and this should be facilitated by encouraging self-talk and promoting self-efficacy.

Review the situation and behavior of clients who are not compliant with your exercise prescriptions, listening carefully and trying a rational problem-solving approach. The problem-solving approach should reexamine priorities, prescription fit, external barriers, alternatives, personal benefits, and incentives.

FORM 2.1   Self-Contract

1. My physical activity goal is _____

_____

2. To achieve my goal, I need to change the following:

_____

_____

_____

3. I am willing to do the following to make it happen:

_____

_____

_____

4. Others will know about the change I am making when _____

_____

5. I might sabotage my plan by _____

_____

6. Therefore, my contract to myself is _____

_____

7. Checkup dates:

_____

_____

_____

_____

_____

Signed:

_____

Client

_____

Appraiser

FORM 2.2 Relapse Planner

How confident are you that you'll keep doing your physical activity during the next 3 months?

Not confident at all	___ 1
Not very confident	___ 2
Somewhat confident	___ 3
Confident	___ 4
Very confident	___ 5

If your score was less than 4, complete the following exercise:

Many people have periods of inactivity. Sometimes these breaks can last for just a few days and sometimes a few years. Planning ahead for the tough times may help you stay active.

1. Have you ever had trouble keeping your physical activity going before? If so, write the reasons.

   _____

   _____

   _____

2. If you have had trouble, what has helped you get back on track (e.g., support from friends, joining a class, setting goals)?

   _____

   _____

   _____

3. What situations do you think would make it tough to keep your physical activity routine? How will you handle these situations to increase your chances of being successful?

   _____

   _____

   _____

   High-risk situations: _____

   _____

   Solutions: _____

   _____

   _____

4. What will help you get started again if you do have a break? Write down your ideas.

   Start-up strategies: _____

   _____

   _____

   _____

From J.C. Griffin, 2015, *Client-centered exercise prescription*, 3rd ed. (Champaign, IL: Human Kinetics). Source: *Canadian Physical Activity, Fitness & Lifestyle Approach: CSEP-Health & Fitness Program's Appraisal and Counselling Strategy,* 3rd edition, © 2003. Reprinted with permission from the Canadian Society for Exercise Physiology.

FORM 2.3   Beat-the-Barriers Plan

• What stands in my way? • What are my potential barriers and how will I meet them?	
• Where is my support?	
• What does success mean to me? • How will I know when I have accomplished my objective?	
• How much do I want this? • Do I believe that this is important in my life?	

Principles of Client-Centered Prescription

Chapter Competencies

After completing this chapter, you will be able to demonstrate the following competencies:

1. Apply the principle that exercise design determines exercise outcomes of exercise prescription.
2. Identify prescription guidelines for health-related fitness.
3. Identify prescription guidelines for general fitness.
4. Identify prescription guidelines for performance-related fitness.
5. Apply the principle that fitness components must be integrated into structural segments of an exercise program.
6. Create a safe, balanced exercise prescription.
7. Apply the principle that exercise modifications and functional progressions personalize the prescription.
8. Apply biomechanical principles to optimize exercise benefits for your clients and at the same time attend to their limitations through biomechanical alterations of the exercise.

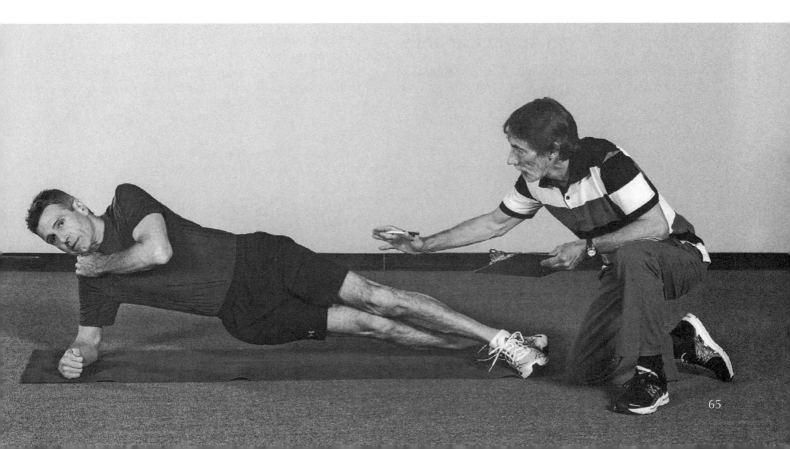

When we formulate a client-centered prescription, we should make decisions by progressing through the issues systematically, making informed selections from a menu of options. As important as the individual exercises within a prescription may be, their chance for success depends on whether we have considered all options and made appropriate decisions.

This chapter examines the three primary principles of client-centered exercise prescription that set the foundation for the recommended guidelines:

1. Exercise design determines exercise outcomes. Exercise is adaptive and can be designed for a number of broad exercise outcomes. We will compare health-related fitness, general fitness, and performance-related fitness prescription principles.

2. Fitness components must be integrated into structural segments of an exercise program. Although there are general fitness components, each of the exercise outcomes (health, fitness, performance) has components that are of particular importance. The second principle addresses how these components are integrated into the structural segments of an exercise program.

3. Exercise modifications and functional progressions personalize the prescription. Finally, we will apply FITT guidelines and principles of biomechanics to learn how to modify and progress the prescription to suit our clients' abilities.

Exercise Design and Outcomes

What has recent research told us about the effectiveness of various types and quantities of exercise? How much do the benefits of exercise depend on the type of client? How much exercise is enough?

Clients today want more than just aerobic fitness and weight control. We must offer more than just the physiological components of fitness! This includes assisting clients in meeting their fitness and health prescription objectives by explaining and orchestrating their lifestyle factors, environment, sport involvement, occupation, and personal attributes.

We can prescribe exercise programs to produce three potential outcomes:

1. Health enhancement
2. Increased general fitness
3. Performance improvements

For years, guidelines for prescribing exercise were based on improvement in athletic ability or physical performance. As overall fitness grew in popularity, led by a surge of interest in aerobics, the guidelines were modified. Intensity levels were reduced, and workouts were structured to include a balance of all fitness components. Exercises were designed to stress the cardiovascular, metabolic, and musculoskeletal systems, thereby creating physiological and structural changes in the components of fitness.

One of the strongest trends in recent history is the adoption of activity as a health-enhancing strategy. Physical fitness and good health are not synonymous, but they are complementary. **Physical fitness** is the ability to carry out daily tasks with vigor and alertness, without undue fatigue, and with ample energy to enjoy leisure pursuits and to meet unforeseen emergencies. **Good health** is not merely the absence of disease—it is a capacity to enjoy life and withstand challenges. It has social, physical, and psychological dimensions, each characterized on a continuum with positive and negative poles. Health benefits may occur in conjunction with improvements in aerobic power or muscular endurance or with improvements in physical performance capacity. However, some health benefits appear to be achieved by exercise that does not always lead to improved physical fitness (International Federation of Sports Medicine [IFSM] 1990).

It is becoming increasingly common to see primary care physicians working with the fitness community because they believe that exercise is good medicine. In a collaborative exercise program with personal trainers, Dr. Neda Amani Golshani said, "The best outcome of (our) program is that I have been able to successfully treat many medical conditions—arthritis, diabetes, hypertension, dyslipidemia, depression, insomnia, pain from various musculoskeletal conditions, PMS, menopause, etc.—either partially or completely with exercise" (Golshani 2006).

How Do Clients' Needs Affect Their Goals?

The details of each exercise prescription vary with the client's goals, desired outcomes, and risks. Skinner (1987) offered a schematic representation of the goals most common for different populations (figure 3.1).

For the athlete, **performance** is usually the central focus of a physical activity program, and health and fitness are secondary goals. However, sometimes an athlete will want to recover from an injury (health goal) or build a strong off-season base (fitness goal). Skinner (1987) suggested that the average client gets involved in activity for **fitness,** with perhaps an added interest in recreational sport performance. Quality of life and reduction of risk factors (health goals) are still in the minds of these clients. Clients with certain health risk factors or with musculoskeletal injuries obviously are most concerned about improving their **health** and are less oriented toward performance.

You will benefit from understanding the interrelationships among lifestyle, environment, genetics, occupation, personal attributes, fitness, and health. By helping to orchestrate these factors, you can assist your clients in meeting their prescription objectives. How do regular physical activity and fitness contribute to health? Figure 3.2 presents Bouchard's model that defines these interrelationships.

The model demonstrates how physical activity and fitness influence each other. The components

of fitness—particularly health-related fitness—are determined by heredity, diet, and patterns of habitual physical activity. Health status also influences both fitness and physical activity. For example, an injury or illness will limit a client's physical activity and eventually will affect her level of fitness. Wellness is a holistic concept of positive health influenced by social and psychological factors, lifestyle habits (e.g., smoking, stress, diet), the environment, and physical well-being. The model also shows that wellness is related to fitness and physical activity.

A purely physiological approach to exercise prescription would ignore many factors in Bouchard's model. To be client centered, you must first establish whether your client's main concern is activity, fitness (performance), or health. Then consider how the surrounding factors may directly or indirectly affect him. Spend time with your client in these earlier stages so both of you develop a clear vision of what he wants to achieve. The relationships in the model will influence how you reach those objectives and how you package the prescription.

For example, you have a client whose health-related fitness **goal** has already been established. The area of **priority** is appearance and a healthy weight. The specific **objectives** include reduction of body fat (especially in the trunk area) and reduction of blood lipids. These objectives are linked to the health-related fitness components of metabolism and body composition. The purely physiological approach may provide a very sound aerobic exercise prescription, but this would fail

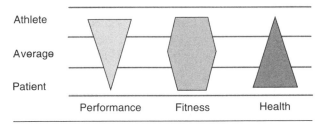

Figure 3.1   Changes in component goals with different clients.

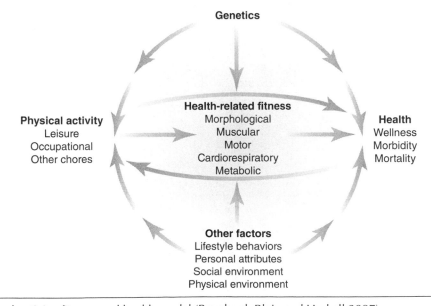

Figure 3.2   Physical activity, fitness, and health model (Bouchard, Blair, and Haskell 2007).

Adapted by permission from Bouchard, Blair, and Haskell 2012.

to serve all your client's needs. Bouchard's model indicates that your client also will benefit from initiatives in the areas of diet, stress management, social environment, occupational activity, and household chores (that provide continuous moderate activity). You will achieve greater success and a more balanced program if your prescription for one area is made in light of how that area interacts with the other areas. This holistic approach is beneficial for athletes, fitness enthusiasts, and health-conscious clients.

How Much Exercise Is Enough?

"I've been walking, but I hear that to be fit I should be jogging." "Recently I read that living actively, like taking the stairs and walking the dog, will make me fit." "As a distance runner, should I be doing the same weekly mileage even though I am working in intervals?" These are typical client concerns. How much exercise is enough? Enough for whom? Enough for what goal or objective?

The question may not be "How much is enough?" but rather, "What constitutes an exercise benefit, and how much exercise is required before I see benefits?" Figure 3.3 contrasts two models of the relationship between the acquired benefits of exercise and the amount of exercise performed.

Exercise physiologists traditionally have held that cardiovascular fitness occurs only after a person reaches a threshold of exercise activity. According to this view, there is little or no benefit until the threshold for fitness is exceeded. Benefits continue to accrue as the level of exercise increases beyond this threshold. At an upper limit, the benefits level off (figure 3.3a).

Figure 3.3b shows that some improvements in fitness occur at low levels of exercise, even though the increases are small. At higher exercise levels, benefits accrue at an accelerated rate

until an upper limit is reached, beyond which the potential for injury and overuse detracts from the positive effects of training. Proponents of the need for some exercise, even at low levels, believe this gradual increase in benefits is typical of many adaptive responses.

Are the Mechanisms of Change the Same for Health and Fitness?

Improvement in health may be attributable to biological changes different from those responsible for fitness. For example, endurance training will increase endurance capacity and may help prevent coronary artery disease (CAD). The increase in endurance capacity most likely results from an increase in oxygen transport to and utilization by the skeletal muscles. The reduction in CAD risk may result from alterations in lipoprotein metabolism or blood clotting activity (Haskell et al. 2007; La Forge 2001). The accelerated rate of energy production during exercise increases the rate of functioning of other biological systems. With repeated stimulus, these systems will increase their capacity or efficiency, providing many of the health-related benefits of exercise (Haskell et al. 2007; La Forge 2001). This information can be extremely motivating to a client who sees no immediate changes in other measures.

In some circumstances, the mechanism for health benefits may relate more to physical or mechanical stress placed on the muscles, connective tissue, or skeleton than to increased energy expenditure. For example, retention of postmenopausal muscle tone and bone calcium through exercise probably results from mechanical stress on muscles and bones from weight-bearing activity or resistance exercise (Ross et al. 2000). Joggers may benefit more from the weight-bearing nature of their steps than from elevated heart rates.

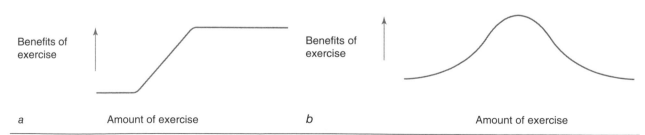

Figure 3.3   Schematic models of the benefits versus amount of exercise. (a) The plateau model notes that when exercise amounts increase, the exercise benefits remain steady after peaking, while (b) the hill model predicts gradual increases in benefits and then adaptation.

Do Health Benefits Build Up or Do They Come and Go?

Although most fitness benefits are somewhat cumulative, this is not always the case with health benefits, which dissipate quickly and require lifelong regularity of exercise (Haskell et al. 2007).

Numerous biochemical changes occur during or immediately after a workout. Although these changes may be transient, they can favorably alter the progression of a specific disease if they occur often enough. For example, a single bout of endurance exercise will decrease elevated plasma triglycerides. Exercise on consecutive days further lowers the triglyceride concentration for 48 to 72 h, but if exercise is not performed for several days, the concentration will return to its elevated level (Haskell et al. 2007). Minimum daily exercise may give rise to discernible health benefits for many clients. Nieman (2009) has shown that a brisk walking program 5 days a week for 12 weeks lowered sick days with the common cold by more than one-half. During each walking bout, important immune cells were increased temporarily in the body, providing enhanced protection from viruses—implying that near-daily activity is optimal for acute immune benefit. Martin, Pence, and Woods (2009) provided evidence to support the process by which short-term and long-term moderate-intensity exercise reduces inflammation and improves the immune response to respiratory viral infections. They recommend this training as a preventive measure against respiratory tract viral infection. In contrast, intense exercise before or during viral infection has been associated with greater morbidity and mortality.

Some of the health benefits of physical activity can be seen right away. Other benefits may take more time and perseverance. The Alberta Centre for Active Living (2011) provides a timeline of some health benefits (table 3.1).

Prescription Guidelines for Health, Fitness, and Performance

Physical fitness and health-related fitness, although not synonymous, are complementary. Although your client may experience the health benefits of exercise along with improvements in fitness and performance (Blair et al. 1989), health benefits also may come from frequent performance of low-intensity exercise that has no fitness training effect. Light- to moderate-intensity exercise

Table 3.1 Health Benefits Timeline

Short term (one session to a week of physical activity)	Moderate term (4-8 weeks of regular activity)
Increases in: • Mood and energy • Self-esteem • Sleep • Concentration • Good cholesterol • Calories used	Increases in: • Muscle strength • Bone and joint strength • Balance and posture • Heart health • Insulin sensitivity
Decreases in: • Stress • Depression • High blood sugar • Bad cholesterol • Blood pressure	Decreases in: • Body weight and body fat • Joint pain and swelling • Falls

on most days of the week produces significant health benefits including primary and secondary prevention of several chronic diseases. There appears to be a graded linear relation between the volume of physical activity and health status. Most physically active people are at the lowest risk; however, the greatest improvements in health status are seen with people in the least fit category. Clients who exercise above recommended guidelines (see later in this section) are likely to gain even greater health benefits.

Health Benefits of Moderate Exercise

Recent guidelines (Haskell et al. 2007; Pate et al. 1995; Wilmore 2003; Warburton et al. 2006) place less emphasis on vigorous exercise than on moderate-intensity exercise (55-75% maximum heart rate [maxHR] or 40-60% $\dot{V}O_2$max), particularly for sedentary adults. Low-intensity dynamic activity (<50% $\dot{V}O_2$max) may reduce stress, contribute to weight loss, or improve certain biochemical reactions such as the release of endorphins. Performed 30 min or more at least three times per week, low-intensity activity significantly improves blood pressure, lipid metabolism, glucose tolerance, and blood clotting—especially in middle-aged and older persons (Haskell et al. 2007; Malkin 2002). Other metabolic changes, like increases in high-density lipoproteins, appear to respond more to increases in the volume of exercise (amount of time spent) than to intensity. Several studies (DeBusk et al. 1990; Ebisu 1985; Kesaniemi et al. 2001) show that multiple periods of moderate-intensity exercise of about 10 min duration spread throughout the day can improve metabolism and body composition. Paffenbarger and colleagues (1986) found that short periods of stair climbing, walking, or light sports provided protection against heart disease. Warburton and colleagues (2006) summarized that for health benefits, physical activity can be accumulated throughout the day, even with short 10 min bouts of exercise totaling about 1000 kcal energy expenditure per week.

One of the most valuable findings of recent research on physical activity is that it produces such health benefits as reduced blood lipids, lowered resting blood pressure, protection from type 2 diabetes, increased metabolic rate (weight loss), and an increased quality of life and independent living in the elderly (Kesaniemi et al. 2001). Exercise is a therapeutic intervention that requires a customized dose (frequency, intensity, time or duration, and type). A dose–response effect exists between exercise and a specific health outcome if there is a consistent relationship between the

volume or intensity of the exercise and the health outcome (La Forge 2001). As personal fitness trainers, we must prescribe the appropriate dose of exercise. Like a drug, a prescription that is not client centered can create adverse effects; these can include overuse strains, fatigue, and immune system dysfunction, resulting in loss in motivation or compliance. The best response will be achieved with a dose-specific health-related exercise prescription based on the information gathered during counseling.

Figure 3.4 (Gledhill and Jamnik 1996) illustrates health gains as related to the volume of physical activity. Lower volumes of physical activity (duration × frequency) show more rapid initial improvement in triglycerides and blood pressure. Improvements in several other health benefit indicators come at higher volumes of participation. Aerobic fitness depends on the intensity of participation, not just its duration and frequency. The other health benefit indicators, however, depend primarily on duration and

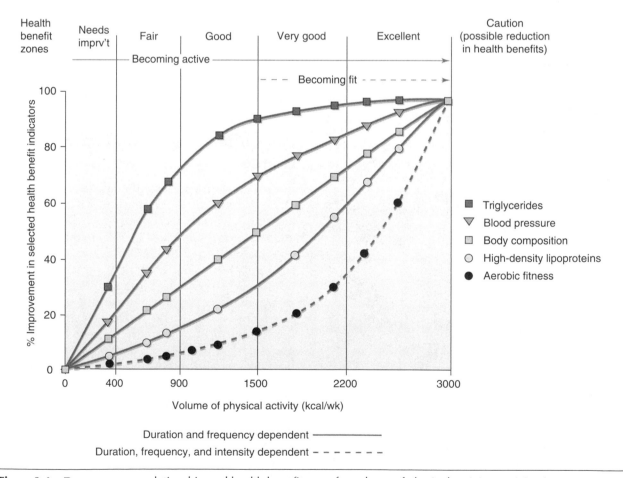

Figure 3.4 Dose–response relationship and health benefit zone for volume of physical activity participation.
Reprinted by permission from the Canadian Society for Exercise Physiology 2003.

frequency of participation. The authors note that figure 3.4 reflects **general** interpretations of the related scientific literature and is meant to show the **collective** improvement in selected health benefit indicators. The health benefit zones in figure 3.4 will help your client determine the benefits of his level of activity.

The relative risk of all-cause mortality declines sharply from a sedentary client (fewer than 30 min of moderate to vigorous leisure-time activity per week) to a client who exercises 90 min per week (figure 3.5). This positive effect continues but flattens out after approximately 2 or 3 h of moderate to vigorous leisure-time activity per week (figure 3.5). These findings help form the basis of the minimum recommendation of 150 min per week; greater activity confers greater benefits, as seen in the lower risk levels found when exercising between 6 and 7 h per week (figure 3.5) (Jonas and Phillips 2009). The recommended activity levels can be translated into caloric expenditures on a weekly basis. The average person walking 3 mph (4.8 kph) burns approximately 100 kcal per mile or 300 kcal per hour. At the recommended 150 min (or 2.5 h per week), our client will expend approximately 750 kcal in physical activity per week. The general goal of 1000 to 2000 kcal/week assists with maintaining weight loss and improving longevity.

Similar to the situation with cardiovascular fitness, there is a dose–response relationship for improvements in health status from better musculoskeletal fitness (Payne et al. 2000). Enhanced musculoskeletal fitness improves bone health, decreases pain in those with chronic low back pain, promotes independent living, and pre-

vents falls and associated injuries (Katzmarzyk and Craig 2002; Warburton et al. 2001). Strength training may preserve bone mineral content and improve psychological well-being. Resistance training may increase high-density lipoproteins, decrease diastolic blood pressure, and increase insulin sensitivity (Goldfine et al. 1991; La Forge 2001). Flexibility exercises will improve muscle balance, posture, and musculoskeletal integrity as your client ages. Women and elderly people have the greatest potential for gains in health status and quality of life. Martin and colleagues (2009) examined the effect of a 6-month trial of 50%, 100%, and 150% of the physical activity recommendations on quality of life (QOL) in a large well-controlled study. They found that changes in all mental and physical aspects of QOL, except bodily pain, were dose dependent and were independent of weight loss. Higher doses of exercise were associated with larger improvements.

Prescription for General Fitness

Intensity is probably the most important variable for improving cardiovascular fitness. If overall fitness is the primary objective for your client, you must progressively raise the intensity to the recommended level. For instance, if your client is of average capability, the intensity will need to build up to around 70% of his maximum heart rate for substantial cardiovascular improvements.

Wenger and Bell (1986) found intensity and duration of training to be interrelated: Total caloric expenditure (energy cost), which is a direct result of intensity, duration, and frequency, may be the most important factor for cardiovascular and body composition improvements (assuming a minimum intensity of 60% of maximum heart rate). The total energy cost of a client's exercise program, based on a body weight of 70 kg (154 lb), should be approximately 900 to 1500 kcal per week or 300 to 500 kcal per exercise session (Donnelly et al. 2009).

Even if you do not have the resources to measure changes attributable to training, you can be reasonably sure that if the American College of Sports Medicine (ACSM) guidelines are followed, fitness will improve. The proper combination of intensity, duration, and frequency will improve your client's aerobic capacity 15% to 30% over a period of 4 to 6 months (Wilmore and Costill 2004). Programs of lesser intensity, duration, and frequency may produce improvements in the 5% to 10% range (Wenger and Bell 1986); this level of improvement might also result if the client has

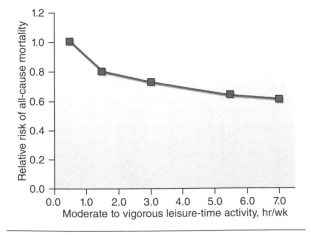

Figure 3.5 "Median" shape of the dose–response curve.

Reprinted from the U.S. Department of Health and Human Services Physical Activity Guidelines Advisory Committee Report, 2008.

a high level of initial fitness. If your client stays with the program, he can expect long-term benefits; middle-aged and elderly men who train consistently show less than 5% reduction in aerobic capacity per decade (Wilmore and Costill 2004). Your client may expect slight decreases in his total body weight and in fat weight and increases in fat-free weight (Hagan 1988). The magnitude of these changes will vary directly with the intensity and duration of the activity and the total caloric expenditure (see chapter 9).

The Canadian Physical Activity Guidelines (Canadian Society for Exercise Physiology [CSEP] 2011) for adults aged 18 to 64 years suggest the accumulation of at least 150 min of moderate- to vigorous-intensity aerobic physical activity per week, in bouts of 10 min or more. They also suggest muscle and bone strengthening activities using major muscle groups at least 2 days per week.

Prescription for Performance-Related Fitness

Optimal training for peak performance can be achieved only with a fine balance between intense training and rest. Client-centered prescription for athletes includes training in those components that constitute performance-related fitness: motor skills (e.g., speed, agility, balance, and coordination), cardiovascular endurance, muscular power, strength, endurance, body composition, skill acquisition, and motivation. You can maximize your client's training efficiency only by prudently selecting training methods and appropriately changing the prescription factors of his program as the need arises. Training should be designed with the principles of periodization (Bompa 1999). Flexible periodization methods can combine strength and energy systems for maximum results (Jensen 2010). This training program should include at least 1 day a week of complete rest to allow for recovery. Monthly schedules should include 1 week that is lighter or is used to taper before or recuperate after a competition.

Because most athletes are highly motivated and tend to overstress themselves, they most frequently err on the side of overtraining rather than undertraining. Both you and your athletic clients must be aware of this problem, because overtraining will deny them their full potentials. Hawley and Schoene (2003) referred to the state of persistent muscle soreness, decreased coordination, and frequent upper respiratory infections as "overreaching" and described it as an expected part of vigorous training. These symptoms usually resolve if followed by a period of lighter training. Your client's performance will increase during this "supercompensation" response. However, if overreaching continues, there will be a decrease in performance and prolonged symptoms characteristic of overtraining (figure 3.6).

But how much exercise is too much? More exercise can be a double-edged sword: It can be helpful or, if poorly directed, harmful. The reinforcement your client receives from his rigorous training regimen can easily cross the line to decreased performance and nagging injuries. It is hard to tell such a motivated athlete that he must slow down or change what so far has been

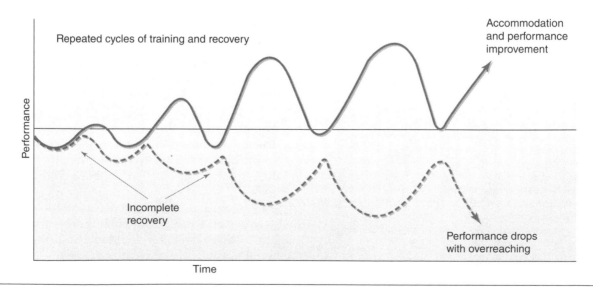

Figure 3.6 Overtraining syndrome.

a successful prescription. Yet all athletes experience periods when their performance levels off or decreases. This overtraining results from failure to tolerate or adapt to the training load. Stone, Keith, and colleagues (1991) observed two types of overtraining: monotonous program overtraining and chronic overwork overtraining.

• **Monotonous program overtraining** demonstrates a loss or plateauing of performance attributable to the consistent, unvarying use of the same type of exercise. It is not caused by excessive fatigue. It is akin to a batting slump or a goal-scoring void for athletes, a feeling of "the blahs," or a lack of energy in the fitness enthusiast. Stone and colleagues (1991) believe that this type of overtraining may be the central nervous system's adaptation to a lack of appropriate stimulation from different movement patterns.

• **Chronic overwork overtraining** also can result in a plateauing or loss of performance. You need to distinguish the differences between chronic and short-term overwork ("overreaching"). Decreased performance as a result of a few sessions of high-intensity or high-volume training (short-term overtraining) is recovered within a few days. For example, a middle-distance runner may experience slower times after doing cross-country training for a few weeks. The recovery period may range from 24 to 72 h. Likewise, after an intense bout of weight training, the athlete's body generally requires 48 h to repair the microtrauma to the muscles and connective tissue, to remove waste products (e.g., lactic acid), and to replace energy stores (e.g., muscle glycogen) in the cells (Westcott 1989). Chronic overwork occurs when the overwork is sustained too long or repeated too frequently and the client no longer responds adaptively to training (figure 3.6). This type of overwork can lead to chronic fatigue, exercise burnout, and higher rates of injury. Recovery from chronic overwork may take several weeks or even months (Kuipers and Keizer 1988).

Prevent overtraining by insisting on the following:

• **Adequate short-term recovery.** If your client performs a 45 min light aerobic workout with some stretching, he will be able to train harder within 24 h. If the workout is 90 min and is more vigorous and high impact, he may need to wait 2 or 3 days before a similar workout. Treatment of overtraining may include relative rest that consists of light aerobic exercise using a modality not related to the athlete's sport. Competitive athletes usually prefer a treatment plan based on therapeutic exercise rather than complete rest. Eating well will give the body fuel for healing, and the client might enjoy massage or whirlpool baths.

• **Proper variation.** Varying volume, intensity, and mechanics of training can reduce the likelihood of overtraining. Such variation also encourages "peaking" at the appropriate time and helps maintain a high level of performance (Kuipers and Keizer 1988). Adjust the training according to your client's levels of physical or emotional stress. Adjustments often take the form of decreased training volume with normal intensities. Sudden changes in intensity and volume may create short-term delays in performance gains, but periodic changes in training technique, venue, or stress management techniques can prove rejuvenating. Combining more than one type of exercise into a weekly training program (cross-training) can add variety and keep the program stimulating; and by using different muscles, it lessens the chance of developing overuse injuries.

• **Careful monitoring.** Recognition of overtraining is critically important, yet difficult. Symptoms of monotonous, short-term, and chronic overwork often overlap. By the time they are recognized and differentiated, the client has progressed to a stage where rest is imperative. Keeping a diary

How to Avoid Runner's Overtraining

The editor of *Runner's World* (Burfoot 1995) provided some practical recommendations:

• Run less when you are tired, more when you find that perfect forest trail.
• Run less when you have a cold, more when you feel strong.
• Run less when your knee hurts, more when you are training for a marathon.
• Run less when you are starting a new job, more when your kids head off to college.
• Run more during some weeks and less during others. Make running fit into everything else you do. Look at the big picture.

or log is essential for the serious performer (see chapter 6). Simple diaries can include quantifying exercise volume and intensity, body weight, diet, and sleep patterns, as well as subjective feelings of general health, fatigue, mood, and ratings of training difficulty. You can provide readings of blood pressure and heart rate, both at rest and postexercise. If your athletes can learn to listen to the messages their bodies are sending them, they can be effective in minimizing injuries. If familiar training is particularly difficult on a given day or produces unusual fatigue or nagging discomfort, this may indicate that your client is overtraining, that the body is in need of rest, or that the athlete is getting sick. See that infections are treated, with your client gradually returning to normal training levels. Remember, formal monitoring methods are no substitute for good communication between you and your client.

Components and Structural Segments of an Exercise Program

Although there are general fitness components, each of the exercise outcomes (health, fitness, performance) has components that are of particular importance. This second principle has to do with how these components are safely integrated into the structural segments of an exercise program.

Health, Fitness, and Performance Components

The essential physiological components of physical fitness are cardiovascular endurance, flexibility, strength, muscular endurance, and body composition.

• **Cardiovascular endurance** is the ability to perform physical work involving large muscle groups continuously for an extended period. This component depends on the efficiency of the oxygen transport system. In the lungs, oxygen moves across a membrane (diffusion) into the red blood cells; it is transported through the arteries to working muscle cells (diffusion and utilization). End products of cellular metabolism (carbon dioxide and at times lactic acid) are transported back through the veins to the heart and lungs. The heart is the key to the oxygen transport system, because it must continuously pump blood to all bodily systems as well as larger quantities to more active tissues.

• **Flexibility** is the capacity of a joint to move freely through a full range of motion without undue stress. For most joints, the limitation of movement is imposed by the soft tissues, including the muscle and its fascial sheaths; the connective tissue, with tendons, ligaments, and joint capsules; and the skin (Wilmore and Costill 2004).

• **Strength** measures the maximum ability of a muscle or muscle group to exert force against a resistance. For example, a person who can maximally curl a barbell weighing 150 lb (68 kg) is twice as strong as the client who can curl only 75 lb (34 kg). Lifting as much as possible in one lift is referred to as one-repetition maximum (1RM).

• **Muscular endurance** is the ability of a muscle or muscle group to exert a force repeatedly or to sustain a contraction for a period of time. A simple measure of muscular endurance involves determining the number of repetitions clients can complete while lifting a fixed percentage of their 1RM.

• **Body composition** refers to the relative amounts of fat and lean body weight in the body. Exercise often decreases total body weight and fat weight and increases fat-free weight (Quinney et al. 1994).

Performance-related fitness components are those necessary for sport performance or optimal work performance. The components include motor skills (e.g., speed, agility, balance, and coordination), cardiovascular endurance, muscular power, strength, endurance, size, body composition, skill acquisition, and motivation.

Health-related fitness components include body composition (e.g., subcutaneous fat distribution, abdominal visceral fat, body mass relative to height), muscle balance (strength, endurance, and flexibility—particularly of postural muscles), cardiovascular functions (e.g., submaximal exercise capacity, blood pressure, lung functions), and metabolic components (e.g., blood lipids, glucose tolerance). Very inactive people benefit from even low-intensity exercise, because the detrimental health-related consequences of extreme inactivity are rapidly reversed.

Creating a Balanced Prescription

We are at a point in the prescription journey where a performance, fitness, or health goal has been established. Each specific objective is linked to one or more fitness components. How to reach those objectives and how to package their prescription make up the next stage. If your prescription is to be effective, it must be both balanced and safe.

Chapters 6, 7, 8, and 9 describe the many tools at our disposal for designing activity programs. They present the physiological bases and advantages of specific methods of training. Effective exercise prescription depends on our ability to achieve selected benefits for specific clients, using popular methods such as weight, flexibility, aerobic, and anaerobic training.

You must integrate the various components of fitness into a balanced workout. There are innumerable ways you can tailor each client's prescription to current needs and wants, as well as key things to keep in mind when deciding how to approach the segments of the workout. To improve or maintain your client's cardiovascular endurance, flexibility, strength, muscular endurance, and body composition, include all the following segments in the prescription:

- **Order.** There is some room for personal preference in the order of the phases of a workout. Regardless of the order, follow the principle of progressive overload as your client enters the aerobic and the muscular conditioning phases. A gradual increase in intensity will prepare the body for the demands of that segment. The order presented previously allows the tissue temperature to be high when your client works on flexibility. It also stretches muscles tightened during the aerobics, in preparation for the resistance training to follow. However, many clients may feel more comfortable doing their flexibility training before aerobic activity or integrating it with their muscular conditioning. For those concerned with weight management, it was found that the excess postexercise oxygen consumption was no different when the order of completing aerobic and resistance segments differed (Oliveira and Oliveira 2011).

- **Warm-up.** The ACSM (Haskell et al. 2007) recommends at least a 5 to 10 min warm-up period at the beginning of each workout session. The more intense the exercise, the longer and more important the warm-up. Often the warm-up consists of the same exercise, for example running, done at a lower intensity. Warming up prepares the muscles that will be used in the workout. When a muscle contracts, not all the individual fibers contract at once. So tension is created among the fibers and the connective tissues between the fibers (Malkin 2004), which can lead to microtears. Warm tissues are less likely to suffer microtears. The initial warm-up activity often perfuses sufficient warm blood to the active muscles to increase tissue suppleness and allow for more effective stretching in the later part of the warm-up. Stretching the warmed muscles and tissue improves range of motion and physical function (Jonas and Phillips 2009).

- **Aerobic conditioning.** Both continuous and discontinuous aerobic training can improve cardiovascular fitness (Åstrand and Rodahl 2003). Interval (discontinuous) training consists of a repeated series of exercise bouts with intermittent relief periods. Because interval training permits a variety of activities, it is popular in many sports and has been recommended for symptomatic clients whose primary goal is health (ACSM 2006). Manipulation of the interval prescription factors, such as duration of effort, time of relief, and number of repetitions, can make prescriptions very precise (chapter 6).

- **Body composition.** Body composition changes are achieved through a combination of aerobic and muscular conditioning.

- **Flexibility.** Flexibility through stretching plays a major role in the maintenance of muscle balance. Your client's objectives will determine how, where, and through what technique you integrate flexibility into the prescription (chapter 8).

- **Muscular conditioning.** You can match strength training programs to your clients' objectives. Almost any form of resistance exercise will stimulate some degree of strength gain, especially if your client is unconditioned. Comfort, convenience, and safety therefore become as important for many clients as results. Again, considering the goals of your clients (performance, fitness, or health) will help you select the appropriate resistance training methods.

- **Cool-down.** At the end of aerobic work and to a lesser degree during muscular work, heart rate and blood volume (cardiac output) remain elevated. The return of blood through the venous system requires the rhythmic contraction of muscles to pump blood back to the heart and then to the lungs to oxygenate vital organs and tissues. This can be accomplished by continuing a weight-bearing activity such as walking until the heart rate returns to within about 20 beats/min of the starting rate (3-5 min). An added benefit of an effective cool-down is to help remove metabolites (e.g., lactic acid). With elevated metabolites and fatigue, muscles may feel tight or sore (from earlier eccentric work) and may go into spasm. Stretching while warm will relieve some of these symptoms, promote relaxation, and improve range of motion.

- **Safety.** A workout plan, no matter how balanced and client centered, is appropriate only if it is safe. What is the safest route through the series of physical stresses presented by each segment of the program? Table 3.2 identifies safety issues prominent during the various segments of a program.

Exercise Modifications and Functional Progressions

Every exercise and activity can be modified to change its degree of difficulty. This has obvious advantages in terms of finding a modification that is an appropriate starting level for your client. It also allows for progressive design changes to meet your client's changing physical condition. These fundamental principles of exercise design are often based on biomechanics of the movement.

Physiotherapists and other health care professionals have long known that muscles, joints, and other body tissue must be stressed gradually according to the manner in which they function. You need to teach your clients to take responsibility to determine the degree of difficulty and the change parameters of their exercise program.

A functional progression is a series of basic movement patterns used in active daily living, in sport or recreation, or in both that is graduated according to the difficulty of the exercise and the tolerance of the client. The functional progressions proceed from simple, safe exercises to more complex skills that mimic functional activities and sport skills and place the same demands on the client that the task will confer. Specific exercises and their progressions should vary depending on clients' needs, abilities, injuries, and goals.

Once you have selected a functional movement pattern that suits the client's needs and places the demand on the appropriate component(s), you can modify the exercise to create levels of difficulty based on the following criteria:

- Level 1 is for people who need the basics and are in poorer shape for the given component. More careful monitoring is needed.
- Level 2 is for the general public wanting to improve but not wanting anything too strenuous. Jarring movements are avoided.
- Level 3 is for people who are currently active and need to make sure they are covering all areas. Tasks are at a "training" level.

Functional progressions may involve gradual changes in intensity, duration, or number completed; overloads; or alternate exercise designs. The rate at which clients can and will progress depends in part on their medical history and their current health and fitness status. As a general rule, clients should increase their exercise program in any of the relevant FIT components (frequency, intensity, or time [duration]) at a rate of no more than 10% per week (Jonas and Phillips 2009). With the exception of the type of exercise, increases should focus on only one of these elements at a time. For example, if your client is increasing the duration of his exercise sessions from 30 to 33 min, he should avoid simultaneous increases in the frequency or intensity of the exercise.

Effective client-based progressions and modifications can be designed through the application of biomechanical principles such as mechanics or leverage changes, alignment and direction of forces, movement variations, or joint–muscle summation. The application of a number of these basic biomechanical principles to modify exercise will greatly enhance your skill and adaptability as a trainer. You will be able to modify the difficulty or intensity of an exercise to suit the condition of your client or to design an effective progression. Your application skills will also allow you to make immediate changes on the floor with your client to alter the focus of the exercise (e.g., primary muscles) or to allow for an effective compensation in the exercise execution.

Biomechanical Principles of Exercise

Biomechanical analysis examines the method of execution of an exercise. We can apply biomechanical principles to optimize exercise benefits for our clients and at the same time attend to their limitations through biomechanical alterations of the exercise. Such analyses enable us to advise our clients concerning

- choosing the best starting position for an exercise,
- finding the optimal speed for their objectives,
- determining the position of joints to isolate specific muscles,
- aligning the movement to the muscle,
- combining muscles for optimal results, and
- modifying the leverage to gain a greater strength output.

The next section is guided by a number of biomechanical principles. The purpose, effectiveness,

Table 3.2 Safety Issues for Program Segments

Prescription	Safety issues
Preparation (warm-up)	
Range of motion (moving major joints)	• Increase joint lubrication and synovial fluid (protect joints) through warm-up. • Have client check on how body feels before work. • Use warm-up to provide some flexibility gains.
Circulatory warm-up (light aerobic; same mode as cardiovascular work)	• Continue warm-up to increase tissue temperature and synovial fluid in preparation for stretching. • Use segment to gradually prepare heart and circulatory system. • Simulate joint mechanics with low trauma.
Stretching (emphasizing static stretching)	• Promote gains in flexibility. • Target muscles used, especially if used eccentrically. • Use dynamic stretches for sport preparation.
Transition (easing into next segment)	• Add a light overload in the activity to follow (start of progressive overload).
Aerobic segment	
Progressive prescription	• Build up gradually whether continuous or intervals. • Provide adequate relief during intervals. • Tier down gradually, avoiding final sprints or sudden stops (better cardiovascular adaptations permitted).
Monitoring	• Monitor heart rate, perceived exertion, talk test, and logging. • Include stretching for muscular tightness.
Sport-specific segment	
	Try to include the following: • Mini warm-up and skill practice (especially in intermittent sports such as baseball) • Stretching tight muscles • Tending immediately to minor injuries
Resistance segment	
Progressive prescription	• Include progressive overload and adequate relief (depends on training method). • Incorporate warm-up sets (e.g., 60% of training). • Follow safety rules of the weight room (especially spotting guidelines).
Specific training method (chapter 7)	• Follow method guidelines as prescribed.
Muscle balance	• Check the balance (agonist and antagonist) of the program (i.e., need for specific muscle stretch or strengthening).
Monitoring	• Have client stretch as needed for muscular tightness. • Teach client to differentiate between fatigue, soreness, and inflammation. • Modify the exercise around minor injuries (including avoidance). • Constantly check for correct breathing, speed of movement, base of support, and alignment such as pelvic stabilization and avoidance of extreme range of motion.
Cool-down segment	
Stretching (emphasizing static stretching)	• Take advantage of warm tissue for greatest flexibility gains. • Use target muscles, especially if used eccentrically. • Consider proprioceptive neuromuscular facilitation (PNF) if flexibility is a priority.
Self-check	• Make sure cardiovascular indicators (e.g., heart rate, depth of breathing, blood pressure) are reduced. • Ensure that muscles feel worked but not sore or tight. • Ice any "hot spots" or minor injuries. • Don't underestimate the therapeutic effect of a relaxing shower.

and risk of an exercise or sport skill may be modified by any of the following:

- Muscle length and force
- Biarticular (two-joint) muscle action
- Composition of forces
- Leverage and strength
- Direction of force application and muscle alignment
- Alignment of external resistance

Muscle Length and Force

The amount of force produced by a muscle is related to the physical length at which the muscle is held. You can use this information to direct your prescription and optimize the results when you understand the answers to the following questions.

What Causes the "Sticking Point" in Weightlifting?

A person working with weights will begin to feel weak at some point during the exercise. Getting the weight started is the first sticking point, and completing the last few degrees is the second sticking point. The maximum tension (force) that can be generated in the muscle will occur when the muscle is activated at a length slightly greater than its resting length—up to about 120% of the resting length. When a muscle is shortened to about 50% to 60% of its resting length, its force is minimal because actin and myosin filaments are doubled over and few cross-bridges are formed (first sticking point). The second sticking point occurs as the muscle is elongated beyond 120% of the resting length and there is slippage of the cross-bridges (fewer are formed) and less force is generated (Edman 1992). In addition, the angle of pull of the muscle on the bone changes as the joint moves through its motion. Maximal force occurs when the angle of pull of the muscle is at 90° to the long axis of the bone. As a result of both factors, your clients will feel weak at the ends of the range of motion.

✅ Application

Select weights that your client can lift through a full range of motion for the prescribed repetitions or assist her through the sticking points.

How Can Your Client Tap an Energy Reserve?

If your client is working with weights, a slight increase in the stretch of the muscle before the contraction will summon an energy reserve for increased performance. The reason is that the total tension or force generated in a shortening muscle receives a contribution from the passive (stretch) tension of the tendon and the connective tissue in the muscle (figure 3.7). This stored elastic energy or passive tension plus the voluntary muscular tension provides the total tension or force output.

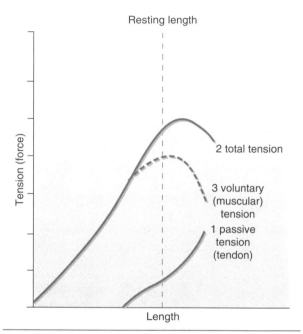

Figure 3.7 Relationship between muscle length and tension.

✅ Application

Your clients can apply this principle in training or in athletic activities by placing the joint in a preparatory phase (prestretched) before the power phase (e.g., the backswing of a batter or the squat of a volleyball spiker). This stored energy can be used only if the shortening contraction occurs within 0.0 to 0.9 s after the stretch and if the muscle is not lengthened too much (Komi 1992). With eccentric training, the force increases as the velocity of the lengthening contraction increases, up to a point where control is lost. These principles are the basis for plyometric training (chapter 7).

Biarticular Muscle Action

Biarticular muscles are those that cross two joints and affect movement at both joints. You can apply this understanding to help clients stretch muscles from both ends, isolate muscles for conditioning, and perform aerobics more efficiently.

How Can a Biarticular Muscle Stretch From Both Ends?

Biarticular muscles are not long enough to allow a full range of motion simultaneously at both joints. If one of the two joints is moved to the end of its range of motion, the attempt to move the second joint to the end of its range will stretch the biarticular muscle nearer the second joint.

Application

For example, the hamstrings attach above the hip and below the knee. Once the knee is pulled tight to the chest, it is not possible to fully extend the knee because the hamstrings are too short. Attempting to extend the knee, however, will stretch the lower hamstrings. To stretch the upper hamstrings, extend the knee and rotate the pelvis forward as the trunk flexes. Hamstring strains are more common in the upper area of the hamstrings, suggesting that stretching this area may be of greater value for prevention or rehabilitation. "Feeling" where the stretch is centered provides feedback that the biarticular principle is being used effectively.

Other biarticular muscles (and the joints they cross) that can be effectively stretched in this manner include these:

- Gastrocnemius (ankle and knee)
- Rectus femoris (knee and hip)
- Iliopsoas (hip and pelvis)
- Erector spinae (pelvis and spine)
- Levator scapulae (shoulder girdle and cervical spine)
- Triceps (shoulder joint and elbow)

Check the JAM charts in chapter 5 for joint movements.

How Can We Isolate a One-Joint Muscle for Conditioning or Stretching?

If the two ends of a biarticular muscle are brought closer together, the muscle is too short to exert a maximum force output, and therefore single-joint muscles can be isolated. This method of isolation will also help you to analyze flexibility exercises. With the example of the gastrocnemius (two joints) and soleus (one joint) that follows, both muscles are stretched when the ankle is dorsiflexed. When the knee is straight, the gastrocne-

mius is maximally stretched; when the knee is flexed, the two-joint gastrocnemius is slack and the soleus stretch is optimized.

Application

This principle is used to isolate the abdominal muscles in a curl-up. When the knees and hips are bent, the biarticular hip flexors (rectus femoris) are short and slack and do not contribute appreciably to the action. The work feels more difficult because the abdominal muscles are being isolated. Adjustment of even one joint can shorten a muscle and decrease its involvement.

Similarly, as the knee flexes during a resisted leg flexion exercise (figure 3.8), the hamstrings lose their force as their origin and insertion come closer together. The individual therefore seeks help from the assistant movers for knee flexion. The JAM charts (see chapter 5) indicate that these include the sartorius, gracilis, and gastrocnemius muscles.

Application

The biarticular gastrocnemius (which attaches above the knee) is more heavily activated during a standing calf raise than when it is shortened during a seated calf raise, thereby isolating the soleus (figure 3.9).

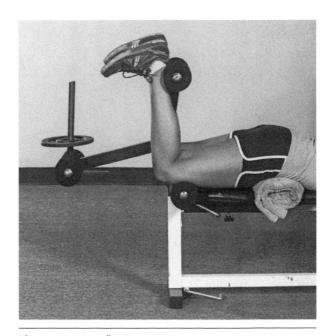

Figure 3.8 Leg flexion.

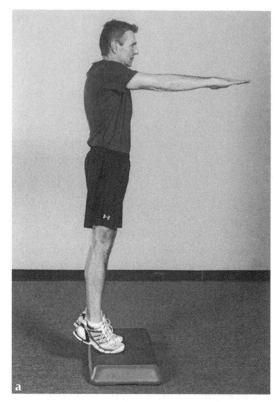

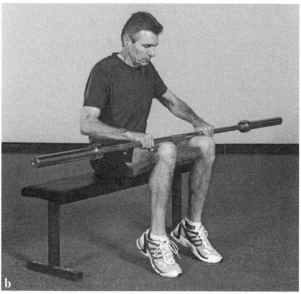

Figure 3.9 Calf raises: *(a)* standing and *(b)* seated.

How Do You Get More Force From a Biarticular Muscle?

Prestretching a biarticular muscle can significantly improve its force output.

Application

The flexor muscles of the wrist act as assistant movers for elbow flexion. When the wrist is slightly hyperextended during elbow flexion,

the increased tension in these muscles contributes to the force of the movement. This is also seen in the leg flexion exercise (figure 3.8), in which the force of the hamstrings is improved when the pelvis is rotated forward and the muscle is elongated. Because greater resistance can be applied, the training results are increased. Caution your clients about excessive pelvic rotation in this exercise, which can increase the lumbar curve and force the low back muscles into contracture.

How Do Biarticular Muscles Increase Efficiency?

Two-joint muscles, particularly in the lower extremity, save energy by allowing concentric work at one joint and eccentric work at the adjacent joint. This mechanical coupling of joints allows for a rapid release of stored elastic energy (passive tension) (Hamill and Knutzen 1995).

Application

In a vertical jump, the gastrocnemius concentrically plantar flexes the ankle. At the knee, which is extending, the gastrocnemius is eccentrically storing elastic energy. These joint couplings occur frequently in walking and jogging and reduce the work required from the single-joint muscles. **Closed kinetic chain exercises** (see chapter 7) that involve direct weight bearing use this mechanical coupling. They are quite useful, and clients wanting to strengthen their knees would benefit from closed kinetic chain leg exercises.

Composition of Forces

Try to visualize the combination of muscles involved in a particular joint movement. Teach your clients to use this visualization to direct their focus to the right muscles and provide helpful sensory feedback.

It is often possible to modify a movement to isolate a targeted muscle or muscle part. Joints do not always follow traditional movements. For instance, they may move halfway between flexion and abduction. Many sport skills or work tasks involve similar oblique movements. Think of a muscle as a string on a mannequin causing joint movement in the direction of the pull of the string. Each muscle acting on that joint is like a string pulling at a different angle. When more than one force is acting on the joint, you can apply the technique of **composition of forces** to help visualize the relative contribution of those muscles to the final movement.

✅ Application

The pectoralis major has two parts, combining the sternal (S) and clavicular (C) forces to produce a resultant force (R) that produces movement in a different direction from that caused by either part of the muscle by itself. This resultant force causes shoulder joint horizontal adduction (figure 3.10).

To use this technique, try the following:

1. Draw (or visualize) the movement as an arrow. This is called the resultant force.

2. Select, from the anatomical analysis, the two primary muscles causing the movement.

3. Represent these muscle forces with arrows, where the arrowheads indicate the direction of pull of the muscles and the length of the arrow depicts the relative strength of that muscle's involvement.

4. Place the base of the two forces (S and C in this example) together on or near the point of attachment of the two muscles.

5. Draw a parallelogram from the arrows.

The diagonal of the parallelogram represents the composition of the forces—that is, the **resultant force**.

The final stage of this technique involves identifying which muscle you want to isolate. Alter the direction of the resultant force closer to the direction of that muscle. You can see in figure 3.10b that as the movement (R_2) is angled more upward, the clavicular arrow becomes larger (C_2). This means that the clavicular part of the pectoralis major is generating more force, effectively isolating it.

Here are more examples of the composition of forces:

• Acting alone, the anterior (A) and posterior (P) parts of the deltoid flex and extend the shoulder joint, respectively (figure 3.11). Their combined action (resultant, R) is shoulder joint abduction. When someone lifts an object by abducting the shoulder joint, she calls into play the anterior deltoid more heavily because the object is in front of the body. If she has a rounded shoulder posture, how would you modify the shoulder joint abduction to emphasize the posterior deltoid? Recall that the posterior deltoid is a prime mover for shoulder joint extension and horizontal abduction (see form 5.1). Shoulder joint abduction slightly behind the midline of the body with a retraction (adduction) of the shoulder girdle will increase the size of the posterior force.

• The two heads of the gastrocnemius, pulling in lateral (L) and medial (M) directions, together exert an upward force (R) on the Achilles tendon and cause plantar flexion of the ankle (figure 3.12). Toeing in will slightly prestretch the lateral head of the gastrocnemius, allowing a small increase

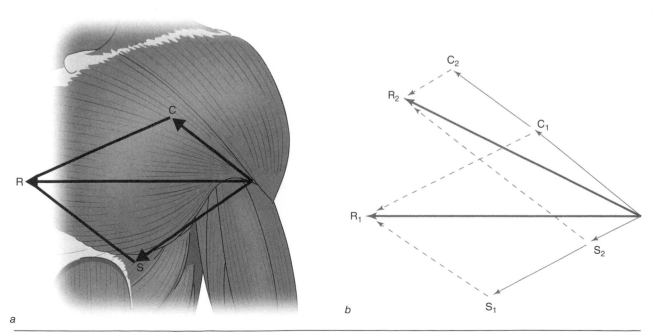

a

b

Figure 3.10   Resultant force: pectoralis major. S = sternal; C = clavicular; R = resultant force.

in the force output of that head during plantar flexion. Only the most avid bodybuilders would want this advantage during an exercise such as a calf raise (figure 3.9).

• The pull of the quadriceps on the patella guides the patella through the path of motion (figure 3.13*a*). Sometimes (figure 3.13*b*) the patella is directed laterally (R) by the quadriceps (Q) and patellar tendon (P)—particularly if the vastus medialis (M) is weak. This muscle imbalance can lead to inflammation on the posterior side of the patella.

• A resultant force acting on the knee in a different direction (figure 3.14) is the pressure

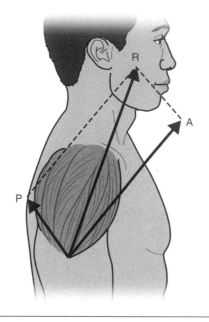

Figure 3.11   Resultant force (R): deltoid.

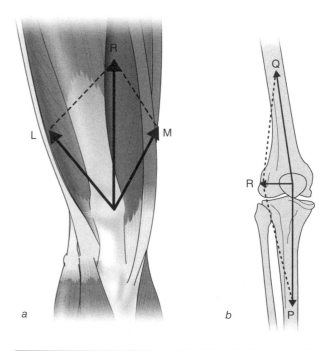

Figure 3.13   Resultant force: quadriceps. R = resultant force; Q = quadriceps; P = patellar tendon; M = vastus medialis; L = vastus lateralis.

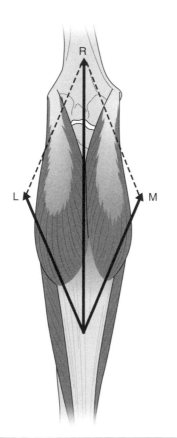

Figure 3.12   Resultant force (R): gastrocnemius.

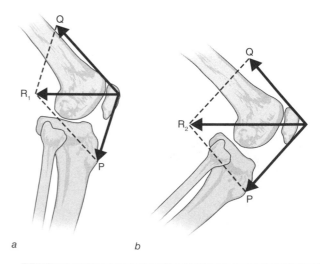

Figure 3.14   Resultant force: patellar pressure.

exerted on the back side of the patella from the quadriceps muscles (Q) and patellar tendon (P). As the knee flexes (as in a squat or a lunge), the resultant force increases (R_1 vs. R_2).

✔️ Application

Have your clients take precautions with the depths and applied loads during these types of exercises.

Leverage and Strength

Lever systems can help you modify exercises to optimize your clients' efforts. If a client is having difficulty with an exercise or wants to make it more challenging, you can adjust the intensity by changing the lever system.

How Do You View the Body as a Series of Lever Systems?

To view the body as a series of lever systems, consider the joint as the fulcrum and the bones as lever arms that move around the fulcrum. Muscle contraction is the force applied to the lever (at the point where the tendon attaches to the bone), whereas the weight of the body parts plus any external weight being lifted is resistance to the force (figure 3.15).

The majority of levers in the body are third class, which means that the force is applied between the resistance and the fulcrum. The biceps acting around the elbow joint is an example of a third-class lever. In figure 3.15, the elbow is

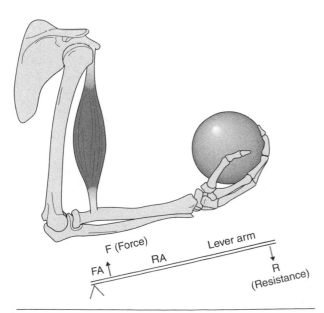

Figure 3.15   The arm as a lever system (e.g., third-class lever). FA = force arm; RA = resistance arm.

the fulcrum, the radius is the lever arm, the biceps exerts the force, and the weight of the ball and the forearm is the resistance.

The tendon of the biceps inserts to the radius just below the elbow. The distance from the fulcrum (elbow) to the force (biceps insertion) is called the force arm (FA). The distance from the fulcrum (elbow) to the resistance is called the resistance arm (RA) (figure 3.15).

How Can You Adjust a Lever System to Modify the Difficulty of an Exercise?

You can modify the intensity or difficulty of an exercise by changing aspects of the lever system.

- **Resistance.** If your clients are lifting weights or have load adjustments on their machines, it is easy to change the resistance. You can introduce (or change the thickness of) tubing or elastic bands. Water offers increased resistance and an added safety element for joints. Increased resistance is the overload of choice when your client's goal is strength.

- **Force.** Force is the strength or the speed of the muscular contractions that cause a movement. Sometimes performing an exercise slowly demands more control and is more difficult than doing it more quickly. As your clients' muscular condition improves, they can generate greater forces in a more coordinated manner. Increased speed of movement is the overload of choice when your client's goal is muscular power. The speed adjustments on isokinetic and hydraulic machines (chapter 7) change the potential force outputs. Even aerobic machines like stair climbers have similar setting options (i.e., slower speed settings generate greater force). With certain flexibility training methods, the isometric contraction phase of a proprioceptive neuromuscular facilitation (PNF) stretch (chapter 8) can modify the force of contraction, changing that element of the lever system and ultimately the effectiveness of the stretch.

- **Force arm.** The distance between the joint and the insertion of the muscle (FA) cannot be changed, but it partially explains differences in performance among clients whose muscular conditioning (force) appears to be equal.

- **Resistance arm.** Changing the distance between the joint and the resistance arm (RA) is the easiest way to adjust the body's lever systems. As the resistance moves closer to the joint, the muscle will need less force to move the resistance. The challenge is to recognize the parts of the lever system in question: Which joint is the acting fulcrum? What represents the resistance? What is the best way to shift the resistance arm? There are often multiple lever systems working at once, and you must identify the one most appropriate to adjust (see table 3.3).

Application

Depending on your client's situation, you can adjust the resistance, force, force arm, or resistance arm.

Direction of Force Application and Muscle Alignment

Tension or force from a muscle is transferred through the tendon to the bone. The angle of attachment of the muscle dictates the direction of force application, which produces the movement (figure 3.16). Near the middle of the range of motion, the angle of insertion of the tendon usually directs more of the force perpendicular to the bone, resulting in its strongest position.

Force application is optimized when the muscle–tendon unit is directly aligned with the plane of movement. This can be seen with the prime movers for specific joint actions. In fact, careful alignment of the movement can emphasize the contribution from particular parts of a given muscle. With this information, you can personalize exercises for your clients. For example:

• **Crossovers** (figure 3.17) using pulleys, tubing, or elastic bands are versatile exercises

because the angle of the pull is easily changed to suit the targeted muscle or the sport skill.

• The **pull-down** exercise uses the latissimus dorsi. Different secondary muscles are pulled into play, however, if the bar is pulled down in front of or behind the head. In front, the pectoralis major is used because of the slight flexion. Pulling behind the head forces the shoulder joint backward and activates the posterior deltoid.

• The **bench press** uses a horizontal movement of the shoulder joint and uses the sternal or hor-

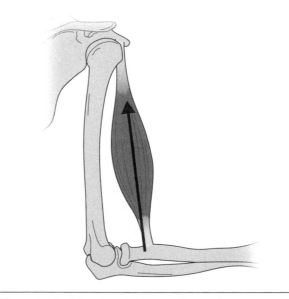

Figure 3.16 Direction of force application. Force increases as the angle between the tendon and the bone approaches 90°.

Table 3.3 Adjusting the Resistance Arm (RA)

Exercise	Fulcrum	Resistance (R)	RA adjustment
Curl-up	Low back	Upper body weight	Arms above the head move R away from the fulcrum—harder
Push-up	Shoulder joint	Weight of entire body	Done from the knees moves a reduced R closer to the fulcrum—easier
Dumbbell fly	Shoulder joint	Dumbbell and arm	Changing the angle of the elbow moves the R
Leg (knee) flexion and extension (machine)	Knee	Assigned weight and lower leg	Adjusting the position of the pad lower—harder
Standing knee lift	Hip	Weight of leg (could use ankle weight or tubing)	Lifting leg with an extended knee; R farther from hip—harder
Bent-over rowing	Low back (not shoulder joint)	Weight of upper body and barbell	Upright rowing brings R closer to lower back—less load on back structures

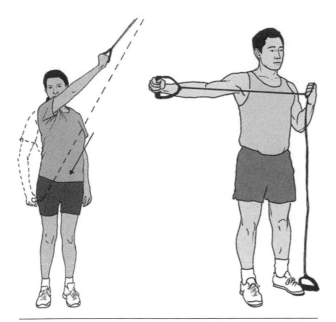

Figure 3.17   Crossovers with different directions.

izontal fibers of the pectoralis major. With the incline bench press, the shoulder joint is angled upward and activates the upper clavicular part of the pectoralis major.

- **Rowing** action with any device may be done with elbows in or out. With elbows in, the shoulder joints extend to involve the latissimus dorsi and pectoralis major as prime movers. With the elbows up, the shoulder joints horizontally abduct through contraction of the posterior deltoid, infraspinatus, and teres minor. A small change in alignment can significantly change the purpose of the exercise.

✅ Application

The external obliques are a good visual example. The muscle fibers run diagonally and therefore are most effective when pulling the trunk in the diagonal direction (such as in a curl-up with a rotation). In a straight curl-up, the external oblique muscle is not as effective—with spinal flexion, the pull of the muscle is at an angle to the action and the entire force is not used for the movement.

Hand in hand with force application is the alignment of muscle action. For example, you should ask yourself which muscles are working in a side leg raise. The hip abductors lift the leg in a side leg raise, and this should affect how you instruct your client. What changes take place if the toe is pointing upward? (Remember, the line of pull of a muscle across a joint will determine the functions of that muscle.) When the toe is pointed upward, the task of lifting the leg has shifted to the hip flexors, which are directly in the line of pull.

Alignment of External Resistance

Do not leave the interface between your client and his equipment to chance. It is not the machine's job to know the proper alignment, stabilization, range of motion, and application of resistance—it is yours. Ask yourself the following questions.

Is the Path of Motion Defined by the Machine the Same as Your Client's Path of Motion?

Many machines have a guided range of motion that may cause problems for smaller or larger clients. If seats and lever arms cannot be adjusted and your client looks or feels unnatural throughout the movement, the machine path is probably unsuitable.

Always ascertain the following:

- A correct position of the joint before the exercise begins
- A safe end point to the range of motion (the machine may have a range-limiting device)
- A smooth arc of motion of the joint

Monitor your client carefully for these three checks, especially during spinal movements and shoulder rotations. New technology is addressing this issue. Some pec decks (e.g., Cybex) now use a dual-axis technology that allows clients to determine their own optimal arc of movement and range of motion. You should monitor the path of motion even when using low-tech body weight resistance. For example, take care that your client does not go too low during dips and excessively hyperextend her shoulder.

The ankle, knee, and hip joints form a kinetic chain. When the foot is stabilized or fixed, this kinetic chain is closed. An open kinetic chain exists when the foot is not in contact with the ground or some other surface. Knee flexion and extension using a machine are examples of open kinetic chain exercises. In a closed kinetic chain, the foot is weight bearing: The forces begin at the ground and work their way up through each joint.

✅ Application

There is an advantage in having forces absorbed by various anatomical structures rather than simply dissipated as in an open chain path of motion.

Is the Direction of the Force Application Safe and Optimal?

There is a direction of movement that generates maximal muscular force. Always determine if the force angle allows for the maximum resistance to be lifted. In many sport skills, if force is divided into sideward or vertical movements when desired direction is forward, there will be a reduced speed (forward velocity).

With pulley systems, tubing, or water, your role involves establishing the correct body position for your client. The purpose of the exercise will significantly affect the line of pull and the position of the joints. This concept is discussed in more detail in chapter 5; look at the example in figure 5.2, which shows that the line of pull and the position of the shoulder are considerably different in two similar exercises. Similarly, various angles on an incline bench can be used to isolate targeted muscles when using free weights.

✅ Application

A 10° decline on the bench when a bodybuilder is doing flys can help him focus on the lower fibers of the sternal section of the pectoralis major. A 45° incline will swing the emphasis to the clavicular section of the pectoralis major.

Does the Equipment Allow Proper Alignment Between the Machine's Fulcrum and the Center of the Moving Joint?

If the fulcrum of the machine does not align with the center of the moving joint, that joint will experience additional shearing force (making it slide apart) that increases more rapidly than the resistance on the machine (Hamill and Knutzen 1995). Clients with previous injuries to that joint are at significant risk.

The following examples illustrate this problem on various pieces of equipment.

• Many pec decks have their pivot points in front of the shoulder, forcing the shoulder girdle to abduct significantly and decreasing the effectiveness of the exercise.

• The knee is particularly vulnerable to shearing forces. Joint alignment on leg extension machines is critical. Correct placement of shin pads (not too low) and a resistance varied by a cam reduces knee stress and optimizes strength gains.

• The leg curl machine involves similar issues. An angled bench that elevates the pelvis will help maintain alignment of the low back as the knee flexes.

• Hack squat machines keep the pelvis and back quite stationary (unlike a regular squat), so

that the knees are placed under greater shearing stress.

• Abdominal machines are particularly difficult because multiple pivot points change throughout the range of motion. Actions that have the trunk flexed well forward creating an L position increase low back stresses (Hamill and Knutzen 1995). Crunching downward or bringing a tucked lower body upward is a preferred movement if no pain is present. Some say that this movement focuses the intensity of contraction to the lower abdominal muscles. More important for people with low back problems, this movement appears to present less compression on the discs of the lower back.

How Are External Forces Affecting Demands on the Muscles?

External forces act on an object. They may be contact or noncontact forces. Gravity is an example of a noncontact force. The force of gravity acting on an object is often considered to be its weight.

Contact forces occur between objects in contact with one another, for example, air or water resistance (fluid) and solid contact forces such as with a piece of resistance equipment, another athlete, or an object. Jumping and running involve reaction contact forces from the ground pushing against you.

External forces such as gravity and momentum demand a reaction from internal forces (muscle contraction). For example, loss of control with ballistic actions (momentum) causes high-intensity eccentric contractions and potential soft tissue strain in order to slow the joint action.

✅ Application

The vigorous actions with added implements such as rackets or weights increase the demand for internal force control.

Case Studies

There are specific prescription guidelines for each client goal. Client 1 has a number of cardiovascular risk factors and has set a goal of health-related fitness. Client 2 is interested in overall fitness and staying in shape. Client 3 is an athlete interested in performance-related fitness and injury prevention.

Case Study 1: Health-Related Fitness Client

Most new clients are interested in the health benefits that are provided by regular exercise. They may express a general desire to feel better or present a

Biomechanics in the Design and Modification of a Lateral Arm Raise

The middle deltoid and supraspinatus have a direct line of pull for shoulder joint abduction. As the deltoid lifts the arm near the horizontal, the deltoid is shorter and not as strong. At this point, the shoulder girdle muscles play a more significant role.

The anterior deltoid assists with shoulder joint abduction. As the client begins to fatigue, she may lift the weights a little more in front of her body to recruit more of the anterior deltoid. This change in alignment alters the composition of forces. By using a thumbs-up position, the starting position of the shoulder is rotated, involving two more of the rotator cuff muscles (infraspinatus and teres minor). This change in alignment is not only a safety feature—it makes the lateral arm raise into a conditioning exercise for the rotator cuff.

A lateral raise (figure 3.18) is a third-class lever where the fulcrum is the shoulder joint, the lever arm is the humerus, the primary force is the deltoid, and the resistance is the weight of the arm and the dumbbell. Increasing the bend of the elbow brings the resistance closer to the fulcrum, reducing the resistance arm and making the exercise easier, a

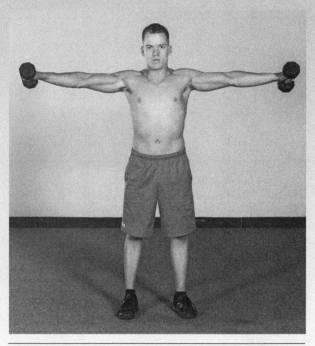

Figure 3.18 Lateral arm raises.

good starting position. As your client progresses, have her straighten her elbows somewhat before changing the weight.

Effective exercise analysis allows the desired purpose of the exercise to be achieved and to meet our clients' needs. You should always alter exercises—anatomically and biomechanically—to account for your client's limitations.

specific concern such as weight loss or blood pressure control.

Health-Related Prescription

- The ACSM recommends moderate-intensity exercise (55-75% maxHR or 40-60% $\dot{V}O_2$max) a minimum of 30 min on 5 days each week (Jonas and Phillips 2009).

- Alternatively, have the client perform less intense exercise 7 days per week or 10 min bouts of moderate-intensity exercise several times per day, most days of the week (goal: 150 min/week).

- For resistance training, have her use large muscle mass exercises, use higher-volume training (i.e., multiple sets, moderate intensity), and avoid exhaustive sets (Feigenbaum and Pollock 1997; Stone, Fleck, et al. 1991; Jonas and Phillips 2009).

- Bear in mind that given equal total energy costs, lower-intensity and longer-duration exercise will

benefit your older or less fit clients as much as higher-intensity and shorter-duration exercise.

- Also remember that moderate-intensity exercise carries lower cardiovascular risk and lower probability of orthopedic injury, and it enjoys higher compliance.

- If your client is concerned about weight loss, have her exercise at a moderate intensity for 150 to 250 min per week (Donnelly et al. 2009). Using frequent short bouts of moderate activity, your client may progress up to a target of 1500 kcal/week (see table 9.5). To keep abreast of any changes in exercise recommendations, periodically check the ACSM website (www.acsm.org).

Case Study 2: General Fitness Client

Client 2 wants to be able to perform moderate to vigorous levels of physical activity without undue fatigue and to maintain such ability throughout life. More specifically, he wants to see improvements in cardiovascular condition ($\dot{V}O_2$max), body composition, flexibility, and muscular strength and endurance.

Consider an inactive 45-year-old. With his doctor's approval, you design an aerobic program with progressively increased intensity. Over a 6-week period, he works up to exercising at 122 to 125 beats/min (70% maxHR) and maintains that intensity regularly for another 16 weeks. The increase in his aerobic capacity is 20%. At his age, on average, 0.5% of his capacity is lost per year—so in effect, this client's improvement amounts to a 10-year rejuvenation!

Weight training can increase your client's muscular strength and cause some changes in body composition, but it will yield only a slight improvement in aerobic capacity. Moderate-intensity programs appear superior to high-intensity ones in preventing musculoskeletal injuries and improving adherence to endurance training (Wilmore and Costill 2004).

Exercises for muscle balance (including strength and flexibility) can prevent poor posture, low back complaints, and osteoporosis. Your client's flexibility will increase with static or dynamic stretching or proprioceptive neuromuscular facilitation stretching (chapter 8).

General Fitness Prescription

The ACSM (2009) recommends the following for healthy adults:

- **Frequency** of training: 3 to 5 days/week.
- **Intensity** of training: 55% to 90% of maximum heart rate or 40% to 85% of oxygen uptake reserve or heart rate reserve. The Canadian Physical Activity Guidelines (CSEP 2012) describe moderate-intensity physical activities as those that cause adults to sweat a little and to breathe harder, such as brisk walking and bike riding. Vigorous-intensity physical activities will cause adults to sweat and be 'out of breath' with activities like jogging and cross-country skiing.
- **Duration** of training: 20 to 60 min of continuous aerobic activity. Duration depends on intensity: For example, lower intensity activity should be done for a longer period of time.
- **Mode** of activity: Any activity that uses large muscle groups, can be maintained continuously, and is rhythmic and aerobic—for example, walking–hiking, running–jogging, bicycling, cross-country skiing, dancing, skipping rope, rowing, stair climbing, swimming, skating, and various endurance game activities.
- **Rate of progression:** Proportional to the initial level of fitness and dependent on age and goals. Clients starting an aerobic training program might achieve a 3% increase per week for the first month, 2% per week the second month, and 1% per week thereafter (Heyward 2010).
- **Resistance** training: Strength training of a moderate intensity, sufficient to develop and maintain fat-free weight (FFW). One set of 8 to 12 repetitions of 8 to 10 exercises that condition the major muscle groups at least 2 days per week is the recommended minimum.
- **Initial level of fitness:** High = higher workload; low = lower workload.

Case Study 3: Performance-Related Fitness Client

For client 3, the serious exerciser or athlete, you will prescribe the upper levels of intensity and volume of exercise. Understanding your client's sport demands will guide your prescription. Whether you have played the sport or not, you must analyze the demands on the body and design similar experiences to effectively adapt and enhance performance.

1. Determine the relative contribution from the metabolic energy systems: aerobic (oxidative-ATP [adenosine triphosphate]), glycolytic (lactic-ATP), phosphocreatine (alactic-ATP) (for more detail, see chapter 6).

2. Determine neuromuscular demands: recruitment (primary muscles used), firing frequency or rate, pattern (synergy), reflex (proprioception) (for more detail, see chapters 7 and 8).

3. Do a biomechanical analysis (more detail earlier in this chapter) of the most important skills within the sport, for example throwing in baseball. Break the skill down into the preparatory phase, force-producing phase, and follow-through phase. Identify the key elements within each of the phases, such as most rapid acceleration, point of impact, or any extreme ranges of motion.

Preparatory phase:

- Preload or prestretch of prime movers
- Example: A pitcher having above average external rotation in order to pitch through greater range of motion

Force-producing phase:

- Generation of force (summation of forces in kinetic chain) to produce movement impact (usually concentric)
- Right force at right time, which affects skills effectiveness (vaulting at right time, snowboarding half pipe)

Follow-through phase:

- Deceleration or recovery
- Example: follow-through of a pitch
- Allows forces to be dissipated or absorbed over as much time as possible and with as many joints as possible (prevents injury)

Once the sport analysis has been done, training priorities will be quite clear. It will be a relatively smooth step into the prescription, including selection of the following:

- Primary fitness or performance components
- Intensity and time of exertions
- Primary muscles and types of contractions
- Joint-specific range of motion
- Critical elements of higher risk

Summary

Client-centered exercise prescription is anchored upon three primary principles:

1. Exercise design determines exercise outcomes. Exercise is adaptive and can be designed to produce three potential outcomes: increased general fitness, health enhancement, or performance improvements. Clients interested in general fitness may want to perform appropriate levels of physical activity without undue fatigue and to maintain such ability throughout life. The average client gets involved in activity for fitness, with perhaps an added interest in recreational sport performance. Quality of life and reduction of risk factors (health goals) are still in the minds of these clients. One of the most valuable findings of recent research is that physical activity of even low intensity reduces blood lipids, lowers resting blood pressure, protects from type 2 diabetes, increases metabolic rate (weight loss), and increases QOL and independent living in the elderly. Exercise prescription can influence the mechanism for health and fitness benefits and should be viewed as a therapeutic intervention that requires a customized dose (frequency, intensity, duration, and type). Client-centered prescription for athletes requires individualized training in those components that constitute performance-related fitness: motor skills (e.g., speed, agility, balance, and coordination), cardiovascular endurance, muscular power, strength, endurance, body composition, skill acquisition, and motivation. You can maximize your client's training efficiency only through prudent selection of training methods and by appropriately changing the prescription factors of the program as the need arises.

2. Fitness components must be integrated into structural segments of an exercise program. Although there are general fitness components, each of the exercise outcomes (health, fitness, performance) has components that are of particular importance. The various components of fitness must be integrated into a balanced workout. The average fitness client may want to see improvements in cardiovascular conditioning ($\dot{V}O_2$max), body composition, flexibility, and muscular strength and endurance. To improve or maintain these components, include all the following phases in your client's prescription: warm-up, aerobic conditioning, body composition, flexibility exercises, muscular conditioning, and cool-down. A balanced workout plan is appropriate only if it is matched to the client and identifies safety issues prominent at the various phases of a program.

3. Exercise modifications and functional progressions personalize the prescription. FITT guidelines and principles of biomechanics should be used to modify and progress the prescription to suit our clients' abilities. Biomechanical analysis examines the method of execution of an exercise. The purpose, effectiveness, and safety of an exercise or sport skill may be affected by any or all of the following biomechanical principles: muscle length and force, biarticular (two-joint) muscle action, composition of forces, leverage and strength, direction of force application and alignment, and alignment of external resistance. Applied biomechanics can optimize exercise benefits for your clients and at the same time address their limitations through alterations of the exercise.

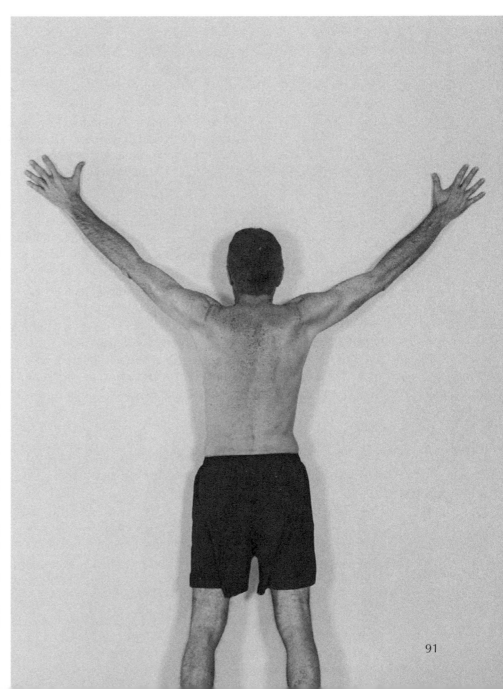

Client-Centered Assessment

Chapter Competencies

After completing this chapter, you will be able to demonstrate the following competencies:

1. Be client centered in your approach to assessment.
2. Use lifestyle appraisal tools to change behavior.
3. Screen your clients for risk factors and symptoms.
4. Consider client issues in selecting specific field tests.
5. Select a cardiovascular exercise mode and test protocol that are suitable for your client's age, sex, anticipated mode of exercise, and health and fitness status.
6. Identify the advantages of field-based cardiovascular assessment.
7. Identify the strengths, weaknesses, and sources of measurement error of laboratory and field-based body composition assessment tools.
8. Describe the factors to consider in selecting field-based musculoskeletal assessments.
9. Identify the objectives of selected field-based strength and endurance assessments.
10. Identify the objectives of selected field-based flexibility and muscle tightness assessments.
11. Screen your client using static and dynamic postural analyses.
12. Select and identify the objectives of appropriate assessments of your client's muscle balance.

91

In client-centered assessment, we look for things our clients want to do that will satisfy their most important needs and complement or at least accommodate their lifestyles. The practice of using a predetermined battery of tests that cover most fitness components, although appropriate for some assessment settings such as job applications or team selection, is not encouraged as a client-centered approach. As well, every client is at a different stage of readiness to make changes,

Assessment Resources

The following is a list of assessment resources, including their emphases:

- **American College of Sports Medicine.** 2009. *Guidelines for Exercise Testing and Prescription.* 8th ed. Philadelphia: Lea & Febiger. As an industry standard, this manual provides quick access to the essential details. Chapter 4: Laboratory cardiovascular treadmill and bicycle ergometer protocols and body composition assessments.

- **Baechle, T.R., and R.W. Earle.** 2008. *Essentials of Strength Training and Conditioning.* 3rd ed. Champaign, IL: Human Kinetics. This substantial text is used in conjunction with the National Strength and Conditioning certification. It has some good norms and is somewhat performance oriented. Chapter 15: Musculoskeletal field-based strength and power protocols.

- **Canadian Society for Exercise Physiology.** 2013. *Physical Activity Training for Health (CSEP-PATH).* Ottawa: CSEP. This update from the 2003 CPAFLA manual is the reference for the Certified Personal Trainer and the Certified Exercise Physiologist in Canada. B2. ASSESS: Physical Activity, Fitness & Lifestyle: Field-based body composition, aerobic, musculoskeletal, and back fitness appraisal measures.

- **Heyward, V.H.** 2010. *Advanced Fitness Assessment and Exercise Prescription.* 6th ed. Champaign, IL: Human Kinetics. This is one of the leading references for broad-based assessment protocols for most fitness components. Chapter 4: Cardiorespiratory maximal and submaximal laboratory and field-based test protocols. Chapter 6: Strength and muscular endurance laboratory and field-based test protocols. Chapter 8: Laboratory and field-based methods for assessing body composition. Chapter 10: Protocols for assessing flexibility.

- **Hoeger, W., S. Hoeger, M. Locke, and L. Lauzon.** 2009. *Principles & Labs for Fitness & Wellness.* Toronto: Nelson Education. This first Canadian edition is a practical text with many easily administered assessments. Field-based testing for body composition (chapter 4), cardiorespiratory endurance (chapter 6), muscular strength (chapter 7), and flexibility (chapter 8).

- **Kaminsky, L.A., American College of Sports Medicine.** 2010. *ACSM's Health-Related Physical Fitness Assessment Manual.* 3rd ed. Philadelphia: Wolters Kluwer/Lippincott, Williams & Wilkins. The many charts and figures and the health-related approach make this 172-page resource very useful.

- **Kendall, F.P., E.K. McCreary, and P.G. Provance.** 2005. *Muscles, Testing and Function: With Posture and Pain.* 5th ed. Baltimore: Williams & Wilkins. Kendall has long been a respected author in the area of physiotherapy with an excellent approach to the assessment of muscle balance. Tests for muscle length and flexibility, tests for posture (chapter 2), and numerous muscle strength tests typically used by physiotherapists.

- **Nieman, C.** 2010. *Exercise Testing and Prescription: A Health-Related Approach.* 7th ed. Mountain View, CA: Mayfield. Nieman uses a health-related approach to test protocol selection. Laboratory and field-based methods for assessing cardiorespiratory fitness (chapter 4), laboratory and field-based methods for assessing body composition (chapter 5), and field-based methods for assessing musculoskeletal fitness (chapter 6).

- **Page, P., C. Frank, and R. Lardner.** 2010. *Assessment and Treatment of Muscle Imbalance: The Janda Approach.* Champaign, IL: Human Kinetics. Using a strong scientific approach, part II in the text outlines posture and other functional evaluations of muscle imbalance.

- **Reiman, M.P., and R.C. Manske.** 2009. *Functional Testing in Human Performance.* Champaign, IL: Human Kinetics. Presented as a hardcover manual, this text describes 139 tests (40 on DVD) for sport, fitness, and occupational settings.

and it is important to establish our client's priorities before selecting or performing an assessment.

This chapter introduces laboratory and field-based tests for cardiovascular, body composition, and musculoskeletal components of fitness. The focus is on the selection of field-based assessments; normative values; specificity, reliability, and validity; client needs; human error; and equipment availability. We discuss client issues in the selection of test items and describe specific field tests for determining the client's distinct needs. Other laboratory protocols outside of the scope of this book can be found in several texts listed in "Assessment Resources."

Fitness testing is not an end in itself but rather is part of the overall exercise program (Nordvall and Sullivan 2002). The client-centered prescription model is flexible, allowing you to verify your client's needs by using selected assessment items that relate to your client's priorities and closely simulate her current training activity. Ultimately, you will validate your client's exercise prescription by using appropriate assessment tools and the baseline values for selected components of fitness. But also remember that first impressions are strong and lasting. If the first thing you do is probe and prod and induce fatigue, clients with low self-esteem may leave with less resolve to change than they had when they entered. Take sufficient time to establish clients' commitment, question them carefully, and focus on their areas of concern.

Health Screening and Lifestyle Appraisal

The human body does not function optimally when it is abused. The major causes of disability and death are no longer infectious diseases but rather diseases of lifestyle. Behaviors that contribute to various chronic illnesses include alcohol and drug abuse, smoking, inappropriate diets, and insufficient physical activity. Elements of a healthy lifestyle include positive attitude toward self and others, ability to cope with stress, a zeal for life, and the practice of healthy behaviors. Early recognition of and empathy with our clients' lifestyles help us set priorities and plan well-rounded fitness programs. It is preferable to assess a client's health status and lifestyle during the early phase of counseling, before other assessments.

Screening is done before any assessment or exercise program to identify chronic disease, acute illness or injury, pains, impairments, medications, cardiovascular risk factors, overall health status, physical activity and exercise patterns, readiness to exercise, procedures, and consent. Pertinent information can be obtained from interview, forms, or questionnaires administered before the assessment or activity or some combination of these. Useful lifestyle appraisal screening tools can be found in the American College of Sports Medicine Guidelines (2009) and the book by Kaminsky (2010). You can use information from the health and lifestyle appraisals to assist in the classification and screening of clients by health status before exercise assessment or prescription. The interview process (also see chapter 1) is a comfortable way to begin gathering this information and establishing a relationship.

Regardless of the type of preparticipation screening you use, information should be interpreted by the appropriate health care professional, and results should be documented (American College of Sports Medicine [ACSM] 2009). This screening information helps you to choose appropriate functional testing suited to your client's abilities and interests.

A health risk appraisal, or, more positively, a health and lifestyle appraisal, may be a client's first step to behavior change. It may be just the extra nudge that a client preparing to take some action needs. Its greatest value is as a tool that leads to healthy lifestyle intervention. Inactivity is so common that we have a critical role to play as providers and promoters of health care. There are three useful lifestyle appraisal tools: RISK-I, Physical Activity Index (PAI), and the FANTAS-TIC Lifestyle Checklist.

- **RISK-I.** RISK-I (pronounced "risky"; form 4.1) can be self-administered and involves selecting the appropriate numerical value in each of the risk categories on the chart (Canadian Society for Exercise Physiology [CSEP] 2003; Getchell and Anderson 1982; National Institutes of Health, National Heart Lung and Blood Institute [NIH, NHLBI] 1998). The first five categories (age, family history, smoking, body mass index, and exercise) are risk factors for coronary heart disease. The last two categories (back and knees) are areas of musculoskeletal risk. You can use the total score, which represents overall risk, to screen clients for a medical referral. RISK-I application is broader than for most tools because of the inclusion of musculoskeletal risk. Although the scoring is not precise, it opens the opportunity to talk to clients about a broad spectrum of issues that may need attention in their exercise prescription.

• **Physical Activity Index (PAI).** Physical activity and fitness reinforce each other. Just as the most fit people tend to be the most active, the most active are frequently the most fit, and the components of fitness are determined by patterns of habitual physical activity. Appraisal tools such as the Fantastic Lifestyle Checklist or RISK-I may have identified lack of physical activity as a habit in need of change. Yet an intense cardiovascular appraisal may not be appropriate for some clients. The PAI (form 4.2) will help you assess the activities in which your client already participates. For example, if your client exercises at a moderate intensity (3 points) for 40 min (5 points) four times per week (4 points), her physical activity index is $3 \times 5 \times 4 = 60$. This "good" rating is a level of physical activity with considerable health benefits, such as lowering blood lipids, blood pressure, and body fat (Shephard and Bouchard 1994). You can administer the PAI periodically to show improvements and help motivate your client.

• **FANTASTIC Lifestyle Checklist.** This tool is presented in chapter 1 (form 1.1) because of its value in lifestyle coaching. The checklist allows clients to understand the effects of various lifestyle habits on their health. It identifies lifestyle areas that need attention and provides help to make the appropriate changes.

PAR-Q and Medical History

Older individuals and people with high-risk symptoms should obtain medical permission before proceeding with vigorous exercise. All maximal exercise tests should include supervision by a physician.

The Physical Activity Readiness Questionnaire (PAR-Q) and now the new PAR-Q+ can help determine whether a client should provide a detailed medical history before entering an exercise program. You can use PAR-Q+, which is online at www.csep.ca/forms.asp, as a screening instrument both for submaximal aerobic assessment and for beginning moderate and progressive exercise programs (CSEP 2013; Shephard 1988; Warburton et al. 2010).

PAR-Q+ helps to identify clients for whom certain physical activities might be inappropriate or who should receive medical advice concerning the type of activity most suitable for them. To ensure the validity of the test as well as to protect yourself legally, administer the PAR-Q+ without providing any interpretation to your clients. All judgments must be their own. If they give one or more "yes" responses, direct them to their doctor for a review of their medical history before permitting them to complete active test components such as aerobic, strength, or endurance tests.

The Canadian Society for Exercise Physiology (Warburton et al. 2010) used an evidence-based consensus process to revise the PAR-Q form (now called the PAR-Q+). The Physical Activity Readiness Questionnaire-Plus (PAR-Q+) is a 4-page form for prescreening before physical activity participation and includes additional questions on chronic conditions for further probing by the CSEP Certified Exercise Physiologist (CEP). The first of the 4 pages includes a section that provides an idea of how the client is directed through the full form. The Canadian Society for Exercise Physiology has also created a new online screening program for individuals with chronic conditions (the e-PARmed-X+). For copies, visit www.csep.ca/forms.asp or go to www.csep.ca/publications.

In contrast to the PAR-Q, the PAR-Q+ is considered more appropriate for today's audience because

• it has been devised off the back of a huge research project;

• it incorporates hypertension and diabetes, which the PAR-Q does not;

• it is not limited to participants aged 15 to 69;

• it acknowledges that the risks of inactivity are considerably greater than the risks of acute exercise in participants who have controlled medical conditions or those who are asymptomatic;

• for most populations living with a chronic medical condition, the risk of premature death is much greater than the acute risks of a structured and supervised program of exercise;

• the PAR-Q+ clearly adopts the position that physical activity and exercise in the right dose, intensity, and environment are good for everyone, especially those with chronic medical conditions;

• it doesn't seek to exclude people quite so quickly as the original PAR-Q document.

Personal Observation

The questionnaires discussed here identify most concerns that can make a fitness assessment inappropriate. It is advisable, however, that you make some general observations within the screening process (CSEP 2003). Cancel or postpone the appraisal if clients

- demonstrate difficulty in breathing at rest;
- are ill or have a fever;
- have swelling in their lower extremities;
- are pregnant and do not have the consent of their physicians;
- cough persistently;
- are currently on medication for cardiovascular or metabolic problems;
- have clearly ignored instructions about eating, drinking, and smoking before arrival; or
- exhibit any other trait that you believe may predispose them to unnecessary discomfort or risk.

For some of these observations (e.g., coughing, swelling), direct clients to their physicians; for others (e.g., illness, eating, drinking), instruct them to return once the concern no longer exists.

Informed Consent

Any client who is exposed to possible physical or psychological injury must give informed consent before participation in an assessment or exercise program (CSEP 2013). The informed consent form should provide clients with an adequate explanation of the tests and program, the potential risks and discomforts that may be involved, and their rights and responsibilities. The client should read, understand, and sign this form before administration of the active appraisal, and you should retain the form as an official record. Filling out the form may prompt questions from your client that provide an opportunity for dialogue and a chance to gather information and build rapport.

Informed consent does not absolve you from negligence in the administration of an assessment or the prescription of exercise. Although the form should be individualized for each facility or business, the following components should be in every informed consent form (Nieman 2010):

- A general statement of the background and objectives of the program
- An explanation of the procedures to be followed
- A description of any risks or discomfort that may be experienced
- A description of the benefits that can reasonably be expected
- An offer to answer any of the client's questions

- An instruction that the client is free to withdraw consent and to discontinue participation at any time
- An explanation of the procedures to be taken to ensure the confidentiality of the information requested

In general, most clients who are found to have low to moderate risk do not need a current medical examination or a stress test before beginning a low- to moderate-intensity exercise program (Morrison 2001). However, 4 out of 10 adults over 65 have a chronic disorder that may result in a functional limitation. These problems, with any client, must be identified through the preexercise screening process. Any medical conditions that would cause the client to be at risk during exercise or physical assessment should require specific consent from the client's physician. Providing information about how to know when it is safe to begin an exercise program further empowers individuals to be responsible for their health. For even the healthiest of clients, you can encourage personal accountability by instructing them in this way: "You are encouraged to do the best you can on all tests, but never push yourself to a point of overexertion or beyond what you think is safe."

Fitness Test Item Selection

You do not have to know up front everything there is to know about your client's condition: The client-centered model is flexible, allowing you to loop back at any point and verify needs by assessing your client's current priorities and situation. It's all right to use certain tests, such as standard screening tools, for all first-time clients. But when your client has expressed a specific interest or need, be sure to include test items for that component. If your client is intimidated by the idea of exercise, you can gather information from simple field-based tests that may be less threatening to him than more complex assessment tools but that can enable you to design an initial prescription suitable to his immediate needs.

Retest sessions need not include all of the initial test items, especially if you used a generic battery of tests. Select only the components that your client has been working on or those in which you anticipate a change. Monitoring throughout the program both shows improvement and indicates when progressions should be made. This may also decrease the need for regular, formal reassessment in areas such as muscular strength.

The closer an assessment comes to simulating your client's training activities, the greater the test's sensitivity and validity.

Learn to view assessment in terms of stages of change. Many first-time clients will not be ready to move much beyond an initial counseling and lifestyle appraisal: Pushing on to a full battery of exhaustive tests can destroy what little motivation they have. On the other hand, athletes after preseason training may be very eager to challenge their limits.

Before developing a detailed exercise prescription, assess baseline values for selected components of fitness. Sometimes trainers sample most of the components of fitness (e.g., cardiovascular, body composition, flexibility, muscular strength, and endurance). At other times, we may assess only high-priority components. Where appropriate, we may use less expensive and more easily administered field-based tests as supplements to or even as substitutes for laboratory tests.

Here we discuss a number of assessment tools, and you can readily find details about a variety of assessment protocols (ACSM 2009; CSEP 2013; Heyward 2010; Hoeger et al. 2009; Reiman and Manske 2009). You are encouraged to use these resources when establishing personal assessment batteries. The appropriateness and the limitations of the lab and field-based tests are discussed throughout the chapter. Table 4.1 categorizes a number of assessment tools into laboratory and field-based measures.

The very process of administering a fitness assessment draws attention to the client-centered nature of our relationship. The test process and the test results help to educate and motivate clients and stimulate their interest in exercise and other health-related issues. However, the primary function of measurement is to determine status.

Any fitness assessment protocol should meet the following criteria (Hoffman 2006):

- Content validity concerns the degree to which a test item represents the content that the test is designed to measure. An example involving physical assessment is use of an isometric measurement to assess strength in a client who participates in a dynamic recreational activity.

- Construct validity measures the extent to which a particular test can measure a hypothetical construct. For instance, intelligence, anxiety, and creativity are all hypothetical constructs because they are not directly seen but are rather inferred by their observable effects on behavior. However, some researchers have used construct validity to assess endurance runs as tests of aerobic capacity.

- Reliability is the ability of a test to produce consistent and repeatable results. Tests with proven reliability can reflect even slight changes in performance when you are evaluating a conditioning program. When error is high, the reliability of the test is low. Several factors can influence reliability, including the type of test, the test length, and the range of abilities and ability levels of the individuals being tested. Unfamiliarity with certain movement patterns or skills has a large effect on test reliability. Rapid improvements often relate more to a learning effect than to any physiological adaptations. Results of performance tests may vary due to differences in how testers assess the same test. This variability is known as objectivity or intertester reliability. If a test is truly objective, then regardless of who assesses the skill, the results should be similar. Intertester variability is minimized if several factors are controlled, such as following standardized procedures to properly administer tests.

- Economy of the protocol means that it is relatively inexpensive, efficient, and easy to administer.

Test results are a means to an end. They should not distract you from the purpose of serving your

Table 4.1 Laboratory and Field-Based Assessment Tools

	Laboratory	Field based
Cardiovascular	• Treadmill (e.g., Bruce, Balke) • Bicycle ergometer • Arm ergometer	• Åstrand-Rhyming bicycle test • 1.5/2.0-mile run • Canadian Aerobic Fitness Test • Physical Activity Index
Body composition	• Hydrostatic weighing • Bioelectrical impedance • Air displacement plethysmography	• Skinfolds • Circumferences • Height and weight • Body mass index • Bioelectrical impedance

clients. It is better to undertest than to overtest so that you can devote more time to counseling and demonstrating the program. Once your client has begun implementing your initial prescription, careful monitoring under standardized conditions can allow her to continue her workout program while you gain information about her status.

Cardiovascular Assessment

Your own experience, training, and educational background will affect the type of test you select. But because you are following the client-centered approach, client factors will be equally important. The following section will help you select laboratory protocols.

To optimize the efficiency of testing administration and to ensure accuracy and reliability, attention should be given to briefing of the coexaminers. Assuming that technical training and preparation have already taken place, a brief meeting of staff before the event is important. It should cover any procedural inquiries, review equipment being used, review forms and client flow, and overview any handouts or booklets being used for the session. Performing a test incorrectly leads to false results and bad conclusions; if you are going to take the time to do the testing (and you should), take the time to do it right.

Laboratory Tests

You can readily find details for a variety of laboratory-based protocols in "Assessment Resources." Table 4.2 compares the four major assessment devices for a number of criteria. You must be able to select an exercise mode and test protocol that are suitable for your client's age, sex, anticipated mode of exercise, and health and fitness status.

The three most common modes used for laboratory cardiovascular assessments are the treadmill, bicycle ergometer, and box step. There are advantages and client suitability for each of these protocols.

Treadmill protocols (ACSM 2009; CSEP 2013; Heyward 2010) are best suited to clients who

- want a walking, jogging, or running prescription;
- want to achieve their highest measurable oxygen uptake; or
- are familiar with running on a treadmill.

Specific protocols (e.g., Balke) use small grade changes each minute with a constant speed and are better suited for sedentary adults who may have trouble jogging. Other protocols (e.g., Bruce) increase grade and speed and may pose limitations to sedentary or older clients due to calf fatigue (Heyward 2010).

Bicycle ergometer protocols (ACSM 2009; CSEP 2013; Heyward 2010) are best suited to clients who

- want a cycle or stationary bicycle prescription,
- already cycle frequently,
- prefer less joint trauma, or
- are overweight and unfamiliar with the treadmill.

Pretest Instructions for Participants

To ensure maximum safety and performance, ask participants to adhere to the following conditions:

- Avoid strenuous physical activity on the day of the testing.
- Wear clothing and shoes appropriate for participating in physical activity.
- Running shoes are the recommended footwear.
- Eat a light meal one to two hours before testing.
- Avoid alcohol use for six hours before testing.
- Do not smoke for two hours before testing.
- Bring reading glasses (if needed) for completing forms.
- Bring medical clearance forms, if required.
- Inform the test administrator of any medical conditions or medications that could affect performance.

Table 4.2   Client-Centered Selection of Assessment Method

Performance factor	Treadmill	Bicycle	Step	Arm ergometer
Familiarity and skills required	****	***	**	*
Adjustment of work-load	****	** (friction)	*	** (friction)
Instrument calibration	**	*** (friction)	****	*** (friction)
Ability to achieve highest oxygen uptake	****	**	***	*
Ability to obtain blood pressure	***	****	**	*
Ability to obtain $\dot{V}O_2$	***	****	*	**
Ability to obtain ECG	***	****	**	*
Ability to obtain heart rate (stethoscope)	***	****	*	**
Local muscle fatigue	****	**	***	*
Cost and maintenance	*	***	****	**
Client compliance	****	**	***	*

Note: Each mode is rated from * (poorest) to **** (best) in the various performance factors. ECG = electrocardiogram.

Step test protocols (CSEP 2013; Heyward 2010; Hoeger et al. 2009) have the following advantages and disadvantages:

- They predict cardiorespiratory fitness by measuring postexercise recovery heart rates to one or more step rates or step heights.
- They require little equipment and are both time and cost efficient.
- They are easy to explain to clients. For example, the modified Canadian Aerobic Fitness Test (CSEP 2013) provides an aerobic fitness score linked to health benefit zones to assist in interpretation and guidance.
- They may require special precautions for those who have balance problems or are extremely deconditioned.

Submaximal or Maximal

Maximal testing is important in a clinical setting, for research purposes, and in high-performance settings (sport and occupational). It has more limited appropriateness in most fitness settings because risks are higher, client discomfort may be experienced, and the qualifications or supervision required for the staff may be limiting.

Predictive maximal cycle ergometer tests estimate maximal oxygen uptake from the highest power output completed. These tests are better measures of exercise tolerance than those that simply measure aerobic power, because anaerobic capacity can significantly contribute to perfor-

mance during the final workload. Submaximal tests are useful tools for tracking training programs and for monitoring blood pressure and heart rate. This added control is suited to older clients. Although the standard error may be about 15%, the measured responses to reproducible workloads provide information for the prescription of cardiovascular intensity (Heyward 2010).

Submaximal tests on the treadmill or bicycle ergometer or with bench stepping are similar to maximal tests but are terminated at a predetermined heart rate. Most submaximal exercise tests determine heart rate at one or more submaximal work rates and use the results to predict $\dot{V}O_2$max or establish a starting intensity. The submaximal test assumes a linear relationship between oxygen uptake, heart rate, and work intensity. In other words, as the workload increases, the oxygen cost of the activity and the heart rate will increase at the same time. Variability in maximal heart rates and mechanical efficiencies usually results in overestimation for highly trained individuals and underestimation for untrained, sedentary clients (Heyward 2010). However, repeated submaximal tests over a period of weeks showing decreased heart rates at a fixed workload can reflect improvements in cardiorespiratory fitness regardless of the accuracy of the prediction of oxygen uptake.

Matching Tests to Client Limitations

It is a challenge to select suitable assessment items for many clients. Conditions such as musculoskeletal problems, overweight, lack of conditioning, advanced age, or high health risks may require that you modify the tests.

Consider the following:

- It is more appropriate to use a bicycle than a treadmill, step, or arm ergometer with clients who need increased monitoring of heart rate or blood pressure.
- Total test time should be less than 15 min for clients who are easily fatigued.
- For clients with poor leg strength, a treadmill is preferable to a bike or step; for those with poor balance, a bike is better than a treadmill or step.
- Clients suspected to have a low oxygen uptake should start at a lower intensity; those who are regularly active can start at a higher intensity.
- Longer warm-ups and smaller increases in workloads are appropriate for those requiring more time to reach steady state.
- Step testing has some technical limitations, such as the client's size and ability to maintain good form.
- Arm ergometry offers a suitable means for testing clients with lower extremity impairment.

Field-Based Tests

Results from relatively simple field-based tests may be adequate for identifying and quantifying your client's needs. Field-based tests are usually less expensive and more easily administered than lab tests. For the personal trainer or small-facility director, field-based tests may be the only option. They can be very helpful if the regular method of monitoring is similar to that used for the field tests (e.g., minutes per mile, miles per hour, heart rates, or perceived exertion—all easily measured—can be quick indicators of progress).

Walking test protocols can be used for relatively inactive clients who are comfortable with walking but for whom jogging is inappropriate. For participants who are overweight, are older, or have scored less than 40 on the PAI, the Rockport One Mile Walking Test (Rockport Walking Institute 1986; Kline et al. 1987; CSEP 2013) may be a useful alternative to laboratory assessments.

All that is needed for this test is a timing device, a track or measured distance of 1 mile (1.6 km), and appropriate shoes and clothing. Have your client do warm-up stretches (5-10 min) and then walk as briskly as she can (no speed walking or jogging). Record heart rate (HR) using a 15 s count or a heart rate monitor immediately upon completion of the mile. Of course, if any signs of intolerance to the exercise start to appear, terminate the test and have your client cool down. Estimate your client's $\dot{V}O_2$max using the following formula, which incorporates body weight (pounds), age (years), sex (male = 1, female = 0), time to complete 1 mile (min), and postexercise heart rate (beats/min):

$$\text{Estimated } \dot{V}O_2\text{max (ml} \cdot \text{kg}^{-1} \cdot \text{min}^{-1})$$
$$= 132.853 - 0.0769 \text{ (Weight)} - 0.3877 \text{ (Age)}$$
$$+ 6.315 \text{ (Sex)} - 3.2649 \text{ (Time)} - 0.1565 \text{ (HR)}$$

Other walk–run field test protocols (Heyward 2010; Hoeger et al. 2009) consist of covering a certain distance in a given period of time (i.e., 12 min run test, 1- or 2-mile walk test, 1.5-mile run test for time). Because more than one client can be assessed at one time, the run protocols are frequently used with sport teams. Careful visual monitoring is suggested because these tests can be near maximal for some individuals. Maximum oxygen uptake or metabolic equivalent (MET) levels can be estimated from the tests.

Body Composition Assessment

Considering the profound health problems associated with body fat and the public's obsession with body image, the assessment of body composition has become very popular. Most assessment methods assume that the body is made up of fat and fat-free components. Percent body fat (%BF) can be obtained by dividing fat mass by total body weight. The recommended %BF values for adults (18-34 years) are 13% for men and 28% for women, and the standard for obesity is more than 22% BF for men and more than 35% BF for women (Heyward and Wagner 2004). Values vary with age, sex, and activity status. However, comparing clients with norms is often less effective than comparing each client's progress over time with his own individual measurements (e.g., girths or individual skinfold sites). Some assessment models have combined skinfold measures, waist girth, and body mass index (BMI) to provide the client with a composite score and health benefit rating (CSEP 2003).

The techniques used for assessing body composition are hydrostatic weighing (densitometry), air displacement plethysmography, bioelectrical impedance, and anthropometry (e.g., skinfold and girth measures). Specific protocols can be found in several of the books listed in "Assessment Resources." These analyses are based on measuring the ratio of fat to fat-free mass. Table 4.3 compares these three methods for cost, ease of use, and accuracy in measuring body fat.

Underwater weighing was for many years the gold standard for laboratory assessment of body composition; however, the assumption of a constant density for fat-free mass introduces some error. As well, the time, expense, and expertise needed are often prohibitive. Air displacement plethysmography is based on the same principle but uses air instead of water and has similar practical shortcomings.

Bioelectrical impedance is based on the stature of the body and the resistance to the flow of electrical current (impedance). Because fat-free mass has higher water and electrolyte content, the impedance through fat-free mass is less than it is through fat mass. The variability of the analyzers and the specificity of the equations (age, sex, obesity, activity) are the weaknesses of bioelectrical impedance (Anderson 2003). As better equations are developed and appropriate pretest conditions are followed, bioelectrical impedance should prove to be a most convenient, safe, accurate, and rapid method. It may also have advantages over the skinfold techniques for clients who are overfat or heavily muscled or who have thick, tight skin (Kravitz and Heyward 1997).

Body composition determined from skinfold measurement correlates well with underwater weighing (ACSM 2009). Performed by an experienced exercise specialist, the method has several advantages:

- The equipment is inexpensive and portable compared with popular laboratory tests.
- Measures are made quickly and easily.
- Measures correlate highly with body density and provide more accurate estimates of body fat than height–weight ratios (Nieman 2010).

Several studies (e.g., Heyward and Wagner 2004; Ross et al. 1996) have shown that fat mass located in a centralized area (usually the trunk) versus a generalized pattern of subcutaneous fat distribution is more directly associated with metabolic disorders, overweight, and possibly hypertension. That is, the visceral distribution of adipose tissue, independent of total body fat, is the critical factor in the health risk of obesity. A relationship has been shown between measures of total, abdominal, and visceral obesity and the measures of BMI, sum of five skinfolds, and waist girth (Janssen et al. 2002).

One of the greatest values for clients is the interpretation and education that you provide when explaining body composition measures. These results can be an excellent motivation tool and a useful basis for goal setting and program monitoring. Field-based tests provide supportive information to estimate body composition and determine a relative health risk. Body mass index and the waist girth measure are estimates of body composition and, along with skinfold measures, can be effective monitoring measures for individual progress.

Skinfold Measures

Any skinfold protocol's predictive formula is specific to the population with which it was developed. To be more effective and fair to your client, select a protocol suited to her. Many equations have been developed for specific types of people. Heyward and Wagner (2004) discussed the major methods of assessment and ways to apply these methods to different ethnic and age groups as well as clinical populations. The recent trend has been to use generalized rather than population-specific equations. These equations apply to a large range of people, with some loss in predictive accuracy. The error associated with generalized skinfold equations is only slightly greater (3.7% vs. 2.7%) than that of the hydrostatic weighing technique (Nieman 2010). For example, if the estimated %BF is 25%, then a 3.7% error provides a range of accuracy of 21.3% to 28.7% body fat. Another major source of error in skinfold measurements is the variability among technicians. Good training in standardized procedures can reduce this significantly (Heyward 2010).

Table 4.3 Methods of Body Composition Assessment

Method	Cost	Ease of use	Accuracy
Skinfold	Low	Moderate	Moderate
Hydrostatic weighing	High	Low	High
Bioelectrical impedance	Moderate	High	Moderate

Based on Baechle, Earle, and Wathen 2008.

Body Mass Index

The BMI is an indicator of proportional weight or obesity. It is more precise than weight tables, is simple to perform, and allows for comparisons of large groups. Calculate BMI by dividing body weight (in kilograms) by the square of height (in meters).

Example:

Weight = 80 kg, Height = 175 cm = 1.75 m

$$BMI = Weight/Height^2$$
$$= 80/1.75^2 = 80/3.06 = 26.1$$

The BMI has the following recommended classifications (NIH, NHLBI 1998):

- <18.5—underweight
- 18.5-24.9—normal (desirable range for adult men and women)
- 25.0-29.9—overweight
- 30.0-34.4—Grade I obesity
- 35.0-39.9—Grade II obesity (medically significant)
- ≥40—Grade III obesity

In the example, the client would be classified as overweight. The BMI is most useful when used in conjunction with skinfold measures. A high BMI could be the result of elevated muscle mass, as with a football player, or excessive body fat. If the skinfold measures are high, this is a definite indication of too much body fat and corresponding health risk.

Waist Girth

Excessive fat in the trunk area is associated with increased morbidity and mortality rates. Some sources (Hoeger et al. 2009; Ross et al. 1996; NIH, NHLBI 1998) have suggested that the waist (abdomen) girth measure provides a valid representation of this pattern of fat distribution.

To measure waist girth, hold the tape horizontally at the level midway between the bottom of the rib cage and the iliac crest and take the measurement at the end of a normal expiration. Maintain tension but do not indent the skin.

Some sources (CSEP 2013) describe waist girth "health benefit zones" based on age and sex. The National Institutes of Health (NIH, NHLBI 1998) acknowledges that waist girth provides a clinically acceptable measure of a client's abdominal fat content and has identified levels at which relative risk increases:

- Men: >102 cm (>40 in.)
- Women: >88 cm (>35 in.)

Monitoring changes to this measure is simple and can be very encouraging, particularly at the start of an exercise program.

Using BMI, Skinfold, and Waist Girth Measures

If your client has a high BMI, use skinfold measures to determine if it is high because of muscle mass or because of excessive body fat. Next, examine the pattern of fat distribution by measuring waist girth or trunk skinfolds. Even with an acceptable BMI and moderate skinfold measures, there may still be health risks if the waist girth is high and the skinfolds are excessive. These anthropometric measures have been used to establish a health benefit rating and a method of counseling clients to reduce health risks (CSEP 2013).

Heyward and Wagner (2004) summarize a number of key points with regard to field-based body composition methods:

- The same calipers should be used when one is monitoring changes in skinfold measures (SKF).
- SKFs should not be measured immediately after exercise.
- Skinfold measurement and anthropometric method error may come from technician skill, client factors, and the prediction equation used.
- Total body fat and regional fat distribution are related to disease risk.
- Waist circumference can assess intra-abdominal (visceral) fat deposition in field and clinical settings.
- The bioelectrical impedance (BIA) method may be more suitable than the SKF method for measuring body composition of clients who are obese.
- Low-cost lower body and upper body BIA analyzers provide reasonable group estimates of %BF, but the individual prediction error is greater than for whole-body BIA analyzers.

Musculoskeletal Assessment

In this section we examine laboratory and field-based tests for each of the major musculoskeletal components of fitness: strength and muscular endurance, flexibility, and muscle balance. Related components such as muscular power, muscle hypertrophy, or neuromuscular performance are examined in this chapter; please see "Assessment Resources" at the beginning of the chapter. The fitness assessments for strength, muscular endurance, and flexibility presented in the following pages can be helpful tools in the assessment of muscle balance. Any misalignments seen in a postural assessment may be attributable to relative tightness or weakness of related muscles.

Specialized aspects of musculoskeletal assessment are examined in later chapters. Chapter 13, "Exercise Prescription for Older Adults," has a section on physical fitness and functional assessments for a client over 50 years old or someone younger with some impairment. Chapter 14, "Functional Mobility and Aging," includes a focus on the assessment and development of musculoskeletal elements of mobility. Functional mobility not only is relevant for an aging population but also is critical in the preparation of an athlete for a wide variety of activities. Therefore, at the end of this chapter, we also examine a popular athletic preparticipation screening protocol called the Functional Movement Screen (FMS) (Cook et al. 2006a, 2006b).

We discuss factors to consider in the selection of field-based tests, client issues in the selection of test items, and specific field tests for determining the distinct needs of the client. An exercise prescription for a client should be validated using the baseline values for selected components of fitness through use of appropriate assessment tools.

A variety of assessment tools can be used to measure musculoskeletal fitness. Table 4.4 categorizes a number of such tools into laboratory and field-based measures. Because laboratory tests are expensive and more complex to administer, we deal almost entirely with field-based tests. Field tests are less clinical, more practical, and often functional or performance oriented. Details of the laboratory protocols can be obtained from the publications listed in "Assessment Resources."

Factors to Consider in Assessment Selection

A plethora of field-based assessments are available. When selecting tests, consider several factors:

- **Joint–muscle relationships.** Strength and endurance are specific to the muscle group, the type and speed of contraction, and the joint angle or range of motion. Always consider how your client will be training, the nature of any primary sport participation, the demands of her work environment, or her stated priorities. For example, if your client would like to significantly improve her squash game, you may wish to establish baseline levels of the following:
  - Dynamic strength for shoulder medial rotators through a full range of motion (the power of a forehand shot comes from a rapid contraction of the shoulder medial rotators).
  - Static grip strength (a general indicator of strength and important for racket stability).

Table 4.4   Musculoskeletal Assessment Tools

	Laboratory	Field based
Muscular strength and endurance	• Isokinetic dynamometer (e.g., Cybex, Kin-Com) • Cable tensiometer • Load cell	• Grip dynamometer • Free weights and exercise machines (percentage of one-repetition maximum) • Calisthenics (e.g., sit-ups, push-ups)
Flexibility	• Leighton flexometer	• Goniometer (e.g., ankle, hip) • Sit-and-reach • Indirect measures (e.g., back hyperextension, shoulder flexion)
Muscle balance	• Fullerton Advanced Balance Scale • Berg Balance Scale (BBS)	• Postural assessment • Muscle tightness tests • Back fitness test • Functional Movement Screen (FMS)

- Dynamic endurance of the knee and hip extensors (extension from a partial crouch position, such as the FMS in-line lunge, is a movement pattern repeated at high intensities throughout a squash match).

- **Maximal effort.** Most tests require maximum effort. Your client may not be at a stage where this will be accurate or safe. Factors such as time of day, sleep, drug use, and anticipation may also affect a maximum performance. Use caution in pushing clients to their maximum. Flaws in technique usually precede fatigue: Watch clients carefully, and stop the test when they start to struggle.

- **Strength level.** Performance on some endurance tests is highly dependent on strength. Use tests that are proportional to a percentage of the client's maximum strength or proportional to her body weight such as the five-level sit-up.

- **Normative values.** Although some age- and sex-based norms exist (see "Assessment Resources"), many tests lack up-to-date norms against which you can compare your client's results—especially for adults over 25 years. However, test results may serve other functions: Use them to establish baseline levels for measuring improvement (especially if the test resembles the training) or to determine starting points for exercise prescriptions.

- **Specificity, reliability, and validity.** Some very reliable laboratory methods have limited usefulness because they are too specific. For example, the sophisticated isokinetic dynamometers normally measure only one joint action. Yet compound movements involving two joints, such as a leg press action, are common in sports. Another example is the cable tensiometer, which is a good measure of isometric strength but is specific to the angle of contraction and may not reflect dynamic strength.

- **Body weight test items.** Calisthenic tests produce highly variable results. People with high body fat have relatively less muscle and therefore a lower strength level for their body weight. Because the resistance is the client's weight or a portion of that weight, these clients are lifting a relatively higher load (expressed as a percent of their maximum strength). Distribution of body weight affects the results of sit-up tests, because those with relatively more weight in their lower bodies have less resistance with their lighter upper body. On a positive note, calisthenics are cheap, they usually require no equipment, and they can be modified to vary the resistance by changing body and limb positions.

- **Client needs.** Strength testing can be used to effectively monitor rehabilitation after injury and provide objective criteria for the resumption of activity. Many nonathletes use strength training for aesthetic as well as functional reasons. Postural misalignment or compensatory movement patterns may indicate a need for muscle balance assessment. Testing can also provide a guideline for prescription and provide a means of monitoring progress.

- **Human error.** A source of error in muscular fitness testing is the human factor. Our clients must be familiar with the testing procedures and the equipment. They may need time to practice to control for the effects of learning on performance. We need to motivate our clients during and after their trials to encourage maximal performance (using caution, as noted previously). To obtain accurate results, follow the standardized starting positions and testing procedures. Clients may inadvertently modify a position or technique particularly as they fatigue. Observe and spot your clients accordingly.

- **Equipment availability.** Many personal fitness trainers are mobile and travel light or for other reasons do not have assessment equipment readily available to them. Large or expensive equipment is often not necessary. In fact, more than 20 assessments are described in this chapter, and all but one can be performed with only a tape measure, watch, goniometer, aerobic step, or plumb line.

Test Limitations

Many traditional physical fitness tests have long been accepted as measures of muscular strength, endurance, or flexibility. Unfortunately, these tests have become evaluations of performance rather than measures of physical fitness. Emphasis is on speed of performance, number of repetitions, or extent of stretching rather than on quality and specificity of movement. These are some examples:

- **Push-ups.** Properly executed push-ups involve scapular abduction during the up phase. When the serratus anterior is weak, the scapulae do not move—and yet the push-up may still be performed. Because other muscles can compensate for this weakness, you may fail to note small changes in body mechanics, such as incomplete flexion of the elbow or an unacceptably wide hand position. The purpose of push-ups is to test the strength or endurance of arm muscles. Winging and lack of abduction of the scapula reveal a weak serratus anterior. If such weakness is not noticed, the test's validity is reduced, and push-ups are not a good index of muscular endurance of the arms.

• **Bent-knee sit-ups.** Exercise specialists often measure endurance of abdominal muscles by having clients perform as many bent-knee sit-ups as possible in 60 s. The curled trunk requires a strong contraction of the abdominal muscles to hold this position. Many people start the test with the trunk curled, but their backs begin to arch because their abdominal muscles are not strong enough to maintain the position. Because the speed and length of the test magnify the problem, the low back is strained. The result is that clients with weak abdominal muscles may pass this test using poor mechanics of the low back and possibly assistance from the hip flexors. Evidence (Chen et al. 2002) shows that curl-ups recruit high abdominal muscle activity, whereas sit-ups do not challenge the obliques; the latter have higher psoas activity and are ill advised for an unstable back.

• **Trunk flexion.** One of the most common tests for flexibility is forward trunk flexion, or **sit-and-reach.** Sitting with knees extended, the participant reaches forward toward or beyond the toes. Designed to measure flexibility of the low back and hamstrings, the test focuses on how far the person can reach. The test fails to consider variables that can affect the results, such as limitations attributable to imbalances between length of back and hamstring muscles. Also, poor flexibility in the low back may go undetected if hamstrings have excessive flexibility. Clients with such imbalances may do well on the test, whereas people with normal flexibility may not do well. Moreover, some trainers would wrongly prescribe therapeutic exercise to increase spinal flexibility or stretch hamstrings when it is unnecessary or contraindicated.

Field-Based Tests

The term **muscular fitness** has been used to refer to the integrated status of muscular strength (maximal force of a muscle) and muscular endurance (ability of a muscle to make repeated contractions or resist muscular fatigue) (ACSM 2009). Assessing muscular fitness involves a continuum of tests that allow few repetitions to measure strength and a greater number of repetitions or longer time held to measure endurance.

Unlike laboratory-based tests for muscular strength and endurance, field-based tests often closely simulate the training activity of your clients, thereby increasing the validity and sensitivity of the assessments. The tests are usually inexpensive and easy to administer and often can be modified to suit desired resistance levels (see form 4.3, Strength and Endurance Testing). They can help you establish starting prescription levels if the tests closely resemble the exercise.

Strength Test 1
Relative Muscular Endurance in RM Weightlifting

To test for relative muscular endurance, assign a submaximal load—that is, a percentage of one-repetition maximum (1RM, a weight the client can lift only once). The load should be specific to the objective of the client: a particular sport, a work task, a rehabilitative goal. The exercise used for the test should also reflect the client's objective and reflect a muscular balance between agonist and antagonist. More easily standardized exercises include bench press, latissimus dorsi pull-down, leg curl, leg extension, leg press, arm curl, and triceps extension.

A modification of the 1RM test involves lifts to fatigue between 2RM and 10RM. Estimates of 1RM can be made from the results without having to reach an exact number of repetitions. Figure 4.1 illustrates the average number of repetitions possible when compared with 1RM (Sale and MacDougall 1981). This graph may be used to evaluate results of relative load tests. It shows the percentages of the 1RM that you can try with your client when prescribing at an 8- to 10RM level or a 1- to 3RM level. Baechle and Earle (2008) combined similar data to provide a relationship between percentage 1RM and repetitions (table 4.5). To estimate 1RM from results obtained between a 2RM and 10RM, divide the weight lifted by the corresponding %1RM.

For example:

Weight lifted = 140 lb (63.6 kg)
Number of repetitions = 8
1RM: 140 lb/0.80 = 175 lb (79.5 kg)

These estimates are helpful guidelines when prescribing training loads but may vary depending on age and sex, size of muscle group (smaller muscle groups may not produce as many repetitions as predicted), number of sets performed, and type of machine or free weights (Baechle and Earle 2008).

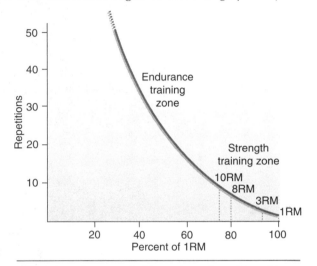

Figure 4.1 Percent of 1RM and number of repetitions.
Reprinted by permission from the Canadian Society for Exercise Physiology 2003.

Table 4.5 Percent of the 1RM and Repetitions Allowed (%1RM–Repetition Relationship)

% 1RM	Number of repetitions allowed
100	1
95	2
93	3
90	4
87	5
85	6
83	7
80	8
77	9
75	10
70	11
67	12
65	15

Reprinted by permission from NSCA 2008.

Strength Test 2
Biering–Sorenson Back Endurance

Following screening for back pain, the client lies prone, with legs on a table or portable steps and trunk hanging at a right angle. The iliac crest is positioned at the edge of the table, and the appraiser secures the lower thighs. The client raises her trunk to a horizontal position, crosses her arms on the chest, and then maintains that position as long as possible to a maximum of 180 s (figure 4.2). Details of the procedure and interpretation of the Biering–Sorenson back endurance test are in the *CSEP-PATH* manual (CSEP 2013).

Back extensor endurance has been positively related to back health. When coupled with other test results that indicate low abdominal endurance and hip flexor and low back tightness, a Biering–Sorenson finding of poor back extensor endurance has a very strong association with the development of low back pain (Albert et al. 2001).

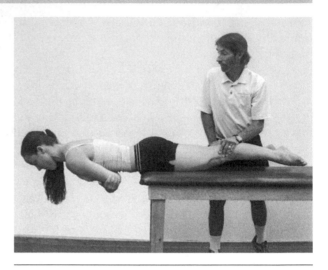

Figure 4.2 Back extensor endurance is associated with back health.

Strength Test 3
Five-Level Sit-Up

With calisthenics, you can use simple biomechanics to change the position of certain body segments and create changes in loading. The five-level sit-up test uses a modified arm position to change the resistance. The knee is at 90° to minimize the involvement of the hip flexors. Figure 4.3 illustrates the procedures for the five levels from least difficult (level 1) to most difficult (level 5). The client executes each level one at a time starting with level 1. If the execution is appropriate, allow a brief rest and then attempt level 2, and so on (Griffin 2006).

Scoring: If your client visibly strains on the attempt but does manage to perform it correctly, this is considered her "strength level." If she has to modify her technique to complete the sit-up (such as extending her legs or using momentum), the previous level is considered her strength level. To assess her "endurance level," select the sit-up one level below her strength level. To test for muscular endurance, have your client complete

as many correct repetitions as possible for 1 min or to the point of fatigue. The test may also be terminated when she performs a second technical flaw (any flawed repetitions are not counted).

Before using the results of the tests to prescribe an exercise program, determine your client's objectives: strength, strength-endurance, or endurance. From the results of the strength and endurance tests, you can prescribe the level of sit-ups and the number of repetitions to suit her objective (also see chapter 7). By having her move her heels 2 to 4 in. (5 to 10 cm) closer to the buttocks, you can make the level slightly more difficult and fine-tune her prescription.

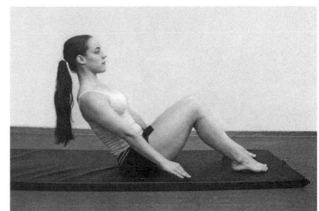

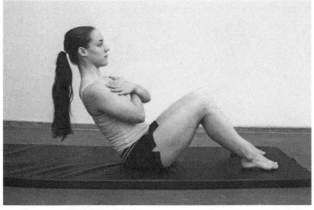

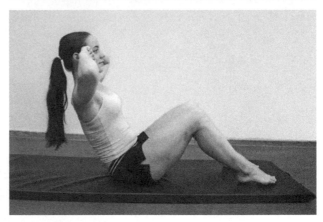

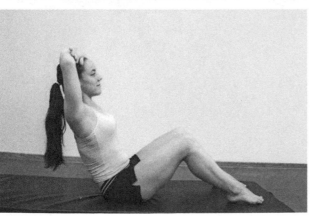

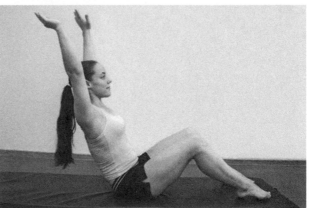

Figure 4.3 Five-level sit-ups provide a starting point for the prescription.

Strength Test 4
Lower Abdominal and Pelvic Stabilization

The client lies supine on a hard surface with her knees bent (figure 4.4). The examiner places one hand, palm up, under the low back. The client straightens her legs directly up in the air (90°) and then slowly lowers her extended legs, trying to keep the pressure on the appraiser's hand. The test is terminated when the spine begins to rise off the appraiser's fingers. The angle between the legs and the floor at this point represents the stabilizing strength of the abdominal muscles as they counter the eccentric pull of the hip flexors. An angle of 75° is poor strength, 60° is fair, 30° is good, and 5° is excellent (Ellison 1995).

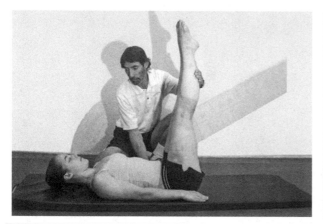 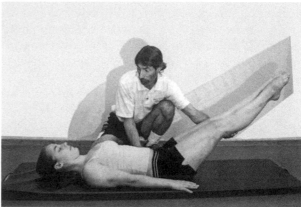

Figure 4.4   Lower abdominal strength is important for core stability.

Strength Test 5
Lateral Lift Test

The lateral lift test assesses the quadratus lumborum, which is part of the back extensor group but is also a prime mover for lateral flexion and provides lateral support to the spine and pelvis.

The client lies on her side with arms folded across the chest and feet stabilized (figure 4.5). While maintaining the body straight with no twisting, the client raises her shoulder off the floor as high as possible and holds it briefly. She should avoid jerking movements or pushing off with the elbow. The scoring is shown in form 4.3, Strength and Endurance Testing (Imrie and Barbuto 1988).

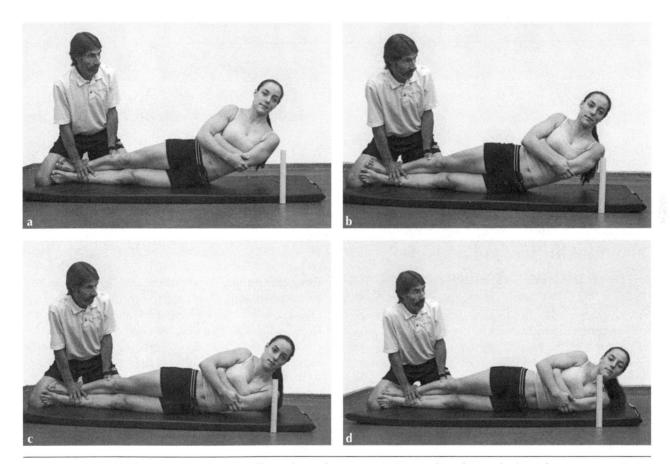

Figure 4.5   Lateral lift test: *(a)* grade 1: excellent, *(b)* grade 2: average, *(c)* grade 3: fair, and *(d)* grade 4: poor.

Strength Test 6
Serratus Anterior (Push-Up)

Push-ups are commonly performed as part of a musculo-skeletal test battery (figure 4.6). An indication of a weak serratus anterior is a winging of the scapulae when your client executes the down phase of a push-up (Michaelson and Gagne 2002).

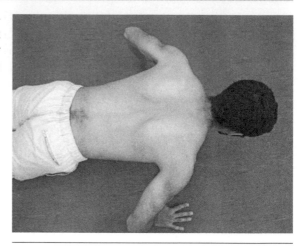

Figure 4.6   Winged scapulae: weak serratus anterior.

Flexibility and Muscle Tightness Assessment

You can determine flexibility directly by measuring the range of motion of a joint or series of joints in degrees with devices like goniometers or flexometers. The Leighton flexometer has a test–retest reliability ranging from 0.90 to 0.99 (Heyward 2010). With goniometers, locating and maintaining the true joint center is critical to obtaining true readings. Goniometer test–retest results with the same appraiser are stronger than between different appraisers (Norkin and White 1995). Indirect assessment methods, using measuring tapes, are often criticized as crude and lacking normative data. As well, because the length or width of body segments can affect the results of some tests, such as the sit-and-reach, comparing individuals may not be highly valid with these tests. These tests nevertheless can be effective monitoring tools for individuals. No single test predicts overall body flexibility.

The range of motion of a joint may be limited by a number of factors including skeletal contact and ligaments as well as tight muscles. There are a number of excellent field tests for muscle tightness that do not involve putting the joint through a full range of motion. For this component of flexibility, it is particularly important to be client centered. Each joint and range of motion are unique. Careful questioning can help you focus on the areas of potential concern. Test joint range of motion to determine if it is limited, excessive, or within normal limits. A summary of the results of these assessments can be recorded in form 4.4, Flexibility and Muscle Tightness Testing.

Examine the needs and demands of your client. Has a joint area been overworked, possibly causing muscle tightness? For example, clients who play a weight-bearing sport or who regularly perform a weight-bearing locomotor activity should have ankle flexibility assessed. Clients who sit for long periods of time should be checked for tightness of the hip flexors and in some cases the trunk extensors. Many manual workers tend to have tight anterior chest muscles such as the pectoralis major and minor. Overuse or underuse of back muscles may leave them tight and the joints inflexible. A horizontal bench or one of the longer portable aerobic steps may substitute for an examination table for the muscle tightness assessments.

Flexibility Test 1
Sit-and-Reach

The client sits, legs extended, with soles of feet (bare) vertical against the flexometer, 6 in. (15 cm) apart and at the 10 in. (26 cm) mark of the ruler (figure 4.7). Instruct her to bend and reach forward gradually with arms even, palms down, and knees straight. She lowers her head and holds at a comfortable distance near maximum for 2 s. Complete details of the test procedure and scoring are in the *CSEP-PATH* manual (CSEP 2013).

Normal: "Good" scores range from 11 to 13 in. (28 to 33 cm) (males) and 13 to 15 in. (32 to 37 cm) (females) for those up to 40 years of age (CSEP 2013). However, this test does not indicate where limitation or excessive motion has taken place (Alter 2004). Various combinations of short hamstrings, back muscles, shoulder muscles, or gastrocnemius may be the cause of poor performance. Watch your clients carefully while they execute this test to identify where movement is restricted (e.g., flat back).

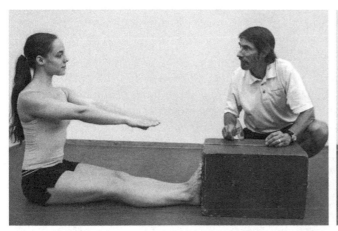 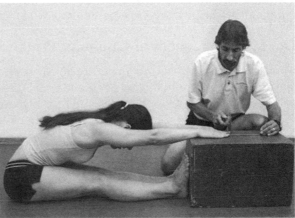

Figure 4.7   Sit-and-reach test may indicate back or hamstring tightness.

Flexibility Test 2
Ankle Range of Motion

The full range of motion for the ankle is conservatively 65° to 70°. These field-based tests are more sensitive to where the muscle tightness may be restrictive. Armed with the information, you can be more client centered with your prescription (figure 4.8).

Plantar Flexion (Length of Dorsiflexor Muscles)

Have the client sit on the edge of a table with knees at 90° and legs dangling. Align the center of the goniometer with the center of the lateral malleolus. Next, align one arm of the goniometer with the head of the fibula, and set the other arm at 90°. The neutral position of the ankle has the lateral sole of the foot parallel to the lower arm of the goniometer. Ask your client to actively plantar flex the ankle. An average range of motion should be 45° to 50° (Kendall et al. 2005). A range of motion much less than 40° may affect your client's ability to buffer the trauma of bearing weight—particularly when running or engaging in other locomotor activities.

Dorsiflexion (Length of One-Joint Plantar Flexor Muscles)

Client and instrument are set up as previously described. Ask the client to actively dorsiflex the ankle. An average range of motion should be 20° (Kendall et al. 2005). Clients with a range of motion less than this have tight soleus or tibialis posterior muscles and possibly weak dorsiflexors. Runners and other aerobic exercisers may experience lower leg rotation or overstretching of the Achilles tendon if these plantar flexor muscles are tight.

Dorsiflexion (Length of Two-Joint Plantar Flexor Muscles)

Have client sit on a table or the floor with knees straight. Align the goniometer as described previously. Ask client to actively dorsiflex the ankle. An average range of motion should be 10° (Kendall et al. 2005). Clients with a range of motion less than this have a tight gastrocnemius muscle. This muscle crosses over the back of the knee; when the knee is extended, the gastrocnemius pulls tight and further restricts the ankle in dorsiflexion. With practice, the angle from the neutral position can be estimated quite accurately without a goniometer.

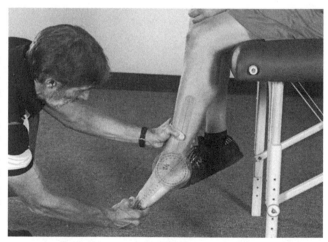

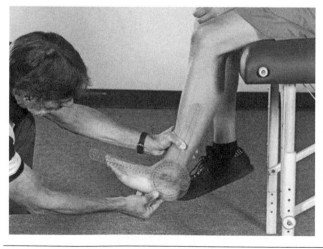

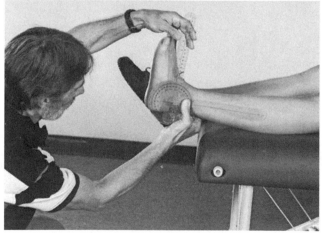

Figure 4.8   Ankle range of motion is important for clients involved in running activities.

Flexibility Test 3
Shoulder Internal and External Rotation Range of Motion

Have the client supine on a table, with knees bent and the spine in a neutral curve (figure 4.9). Arm is abducted to 90°, elbow is at 90° and off the table, and forearm is perpendicular to the floor. The goniometer axis is aligned with the humerus, the stable arm is perpendicular to the floor, and the moving arm is aligned with the styloid process. Internal (medial) rotation movement should be 70° (measuring infraspinatus and teres minor tightness). The external (lateral) rotation should be 90° (measuring subscapularis tightness). Instruct your client to avoid protracting shoulder girdle, rotating trunk, lifting shoulder, and changing angle at shoulder or elbow (DeLisa 1998).

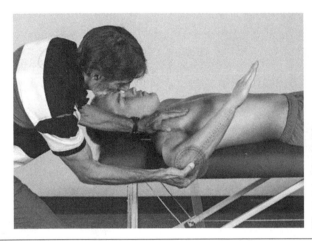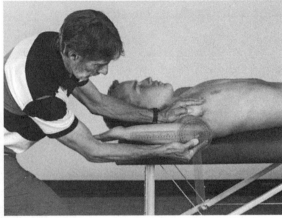

Figure 4.9   Shoulder rotation is important for clients involved in throwing activities.

Flexibility Test 4
Hip Internal and External Rotation Range of Motion

Have your client sit with knee flexed at 90° and leg dangling (figure 4.10). The center of the goniometer is on the patella, aligned with the femur. The stable arm is perpendicular to the table, and the moving arm is aligned with the middle of the anterior ankle. Internal (medial) rotation movement should be 35° and external (lateral) rotation should be 45°. Avoid rotating trunk or lifting thigh from the table (DeLisa 1998).

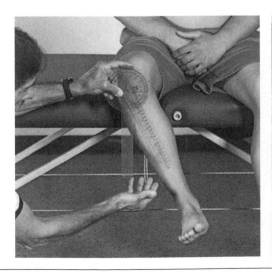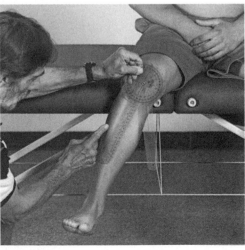

Figure 4.10   Lack of hip rotation can increase strain on knees and low back.

Flexibility Test 5
Spinal Rotation Range of Motion (Cervical and Lumbar-Thoracic)

Have the client sit with arms folded across her chest or with hands on anterior thighs. The goniometer is horizontal with the axis over the center cranial head with the examiner standing behind and looking down (figure 4.11).

Cervical Rotation

The stable arm is aligned parallel to an imaginary line between the two acromial processes. Align the moving arm with the nose. Rotation to the right and left should be 65° to 70° each. Have the client stabilize his shoulder girdle on the back support of the chair to prevent rotation of the thoracic and lumbar spine.

Lumbar and Thoracic Rotation

The stable arm is aligned parallel to an imaginary line between the two anterior iliac spines. Align the moving arm with the nose. It must remain aligned with the sternum (i.e., the cervical spine does not rotate). Rotation to the right and left should be 45° each. Check that the client stabilizes his pelvis to prevent any other spinal movement (Norkin and White 1995).

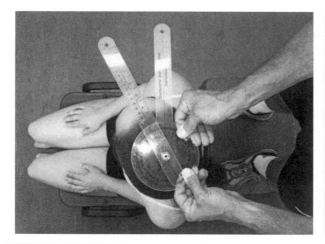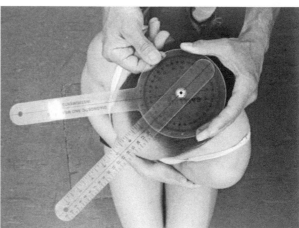

Figure 4.11   Many functional activities are dependent on good spinal rotation.

Tightness Test 1
Length of Pectoralis Minor

(Kendall et al. 2005)

1. Have the client lie supine, knees bent and low back neutral, palms up (figure 4.12).
2. Look from above the head; determine whether the shoulders are significantly off the table and are equal.
3. Gently push the shoulders to judge the resistance and to see if muscle tightness is slight, moderate, or marked.

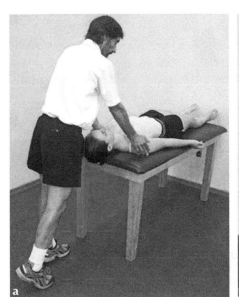
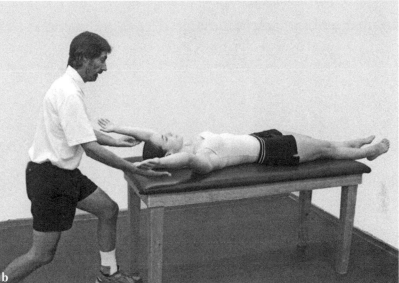

Figure 4.12   Muscle length assessments of the shoulder: (a) pectoralis minor and (b) pectoralis major (sternal).

Tightness Test 2
Length of Pectoralis Major (Sternal)

(Kendall et al. 2005)

1. Have client lie supine, knees bent, and low back neutral.
2. Assist client to slowly lower arm at 135° abduction.
3. Be sure shoulder is laterally rotated (thumbs pointing back) and elbow is straight.
4. Normal: Arm should rest, relaxed on the table.

Tightness Test 3
Length of Hip Flexors (Thomas Test)

(Kendall et al. 2005)

1. With the client seated at the very edge of the table, help her roll back to a tucked supine position. Appraiser has one hand behind client's back and the other under her knee.
2. Have the client pull one thigh toward the chest only enough to flatten the low back and sacrum to the table.
3. The opposite thigh is allowed to slowly lower over the edge of the table with the knee freely relaxed (figure 4.13a).
4. Note the angle of thigh and knee.
   - Normal one-joint hip flexor (e.g., iliopsoas): thigh remains on the table (any lift is measured in degrees).
   - Normal two-joint hip flexor (e.g., rectus femoris): knee flexion of 80°.
   - If the hip abducts and internally rotates with some knee extension, the tensor fascia latae are probably tight.

Tightness Test 4
Length of Hamstrings

(Kendall et al. 2005)

1. Have client lie supine on the table or floor.
2. See that client's legs are extended, with low back and sacrum pushed flat on table.
3. If low back is not flat (short hip flexors), use a rolled towel under the knees just enough to flatten the back.
4. Hold one thigh down and assist client to gently raise the test leg (figure 4.13b).
5. Be sure the knee is straight and the foot is relaxed.
6. Have the client raise his leg until restraint is felt (normal: 80° to 90°).

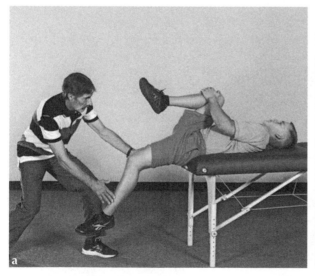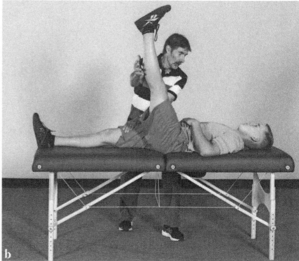

Figure 4.13 Muscle length assessments of the lower body: (a) hip flexors and (b) hamstrings.

Muscle Balance Assessment

Muscle balance does not mean equal strength between agonists and antagonists (e.g., hamstrings and quadriceps). And it means more than a proper ratio of strength or muscular endurance of one muscle group relative to another muscle group. Muscle balance exists when there is a proper relationship between the strength, length, and neural excitation of related muscles. These three factors work together to provide balanced support and movement and represent a holistic approach to muscular fitness. This relationship should exist between agonists and antagonists, between synergistic muscles that work together, and between prime movers and stabilizers. When certain muscles become stronger or tighter than their counterparts, muscle imbalance occurs. Muscle imbalance affects functional performance and is also a major cause of injury from faulty movement patterns (Cook et al. 2006a, 2006b).

The prescription of flexibility and strengthening exercises based on client-specific outcomes from these assessments has been shown to be very effective (Page et al. 2010). Although not a new concept, assessment and prescription for muscle balance is a new approach to solving common problems that is client centered whether the client is an athlete or fitness enthusiast or is recovering from an injury. The assessments—posture, tightness, and weakness—are not meant to be diagnostic. As well, personal fitness trainers should be encouraged to refer to other health care professionals when the situation is beyond their capabilities.

A battery of fitness assessments for strength, muscular endurance, and flexibility, similar to what we have just discussed, can be a helpful tool in assessing muscle balance. However, a more focused client-centered approach is most effective:

1. First, you will probably notice some indication of muscle imbalance: For example, a past injury, a complaint of localized tightness or aching, or an occupation or sport that requires repetitive movement patterns may come up during the preassessment counseling.

2. A closer examination may be afforded with a postural assessment. Any misalignments may be attributable to relative tightness or weakness of related muscles.

3. Further probing with respect to symptoms, history, or lifestyle may shed new light at this point.

4. To verify relative tightness or weakness, select relevant tests outlined in this chapter.

5. With these data in hand, specific to the symmetry of your client, you are much better prepared to set clear objectives and design effective prescriptions.

Postural Assessment

The ultimate goal of the human kinetic chain is to maintain dynamic postural equilibrium. The adaptive potential of posture is limited by poor flexibility, muscular weakness, and inappropriate neural firing. Good posture involves all body parts in a state of balance and the muscles holding the body erect against gravity without fatigue. A misaligned human body does not collapse—rather it twists out of shape to compensate for imbalances and requires extra muscular energy and tension to hold itself up.

Postural assessment is a very effective screening tool (figure 4.14). By carefully observing alignment, we can detect strain produced by faulty relationships of various body parts. For static posture assessment, observe your client standing from three positions—side, back, and front—and based on the standard of appropriate alignment, document any faulty alignments. Dynamic foot and shoulder alignment is also helpful. By keeping

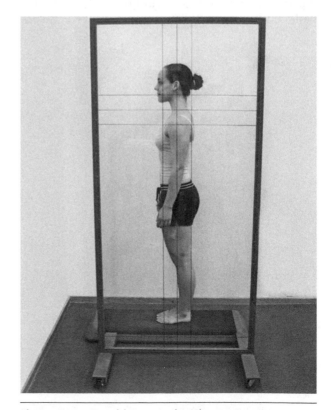

Figure 4.14   Portable postural grid.

the postural assessment simple, we increase the speed of assessment and can go directly to the next stage of muscle balance assessment: muscle tightness and weakness testing.

The body is a series of kinetic chains in which misalignment in one area can set off a number of compensatory adjustments that may be seen, and felt, a distance from the original problem. For this reason, a complete static postural assessment from at least three views should be done. However, because of time or prior knowledge of the problem area, the examiner may elect to do a "segmental" postural analysis. Separate assessments (see forms 4.5, 4.6, and 4.7) may be done for the lower body, upper body, and spine. These forms overlap slightly to reflect muscles extending into adjacent areas that may exert imbalanced forces.

Therefore, the scores for each segment cannot be summed and are merely helpful benchmarks for reassessment.

The left column of each segmental postural assessment form (forms 4.5, 4.6, and 4.7) lists key body areas to be examined. As an ideal standard, there is a column describing "good alignment." The best vantage point for viewing this alignment (A = anterior; P = posterior; L = lateral) is suggested in the preceding column. A description of faulty alignment is included to contrast the good alignment and to cue the examiner toward specific observations. A clear indication of the faulty posture would score a 3. The table allows the recording of left or right sides and any other comments or observations (e.g., "chin forward") or relevant client remarks.

Alignment During Standing

Have your clients remove shoes and socks. Women should wear a two-piece bathing suit, and men should wear trunks, to allow a clear view of landmarks. You will find a plumb line and a horizontal line grid very helpful but not necessary for screening purposes. A brick or cement block wall also is helpful. Assess your client in a standing position from three positions—side, back, and front. Ask your client to stand in an upright, relaxed position, looking forward. Figure 4.14 shows the anatomical structures that coincide with the line of reference. Your observations should be referenced to Segmental Postural Assessment forms 4.5 through 4.7. Figure 4.15 illustrates ideal alignment, and figure 4.16 illustrates common postural faults. Practice in judging good and faulty posture will quickly improve your skill levels.

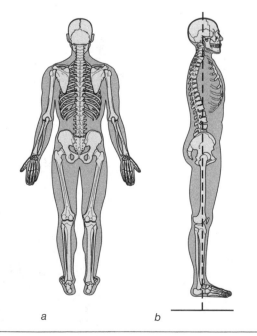

Figure 4.15 Ideal alignment: *(a)* back view and *(b)* side view.

© K Galasyn Wright '94.

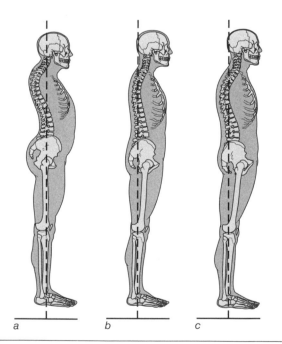

Figure 4.16 Common postural faults: *(a)* kyphosis–lordosis posture, *(b)* flat-back posture, and *(c)* posterior pelvic tilt.

The "standard posture" (Kendall et al. 2005) represents an ideal skeletal alignment that minimizes stress and maximizes efficiency. No one will match the standard in every respect.

Side View

The following points coincide with a vertical line of reference in a lateral view:

- Slightly anterior to lateral malleolus
- Slightly anterior to axis of knee
- Slightly posterior to axis of hip
- Bodies of lumbar vertebrae
- Shoulder joint
- Bodies of most of cervical vertebrae
- Mastoid process (Kendall et al. 2005)

Check alignment of knees, position of pelvis, curves of the spine, head position, and chest position. If the spinal curves appear excessive, have the client stand with heels 3 in. (7.6 cm) from the wall with the buttocks, scapulae, and head touching the wall. Slide your cupped hand, fingertips against the wall, behind his neck to approximate normal cervical lordosis. Place your cupped hand behind his low back to check for excessive lumbar lordosis. If the cupped hand fits easily between the spine and the wall, the lordosis is pronounced.

Back View

Start by observing alignment of the Achilles tendon, angle of the femurs, height of the posterior iliac spines, lateral pelvic tilt, spinal deviations, position of shoulders and scapulae, and angle of the head.

Front View

Observe the following: position of the feet, knees, and legs; height of the longitudinal arch; pronation or supination of the foot; rotation of the femur as revealed by the patella; knock-knees or bowlegs; rotation of the head; or prominence of the ribs.

Static and Dynamic Foot Alignment

For any client who will be running or walking, carefully observe the longitudinal arch as part of a static and dynamic postural assessment.

Longitudinal Arch

While the client is standing, feet shoulder-width apart, have him lift one foot off the floor so you can observe his arch. This assessment may also be done in a sitting position if it is more comfortable. The idea is to assess the arch in a non–weight-bearing position (Griffin 1989). Another alternative is to have your client remove his shoes and immediately stand on a noncarpeted surface. When he steps off, a moist imprint of his foot showing his arch should be visible.

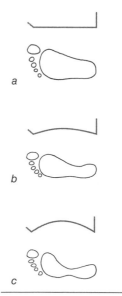

- If the foot appears flat with little or no arch, the client should be cautious of weight-bearing activities (figure 4.17a).
- If the arch looks small, it may be supple and will require extra support (figure 4.17b).
- If the arch looks full it is probably healthy, mechanically sound, and able to support trauma (figure 4.17c).

Figure 4.17 Poor arch support can lead to lower leg overuse injuries.

Dynamic Foot Alignment

Whether pronation or a flattened arch was present during the static postural assessment, you should observe the back and front of the foot for the degree of rolling inward while the client walks or jogs. This assessment is best performed with the client wearing no shoes (Griffin 2006) (figure 4.18).

- If the heel or forefoot rolls inward, "flattening the arch" while the client is walking or jogging lightly, the client pronates.

- If the heel rolls inward somewhat while the client is walking or jogging lightly, the client should avoid overuse.

- If the heel remains stable and the Achilles tendon is vertical while client is walking or jogging lightly, then the ankle is aligned.

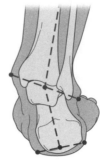

If the heel or forefoot rolls inward, "flattening the arch" while the client is walking or jogging lightly, the client pronates.

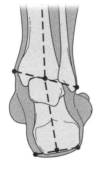

If the heel rolls inward somewhat while the client is walking or jogging lightly, the client should avoid overuse.

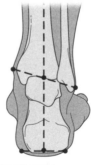

If the heel remains stable and the Achilles tendon is vertical while client is walking or jogging lightly, then the ankle is aligned.

Figure 4.18 Foot pronation should be assessed with all clients involved in running activities.

Dynamic Shoulder Alignment

During the static posture assessment, you may have recognized rounded shoulders, forward head, abducted or winged scapula, protracted head with a cervical lordosis, or backward-facing palms (see form 4.6, Segmental Postural Assessment: Upper Body). Repetitive movements that overemphasize one muscle group, movement compensations perhaps caused by injury, lack of range of motion, or even emotional stress may cause any combination of these misalignments.

A more functional approach examining dynamic shoulder alignment may give us a better idea of muscular or neural imbalances. The shoulder clock test (figure 4.19) will help you observe the dynamic relationship between the shoulder girdle and the shoulder joint. The client is positioned with her head, back, and arms pressed against the wall with her feet approximately 1 ft (30 cm) away from the wall. Ask her to slide her extended arms up the wall, palms forward, in a slow and deliberate manner, as high as she can without her back, head, or arms leaving the wall (Michaelson and Gagne 2002). This may also be repeated with the client facing the wall so you can better observe the scapular movement and trapezius contraction.

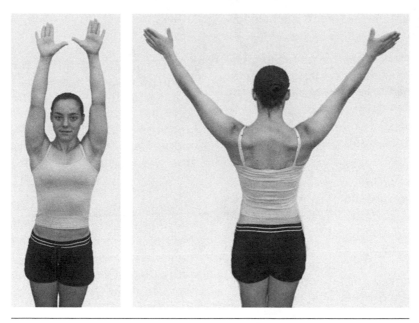

Figure 4.19   Shoulder girdle and shoulder joint should work synchronously.

Watch for a number of things:

- Excessive elevation (shrugging) of the scapula may indicate dominant or neurally facilitated upper trapezius. It may also reflect a weakness in the lower trapezius and serratus anterior if normal upward (lateral) rotation of the scapula is not seen. (*Note:* Weakness of the serratus anterior and possible tightness of the pectoralis minor may be present if your client's scapulae "wing" during the down phase of a push-up.)
- If the arms leave contact with the wall, the pectoralis major or the latissimus dorsi may be tight (Michaelson and Gagne 2002).
- If the client cannot keep his low back in a neutral position and you observe excessive lumbar lordosis while he raises his arms, he may have tight anterior chest or medial shoulder rotators, and his arched back is allowing his arms to remain against the wall.
- The client should demonstrate symmetry: Do his arms rise at the same speed; does one lose contact with the wall; does the head lean to one side; does one scapula rise before or higher than the other?
- Shoulder joint abduction range of motion should approach 180°.
- If pain occurs, perhaps resulting from impingement, note the angle at the onset of the symptom—beyond this range should be avoided.

Tightness and Weakness Assessment

When postural screening reveals faulty alignment or body mechanics, consider the possibility that your client has a muscular imbalance. Confirm those results by applying specific flexibility or muscle tightness tests and strength and muscular endurance tests to the joint areas. The postural analysis will help you determine which musculoskeletal tests you should perform.

Although flexibility is often defined as range of motion of a joint, it is not a simple matter: It involves both the length and strength of muscles. A short muscle restricts the normal range of motion. A shortened muscle may not be a strong muscle because there are fewer cross-bridge sites available with the overlap of the actin and myosin filaments. Muscles that are too short hold the opposite muscle in a lengthened position. Excessively long muscles are usually weak and allow adaptive shortening of antagonists. As the old question goes, "Did the chicken or the egg come first?"

When prescribing to improve muscle balance, use exercise movements that

- **lengthen** short muscles by increasing the distance between the muscles' origin and insertion opposite to the direction of the muscle action, and

- **strengthen** weak muscles that have been elongated by tight antagonist muscles.

You will encounter a large number of clients, particularly middle-aged people, with musculoskeletal injuries or low back problems. Most low back problems are attributable to postural misalignment and a lack of muscle balance. The highest incidence of aerobic and running injuries involves the lower leg, precipitated by muscle tightness and poor range of motion around the ankle. Careful questioning can help you focus on the areas of potential concern.

A preoccupation with instrumentation has left many personal trainers feeling inadequate when faced with the measurement of flexibility and strength. Yet physiotherapists, athletic trainers, and physicians rely successfully on their skills of manual assessment. Although as a personal fitness trainer you are not qualified to diagnose, treat, or directly prescribe treatment for any injuries, you must develop the knowledge and skill base to recognize what exercises will help strengthen weak muscles, stretch tight muscles, or correct negative muscular imbalances, thus aiding prevention or rehabilitation of an injury.

Functional Movement Screen

Sport training and rehabilitation has trended away from isolated assessments and strengthening toward an integrated functional approach. Similar movements occur throughout many athletic activities; and to prepare the athlete, the FMS assesses the ability to perform essential movements. Performance tests such as sit-ups, push-ups, or agility tests are not specific to the task or the basic movement patterns often needed. The discussion of muscle balance has emphasized the important relationship between mobility and stability. Cook and colleagues (2006a, 2006b) designed a series of tests (FMS) that revealed imbalances, weakness, and tightness when appropriate stability and mobility are not used. The FMS examines functional movement deficits that may limit performance and predispose the individual to microtraumatic injury. When used as part of a comprehensive assessment, the FMS can lead to individualized functional recommendations for

other physical fitness assessments or exercise design.

The FMS is composed of seven fundamental movement patterns that require a balance of mobility and stability. The tests include deep squat, hurdle step, in-line lunge, shoulder mobility, active straight leg raise, trunk stability push-up, and rotary stability. The tests place the individual in extreme positions in which weakness and imbalances become noticeable if appropriate stability and mobility are not used. As a result, poor, inefficient compensatory movement patterns are repeated, potentially leading to overuse injury. An alternative explanation for development of poor movement patterns is the presence of previous injuries. The FMS is designed to identify individuals who have developed compensatory movement patterns in the kinetic chain. The negative effect on the kinetic linking system results in altered mobility, stability, and symmetry of forces, eventually leading to compensatory movement patterns. The scores for each test range from 0 to 3. A score of zero indicates pain during the test. A score of 1 is given if the person is unable to complete the movement pattern. A score of 2 represents compensation movement to complete the task, and a score of 3 is a correct movement pattern with no compensation. The FMS is not intended to be used for diagnosis, but rather to demonstrate limitations or asymmetries with respect to human movement patterns and eventually correlate these limitations with outcomes, which may lead to an improved proactive approach to injury prevention (Cook et al. 2006b).

Case Studies

For each new client, you must determine what to assess and how to measure it. The following examples trace these decisions about assessments. More details about the individual assessments are provided throughout the chapter, and you will find further case histories in chapter 9.

Case Study 1: Moderately Overweight Client

Your first client is a 55-year-old man, moderately overweight. He has been doing some outdoor cycling, so he is already in an "action" stage of behavioral change (chapter 1). His doctor has recently encouraged him to get more exercise, and so he has come to your fitness center for guidance.

Is any screening necessary? A number of risk factors become evident in the preliminary counseling, so you select a series of items from the health and lifestyle appraisal (e.g., RISK-I and PAR-Q).

Your client has been cycling outdoors. Considering your preferred mode of assessment, a bicycle ergometer has the advantage of being non-weight bearing, with no balance concerns. Which method of cycle ergometer assessment is most appropriate? There is no need to push your client to exhaustion. You want to determine his response to various intensities of cycling. Your selection is a three-stage submaximal bike test with the results graphed, allowing you to estimate his heart rate at a large range of workloads.

Because your client's concern about weight comes primarily from a health perspective, your choice for body composition is to use BMI, skinfold measures, and waist girth measure.

Case Study 2: Reserved Client

Your second client is a previously sedentary 33-year-old woman whose main objective is weight loss. She appears to be moving from a preparation stage to an action stage of behavioral change. She has made it clear that she does not want to be poked and prodded with "those fat pinchers."

How do you proceed with this level of reservation? A health and lifestyle appraisal is a noninvasive way to gain useful information and to continue building rapport. The FANTASTIC Lifestyle Checklist (form 1.1) takes a holistic approach to weight management; Inventory of Lifestyle and Activity Preferences (form 1.2) gives her some choices.

Can you evaluate body composition without skinfold calipers or invasive equipment? Body mass index uses height and weight measures to provide an indication of relative overweight. You can examine the pattern of fat distribution through the waist girth measure, which also provides a barometer for improvement.

If no significant health risks exist and your client does not want a formal cardiovascular assessment, do you even need to do an assessment? You can use a heart rate reserve calculation (chapter 6) to determine your client's training zone based on her age, resting heart rate, and desired training level. If you regularly monitor heart rate and compare it with measures of perceived exertion, you can initiate a safe program.

Summary

The client-centered prescription model is flexible, allowing you to verify your client's needs by using selected assessment items that relate to your client's priorities and closely simulate her current training activity. Laboratory and field-based tests for cardiovascular, body composition, and musculoskeletal components of fitness should be tailored to the client's distinct needs.

A health and lifestyle appraisal may be the client's first step to behavior change. It may be just the extra nudge that a client needs. Its greatest value is as a tool that leads to healthy lifestyle intervention. An initial screening of your client may include PAR-Q+, personal health history, personal observation, informed consent, and preexercise heart rate and blood pressure. When your client has expressed a specific interest or need, include test items for that component. The very process of administering a fitness assessment draws attention to the client-centered nature of the relationship.

A cardiovascular exercise mode and test protocol should be selected that is suitable for your client's age, sex, anticipated mode of exercise, and health and fitness status. Results from relatively simple field-based tests may be adequate to identify and quantify your client's needs. They can be very helpful if the regular method of monitoring is similar to that used for the field tests (e.g., minutes per mile, miles per hour, heart rates, perceived exertion).

The strengths, weaknesses, and sources of measurement error should be considered for the techniques used to assess body composition: hydrostatic weighing (densitometry), air displacement plethysmography, bioelectrical impedance, and anthropometry (e.g., skinfold and girth measures).

The selection of field-based musculoskeletal assessments should consider joint–muscle relationships, maximal effort, normative values, specificity, reliability, and validity, body weight test items, client needs, human error, and equipment availability. The objectives of selected field-based flexibility and muscle tightness assessments are to determine if flexibility is limited, excessive, or within normal limits or if a joint area has been overworked, possibly causing muscle tightness.

The body is a series of kinetic chains in which misalignment in one area can set off a number of compensatory adjustments that may be seen and felt. By carefully observing alignment, we can detect strain produced by faulty relationships of various body parts. When postural screening reveals faulty alignment or body mechanics, consider the possibility that your client has a muscular imbalance. Confirm those results by applying specific flexibility or muscle tightness tests and strength and muscular endurance tests to the joint areas.

FORM 4.1   RISK-I

Select the number that best describes your situation for each of the following and compare the total score for an overall rating.

	1	2	3	4	5	Score
Age	20s	30s	40s	50s	60s	
Family history	No known heart disease	One relative over 50	Two relatives over 50	One relative under 50	Two relatives under 50	
Smoking	Nonuser	User <5 years ago	<10/day	10-20/day	>20/day	
Body mass index	18.5-23	24-27	28-31	32-35 or <18.5	>35	
Exercise	Active >2 times/week	Active 1-2 times/week	Moderately active 1-3 times/month	Stopped activity <3 months ago	Sedentary	
Back	Healthy	Minor problems in past	Aches occasionally or after activity	Problems in past or current discomfort	Frequent problems/diagnosed condition[a]	
Knees	Healthy	Minor problems in past	Occasional pain after vigorous activity	Problems in past or current discomfort	Frequent problems/diagnosed condition[a]	
Total score						

Family history: Count parents, grandparents, brothers, and sisters who have had a heart attack or stroke.

Smoking: If you inhale deeply or smoke a cigarette right down, add 1 to your score.

Body mass index: This is a measure of body proportion and a better indicator of risk than just weight (CSEP 2003). It is the ratio of body weight (in kilograms) divided by the square of height (in meters).

Example:

Weight = 75 kg

Height = 1.72 m

BMI = $75/1.72^2$

= 75/2.96

= 25.3 (RISK-I score = 25)

Interpretation:

Total score	Rating
7-10	Very low risk
11-15	Low risk
16-20	Average risk
21-25	High risk
26-30	Dangerous risk[a]
31-35	Extremely dangerous risk[a]

[a]Medical clearance necessary.

From J.C. Griffin, 2015, *Client-centered exercise prescription*, 3rd ed. (Champaign, IL: Human Kinetics).

FORM 4.2   Physical Activity Index

Instructions

Select the appropriate points for each of the following three parts.

Part 1—When you engage in sport, fitness activities, or active leisure, which description is most appropriate?

Intensity descriptions	Points
Very heavy: Continuous intense effort resulting in rapid heart rate or heavy breathing for the length of the activity.	5
Heavy: Bursts of effort that cause rapid heart rate or heavy breathing.	4
Moderate: Requires moderate effort and works up a sweat.	3
Light: Requires light effort and is often intermittent.	2
Minimal: Requires no extra effort.	1

Part 2—When you participate in the activity described in Part 1, how long do you keep at it?

Duration descriptions	Points	Duration descriptions	Points
35 min or more	5	5-14 min	2
25-34 min	4	Less than 5 min	1
15-24 min	3		

Part 3—How often do you participate in the activity described in Part 1?

Duration descriptions	Points	Duration descriptions	Points
Daily	5	1-3 times per month	2
3-6 times per week	4	Less than once per month	1
1-2 times per week	3		

PAI Scoring

Multiply your intensity points times your duration points times your frequency points to obtain your health benefits score.

Physical Activity Index = intensity points ___ × duration points ___ × frequency points ___

Health Benefit Rating for PAI Scores

PAI score	Rating	Significance
100 or more	Excellent	This level of physical activity is associated with optimal health benefits.
60-99	Good	This level of physical activity is associated with considerable health benefits.
40-59	Average	This level of physical activity is associated with some health benefits. Increased activity will provide increased health benefits.
20-39	Fair	This level of physical activity is associated with some health benefits and some health risks. Duration or frequency of activity should be increased.
Less than 20	Needs improvement	This level of physical activity is associated with considerable health risks.

From J.C. Griffin, 2015, *Client-centered exercise prescription,* 3rd ed. (Champaign, IL: Human Kinetics).

FORM 4.3   Strength and Endurance Testing

Client: _____ Date: _____

Assessor: _____

Muscle	Test	Rating system	Comments
(1) _____ (2) _____ (3) _____ (4) _____	Weightlifting	Exercise: _____ 5-10RM ___; 1RM ___ Exercise: _____ 5-10RM ___; 1RM ___ Exercise: _____ 5-10RM ___; 1RM ___ Exercise: _____ 5-10RM ___; 1RM ___	
Erector spinae	Biering–Sorenson	Example: Age 20-29 male (M) and female (F) (s) Needs improvement Fair Good Very good Excellent M ≤85 86-98 99-132 133-175 176-180 F ≤65 66-101 102-135 136-179 179-180	
Rectus abdominis	Five-level sit-ups	(1) ___ (2) ___ (3) ___ (4) ___ (5) ___ Number of reps _____	
Lower abdominal muscles	Leg lowers	75° = poor; 60° = fair; 30° = good; 5° = excellent ° = degrees when back arches while lowering legs	
Quadratus lumborum	Lateral lift	**Right shoulder** Grade 1: Shoulder 12 in. off floor without difficulty Grade 2: Shoulder 12 in. off floor with difficulty Grade 3: Shoulder 2-6 in. off floor Grade 4: Unable to raise shoulder off floor **Left shoulder** Grade 1: Shoulder 12 in. off floor without difficulty Grade 2: Shoulder 12 in. off floor with difficulty Grade 3: Shoulder 2-6 in. off floor Grade 4: Unable to raise shoulder off floor	
Serratus anterior	Push-up	Strong = scapulae flat in down phase Weak = scapular "winging" in down phase	

Complete norms and health benefit zones are available for Biering–Sorenson test in CSEP (2013).

From J.C. Griffin, 2015, *Client-centered exercise prescription*, 3rd ed. (Champaign, IL: Human Kinetics).

FORM 4.4 Flexibility and Muscle Tightness Testing

Client: _____ Date: _____

Assessor: _____

Shoulder, chest assessment	Results (observations)	Normal ROM	Pain Y/N
Shoulder internal (medial) rotation: (tightness of infraspinatus, teres minor)	L: _____ R: _____	70°	
Shoulder external (lateral) rotation: (tightness of subscapularis)	L: _____ R: _____	90°	
Pectoralis major (sternal) length		Table level	
Pectoralis minor length	L: _____ R: _____		
Shoulder joint abduction (see dynamic shoulder alignment)		180°	

Interpretation and comments:

_____

_____

_____

_____

Back assessment	Results (observations)	Normal ROM	Pain Y/N
Spinal rotation: Lumbar Cervical	 L: _____ R: _____ L: _____ R: _____	 45° 65°-70°	
Sit-and-reach test: (actual) (visual)		Good: 11-13 in. (28-33 cm) (males) 13-15 in. (32-37 cm) (females)	

Interpretation and comments:

_____

_____

_____

_____

(continued)

(continued)

Hip, knee assessment	Results (observations)	Normal ROM	Pain Y/N
Hamstring length	L: _____ R: _____	80° (males) 90° (females)	
Hip flexors: 1 joint (tightness of ilio-psoas)	L: _____ R: _____	Thigh table level	
Hip flexors: 2 joints (tightness of rectus femoris)	L: _____ R: _____	Knee: 80°	
Tensor fascia latae tightness	L: _____ R: _____		
Hip internal (medial) rotation (tightness of gluteus maximus, piriformis)	L: _____ R: _____	35°	
Hip external (lateral) rotation (tightness of gluteus minimus, anterior gluteus medius)	L: _____ R: _____	45°	

Interpretation and comments:

_____

_____

_____

_____

Ankle assessment	Results (observations)	Normal ROM	Pain Y/N
Ankle plantar flexion: (tightness of tibialis anterior)	L: _____ R: _____	45°-50°	
Ankle dorsiflexion: 1 joint (tightness of soleus)	L: _____ R: _____	20°	
Ankle dorsiflexion: 2 joints (tightness of gastrocnemius)	L: _____ R: _____	10°	

Note: ROM = range of movement.

Interpretation and comments:

_____

_____

_____

_____

_____

From J.C. Griffin, 2015, *Client-centered exercise prescription*, 3rd ed. (Champaign, IL: Human Kinetics).

FORM 4.5   Segmental Postural Assessment: Lower Body

Alignment scale: 5   4   3   2   1
                  (good)   (faulty)   (very faulty)

Joint	View	Good alignment	Faulty alignment	Score	Left/right	Comments
Foot	A	Half dome arch	Low arch, flat foot			
	A/P	Feet toe out slightly	Significant toeing out or in pronation or supination			
Knees and legs	A/P	Vertically aligned	Bowlegs (genu varum) or knock-knees (genu valgum)			
	A	Kneecaps face ahead	Kneecaps inward or outward (rotated femur)			
	L	Knees straight, not locked (lateral view)	Flexed or hyperextended knee			
Spine and pelvis	A/P	Hips level, weight even on both feet	One hip higher (lateral tilt), hips rotated (forward one side)			
			Score	**___/30**		

Note: A = anterior; P = posterior; L = lateral.

Recommendations:

_____

_____

_____

_____

From J.C. Griffin, 2015, *Client-centered exercise prescription,* 3rd ed. (Champaign, IL: Human Kinetics).

FORM 4.6 Segmental Postural Assessment: Upper Body

Alignment scale: 5 4 3 2 1
(good) (faulty) (very faulty)

Joint	View	Good alignment	Faulty alignment	Score	Left/right	Comments
Head	L P	Erect and balanced	Protruding, chin forward Tilted or rotated			
Arms and shoulders	A	Arms relaxed, palms facing body	Arms stiff, away from body Palms facing backward			
	L	Shoulders back	Shoulders rounded or forward			
	A/P	Shoulders level	One or both shoulders up, down, or rotated			
	P	Scapulae: flat on rib cage, 4-6 in. (10-15 cm) apart	Scapulae: prominent winged, far apart			
Score				___/25		

Note: A = anterior; P = posterior; L = lateral.

Recommendations:

_____

_____

_____

_____

From J.C. Griffin, 2015, *Client-centered exercise prescription,* 3rd ed. (Champaign, IL: Human Kinetics).

FORM 4.7   Segmental Postural Assessment: Spine

Alignment scale: 5   4   3   2   1
                    (good)   (faulty)   (very faulty)

Joint	View	Good alignment	Faulty alignment	Score	Left/right	Comments
Spine and pelvis	A/P	Hips level, weight even on both feet	One hip higher (lateral tilt), hips rotated (forward one side)			
	P	No lateral curve to spine (posterior view)	C- or S-curve scoliosis Ribs prominent one side			
	L	Natural lumbar curve	Lordosis: forward tilt of pelvis Flat back: pelvis tilts backward			
	L	Natural thoracic curve	Kyphosis: thoracic rounding			
	L	Natural cervical curve	Cervical lordosis: forward head			
Trunk	L	Flat or slightly rounded abdomen	Lower or entire abdomen protrudes			
	L	Chest slightly raised	Hollow chest or rounded back			
Head	L P	Erect and balanced	Protruding, chin forward Tilted or rotated			
Score				___/40		

Note: A = anterior; P = posterior; L = lateral.

Recommendations:

_____

_____

_____

_____

From J.C. Griffin, 2015, *Client-centered exercise prescription,* 3rd ed. (Champaign, IL: Human Kinetics).

Exercise Analysis, Design, and Demonstration

Chapter Competencies

After completing this chapter, you will be able to demonstrate the following competencies:

1. Anatomically analyze the joint movements, muscles used, and types of contraction for exercises and activities common to fitness programming.
2. Describe and use the five-step musculoskeletal exercise design model.
3. Use the client-centered exercise demonstration model to provide personal exercise demonstrations involving preexercise explanations, trainer demonstration, client trial, performance feedback, and follow-up.
4. Apply teaching cues and resolve common problems during exercise demonstration.

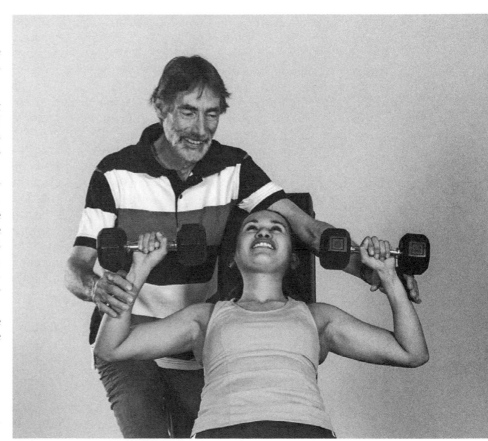

As a personal fitness trainer, there are certain essential skills at which you should excel. This chapter deals with three of those skills: anatomical exercise analysis, musculoskeletal exercise design, and exercise demonstration.

Exercise analysis includes the ability to observe a resistance exercise or flexibility exercise in the gym, understand an example in a book, or see one demonstrated on the Internet and without hesitation determine the primary joint movements, muscles involved, and types of contraction. This ability also transfers to sport; the same determinations can be made in the analysis of a specific sport skill or movement. Applied anatomy skills must be strong; it is only through these skills that you will always be able to determine the validity of the purpose of an exercise. This chapter develops those applied anatomy skills with various phases of movement and also explains the skills of evaluating movement effectiveness and its relative risk.

Exercise design is the quintessential focus of this book. Eventually, you will have detailed exercise prescription models for cardiovascular training, resistance training, muscle balance, and weight management. A prescription will identify training methods, modes, intensity-workload, duration, frequency, and progressions. However, our first step is an exercise design model to target specific muscles. Exercise design provides the starting position, joint movements or changes in position, and any precautions for a specific musculoskeletal exercise. Whether the exercise is to strengthen or to stretch a muscle, this skill set will allow you to respond to any specific need or request for an exercise that targets a specific muscle or group of muscles. Further expanding your skills will help you examine how to effectively modify an exercise and establish its safety with specific reference to the client.

Exercise demonstration provides the opportunity for the personal fitness trainer to teach new exercise skills to clients. Clients need to hear how an exercise will help them, see it demonstrated, and then try it with some expert feedback. This one-on-one time with clients can be a critical point in changing their behavior and in setting the tone for subsequent sessions. Very few texts address the skills of exercise demonstration, and even less research has been done on these skills. This chapter draws on the counseling skills from chapter 1 and an exercise demonstration model that has been used successfully at my college for over 20 years.

The chapter starts with anatomical exercise analysis. Numerous examples of popular exercises are used, and their suitability to client needs is determined. A progressive model for exercise analysis and a five-step approach to client-centered musculoskeletal exercise design are provided as pivotal points in the prescription model. Finally, one of the most frequent tasks of a personal fitness trainer—exercise demonstration—is presented as both a science and an art using a four-step model.

Exercise design is optimized when each exercise is client centered. There are three broad criteria for client-centered exercise:

1. Meeting the client's needs
2. Effectively and safely achieving the purpose for which the exercise was designed
3. Being accepted by the client as something he wants to do

Only if an exercise meets these criteria will it be included in the prescription.

Client personalization comes a step closer with the "selection + modification" approach. Modification molds an exercise to meet exact specifications—for example, to simulate a movement pattern used in a work task or sport skill. Figure 5.1*a* shows a resisted horizontal adduction of the shoulder joint that strengthens the pectoralis major and anterior deltoid. Figure 5.1*b* shows a modification suitable for an athlete whose sport includes throwing. The modified exercise involves the same muscles but works them at a slightly different angle and includes a medial rotation (subscapularis) and some trunk rotation.

We must meet the needs of our clients with appropriate modifications. Most often we recognize the need to modify an exercise during the **demonstration**. At this time, our counseling skills (chapter 1) play a critical role as we observe body language, question the client effectively, provide clarifications, and encourage two-way feedback. We change designs based on answers to a number of questions: Does it work the targeted muscle? Does the joint action suit the purpose? Is the difficulty level appropriate? Does this exercise maintain a balance with the rest of the prescription? Does the client need unique modifications? Are the starting position and range of motion safe and effective? Is the equipment appropriate; is it needed at all? Will the client enjoy or value the exercise? What is the effectiveness versus risk ratio? Do monitoring techniques need to be integrated? How does the client feel about the comfort, difficulty, and effectiveness of the exercise? Our system of exercise design must be simple to use but sensitive enough to deal with these issues.

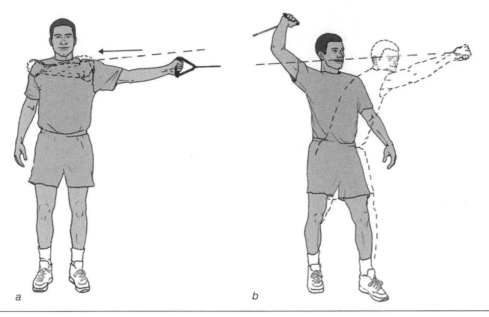

Figure 5.1   Design modifications.

The skills in this chapter involve **breaking down** exercises to determine their purpose (i.e., **analysis**) and **building** exercises based on need (i.e., **design**). These skills are invaluable for

- **exercise analysis** to aid in selection or modification of an exercise;

- **sport skill analysis** to aid in selection of exercises that simulate the movements and muscular patterns of a skill; and

- **work task analysis** to aid in design of exercises that build the required muscular strength and endurance or to balance the overuse effects of repetitive or prolonged tasks.

You should be able to anatomically analyze the joint movements, muscles used, and types of contraction for exercises and activities common to fitness programming. To analyze, design, and demonstrate exercises, you need to understand the anatomy of the targeted area, recognize the degree of risk, know how to deal with alignment or compensation issues, and be able to provide modifications and alternatives.

Anatomical Analysis of Exercise

You must understand the muscular focus of an exercise and know if that focus is appropriate for your client. To the untrained eye, identifying the muscles responsible for various exercises can be confusing. The following should help you judge your current skills of anatomical analysis.

Imagine you are with a client at the local fitness center and he asks what the difference is between the exercises being done by the people in figure 5.2.

Because the movements of the arm look very similar, one might assume that the same muscles are responsible for each exercise. In each case, rubber tubing is providing the resistance in a muscular conditioning exercise for the upper body. However, this is where the similarities end. In figure 5.2, the muscles working are as follows:

- **Exercise *a:*** Middle and posterior deltoid, middle and upper trapezius, and rhomboids

- **Exercise *b:*** Pectoralis major, anterior deltoid, serratus anterior, and pectoralis minor

- **Exercise *c:*** Infraspinatus and teres minor

Even the seasoned exercise specialist must scrutinize an exercise carefully. Watch the exercise several times and perhaps repeat it yourself slowly. Notice which body parts are moving and which are stabilizing without movement. Are joints bending or straightening through a full range of motion or to the end of their range of motion? Are the muscles being stretched or are they contracting, and if so, how? This section on anatomical analysis shows how to determine the targeted muscle group for each exercise.

You should analyze every exercise you prescribe. You should also apply the following steps when critiquing an existing program (written or demonstrated), observing a class or workshop, reading a fitness journal or book, receiving a program from a rehabilitation referral, seeing exercise equipment promotions, or trying new things yourself. With practice, the following simple five-step approach to **anatomical analysis** will become second nature to you:

Step 1: Analyze phases.

Step 2: Analyze joints and movements.

Step 3: Analyze types of contractions.

Step 4: Analyze which muscles are being used.

Step 5: Evaluate purpose, effectiveness, and risk.

Step 1: Analyze Phases

Break the exercise into phases. Most exercises have two discernible phases: up and down, in and out, push and pull, or left and right. For example, exercise *a* in figure 5.2 has "out" and "back"

phases. The phases are not technical terms but are chosen as brief and descriptive. New phases generally are determined by the point when a joint movement stops and a new movement begins. In muscular conditioning exercises such as with free weights or calisthenics, the phases are usually "up" and "down" to take advantage of gravity's opposition on the up phase. In figure 5.3, the side-lying position optimizes the force of gravity in the up and down phases of the exercise.

Some complex sport skills have several phases. The **power phase** is illustrated in the batter example (figure 5.4). The power phase is the time of the greatest force generation and is often the part of the movement that ends with contact (e.g., in batting) or release (e.g., in throwing). The **preparatory phase**, or windup, precedes the power phase—usually in the opposite direction—and

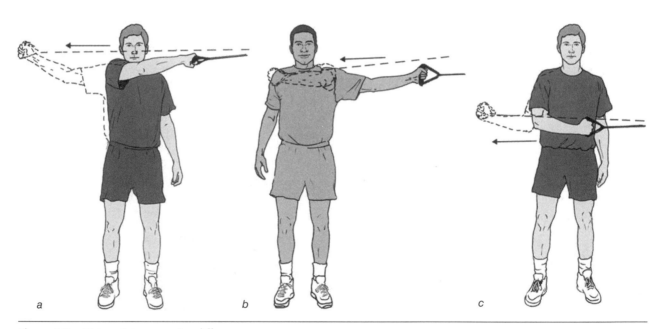

a   *b*   *c*

Figure 5.2   Determining exercise differences.

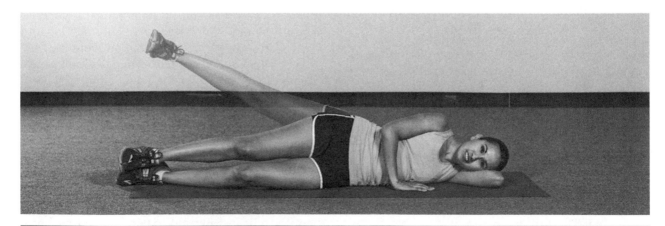

Figure 5.3   Side leg raise with up and down phases.

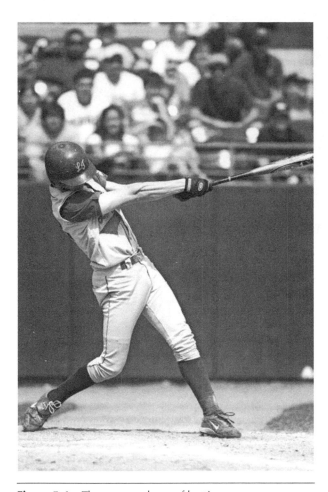

Figure 5.4 The power phase of batting.

serves two functions: to increase the range of motion through which the force can be applied in the power phase and, if done quickly, to prestretch the muscles responsible for the power phase and thereby increase their force.

After the power phase is the **follow-through phase**. By watching the follow-through, you can get a good idea about the direction of force application. This phase has no effect on the amount of force transferred from the body (or bat). These three phases are typical of many sport skills. You will focus your analysis on the power phase—for this is where the client will need the greatest strength or power.

Step 2: Analyze Joints and Movements

Within specific segments of exercise phases, determine which joints are involved and what movements they are performing. Joints move when muscles crossing those joints contract. During concentric (shortening) contractions, the insertion of the muscle moves toward the origin. To be more effective in exercise analysis, review your knowledge of anatomy so that you can accurately describe major joint movements (see figure 5.5).

The following are definitions of the major movements at joints throughout the body (Batman and Van Capelle 1992). All movements are from the anatomical position. The **anatomical position** involves the body standing at an erect position, arms and legs straight, head facing forward, with palms and toes also facing forward.

- **Flexion:** Bending; bringing the bones together; reducing the angle at a joint. The exception is flexion at the shoulder joint, which occurs when the humerus is moved forward.

- **Extension:** Straightening; moving bones apart; increasing the angle at a joint. The exception is extension at the shoulder joint, where the humerus is brought back toward the body.

- **Abduction:** Movement away from the midline of the body—for example, moving the arms and legs away from the trunk in a sideways motion.

- **Adduction:** Movement toward the midline of the body—for example, moving the arms or legs toward the trunk in a sideways motion.

- **Medial (internal) rotation:** Rotation of a limb toward the midline of the body—for example, rotating the arms or legs toward the trunk.

- **Lateral (external) rotation:** Rotation of a limb away from the midline of the body—for example, rotating the arms or legs away from the trunk.

- **Supination:** Lateral rotation movement at the radioulnar joint (below elbow) or a roll to the outside of the heel at the subtalar joint (below the ankle).

- **Pronation:** Medial rotation movement at the radioulnar joint (below elbow) or a roll to the inside of the heel at the subtalar joint (below the ankle).

- **Horizontal abduction:** Movement of a limb away from the midline of the body in a horizontal plane—for example, moving the arm from a front horizontal position to a side horizontal position.

- **Horizontal adduction:** Movement of a limb toward the midline of the body in a horizontal plane—for example, moving the arm from a side horizontal position to a front horizontal position.

- **Circumduction:** Circular movements at a joint; combines many other movements—for example, occurs at shoulder joint, hip joint, and spinal joint.

Figure 5.5 shows actions performed by specific joints. Some movements occur only at one pair of

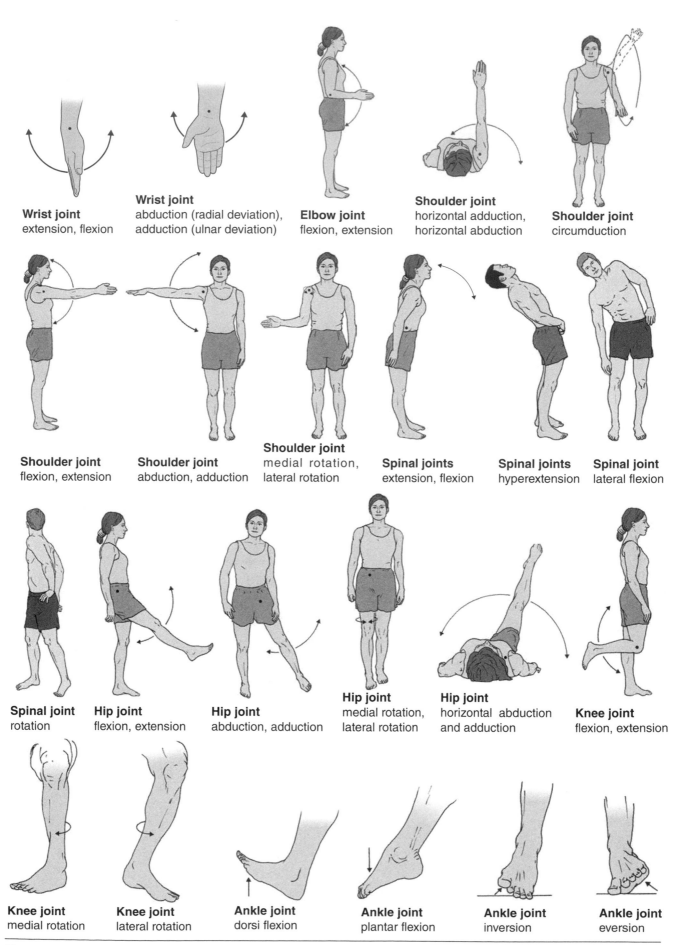

Wrist joint
extension, flexion

Wrist joint
abduction (radial deviation),
adduction (ulnar deviation)

Elbow joint
flexion, extension

Shoulder joint
horizontal adduction,
horizontal abduction

Shoulder joint
circumduction

Shoulder joint
flexion, extension

Shoulder joint
abduction, adduction

Shoulder joint
medial rotation,
lateral rotation

Spinal joints
extension, flexion

Spinal joints
hyperextension

Spinal joint
lateral flexion

Spinal joint
rotation

Hip joint
flexion, extension

Hip joint
abduction, adduction

Hip joint
medial rotation,
lateral rotation

Hip joint
horizontal abduction
and adduction

Knee joint
flexion, extension

Knee joint
medial rotation

Knee joint
lateral rotation

Ankle joint
dorsi flexion

Ankle joint
plantar flexion

Ankle joint
inversion

Ankle joint
eversion

Figure 5.5   Action at specific joints.

138

joints, such as at the shoulder girdle, the pelvic girdle, and the foot.

Shoulder Girdle

This joint is a combination of three joints that work together. The movements are often difficult to see. The following actions describe movements of the shoulder girdle, which comprises the scapula and clavicle.

- **Elevation:** Movement of the scapula upward.
- **Depression:** Movement of the scapula downward.
- **Abduction (protraction):** Movement of the scapula away from the spinal column.
- **Adduction (retraction):** Movement of the scapula toward the spinal column.
- **Upward rotation:** Rotation of the scapula upward. The inferior angle (bottom) moves outward and upward.
- **Downward rotation:** Rotation of the scapula downward. Inferior angle moves down and in.

Although its joints can move independently, the shoulder girdle mainly supports and assists movements of the shoulder joint. The shoulder girdle actions allow the arm (humerus) to move through a wide range of motion. When you analyze shoulder joint and shoulder girdle movements, it might be helpful to use table 5.1 to identify the

Table 5.1   Combined Actions of the Shoulder Girdle and Shoulder Joint

Shoulder joint action	Shoulder girdle action
Abduction	Upward rotation Abduction
Adduction	Downward rotation Adduction
Flexion	Upward rotation Abduction
Extension	Downward rotation Adduction
Medial rotation	Abduction
Lateral rotation	Adduction
Horizontal abduction	Adduction
Horizontal adduction	Abduction

Practicing Steps 1 and 2

At this point, you are able to divide the exercise into phases, identify all joints that are involved for each phase, and determine the movement or movements for each joint.

You should practice these skills. In the following exercises, determine the phases, the joints involved, and the movements taking place at those joints:

- Curl-ups
- Resisted toe points
- Prone scapular retraction

To make your analysis easier, sketch three analysis charts with columns labeled "Phase," "Joint," and "Movement." Leave at least five rows between each chart for your analysis. After you have analyzed these three exercises, compare your conclusions with tables 5.2, 5.3, and 5.4. Using a grid such as these tables will make your analyses easier.

Table 5.2   Exercise: Curl-Up

Phase	Joint	Movement
Up	Spine (lumbar)	Flexion
Down	Spine (lumbar)	Extension

Illustrations adapted by permission from Cook and Stewart 1996.

Table 5.3   Exercise: Resisted Toe Points

Phase	Joint	Movement
Out	Ankle	Plantar flexion
In	Ankle	Dorsiflexion

(With tubing around foot, press foot down.)

Illustrations adapted by permission from Cook and Stewart 1996.

Table 5.4   Exercise: Prone Scapular Retraction

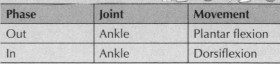

Phase	Joint	Movement
Up	Shoulder joint	Horizontal abduction
Up	Shoulder girdle	Adduction
Down	Shoulder joint	Horizontal adduction
Down	Shoulder girdle	Abduction

(Pinch shoulder blades together with arms out from sides and elbows bent.)

action at the shoulder joint and then look across to the corresponding action of the shoulder girdle.

Pelvic Girdle

The following actions are specifically related to the pelvic girdle.

- **Forward tilt:** Movement of the pelvic girdle forward.
- **Backward tilt:** Movement of the pelvic girdle backward.
- **Lateral tilt:** Movement of the pelvic girdle such that one side drops.

Foot

The following actions are uniquely related to the ankle and foot.

- **Dorsiflexion:** Same as flexion, only at the ankle joint.
- **Plantar flexion:** Same as extension, only at the ankle joint; pointing the foot.
- **Eversion:** Turning the sole of the foot outward, where the weight is taken on the inside of the foot. Occurs at the subtalar joint.
- **Inversion:** Turning the sole of the foot inward, where the weight is taken on the outside of the foot. Occurs at the subtalar joint.

Step 3: Analyze Types of Contractions

To cause a movement, a muscle must produce tension and contract. While under tension, the muscle may shorten during the contraction, lengthen, or stay the same length.

With a **concentric contraction**, the muscle develops tension great enough to overcome a resistance and produces an action by shortening. The "up" phase of calisthenics, free weights, sport skills, and many resistance machines involves concentric contraction of the muscles producing joint movements in that direction. For example, in the up phase of a biceps curl, the biceps shorten under tension (concentric contraction) to produce flexion at the elbow. The biceps are creating enough tension to overcome the resistance of gravity, the weight of the arm, and the external weight.

With an **eccentric contraction,** the tension generated by the muscle is less than the resistance and the muscle will lengthen. Eccentric contractions occur when

- muscles attempt to counter the force of gravity, such as when the body or a limb is lowered, or
- muscles attempt to counter the force of momentum by slowing down the action (e.g., the ballistic action of the follow-through of a batter).

Eccentric contractions do not increase flexibility, because the muscle is producing tension while it is lengthening. In fact, eccentric contraction can generate more tension than a shortening contraction (Wilmore and Costill 2004). The down phase of calisthenics, free weights, sport skills, and many resistance machines involves eccentric contraction of the muscles that produce joint movements in that direction. Remember, the force of gravity produces significant acceleration if an object or limb is allowed to fall freely. In most exercises, the down phase involves eccentric contractions of the muscles that initiated the up movement. We control the speed of the descent with eccentric contractions. For example, the biceps lower the weight in the biceps curl at a rate slower than gravity, thus controlling the free fall.

It is sometimes difficult to understand that the same muscle groups are responsible for both the up and down phases of an exercise. These muscles shorten on the way up with a concentric contraction and lengthen on the way down with an eccentric contraction. Eccentric contractions are a big part of everyday life—for example, the landing phase of each step of a jog, or lowering yourself to sit, walking down the stairs, lowering a fork from your mouth, and bending down.

Eccentric contractions also occur when we slow down something that is moving quickly or that has significant momentum. We are still attempting to control a movement. When a person throws a ball, for example, the anterior shoulder muscles contract concentrically to produce the movement (power phase), but after the ball has been released (follow-through phase), the arm must be slowed down to prevent injury. This control comes from tension in the muscles on the posterior shoulder. The momentum of the arm keeps it moving forward, but the lengthening contraction slows the movement. Many high-power sports and ballistic exercises (such as arm actions with hand weights) involve rapid eccentric contractions. The greatest muscular forces are generated with rapid eccentric contractions, and more strain is placed on connective tissue when it is elongated under tension.

Proper execution of an exercise or skill may involve the stabilization of a joint. If a muscle develops tension but there is no visible movement of the joint, it is called an **isometric contraction**. Although the information is not included on our analysis chart, you should identify the major muscles involved in any isometric contraction where stabilization is a critical part of your client's activity. For example, upper body exercises involving barbells or dumbbells such as the lateral arm raises in table 5.5 require the shoulder girdle to be stabilized. An isometric contraction of the shoulder girdle elevators and adductors will form a strong base for shoulder joint movements. Also note the following:

- There is no movement in the elbows and wrists, which are stabilized (isometric contractions) during both phases of the exercise.

- In the first 60° of shoulder joint abduction, there is little or no movement of the shoulder girdle. Shoulder girdle adductor muscles contract isometrically to stabilize.

- It is useful, then, to expand the analysis chart to include the type of contraction.

Table 5.5 Exercise: Lateral Arm Raises

Phase	Joint	Movement	Contraction type
Up	Shoulder joint	Abduction	Concentric
Up	Shoulder girdle	Upward rotation Abduction	Concentric
Down	Shoulder joint	Adduction	Eccentric
Down	Shoulder girdle	Downward rotation Adduction	Eccentric

(Raise arms out from the body.)

Illustrations adapted by permission from Cook and Stewart 1996.

Step 4: Analyze Which Muscles Are Being Used

Here are two helpful visualizations for exercise analysis:

- Muscles affect movement of the joints that they cross. An obvious example is the biceps at the elbow. Flexion of the elbow is the primary movement, but the biceps also crosses the radioulnar joint and the shoulder joint and can be recruited to cause movements at these joints.

- If alignment of the muscle–tendon unit is in the direction of the movement, the influence of that muscle will be optimal (see the section on biomechanical analysis of exercise in chapter 3).

Once you have determined the joint action and type of contraction, your final and most important step is to identify the active muscles. Determining individual muscles responsible for a movement can be simplified by following this principle: *The muscle group causing the action is named by that joint and action (if the contraction is concentric).* For example, in the up phase of a biceps curl, the elbow flexes—and the muscle group used is the elbow flexors. In lateral arm raises, the shoulder joint abducts in the up phase; therefore, the shoulder joint abductors are responsible. For a more detailed analysis, we will look at a bench press (see table 5.6).

Table 5.6 concisely presents the active joints, their movements, the primary muscles, and how they are contracting during the phases of the bench press. The most challenging part of the anatomical analysis is recalling the specific muscles responsible for the joint actions (Tortora and Grabowski 2003). To facilitate this step, the end of the chapter presents **JAM** charts (forms 5.1-5.7): these are quick references indicating joint, actions, and muscles.

Synergists

Synergists are muscles that act together to create a combined force. They can be separate parts of the same muscle, as when the anterior and posterior parts of the gluteus medius work together for hip abduction or the upper and lower trapezius muscles complement one another in shoulder girdle adduction. Synergists may also be opposing muscle parts that work together for one action but neutralize each other because of opposing roles: For example, wrist muscles that flex and abduct work in synergy with others that flex and adduct. The result is stronger wrist flexion with neither abduction nor adduction. In the foot, both invertors and evertors combine to plantar flex without rotation. A common effect of this synergistic muscle action is greater joint stabilization.

Table 5.6   Exercise: Bench Press

Phase	Joint	Movement	Contraction type	Muscles
Up	Shoulder joint	Horizontal adduction	Concentric	Pectoralis major Anterior deltoid (Shoulder joint horizontal adductors)
Up	Shoulder girdle	Abduction	Concentric	Serratus anterior Pectoralis minor (Shoulder girdle abductors)
Up	Elbow	Extension	Concentric	Triceps (Elbow extensors)
Down	Shoulder joint	Horizontal abduction	Eccentric	Pectoralis major Anterior deltoid
Down	Shoulder girdle	Adduction	Eccentric	Serratus anterior Pectoralis minor
Down	Elbow	Flexion	Eccentric	Triceps

(Press bar up; lower bar near chest.)

Illustration reprinted by permission from Howley and Franks 1997.

Let's apply the JAM charts for anatomical analysis of a partial squat designed to strengthen the lower body—particularly the quadriceps. The exercise is effective in producing gains but does carry some risk. The patellar–femoral pressure increases dramatically as the angle of the knee approaches 90°. Use a light weight and restricted range of motion to begin.

Remember the principle: The muscle group causing the action is named by that joint and action (if the contraction is concentric). This directs us to the JAM chart columns for hip extensors (form 5.4), knee extensors (form 5.5), and ankle plantar flexors (form 5.6). Reading down each column of the JAM chart, select the prime movers (PM) and insert them in the analysis chart (table 5.7). Remember, the down phase is the opposite movement but the same muscles are contracting eccentrically. Notice the advantage in always analyzing the up phase first.

Step 5: Evaluate Purpose, Effectiveness, and Risk

Evaluate each exercise, using the information gained during steps 1 through 4. Having completed the anatomical analysis of an exercise, you know what muscles it will work. Is this what you want for your client? With the client-centered counseling approach, you have established her priorities by considering her needs, wants, and lifestyle. It is time now to evaluate how well the exercise fills its purpose, its effectiveness, and the degree of personal risk it carries.

Purpose

Establish the general purpose of the exercise, that is, which primary fitness component is being challenged. The purpose of the exercise must coincide with the component and body area that the client identifies as an area of priority. Discussion in this chapter will focus primarily on the components of flexibility and muscular conditioning. It is sometimes difficult to differentiate between a flexibility and a strengthening exercise. To assist, try the three simple checks in table 5.8. The checks should verify that a stretch will pull the muscle, extend its length without creating much tension, and leave the muscle more relaxed after the stretch, whereas a strengthening exercise will shorten the muscle, create significant tension, and result in fatigue.

Define the purpose more specifically by referring to the areas of the body targeted by the exercise. For example, the purpose of an exercise may be to stretch the calves, to strengthen the abdominal area, or to develop power needed for a vertical jump.

Effectiveness

Effectiveness refers to how well an exercise fulfills its purpose. No two clients will take exactly the same route to reach an objective. Effectiveness is not just what researchers have said about an exercise or training method—effectiveness varies

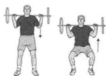

Table 5.7   **Exercise: Partial Squat**

Phase	Joint	Movement	Contraction type	Muscles
Up	Hip	Extension	Concentric	Gluteus maximus Semitendinosus Semimembranosus Biceps femoris
Up	Knee	Extension	Concentric	Rectus femoris Vastus lateralis Vastus intermedius Vastus medialis
Up	Ankle	Plantar flexion	Concentric	Gastrocnemius Soleus
Down	Hip	Flexion	Eccentric	Gluteus maximus Semitendinosus Semimembranosus Biceps femoris
Down	Knee	Flexion	Eccentric	Rectus femoris Vastus lateralis Vastus intermedius Vastus medialis
Down	Ankle	Dorsiflexion	Eccentric	Gastrocnemius Soleus

(Keeping back straight and head up, lower the bar by flexing the knees to 90°. Return.)
Illustrations reprinted by permission from Heyward 1998.

Table 5.8   **Checking for Purpose**

Checks	Stretch	Strength
Attachment points (i.e., origin and insertion)	Pulled farther apart	Moved closer together (concentric contraction)
Muscle tension	Slight	Moderate to high
Gradual feeling	Relief and relaxation	Hardness; fatigue

considerably among clients. The bottom line to effectiveness is "Will the exercise do what I want it to do for my client?" Ask the following questions:

- What is the appropriate overload to challenge the desired fitness component?
- Does the stretch avoid excessive tension, and is the alignment such that the stretch is in the direction of the fibers and elongation of the muscle?
- For a strengthening exercise, is fatigue felt in the targeted muscles, and are they directly resisted by an external resistance such as free weights, equipment, elastic bands, or gravity?
- Is the exercise effective from the physiological point of view?

- What monitoring can be built into the design to track its effectiveness?

For example, would it be an effective stretch if your client were to lie supine on a bench with reasonably heavy weights in her outstretched arms such that the chest and anterior shoulders were supporting the resistance? As she slowly lowered the weights, she would feel the pectoralis and anterior deltoid muscles elongating—certainly this must be an effective stretch. It is true that those muscles are elongating, but they have significant tension because they are eccentrically contracting. The muscles will not relax. In fact, they will eventually fatigue, placing added stress on the shoulder ligaments. Effectiveness is poor according to our evaluation, and there is an inherent risk of injury.

Risk

Careful risk analysis is inherent in any client-centered prescription. Not all exercises are created equal. Some movements or positions actually increase the risk of injury. For example, forward flexion of the trunk should not be performed with the knees locked in full extension. The hamstrings are pulled tight when the knees are locked, restricting the pelvis from rotating forward. As a result, most of the movement will be centered on the lower back, with the anterior intervertebral disc of L5-S1 and those above it being considerably compressed. This position is also contraindicated for those with osteoporosis and older clients because of the risk of vertebral fractures. Exercises like sit-ups, toe touches, and even some back stretches have added risk.

There may be risk in *how* the exercise is executed, and we will examine that in discussing demonstration. Exercise execution and other training errors are called extrinsic risks. Biomechanical risks or structural weaknesses that clients bring with them are referred to as intrinsic risks. Details of how to control these risk factors are discussed in chapter 10, "Causes and Prevention of Overuse Injuries."

Anatomical Analysis of a Weight Training Exercise

Laura worked as a sorter in the post office. She was interested in adding weights to her fitness program. Sometimes her shoulders tired at work, and she wanted to improve her shoulder endurance and prevent the injuries she had seen in some of her coworkers. Their injuries resulted from impingement (chapter 11), where the soft tissue between the head of the humerus and the acromion process of the scapula can be jammed. One of the core exercises I designed for her was a lateral arm raise.

The purpose of the lateral arm raise is to develop the shoulders and upper back. The exercise effectively targets the deltoids and upper shoulder girdle muscles (table 5.9). Heavier weights and arms lifted above the horizontal can magnify the risk of impingement. Keeping the thumbs up provides the largest space for the tissues and a reduced risk (see discussion of impingement syndrome in the chapter 11 section "Rotator Cuff Tendinitis"). Because Laura had no shoulder problems, I expected that application of a progressive overload would bring the desired results with no complications. I advised Laura to avoid rapid movements, especially much beyond the horizontal. If she began to feel any discomfort, she was to stop and ice her shoulder after the workout.

A full and effective anatomical analysis involves all five steps. You must achieve the desired purpose of the exercise, meet your client's needs, account for any limitations, and validate the exercise design. You should always alter exercises—anatomically and biomechanically—to take your client's limitations into account and reduce the risk of injury.

Table 5.9 Anatomical Analysis of Lateral Arm Raises

Phase	Joint	Movement	Contraction type	Muscles
Up	Shoulder joint	Abduction Lateral rotation (thumbs up)	Concentric Isometric	Middle deltoid Supraspinatus Infraspinatus Teres minor
Up	Shoulder girdle	Upward rotation Abduction Elevation	Concentric	Serratus anterior Trapezius 1 and 2 Levator scapulae[a]
Down	Shoulder joint	Adduction Lateral rotation (thumbs up)	Eccentric Isometric	Middle deltoid Supraspinatus Infraspinatus Teres minor
Down	Shoulder girdle	Downward rotation Adduction Depression	Eccentric	Serratus anterior Trapezius 1 and 2 Levator scapulae[a]

[a]Pectoralis minor and trapezius 4 are depressors and less effective in this exercise.

Musculoskeletal Exercise Design Model

Training methods and exercise equipment are the setting for the real actors—the individual exercises. The script for these actors starts with the design of the exercise. Exercise *design* provides the initial body position, how the client needs to move or stabilize, and appropriate precautions for a specific musculoskeletal exercise. Exercise *prescription* continues from the design with adjustment of the prescription factors (FITT—frequency, intensity, time, type of exercise and progression) to suit the client. Our focus in this chapter is exercise design. Models for exercise prescription are presented in part II.

Just as a patient approaches the physician or pharmacist with the request, "Give me something for my . . . ," clients approach personal fitness trainers requesting specific exercises. The proliferation of strength training technique seminars and exercise design workshops for aerobic leaders and personal trainers is a testament to the interest in exercise design. Yet many people in the industry are on the verge of "design template syndrome" where every program they design starts to look the same. In contrast, we should be able to draw on a variety of exercises to personalize our prescriptions—particularly in the component areas of flexibility, muscular balance, and conditioning.

After we analyze possible exercises, we select those that most closely match the needs of our client. We usually need to make modifications to improve the client "fit." And if the fit is still not right, we can build the ideal exercise for our client from scratch.

The following model, which puts together the techniques discussed in this chapter, is a simple five-step approach to guide you through this process of exercise design:

Step 1: Identify the primary component.

Step 2: Target the muscles.

Step 3: Determine the appropriate joint movements or position.

Step 4: Design and modify.

Step 5: Finish with a safety check.

Step 1: Identify the Primary Component

Sometimes you will have to take your client's vision and translate it into a physiological compo-nent. For example, your client may want to make it through his work day without low back pain. This may require exercises for stretching the hip flexors, low back, and hamstrings; muscular endurance for the abdominal muscles and gluteals; and some aerobic work. Your client's objectives may also involve multiple components. For example, someone who wants aerobic work but has a lower leg problem must deal with modifications of the aerobic task while rehabilitating the leg. As the client makes gains, the importance of some of the components may decrease (e.g., lower leg strength) while that of others may increase (e.g., cardiovascular endurance).

Step 2: Target the Muscles

Step 2 identifies the goal area of the body and then targets the primary muscle groups (figure 5.6).

In this step you must consider muscular balance and postural stabilizers. For example, someone who spends many hours at a computer has asked for exercises to help with his baseball throwing ability. The exercise illustrated in figure 5.1*b* will strengthen the anterior chest and shoulder muscles used in throwing. However, these muscles are tight because of the client's constant computer posture. Targeted muscles must strike a muscular balance with their antagonists. Therefore, your design should include stretches for the active chest muscles and strengthening of the upper back and posterior shoulder muscles (i.e., posterior deltoid, latissimus dorsi, and trapezius). Chapter 8 shows you how to analyze and work with muscle balance and posture.

Please note: Narrow targeting with muscle "isolations" is sometimes appropriate, but it may leave gaps in your client's program. Some machines can prevent muscles from working together naturally with other muscles as synergists or cocontractors. For example, there is little correlation between performance on isokinetic knee extension machines and functional performance in a weight-bearing sport or activity that uses the quadriceps (Ellison 1993).

Step 3: Determine the Appropriate Joint Movements or Position

You can read the JAM charts in reverse to determine the movement needed for an exercise design (see the forms at the end of the chapter). Here is an example:

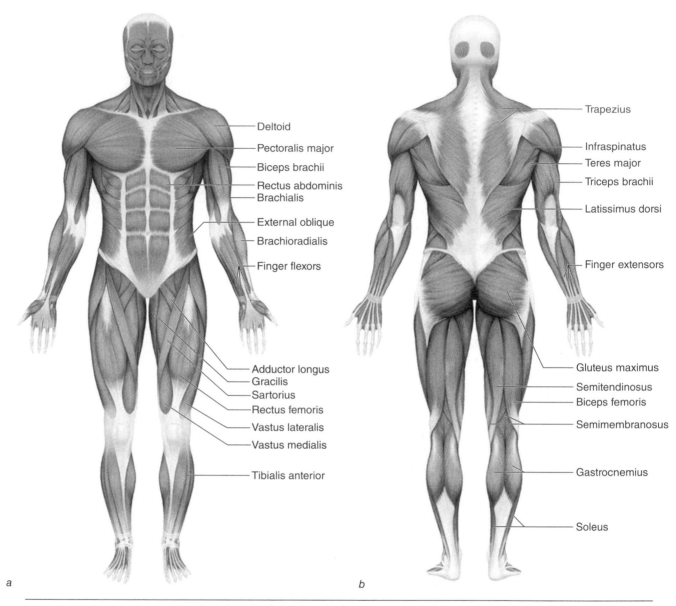

Deltoid
Pectoralis major
Biceps brachii
Rectus abdominis
Brachialis
External oblique
Brachioradialis
Finger flexors

Adductor longus
Gracilis
Sartorius
Rectus femoris
Vastus lateralis
Vastus medialis

Tibialis anterior

Trapezius
Infraspinatus
Teres major
Triceps brachii
Latissimus dorsi

Finger extensors

Gluteus maximus
Semitendinosus
Biceps femoris
Semimembranosus

Gastrocnemius

Soleus

a

b

Figure 5.6   Front and rear view of adult male skeletal musculature.

• The muscle to be targeted is the gluteus maximus. Form 5.4 indicates that the gluteus maximus is a prime mover for hip extension and lateral rotation and an assistant mover for hip abduction. In step 4 you will see how to design three muscular endurance calisthenics that use these hip movements, or a single exercise modified in three ways. The JAM charts are a reminder that multiple movements are required to fully challenge all fibers of a muscle.

• A second example involves a client who has tension in the upper back. Step 2 targeted the upper trapezius muscles, levator scapulae, and the erector spinae of the cervical spine. Step 4 will explain how to design some static stretches for these muscles—but in what positions should the shoulder girdle and cervical spine be placed to stretch all of these muscles? Form 5.2 of the JAM charts shows that the levator scapulae and trapezius 1 and 2 are responsible for shoulder girdle elevation, upward rotation, and some assisted adduction. Taking the opposite position will stretch these muscles, pulling origin and insertion apart. Form 5.7 of the JAM charts shows that the erector spinae would be stretched when the neck is flexed, laterally flexed, or rotated.

Step 4: Design and Modify

This system establishes the requirements before an exercise is selected. Your guidelines are the muscle actions or movements. You are not restricted to a menu of exercises. Let the creative juices flow!

In the first example, figure 5.7 suggests three calisthenics that work the gluteus maximus in *(a)* lateral rotation with extension tubing (dynamic),

(b) extension (isometric), and *(c)* abduction (dynamic). Dynabands could be used in all three exercises; ankle weights could be used from a standing position in exercises 1 and 3; or the range of motion could be increased in all three movements.

In the second example (figure 5.8), the first exercise *(a)* stretches both sides of the erector spinae, trapezius 1, and levator scapulae. The second exercise *(b)* focuses on one side at a time and stretches all four muscles. If your client has tension at his computer work station, you could modify the second exercise to be done in a chair. Grasping the bottom of the chair seat, he would lean to one side with a lateral flex to the neck.

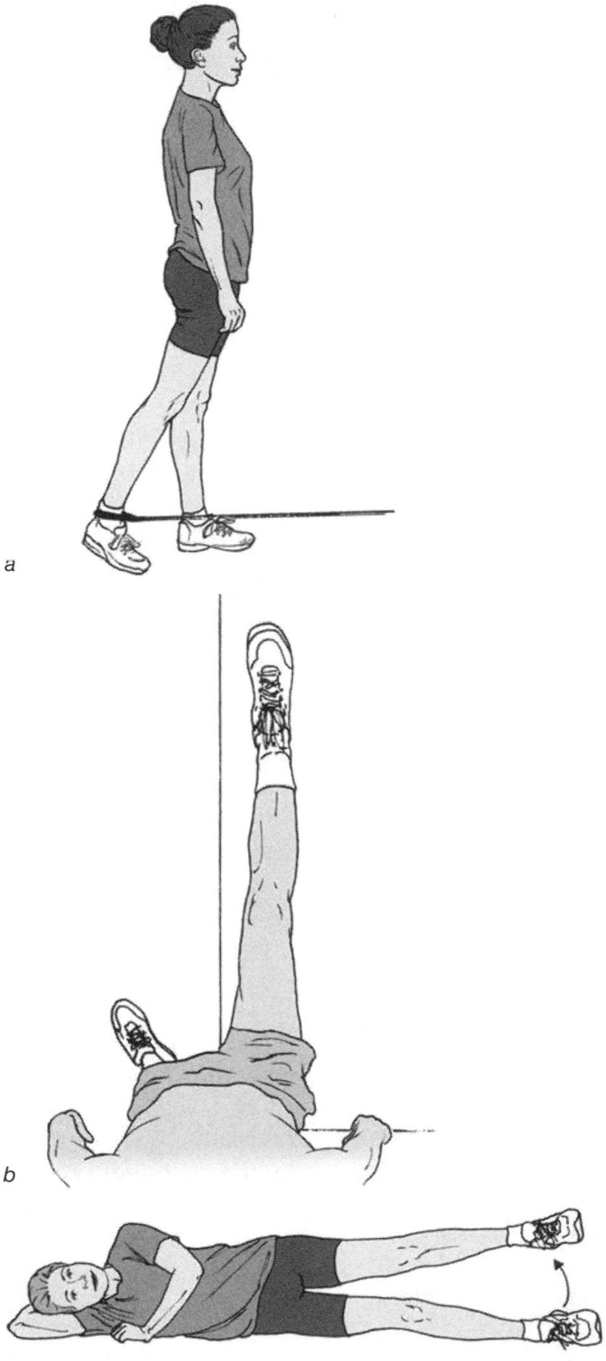

a

b

c

Figure 5.7 Strengthening exercises for the gluteus maximus.

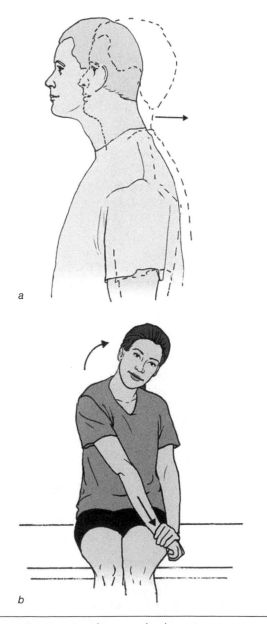

a

b

Figure 5.8 Exercises for upper back tension.

Part II of the book provides sample program cards to record the exercises for your client. Consider the quality and format of the way you present the exercise on the program card. A diagram or photograph will be of immeasurable help at the early stages of the program when you are not around. Provide an exercise name and the primary muscles involved. Select your wording carefully as you describe the exercise, from the initial body position through all sequenced movements. Give helpful cueing such as what to stabilize, and include all relevant safety precautions.

Step 4 may also involve refinement and modification of exercises. To generate creative ideas, consider changes in body position, joint angle, or range of motion; the addition of other body segments, stages of the exercise, or combining movements; or simulation of a work task or sporting skill. Let's work with lateral arm raises (table 5.5) and consider a variety of modifications suited to specific scenarios. You are training at a home and only have 10 lb (3.7 kg) dumbbells, and your client is having some difficulties. Modify the exercise by having your client slightly bend his elbows to bring the resistance closer to the joint. Another client is a water polo player and needs core stability while using the shoulders. Have this athlete perform the exercise while sitting on a stability ball with varying degrees of leg support. Or you may have a recreational tennis player who feels weak on her backhand topspin. Have this client start the lateral lifts from a bent elbow position and, as the arm is raised, lift the weight to point straight up (lateral rotation of the shoulder joint). This compound movement simulates a backhand topspin.

Step 5: Finish With a Safety Check

After creating your design, scrutinize it for safety. Check for risk in the design and later in the execution. Look for repetitive forces contributing to overuse, excessive force in the development of momentum, or forces applied when joints are not aligned. Modify the design further if the exercise has high injury risk (see table 5.10). During an exercise program demonstration, you present a lot of information for your client to retain. One of the real values of a personal fitness trainer is that you provide ongoing safety checks.

Your client may already have some areas of weakness to which you need to be sensitive, such as muscle imbalances, joint instability, muscle tightness, or previous injuries. I recall demonstrating a program to a strong, very fit client who followed my instructions and demonstration with good safe form. After a few sessions, I left him on his own for a few weeks and when I returned, he was doing one exercise with a form that was contraindicated. I had given him wall squats with a

Table 5.10   Exercise Design Safety Check

Component	Design safety issue
Flexibility (in the warm-up)	• Avoid static stretching until increases in tissue temperature and joint synovial fluid occur. • Low-trauma dynamic stretches may precede static stretches. • Target muscles, especially those to be used eccentrically. • For sport preparation, simulate joint mechanics.
Flexibility (in the program)	• Have client stretch as needed for muscle tightness. • For sport, do stretching (dynamic, static) in intermittent sports such as baseball. • Have client stretch as needed between resistance exercises.
Flexibility (in the cool-down)	• Take advantage of warm tissue for greatest flexibility gains. • Target muscles used, especially if used eccentrically. • Don't underestimate the therapeutic effect of a relaxing shower.
Resistance exercise (strength, muscular endurance, power)	• Emphasize the precautions specifically outlined for the given exercise. • Ensure that both agonist and antagonist have been targeted. • Muscle imbalances may require specific muscle stretch and opposite muscle strengthening. • Have client stretch as needed for muscle tightness. • Differentiate between fatigue, soreness, and inflammation. • Ice any "hot spots" or minor injuries. • Modify the exercise around minor injuries (including avoidance). • Conduct ongoing checks for alignment such as pelvic stabilization and avoidance of extreme range of motion. • Ensure that muscles feel worked but not sore or tight. • Follow the training method guidelines as prescribed (chapter 7).

stability ball behind his back, but he had adjusted his feet well back toward the wall with his toes pointing outward. He said he made the changes because he developed some shin splints from running and this position gave him some relief. I knew at a glance that the shear and torque on the knee were not safe and eliminated that exercise until he could perform the squat correctly without shin pain.

Client-Centered Exercise Demonstration

First impressions about the prescription form in the demonstration stage and continue to be reinforced through subsequent workouts and all the stages of monitoring. There is a relative paucity of articles concerning the teaching and demonstration of new exercise skills, despite the fact that this often constitutes a vast majority of the time of a personal fitness trainer. Teaching behaviors such as exercise explanations, demonstrations, positive reinforcement, and performance feedback increase the level of exercise focus.

Clients need to understand how an exercise will help them. They need to see it demonstrated and then try it with some expert feedback. Finally, the exercise may need to be modified or integrated into a full prescription. These are the steps involved in form 5.8, Exercise Demonstration Model Checklist. Adapt this model to suit your client and situation.

The one-on-one exercise demonstration is a core element of your client-centered services. The exercise demonstration model (presented in the highlight box here, and as a checklist in form 5.8) identifies more than two dozen critical behaviors that make up a single demonstration. The items on the checklist guide you through this process. For many of the items, the checklist provides examples of behaviors or methods of showing that item. They are merely suggestions that may guide your actions or dialogue with your client.

There are four distinct steps.

1. The **predemonstration** sets the scene, in which you ensure that the client is comfortable, find out about the client's previous experience, and provide an idea of what is to come and why.

2. The actual **demonstration** stage teaches the client how to perform the exercise correctly and safely. Effective use of verbal and physical techniques adds clarity to the teaching.

3. The third stage is the **client trial,** in which you observe carefully and provide specific feedback.

4. The **follow-up** allows you to gather feedback from the client and provide client-centered prescription guidelines.

Demonstrating an exercise is both a science and an art. It requires a balance between your technical knowledge and your people skills. With practice, you will learn to alter the technical aspects to suit each client's personality and learning style.

You should always observe, analyze, and modify technique. You must have a sound knowledge of the biomechanics of the exercises and an ability to design multiple variations in technique to suit the abilities of your clients. In addition to designing appropriate exercises, you must reinforce good technique both by demonstrating new exercises and by observing your client as she attempts to duplicate your demonstrations.

These are key technical issues on which you must focus to provide effective exercise demonstration:

- **Initial body position.** Focus on overall body posture. Instruct your client to "set" herself into a good body position before any exercise. Focus on exactly where you want your client to begin.

Weekend Warrior

A word of caution about the "weekend warrior," the impetuous client who charges from his week of sedentary living directly to the competitive playing field. He is a prime candidate for muscle or connective tissue injury caused by a rapid or forceful eccentric contraction. Avoidance is not the message he wants to hear, and a few cold stretches do little to prepare his body for the trauma. A longer warm-up integrating progressive eccentric actions similar to those in the sport will help. Also add a supplemental program to strengthen (eccentrically) the muscles used in the sport, particularly in preseason. Always critically evaluate eccentric contraction patterns within your client's activity prescription. What other counseling would be appropriate for this type of client? Why?

Design Faults or Execution Faults?

When you assign "cookbook" exercises to your clients, the chances of missing important individual differences in the mechanics of the movement are high. Another significant source of design faults is the failure to watch for execution errors during the demonstration. A client's errors may not simply be a learning issue; it may be that an area of instability is causing the altered mechanics. For example, during a lying hamstring curl, watch for the buttocks rising and the hip flexing. This may be caused by one of three things: (1) the weight is too high; (2) the rectus femoris is too tight, pulling to rotate the pelvis; or (3) the abdominal muscles are too weak to hold a neutral spine position. Modify the design by placing a rolled-up towel under the pelvis to prestretch the rectus femoris or reduce the range of knee flexion. Modify the execution by emphasizing pelvic stabilization and terminating when fatigue starts to affect any change of form.

For example, when beginning a bench press, your client should press her low back into the bench, with feet on the bench (if possible) and hands slightly wider than shoulder-width apart. Establish what will be stabilized and how that will feel (e.g., shoulder girdle or pelvic stabilization).

• **Movement pattern.** From the starting position, describe the sequence of movements and the body or joint position at the end of the exercise.

• **Cueing.** Give alignment and "feeling" cues to assist in the execution phase of the exercise. For example, when your client is doing side-lying lateral leg raises, show how the hips are aligned one on top of the other, raising to approximately 45°, with knees facing forward.

• **Safety and quality.** Using your knowledge of the demands and biomechanics of the exercise, provide appropriate safety guidelines. Focus on quality versus quantity. This refers to the number of repetitions your client performs correctly and the speed at which they occur. When resistance equipment is being used, remember the issues we raised in "Direction of Force Application and Muscle Alignment" in chapter 3:

  • Is the path of motion defined by the machine the same as your client's path of motion?

  • Is the direction of force application safe and optimal?

  • Does the equipment allow proper alignment between the machine's fulcrum and the center of the moving joint?

• **Spotting.** Spotting is an important component of exercise demonstration. Spotting refers to the visual and physical aspects of monitoring clients as they execute exercises. Visual spotting is done for all exercises, whereas physical spotting is used primarily in weight training. Watch for correct body alignment, signs and symptoms

of fatigue, signs of discomfort, control of movements, and the direction of the exercise energy. Assist the client to make technique corrections, attempt more repetitions, or complete the range of motion. For clients who are more advanced, verbal reinforcement cues are effective to correct their technique. Once the neural pattern (motor schema) has been cemented, the cues can prompt fluid modification during the repetition (Baker 2001). The simple use of one or two key words such as *head up, pelvis stable,* or *pinch* provides sufficient feedback based on the client's current knowledge of performance. Spotting the client provides an excellent opportunity to monitor good form. For more detail on spotting, see chapter 7.

• **Positioning.** While you are training or demonstrating to your client, your positioning can help you and affect your rapport with your client. Position yourself for the best view of the client's technique if you are not spotting. From the side or a 45° angle, you should also be able to view her face and most of her body. Match your client's upper body level, and avoid talking down to her. Like an athlete, be in a ready position to assist your client. Being casual by leaning or sitting can make you appear unprofessional.

• **Touching or not touching.** Many personal fitness trainers touch their clients to adjust their position. We must always respect individual boundaries. If you have not received permission to touch your client or are hesitant to ask, you can use a few strategies to help position your client without touching her. Demonstrate the exercise and then point out the adjustments on your own body while the client performs the exercise. Another technique is to provide a mental image such as "squeezing the abdomen like an accordion" (Cantwell 1998).

The skills involved in demonstration are significantly based in the psychosocial domain. Table

Exercise Demonstration Model

1. Predemonstration

- Set climate by making client feel comfortable and being receptive and responsive.
- Provide overview by explaining the purpose of this session and what is to happen in this session.
- Determine client's background and experience by asking, "Have you done this exercise before?" "Have you used this type of equipment before?" "What was your experience?"
- Clarify purpose of exercises by explaining the specific muscles used (major prime movers) and relevance to stated needs and wants.
- Encourage the client to ask questions and provide input.

2. Demonstration

- Provide precise and appropriate verbal instructions.
- Position client appropriately to watch demo.
- Provide clear physical demonstration (4-6 reps before client trial).
- Ensure that overall technical execution was smooth and confident.
- Ensure beginning position alignment and proper grip.
- Isolate the movement (i.e., no compensation or inappropriate movements).
- Stabilize the pelvis and key joints.
- Ensure that terminal points of range of motion are appropriate.
- Demonstrate safety, including controlled breathing and no Valsalva maneuver.
- Demonstrate safety, including controlled speed and no momentum at the end of the range of motion.
- Ensure efficient use of time with descriptions and explanations.

3. Client Trials

- Set client up by positioning and alignment.
- Select appropriate weight (moderately difficult).
- Ensure trial safety by controlling breathing, momentum, and plane of movement and ensuring no joint locking.
- Ensure effective spotting by being in position to observe and assist with starting and finishing positions.
- Have client execute a full set.
- Provide feedback to the client, which may include providing specific information and monitoring, focusing on behavior and not the person, correcting one aspect at a time, and being positive and helpful (providing success).
- Demonstrate verbal skills such as cueing during execution, paraphrasing, summarizing, and questioning.
- Demonstrate nonverbal skills such as using correct body position, being engaged, providing eye contact, and ignoring distractions.

4. Follow-Up

- Obtain feedback from client by asking how it felt (i.e., awkward, comfortable, difficult) and encouraging the client to ask questions and provide input.
- Demonstrate active listening skills by responding to feedback.
- Provide prescription guidelines (including weight, reps, and sets, or frequency, intensity, time, and type) that integrate and interpret information from client trial.
- Suggest a method of progression or encourage self-monitoring and assessment.
- Provide a modification on request (problem solving).

5.11 outlines some of these psychosocial aspects involved in the stages and activities, from the time we meet our clients for the program demonstration until later in the program follow-up.

It is important within the exercise demonstration to adjust your approach to suit each client's learning and personality style. In the beginning stages, focus on giving only the important points. As your client becomes more experienced, offer more alternative exercises, allowing your client to make his own selection. Base the amount of information you share with your client on his current stage of learning as well as on his preferred learning style. These are different learning styles and personalities, each followed by an example of how you would use that learning style with a client:

• **Learning by doing:** Have the client perform a series of abdominal exercises at a very slow and controlled pace, rather than the faster pace to which she is accustomed.

• **Learning by observation:** Demonstrate for your client the difference between a slow and faster pace for the exercise, then have her try it. Ask your client to comment on specific items she observed or felt—for example, "Did I look in full control of my body during the fast pace?" or "How did the slow exercises feel? Was there more energy required to perform the series slow or fast?"

• **Learning by knowing the theory:** This is a combination of your client's experience and observations; ask, for example, "What does this mean about the next time you will do sit-ups?"

• **Learning by applying the information to individual situations:** Have your client consider how this information will apply to other exercises he executes. "What would be the best way to perform muscle endurance exercises? Where else can this information apply?"

Teaching strategies can also be based on clients' personality characteristics. During the initial part of your meeting, try to determine their predominant personality style. Here are three different personality styles, each followed by an example of how you would adapt the demonstration for that client:

• **Technical personality:** Explain the pros and cons of your exercise choice or design. Deliver information at a moderate pace and be specific about your feedback.

• **Sociable personality:** Maintain a relaxed pace, inviting feedback and regularly checking on comfort. Be a good listener.

Table 5.11   Psychosocial Aspects in the Program Demonstration and Follow-Up Model

Step	Activities
1. Predemonstration	• Reassess and discuss client goals, values, motivational interests, and fitness assessment results. • Reconnect: Re-create and further build a positive climate. • Give clients permission to be themselves; show pleasure in what they are doing; provide protection from negative forces (e.g., negative self-talk, interruptions, intimidating atmosphere). • Ensure that clients' needs are being met.
2. Demonstration	• Base delivery of the information on clients' preferred learning styles (see examples that follow). • Approach and pace should reflect the client's personality style (see examples that follow). • Provide precise and appropriate verbal instructions. • Be time efficient with descriptions and explanations.
3. Client trials	• Provide feedback to the client that is specific, positive, and helpful (provides success). • Focus on the behavior, not the person. • Use verbal skills such as cues during execution, paraphrasing, and summarizing. • Use nonverbal skills to show engagement.
4. Follow-up	• Determine level of comfort and understanding. • Obtain feedback from client (specific probing). • Use active listening skills and respond to feedback. • Modify design if necessary; make sure the client accepts the exercise. • Make an appointment for connection in 2 or 3 days. • Move toward using intrinsic motivators.

- **Assertive personality:** Be businesslike, reasonably fast paced (once their execution is successful), and stimulating. You may need to limit the options you present, but be sure to incorporate clients' input.

Teaching Cues and Common Problems During Exercise Demonstrations

Spotting and positioning are technical elements but relate directly to client execution. Poor spotting or positioning could result in serious injury to the client or trainer; good spotting provides a trust-building experience that rivals any counseling technique. Cueing is a prompt or a signal that acts as a reminder to do something. As trainers we are teachers, reminding (cueing) our clients of the correct position, area of stabilization, or movement; but we also have a physical presence through our own positioning and spotting.

The following are three common resistance exercises, one lower body, one upper body, and one for the trunk. Common execution problems and appropriate cueing are presented.

Lower Body Example: Leg Press or Hack Squat

A common fault is bringing the weight too low. When the knee tracks beyond the toes, excessive forces are placed on the posterior cruciate ligament. A tactile range-limiting cue such as a palm of the hand on the knee may be effective. Some clients may turn their feet inward or outward to try to isolate parts of the quads. Assure your clients that there is no consensus that foot position can alter quad muscle recruitment. Encourage them to find the most comfortable foot position that poses the least stress. In many lower body resistance exercises, you should assist the client at the end of the movement or if the speed decreases because of fatigue.

Upper Body Example: Barbell Curl

A common fault is moving the torso or shoulder joint during the execution. Extending the torso in the up phase creates momentum. To deter this habit, you may have your client perform the exercise with the upper back against a wall. Flexing the shoulder joint draws assistance from the anterior deltoid and upper pectoralis major. Placing a finger on the posterior elbows of your client will be a sufficient tactile cue not to lift the arms forward. The faults described are actions that do not allow the elbows to move through a full range of motion and decrease the muscle fiber recruitment of the biceps. In many upper body resistance exercises, you should position yourself close to the client where you have the most effective position for assistance. For dumbbell exercises, position your hands at the joint that is immediately below the weight.

Trunk Example: Exercise Ball Crunch

A common fault is using a position on the ball that does not allow for a range of motion suited to the client strength. A position of support in the middle and upper back will decrease the range of motion and reduce the lever arm length, creating an easier modification. A lower starting position allowing the spine to slightly hyperextend prestretches the abdominal muscles, changes the fulcrum, and increases the lever arm, therefore increasing the contractile range of motion. Initially you may need to stabilize the ball against a wall with your feet or with available equipment. Monitor the position of your client, observing the fulcrum of the movement, the range of motion, and perceived difficulty of the client. With many trunk exercises, you must teach pelvic stabilization to minimize low back curvature and strain. Have clients touch their abdominal area to cue this pelvic stabilization and monitor their breathing.

Reinforcing the Client in the Demonstration

The client trial and follow-up stages are an excellent opportunity for motivation and reinforcement. Baker (2001) described three methods of reinforcing behavior.

1. Achievement reinforcement helps cultivate motivation to achieve preset goals. Recognize even a small improvement, but make sure it is praiseworthy because clients will know if you are sincere.

2. Sensation motivation comes from the feeling of execution excellence and, if reinforced immediately, will remain clear in the kinesthetic memory.

3. Verbal reinforcement should be positive and specific to the performance. To correct a client error, avoid negative phrases such as "No . . . that's not right," "That's too fast," or "Don't lock your elbows." Instead try more positive corrective cues such as "If you adjust that position, you should feel the difference," "Keep that cadence of 1 up and 3 down," or "Keep your elbows soft . . . good."

Reinforcing the client during the trial and follow-up stage is an effective means of motivating him to continue with positive behaviors or to

Connecting With Your Client

Try to get a broad picture of the human side of program demonstration. Imagine that you are demonstrating a modified squat to a novice middle-aged client. In the following, a description of your role in each stage precedes a brief sample statement appropriate for that stage of the exercise demonstration.

Predemonstration

This first step requires a sales technique. You need to sell the benefits and show your client how the exercise is relevant to him.

By doing the squats regularly, you will be better able to climb longer flights of stairs, lift heavier objects from the floor, and walk farther without fatigue.

Demonstration

You are the role model, yet you must be sensitive to your client's style of learning—tactile, auditory, or visual.

Stand with feet shoulder-width apart, knees slightly bent; your back is pushed flat against the wall with your arms on your thighs for support, like this.

Client Trials

Your focus is on your client's behavior. Leave him with a feeling of success and an idea of how to do better.

As you bent your knees to lower your body, your knees moved beyond the line of your toes initially, but then you pressed your hips farther back as you lowered your body and realigned . . . that's good.

Follow-Up

Ask for your client's feelings. If you have rapport with him, you will gain valuable insights. Knowing that you are there for him gives him the confidence for greater autonomy.

Are there any aspects of the exercise you are unsure of or want to clarify? Which part of the program are you most looking forward to?

---

modify incorrect techniques. Westcott and colleagues (2003) found that high levels of focused trainer–client interaction should address major aspects of proper exercise performance without being too technical during the first few weeks of training. They further suggested that comments should not disrupt exercise flow and should be exercise focused, reinforcing the client's training efforts.

Case Study

Part I of the book has established very important foundations needed to develop a client-centered approach to exercise prescription. Let's take a look at how these models and skills could translate into a sample of two 1 h sessions with a new client. Obviously the management structure of each facility will differ, some emphasizing the counseling or the assessment and others encouraging program development and demonstration as soon as possible.

For a personal fitness trainer to accomplish all things outlined in the first five chapters, it would take hours of contact time, which is unrealistic. Each situation and each client are new and unique, and we must glean the most relevant information and use our time effectively. In the example of a two-session format, suggestions are provided for what might be done within a reasonable time frame.

Sample First Two Sessions

The facility manager has scheduled your first 1 h session with the client. Per the facility protocol, the client has already filled out the following forms: Stages of Change Questionnaire (form 1.6), PAR-Q+ (www.csep.ca/forms.asp), a standard facility informed consent, and a health risk appraisal. If time permits, it would be helpful if the client had also completed the Activity Preferences Questionnaire (form 1.4).

Session 1

Initial Counseling (10-15 min)

- Establish a friendly welcome by being receptive and responsive, showing that you care.

- Outline the counseling process and discuss your client's reason for attending. Get your clients talking about themselves; listen carefully and paraphrase when needed.

- Establish desired outcome: fitness, health, or performance (may refer to the health risk appraisal form).

- Review the Stage of Change Questionnaire.

Counseling: Information Gathering (20-35 min)

- Start gathering information. Forms such as Activity Preferences Questionnaire (form 1.4) and Focus on Lifestyle (form 1.5) may be helpful to record key points. Take a look at the sample dialogues and questioning skills in chapter 1 for help with appropriate questions.

- Review past activities enjoyed; then collect FITT for current activities (you may elect to use the Physical Activity Index, PAI).

- Discuss and record:

  - Wants: activity preferences, special interests, or expectations

  - Needs: injury, fitness component, health risk factors, special design, education, or motivational support

  - Lifestyle: facilities, partners, travel, employment, and so on; routines, for example work, activity, sleep, eating, family

Counseling: Activity and Outcome Focus (10-15 min)

- Examine the options and if needed, use the Decision Balance Summary.

- Establish goals consistent with the client's desired outcome (fitness, health, performance).

- Identify key components needed for goals and confirm with the client.

Between Sessions

- Determine a motivation strategy that matches the client's stage of change and lifestyle information.

- Based on the client's objectives, select tests that will reflect the status of your client in the areas of concern. Time in the second session may limit your selection, but further items may be introduced in subsequent sessions. Careful and standardized monitoring can be effective as well at determining status and improvement.

- Select or design the number of exercises that are needed or will fit within a typical workout period. Draft the FITT for each exercise. These can be modified after the tests or during the demonstration.

Session 2

Assessment (20-30 min)

- Confirm the objectives with your client, now expressed as SMART objectives (i.e., including activity and outcome).

- Complete any screening (may vary depending on testing to be done).

- Administer the tests that have been selected.

Assessment Interpretation and Program Overview (5 min)

- Interpret the test results for the client and modify the prescription, if needed.

- Describe the overall program structure (present the program card if available at this time).

Demonstration (20-30 min)

- Perform the key exercise demonstrations. This may take longer if the client is totally unfamiliar with all the exercises.

- Finalize FITT, progressions, and safety precautions based on feedback from the demonstration. Information needed to complete this final item may be in part II or III of this book.

Summary

As a personal fitness trainer, certain essential skills enable you to design and teach exercises: anatomical exercise analysis, musculoskeletal exercise design, and exercise demonstration.

Exercise analysis includes the ability to observe a resistance exercise or flexibility exercise and determine the primary joint movements, muscles involved, and types of contraction. Numerous examples of popular exercises are presented in the chapter, and their suitability to client needs is determined.

A five-step approach to client-centered musculoskeletal exercise design is provided as a pivotal point in the prescription model. Exercise design provides the starting position, joint movements or changes in position, and any precautions for a specific musculoskeletal exercise. We further examined how to effectively modify an exercise and establish its safety in a way specific to the client.

Lastly, one of the most frequent tasks of a personal fitness trainer—exercise demonstration—is presented as both a science and an art using a four-step model. Clients need to understand how an exercise will help them. They need to see it demonstrated and then to try it with some expert feedback. Finally, the exercise may need to be modified or integrated into a full prescription. The chapter discussed useful teaching cues and methods to resolve common problems during exercise demonstration.

Your first session with a new client can be a daunting challenge. The final case study of the first two sessions integrates your acquired skills and provides a template to guide your initial experience.

FORM 5.1 JAM Chart: Shoulder Joint Muscles and Their Actions

Muscle	Flexion	Extension	Abduction	Adduction	Medial rotation	Lateral rotation	Horizontal adduction	Horizontal abduction
Anterior deltoid	PM		AM				PM	
Middle deltoid			PM					PM
Posterior deltoid		PM						PM
Supraspinatus			PM					
Pectoralis major[a]	PM						PM	
Pectoralis major[b]		PM		PM			PM	
Subscapularis					PM		AM	
Infraspinatus						PM		PM
Teres minor						PM		PM
Latissimus dorsi		PM		PM				AM
Teres major		PM		PM	PM			

Note: PM = prime mover; AM = assistant mover.

[a]Clavicular; [b]sternal.

From J.C. Griffin, 2015, *Client-centered exercise prescription,* 3rd ed. (Champaign, IL: Human Kinetics).

FORM 5.2 JAM Chart: Shoulder Girdle Muscles and Their Actions

Muscles	Elevation	Depression	Abduction	Adduction	Upward rotation	Downward rotation
Pectoralis minor		PM	PM			PM
Serratus anterior			PM		PM	
Trapezius 1	PM					
Trapezius 2	PM			AM	PM	
Trapezius 3				PM		
Trapezius 4		PM		AM	PM	
Levator scapulae	PM					
Rhomboid	PM			PM		PM

Note: Large muscles of the shoulder joint can influence shoulder girdle actions. PM = prime mover; AM = assistant mover.

From J.C. Griffin, 2015, *Client-centered exercise prescription,* 3rd ed. (Champaign, IL: Human Kinetics).

FORM 5.3 JAM Chart: Elbow and Radioulnar Joint Muscles and Their Actions

Muscles	Flexion	Extension	Pronation	Supination
Biceps brachii	PM			AM
Brachialis	PM			
Brachioradialis	PM		AM	AM
Pronator quadratus			PM	
Pronator teres			AM	
Supinator				PM
Triceps brachii		PM		
Wrist extensors (posterior forearm)		AM		
Wrist flexors (anterior forearm)	AM			

Note: PM = prime mover; AM = assistant mover.

From J.C. Griffin, 2015, *Client-centered exercise prescription,* 3rd ed. (Champaign, IL: Human Kinetics).

FORM 5.4 JAM Chart: Hip Joint Muscles and Their Actions

Muscles	Flexion	Extension	Abduction	Adduction	Medial rotation	Lateral rotation
Iliacus	PM[a]					AM
Psoas	PM[a]					AM
Rectus femoris	PM[a]					
Pectineus	PM[a]			PM	AM	
Sartorius	AM		AM			AM
Tensor fasciae latae			PM		AM	
Gluteus medius			PM			
Gluteus minimus			AM		PM	
Gluteus maximus		PM	AM			PM
Semitendinosus		PM				
Semimembranosus		PM				
Biceps femoris (LH)		PM				
Adductor longus				PM		
Adductor brevis				PM		
Adductor magnus				PM		
Gracilis				PM		
Six lateral rotators						PM

PM = prime mover; AM = assistant mover; LH = long head.

[a]These muscles may indirectly cause hyperextension of the low back by tilting the pelvis forward.

From J.C. Griffin, 2015, *Client-centered exercise prescription,* 3rd ed. (Champaign, IL: Human Kinetics).

FORM 5.5   JAM Chart: Knee Joint Muscles and Their Actions

Muscles	Flexion	Extension	Medial rotation	Lateral rotation
Semitendinosus	PM		PM	
Semimembranosus	PM		PM	
Biceps femoris	PM			PM
Rectus femoris		PM		
Vastus lateralis		PM		
Vastus intermedius		PM		
Vastus medialis		PM		
Sartorius	AM		AM	
Gracilis	AM		AM	
Popliteus			PM	
Gastrocnemius	AM			

Note: PM = prime mover; AM = assistant mover.

From J.C. Griffin, 2015, *Client-centered exercise prescription,* 3rd ed. (Champaign, IL: Human Kinetics).

FORM 5.6   JAM Chart: Ankle and Foot Muscles and Their Actions

Muscles	Dorsiflexion	Plantar flexion	Inversion	Eversion
Gastrocnemius		PM		
Soleus		PM		
Tibialis posterior[a]		AM	PM	
Peroneus longus[a]		AM		PM
Peroneus brevis		AM		PM
Flexor digitorum longus[a]		AM	AM	
Flexor hallucis longus[a]		AM	AM	
Tibialis anterior	PM		PM	
Peroneus tertius	PM			PM
Extensor digitorum longus	PM			PM
Extensor hallucis longus	AM		AM	

Note: PM = prime mover; AM = assistant mover.

[a]These muscles also support the arch.

From J.C. Griffin, 2015, *Client-centered exercise prescription,* 3rd ed. (Champaign, IL: Human Kinetics).

FORM 5.7   JAM Chart: Spinal Muscles and Their Actions

	Flexion	Extension	Lateral flexion	Rotation (same side)	Rotation (opposite side)
Lumbar and thoracic spines					
Rectus abdominis	PM		AM		
External oblique	PM		PM		PM
Internal oblique	PM		PM	PM	
Psoas	AM	a			
Quadratus lumborum		AM	PM		
Erector spinae group		PM	PM	PM	
Deep posterior group		PM	PM		PM
Cervical spine					
Sternocleidomastoid	PM		PM		PM
Scaleni group	AM		PM		
Erector spinae group		PM	PM	PM	
Deep posterior group		PM	PM		PM

Note: PM = prime mover; AM = assistant mover.

[a]The psoas may pull the spine into hyperextension without balance from the abdominal muscles, especially if the iliacus tilts the pelvis forward.

From J.C. Griffin, 2015, *Client-centered exercise prescription,* 3rd ed. (Champaign, IL: Human Kinetics).

FORM 5.8 Exercise Demonstration Model Checklist

1. **Predemonstration**
   - ❏ Set climate by making client feel comfortable and being receptive and responsive.
   - ❏ Provide overview by explaining the purpose of this session and what is to happen in this session.
   - ❏ Determine client's background and experience by asking, "Have you done this exercise before?" "Have you used this type of equipment before?" "What was your experience?"
   - ❏ Clarify purpose of exercises by explaining the specific muscles used (major prime movers) and relevance to stated needs and wants.
   - ❏ Encourage the client to ask questions and provide input.

2. **Demonstration**
   - ❏ Provide precise and appropriate verbal instructions.
   - ❏ Position client appropriately to watch demo.
   - ❏ Provide clear physical demonstration (4-6 reps before client trial).
   - ❏ Ensure that overall technical execution was smooth and confident.
   - ❏ Ensure beginning position alignment and proper grip.
   - ❏ Isolate the movement (i.e., no compensation or inappropriate movements).
   - ❏ Stabilize the pelvis and key joints.
   - ❏ Ensure that terminal points of range of motion were appropriate.
   - ❏ Demonstrate safety, including controlled breathing and no Valsalva maneuver.
   - ❏ Demonstrate safety, including controlled speed and no momentum at the end of the range of motion.
   - ❏ Ensure efficient use of time with descriptions and explanations.

3. **Client trials**
   - ❏ Set client up by positioning and alignment.
   - ❏ Select appropriate weight (moderately difficult).
   - ❏ Ensure trial safety by controlling breathing, momentum, and plane of movement and ensuring no joint locking.
   - ❏ Ensure effective spotting by being in position to observe and assist with starting and finishing positions.
   - ❏ Have client execute a full set.
   - ❏ Provide feedback to the client, which may include providing specific information and monitoring, focusing on behavior and not the person, correcting one aspect at a time, and being positive and helpful (providing success).
   - ❏ Demonstrate verbal skills such as cueing during execution, paraphrasing, summarizing, and questioning.
   - ❏ Demonstrate nonverbal skills such as using correct body position, being engaged, providing eye contact, and ignoring distractions.

4. **Follow-up**
   - ❏ Obtain feedback from client by asking how it felt (i.e., awkward, comfortable, difficult) and encouraging the client to ask questions and provide input.
   - ❏ Demonstrate active listening skills by responding to feedback.
   - ❏ Provide prescription guidelines (including weight, reps, and sets, or frequency, intensity, time, and type) that integrate and interpret information from client trial.
   - ❏ Suggest a method of progression or encourage self-monitoring and assessment.
   - ❏ Provide a modification on request (problem solving).

From J.C. Griffin, 2015, *Client-centered exercise prescription*, 3rd ed. (Champaign, IL: Human Kinetics).

PART II

Client-Centered Exercise Prescription

The counseling stage of the prescription journey has provided us with a picture of our client's history, needs, and hopes as well as potential sources of motivation. We have helped our clients to clarify priorities by refocusing on what is important. We understand our clients' needs; we have learned about their areas of interests and expectations; we have a very clear picture of what and how our clients want to change; and we have selected assessment items that best match our clients' priorities. We will create exercise strategies based in large part on our interpretation of the counseling and assessment results. The key to a successful program lies in our ability to help clients maintain the conviction that our prescription will bring about the changes they want. Exercise will be a high priority if this personalized connection is maintained. We must provide constant support and reinforcement for this action–benefit relationship.

In this second stage of our journey, we select appropriate exercises and elements of the exercise prescription, from a wide menu of choices, according to how they fit our client's goals. A variety of training methods allow us to match specific benefits to specific clients. It is because of this variety that the client-centered approach to prescription is safe and effective. The details of the personalized exercise prescription are based on two main criteria: the physiological rationale and the client's willingness to accept the program. Knowing this in advance of our prescription design is a powerful tool.

We can prescribe exercise programs to produce three potential outcomes: increased general fitness, performance improvements, or health enhancement. Part II of the book details four prescription models: cardiovascular conditioning, resistance training, functionally integrated exercise including muscle balance and flexibility, and weight management. These models show how adaptation can be manipulated through prudent selection of appropriate exercises, prescription factors, equipment, and training methods.

Although cardiovascular fitness is still the foundation of most exercise prescriptions, the client-centered approach can adjust the outcome to suit more personal goals such as improved performance or reduction of stress or heart disease risk factors. New evidence is reported on high-intensity interval training (HIIT), circuit training, and dynamic warm-ups for highly eccentric workouts.

The challenge with resistance training is to shape the overload to suit your client by manipulating the prescription factors according to the principle of specificity—namely, that gains in muscular fitness are specific to the muscle group, training method, and exercise volume. With a specific focus on training volume, recent research can help us be more client centered for our novice and untrained participants. Exciting new approaches to periodization, instability techniques, and manual resistance will help you expand your offerings.

Our concern with muscle balance is multifaceted: It is not limited to strength, flexibility, or endurance but may involve strength of one muscle group and flexibility of an opposing muscle group following guidelines for functional exercise design. Clients who have muscle imbalances or postural alignment problems can be helped with functionally integrated exercise. New insights into myofascial tissue continuity may help guide our musculoskeletal exercise design.

The unique role of exercise in energy balance is the backdrop for discussion of client issues in weight management. New physical activity recommendations from the American College of Sports Medicine in 2009 are discussed along with a number of special nutritional concerns for active clients.

Each prescription model is similar in format and is followed by case studies, which deal with specific client situations and demonstrate the application of many of the prescription tools. Within each case study, physiological justifications or client-centered (behavioral) justifications are presented for each design decision.

Client-Centered Cardiovascular Exercise Prescription Model

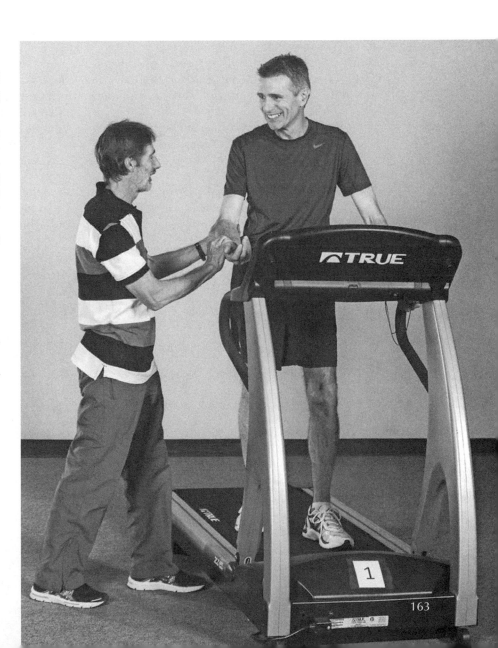

Chapter Competencies

After completing this chapter, you will be able to demonstrate the following competencies:

1. Use a seven-step prescription process to guide you through decisions when designing a cardiovascular prescription. (The remaining competencies reflect the seven steps of the model for cardiovascular exercise prescription.)
2. Review client needs and confirm goals.
3. Select activities and equipment.
4. Select training method.
5. Set intensity and workload.
6. Set volume.
7. Design progression and monitoring.
8. Design a warm-up and a cool-down.

Although cardiovascular fitness is still the foundation of most exercise prescriptions, you can use the client-centered approach to adjust the outcome to suit more personal goals (e.g., reduction of stress or of risk factors for coronary heart disease, improved performance). Explaining to a client that with 4 months of aerobic exercise she can increase her maximum oxygen uptake by 15% may be realistic; but if her goal is to reduce stress, knowing about the oxygen uptake increase will provide scant encouragement. Always explain potential benefits and interpret observed results in terms of the client's goals.

The cardiovascular prescription model uses a seven-step prescription process to guide you through decisions concerning exercise intensity, volume, and progression based on access to test data, past experience, availability of monitoring equipment, and the client's exercise needs and level of fitness. Physiological justifications and client-centered (behavioral) justifications for each choice made in the prescription model are reinforced with several case studies.

Following is the Client-Centered Cardiovascular Exercise Prescription Model, which will serve both as an overview of what is to come and as a useful tool for review (table 6.1). It outlines a seven-step model for physiologically sound and client-centered exercise prescription for cardiovascular fitness. Each step describes a decision that you will face. Many of the choices available for each decision are listed for each step. Following a brief background for each step, sample case studies are presented, including the choices that were made for the client and a justification for those choices. At the end of the chapter is the Client-Centered Cardiovascular Exercise Prescription Worksheet (form 6.1) to help in your final design.

Step 1: Review Client Needs and Confirm Goals

As noted in part I, client needs may be related to medical or high-risk (e.g., elevated blood lipids, hypertension), educational (e.g., shoe features), or motivational (e.g., lack of self-esteem) factors. Client needs also can be determined by results of fitness assessments (e.g., oxygen uptake) or by physical limitations attributable to weight or orthopedics. Chapter 4 identifies a number of laboratory and field-based cardiovascular assessments. It also outlines how careful screening procedures can identify when medical intervention is warranted. Often the client is unaware of emerging needs such as borderline hypertension or lack of core strength. Gathering information on her activity profile can establish current levels of energy expenditure.

Recall that goal setting involves specifying what needs to be done, when and how to do it, and the anticipated outcomes. Integrating needs, wants, and lifestyle will increase the probability of compliance with any prescription. It is often easier to begin with long-term goals that are more global and then direct the client's attention to formulating several shorter-term goals that could be accomplished before major changes in assessment measures. You can play a vital role by helping your client set realistic, measurable goals and posting them for regular review. The client's goal has a direct influence on the design of the program in many ways. The case studies in this chapter demonstrate this diversity dramatically whether the client is concerned about health, fitness, or athletic performance. Explaining to your client how your prescription decisions suit her goals will significantly affect her compliance in the early stages of exercise. Because this step is so important, periodically review part I until you are sure that you have a firm grasp of the principles of counseling, motivating, and enhancing adherence and of client-centered assessment and prescription.

Before continuing on to the next step, review the choices presented in step 1 of the Cardiovascular Exercise Prescription Model (table 6.1).

Step 2: Select Activities and Equipment

Your reflective listening, probes, and clarification will give your client a clearer picture of the type (mode) of activity he would like to do and any equipment he may need. Clients select their activities based on the benefits they see from their own perspective, not necessarily yours. The challenge is to demonstrate clearly how an activity will fill their wants and needs. As outlined in part I, three steps will increase your chances of demonstrating this: (1) Come up with options, (2) analyze the options, and (3) lead the client to commitment. Select the activities of highest priority, determine those that present the best combination of options, and discuss the most effective strategy for integrating the new activity or equipment.

Table 6.1 Client-Centered Cardiovascular Exercise Prescription Model

Decisions	Choices

1. Review needs and confirm goals.	• Screening—medical history: intervention needed (e.g., meds)
	• Limitations (e.g., CV risk, orthopedic issues, injury, test results)
	• Activity profile and history (review current energy expenditure)
	• Design considerations or preferences (e.g., time, equipment availability, location)
	• Priorities: health, fitness, performance
	• Motivational strategy, personality, learning style
	• Stress management issues
	• Assessment interpretation:
	  • Functional capacity (e.g., maximum oxygen uptake, aerobic fitness score) and normative or health rating
	  • Heart rate, blood pressure, and perceived exertion responses (recovery rate, steady states, termination criteria)
	  • Visual signs, symptoms, comments

2. Select activities and equipment.	• Equipment (and brand) pros and cons • Equipment features (e.g., info display, braking mechanism) • Treadmill, run, walk • Bicycle, ergometer • Elliptical trainer • Rower • Stepper • Swim • In-line skating • Group classes, activities, sports • American College of Sports Medicine (ACSM) groups 1 and 2—aerobic • Specific exercises (order)
3. Select training method.	• Continuous • Interval • Circuit • Plyometrics (see chapter 7) • Cross-training, sports • Fartlek • Active living
4. Set intensity and workload.	Recommended training zone: • %$\dot{V}O_2$ reserve, % max METs, %HRR, perceived exertion (e.g., 40/50-85% $\dot{V}O_2$ reserve/HRR—sufficient to complete duration and tolerate the exercise without risk) • Calculate corresponding workload (e.g., ACSM metabolic formulas) or select a workload that elicits an appropriate HR (e.g., 40/50-85% HRR); verify selection during demo client trial • Calculate kcal/min (e.g., chart or L/min × 5 kcal) • Recreational sport and active living (MET/kcal chart) • Manipulate balance with duration and frequency • Confirm consistency with goals and needs
5. Set volume (duration and frequency).	Total work per session (intensity and duration) • Intervals: duration of work and rest • 20-30 min, progressing to 45-60 min • 250-500 kcal/session • Frequency: minimum 2 times/week; recommend 3-5 times/week (daily active living) • Total work/week (intensity, duration, and frequency)—1000-2000 kcal/week • Supplement with active living recommendations

(continued)

(continued)

Decisions	Choices
6. Design progression and monitoring.	• Stage of progression (ACSM: initial, improvement, maintenance) • Stage of training (periodization) • Methods of progression—FITT (e.g., increase time initially) • Rate of progression (1-3%/week; e.g., 10-12% in first month) • Monitoring to cue progression timing • Monitoring to suit client's objectives but avoid overtraining • Monitoring to motivate • Follow-up checks established • Primary safety precautions listed
7. Design warm-up and cool-down.	• CV warm-up and cool-down transitions • Specific joint and muscle stretching before and after • Suits nature of the prescription and client specifics (e.g., mode, time, intensity, monitoring)

Note: CV = cardiovascular; MET = metabolic equivalent; HR = heart rate; HRR = heart rate reserve; FITT = frequency, intensity, time, and type.

Cardiovascular Activities

It is often easier for your client to talk about his needs and goals than it is to select an activity or exercises, because the latter is the start of a specific commitment. Some clients may be so overwhelmed by the whole exercise thing that even basic exercises or the simplest of equipment intimidates them at first. Others may hate the idea of exercising indoors and want only to do sports or aerobic exercise outside. You need to anticipate this reaction and be ready to accommodate those needs. Situations often change as well. Substituting an indoor cardio circuit for an outdoor run during a bad storm, switching to a rower or recumbent bike during a bout of shin splints, or advising a client on breathable rainwear for his new walking program will modify the activity selection and remove those barriers to regular exercise.

Your clients generally will be most satisfied with modes of exercise that allow them to sustain intensity with some variability and with ease of monitoring. These modes include walking, jogging, running, swimming, cycling, cross-country skiing, ice skating, in-line skating, stepping, skipping, and rowing. Cardiovascular improvements are comparable for most modes of aerobic exercise as long as intensity, frequency, and duration of exercise are prescribed in accordance with sound scientific principles (Heyward 2010).

Cardiovascular prescriptions typically include FITT (frequency, intensity, time, type); informed choices and options for different exercise modes are less commonly advised. Rinne, Miilunpalo, and Heinonen (2007) evaluated the motor abilities and physical fitness components of those exercise modes that middle-aged people most commonly practice—information that you need when counseling clients to start a physically active lifestyle. They examined five different motor abilities (e.g., reaction ability) and four fitness components (including cardiovascular endurance). They concluded that when adopting physical activity behavior, inactive people should be counseled to start with exercise modes with fewer motor requirements, such as walking, jogging, cycling, and calisthenics. These authors view skating, downhill skiing, and martial arts as requiring all five motor abilities and for this reason suggest that they might not be preferred exercise modes for beginners. Squash, badminton, and jazz dance involve reasonably high levels of motor abilities and physical fitness.

Aerobic Equipment

Most people will eventually use some form of aerobic exercise equipment. Thus we must understand the features as well as the design, manufacture, safety, cost, and serviceability of a variety of aerobic equipment.

Accurately assessing your clients' needs is the most important part of equipment selection. This is particularly important when your client selects outdoor or sporting activities that you will not attend. You must be prepared to provide guidance on appropriate quality equipment and maintenance: for example, a mountain bike that suits the challenge of the terrain, running shoes that won't cause shin splints, in-line skates that are well made and that fit, or a good quality life jacket for rowing. Have a list of trusted retail stores and experienced proprietors who can assist you with this service. Equipment should suit the anatomy, interests, and fitness levels of your clients. They want equipment that will not cause overuse injuries, is low impact, provides well-rounded fitness, and, most of all, makes efficient use of their time.

Even though the client's preferences and availability of equipment will usually narrow the choices, you probably will need to show your clients how certain equipment can contribute to their goals. Because boredom and lack of comfort are the reasons people give most often for not using aerobic equipment (Dishman 1990), you must be proactive in preventing frustration and providing stimulation (through equipment change or use of video) as you work through questions of equipment use with your client.

Nonportable Equipment

Table 6.2 examines the design and safety features of a variety of common machines and identifies the type of client for which these features are most beneficial (table 6.2). Although comfort, appearance, durability, and cost are important factors in exercise machines, the mechanism that provides resistance and the mechanics of the movement are the most critical features to scrutinize.

- **Treadmills.** In 1994, 16.2 million Americans walked for fitness at least twice a week; nearly half that number jogged or ran (Sillery 1996). This adds up to the largest identifiable group of exercisers. It is not surprising that treadmills have become so popular. Treadmills burn more calories than any other simulator at heart rates of 65%, 75%, and 85% of age-adjusted maximum (Allen and Goldberg 1986).

- **Stationary bicycles.** The choices here include electronic, in which the pedaling effort is controlled electronically, and nonelectronic, in which the resistance mechanism is a belt circling a heavy flywheel. Your clients may choose either an upright or a recumbent-style bike. The upright bike is the most common piece of equipment in most centers.

Table 6.2   Equipment–Client Match-Up

Design and safety features	How does it suit the client?
Treadmills	
Provide alternative to the hazards of outdoor running and walking	Are useful in inclement weather (e.g., too hot, cold, stormy) or unsafe times, locations, health conditions
Allow precise measurement	Are useful for stress testing, rehab, and medical assessments (prescription is more accurate if the treadmill was also used for the assessment)
Provide fingertip control of speed and elevation	Allow personalized fine-tuning
Allow user to set course and pace according to stature and condition	Allow prescription to be fed into the electronic circuitry to control workout
Are easy to learn and use	Can feel awkward to mount and control the panel while using the machine
Provide reduced impact versus outdoors for runners	Are useful for clients with lower extremity or back problems or those who are overweight
Have monitoring features	Are helpful for higher-risk clients or for feedback and motivation
Have preprogramming capabilities	Encourage proper warm-ups and cool-downs because they are part of the program; provide interval and continuous options
Stationary bicycles	
Are long lasting, heavy duty, affordable (nonelectronic bicycles)	Are suitable for home programs; are space efficient and portable
Often have exciting computer graphics (electronic bicycles)	Can increase motivation through immediate feedback (e.g., simulated hills)
Offer option to control pedaling effort by heart rate response to the ride	Optimize training level and a safety feature

(continued)

(continued)

Design and safety features	How does it suit the client?
Allow precise measurement	Are useful for stress testing, rehab, and medical assessments (prescription is more accurate if the bike was also used for the assessment)
Provide preprogramming capabilities on most electronic models	Encourage proper warm-ups and cool-downs; provide interval and continuous options
Offer greater comfort (recumbent bikes)	Are suited to clients with back problems; provide greater loading for gluteals and hamstrings and reduce lower leg weight bearing
Rowers	
Provide low impact, especially for the lower body	Provide good aerobic alternative if weight bearing is a problem
Provide quality simulation via the air and flywheel	Are affordable for home use and comfortable to use
Work muscles of the legs, shoulders, back, and arms	Provide overall muscular endurance benefits for large muscle groups of the body
Cause some compression and shearing forces in the lower back	Are not suitable for clients with low back pain
Can be smaller than other types of equipment (some home models)	Are space efficient and portable
Can have TV, audio, and modulation of workout variables (e.g., competition, time, speed) (some electronic models)	Increase motivation through immediate feedback; provide interval and continuous options
Stair climbers	
Foot platforms must hinge to remain parallel to the floor	Clients with ankle or knee problems will have added stress if platforms don't hinge (e.g., knee hyperextension)
Independent step allows both steps to go up or down whereas dependent step has one go up when the other comes down	Independent takes a little more practice to learn but offers more control and often less weight shifting
Electronic models offer programming and monitoring displays	Provide tracking of floors climbed, floors per minute, calories, and elapsed time, which increase interest and motivation
Motor skill and balance are an issue with some models	May be inappropriate for some seniors or clients with a balance or coordination problem; weight bearing with arms may cause elbow overuse injuries
Some models have an aerobic self-test option	Care should be taken not to place too much confidence in the self-test results
Elliptical trainers	
Provide lower impact forces because feet never leave footpads	Are suitable for clients with higher risk of lower extremity orthopedic injury
Offer wide range of intensities with low impact	Provide a good substitute for jogging
Are able to go backward as well as forward	Backward direction may not burn more calories but it adds variety and appears to involve the hip extensors more actively
At similar ratings of perceived exertion (13), elliptical has heart rates and oxygen consumption values similar to those for running but less than half the ground reaction force (Porcari et al. 2000)	Provide high aerobic benefit with decreased impact-related risks
Shape of ellipse can vary on different machines and change the "feel" of the movement	Clients should always try the machine first, especially if purchasing for home use
Energy expenditure is higher than for walking yet still low impact	Are well suited to overweight clients and fit seniors

- **Rowing machines.** Rowers have come a long way since the squeaky spring-loaded models tucked away in attics and garages. Except for a few designs like the hydraulic resistance rowers, most provide a realistic feel to the rowing action. Most nonelectronic machines use a flywheel for resistance; many people like the feel of the air machines more than the more expensive electronic models. The upper body workout provided by rowing machines is an attractive added benefit for many clients. Because these machines permit such great freedom of technique, however, clients risk injuring themselves. Show your clients how to use their legs to push off, not their backs, and to maintain a smooth pull with the arms in and just below chest level.

- **Stair climbers.** An attractive feature of these machines is that, in addition to providing excellent aerobic benefits, they provide muscular conditioning to the lower body. Many people should begin with a short range of motion and a slow stepping rate. To reduce stress on the knees, clients should not lean into the machine or move their knees forward over their toes during stepping. Leaning forward also increases strain on the low back.

- **Elliptical trainers.** Elliptical trainers involve a lower body motion that is a cross between an upright stationary cycle and a stepper, except that the feet move in an elliptical pattern as opposed to a circular path. The low impact forces and wide ranges of aerobic intensity are good news for clients looking for a high-intensity, low-impact substitute to jogging.

Transportable Equipment

The most effective, versatile, and portable piece of equipment you own is yourself. You are the computer, the feedback display, the variable resistance, the monitor, and the motivation machine. Still, some equipment is needed to enable you to deliver the best possible workout to each client. Whether advising a client about a purchase or building your own collection, strongly consider adding some affordable and transportable pieces of aerobic equipment. The following is not an exhaustive list, but consider the items first from a personal preference perspective; then consider cost versus benefit, portability, need for multiple units (e.g., team training), and space.

- **Bench step.** Steps have probably done more to change the industry than most other equipment. Not only have the inexpensive platforms brought more men into the aerobics circle, but steps have expanded the concept of methods of training. They are effective tools for interval and circuit training, particularly when step training and conditioning exercises are combined (Brooks and Copeland-Brooks 1991). Bench steps are a good alternative for people who would rather not walk or jog or invest large sums of money in aerobic machinery.

- **Slide.** This 8 ft (2.4 m) piece of plastic, with angled bumpers and low-friction slippers, allows for a reasonably intense lower body and aerobic workout. Various slide techniques and arm movements can increase variety and can be combined with step or other exercises for an interval or circuit design. Slides can be adapted for sports such as hockey. Clients with ankle or knee instability should be cautious when using slides.

- **Videos.** Commercial fitness videos have expanded to the point where they are targeting specific groups and needs. Whether your client is a senior, is an athlete, is overweight, or wants to work her heart, buttocks, or thighs, there is something she can buy! Help her screen videos for the appropriate intensity level, style, and degree of safety. Consider videotaping a workout for your client to use during travel, during vacation, or when you can't get together.

- **Recreational and sporting equipment.** Any equipment that helps your client associate fitness with fun will serve you both well. There are many opportunities for bicycling, one-on-one basketball, in-line skating, cross-country skiing, tennis, throwing Frisbees, and even shadow boxing.

- **Home swimming pool.** The buoyancy of water reduces the impact of land-based aerobic exercise. Older adults, obese individuals, clients with arthritis or back pain, and rehabilitating athletes will gain major benefits from aquatic exercise. Basic aquatic exercise movements include walking, jogging, kicking, jumping, and scissors against the resistance of the water. The client may also wear paddles on her hands, devices to increase drag through the water, or flotation devices used in the deep end to keep the head above water while moving.

- **Skipping rope.** Rope skipping is quite intense, can be high impact, and takes some skill; however, various techniques of lower-intensity and lower-impact skipping can make it a viable station within a circuit. The rope also can be used as a source of resistance or as a stretching device.

- **Music.** Building a client's endurance or time at an activity is a challenge. Music does more than distract from sweat and pain. Studies on perceived exertion have shown that music makes an exercise session feel easier and extends the time required to reach exhaustion (Iknoian 1992). Preparing music for your client or downloading from the Internet is greatly simplified by the availability of commercial speed-adjusted recordings from funky exercise to soft stretch.

- **Gaming systems.** Exergaming is a term used for video games that are also a form of exercise. Exergaming relies on technology that tracks body movement or reaction. The Wii has been seen as more physically demanding than sedentary game consoles. However, a study in *British Medical Journal* (Graves et al. 2007) showed that although playing the Wii uses significantly more energy than playing sedentary computer games, the energy used in playing active Wii games is not high enough in intensity to contribute toward the recommended daily amount of exercise in children.

- **Fitness apps.** In the last few years there has been a huge increase in the number of fitness apps for iPhone and iPod Touch (Wachner 2012). With most less than $10 and many free, these are a popular choice for the under-40 crowd. Whether you want to track your running, download an aerobics class, or follow a home cardio workout, the choices seem endless. Buyer or downloader beware regarding quality and safety.

- **Dog leash.** A greater proportion of those who regularly walked their dogs were more likely than those who didn't own dogs to meet the recommendations of 150 min of physical activity per week.

Chapter 7 examines different types of portable home resistance equipment. Many of these items can be used in aerobic or mixed-component circuit training.

Endurance Activities by Intensity

Any activity that uses large muscle groups, can be maintained, and is rhythmic and aerobic can increase cardiovascular endurance. The American College of Sports Medicine (ACSM 2009) classifies cardiovascular endurance activities into three groups:

- **Group 1:** Physical activities in which exercise intensity is easily sustained with little variability in heart rate response: walking, aerobic dancing, swimming, jogging, running, and cycling

- **Group 2:** Physical activities in which energy expenditure is related to skill but for a given individual can provide a constant intensity: figure skating, swimming, highly choreographed dance exercise, cross-country skiing, and skating

- **Group 3:** Physical activities that are quite variable in intensity and skill: soccer, basketball, and racquetball

Group 1 activities are most appropriate for beginning clients who need to carefully control intensity. Group 2 activities are often outside of the gym, providing an enjoyable venue. Combining a group 1 and a group 2 activity can reduce boredom and attrition and improve skill levels. Group 3 activities may be the most fun and provide variety and cross-training opportunities. They are often group oriented, adding a social element. The sporadic changes in intensity demand caution: People should spend time in a group 1 activity (e.g., preseason conditioning) before entering a group 3 activity.

Before continuing on to the next step, review the choices presented in step 2 of the Cardiovascular Exercise Prescription Model (table 6.1).

Client-Centered Tips for Setting Cardiovascular Mode

Whenever possible, the test mode should be specific to the training mode—if your client will be training on a bicycle, test her on a bicycle. Monitor your clients to verify that the workload you prescribed is eliciting the desired heart rate and perceived exertion. This is especially important if no assessment was done or if the training mode is different from the assessment mode.

If the total work (intensity × duration × frequency) and initial fitness status are similar, the mode of activity does not significantly influence the cardiovascular training effect. However, each activity has some local or specific muscle benefits. Therefore, consider selecting a mode that will enhance other objectives such as isolating a body area or pursuing cross-training benefits for a sport.

Consider the possibility of overuse or acute injury when selecting the mode. For athletes, this may mean selecting a fitness mode that provides some rest for overused joints. You can use metabolic calculations and charts (see table 6.7 later in the chapter) to match activities with energy costs, but you will need to monitor and fine-tune the results (see "Metabolic Calculations" in the later section "MET Level Method").

Step 3: Select Training Method

Select a training method based on your conversations with your client about

- stated preferences and interests,
- goals and objectives,
- availability and convenience (facility, equipment, time),
- skills and background,
- suitability (e.g., level of fitness, risk), and
- other desired benefits (e.g., enhanced skills, social opportunities, targeted energy system).

Although some training methods rely mainly on one energy system, usually they use a combination of two or even three (see "Energy Systems Used by the Body"). Consequently, different types of exercises and training methods will be needed to maximize your client's use of the required system. The two broad categories of aerobic methods are continuous and interval training. Research indicates that both are effective in improving cardiovascular fitness (Heyward 2010). The methods differ in their physiological bases, types of demand, and benefits. You must select the method and the training factors that match your client's needs. Although continuous and interval training are two of the most popular training methods, it may be more suitable for your clients to use circuit training, cross-training, fartlek training, or simply active living.

Continuous Training

Continuous training (CT) involves exercise (walking, jogging, in-line skating, cycling, stair climbing, swimming) at a moderate intensity with no rest intervals. Fitness runners often adopt a low-intensity CT program, termed long slow distance training (LSD). However, higher-intensity CT programs have been shown to offer more significant improvements.

There are many advantages to CT for certain clients:

- Low to moderate intensities (e.g., 40-70% $\dot{V}O_2$ or 60-80% maximum heart rate [HRmax]) are safe, comfortable, and able to produce health and cardiovascular benefits for less fit individuals.
- Continuous training is generally well suited for clients initiating an aerobic exercise program.
- Dropout rates for adults may be half those for high-intensity interval programs (Dishman 1990).
- A prescribed exercise intensity is easily maintained in an evenly paced workout.
- Continuous training is generally less taxing physiologically and psychologically and therefore requires minimal motivation.
- Daily workouts are possible, because glycogen is not depleted to the extent that it cannot be replenished within 24 h (Wilmore and Costill 2004).
- Continuous submaximal training is appropriate for athletes during the off-season and during the competitive season as a light day alternating with heavier interval days.
- Benefits to the oxygen transport system from CT are more easily transferred from one mode of training to another or to a specific sport.

Energy Systems Used by the Body

1. Adenosine triphosphate (ATP) is the immediately usable form of chemical energy stored in muscle cells and used for muscular activity. The ATP–PC system is an anaerobic energy system that resynthesizes ATP from energy released when phosphocreatine (PC) is broken down. This energy system is a very rapid but limited source of ATP that is used predominantly during high-power, short-duration activities. Phosphocreatine is restored for reuse during each relief interval (50% in 30 s, 75% in 60 s, 95% in 2 min), thereby reducing reliance on the lactic acid system.

2. The lactic acid (LA) system, also anaerobic, resynthesizes ATP from energy released during the breakdown of glycogen (sugar) to lactic acid. Accumulation of the latter causes muscular fatigue. This system is used mainly during activities that require between 1 and 3 min of maximum effort.

3. The oxygen system uses both glycogen and fats as fuels for ATP resynthesis. By a series of reactions that take place in the mitochondria of the cells, the system yields large amounts of ATP but no fatiguing byproducts. The aerobic system is used predominantly during endurance tasks or low power output activities.

This provides a variety of training activities and is well suited to incorporation of cross-training techniques.

- Fewer injuries are reported in CT than in interval training (Pollock et al. 1977).

Depending on the client and the desired outcome, the optimal prescription can vary considerably based on the following guidelines:

- **Athletes and well-conditioned clients.** Continuous exercise involving large muscle groups at 75% of the client's aerobic capacity or $\dot{V}O_2$ (around 85% HRmax) optimally trains the central oxygen transport system (Wilmore and Costill 2004). Powers and Howley (2009) reported that a work rate at or near the lactate threshold provides excellent improvement in maximal aerobic power.

- **Average client.** Training gains for the average client initiating a program may start at 50% to 70% $\dot{V}O_2$ or 65% to 80% HRmax (Heyward 2010).

- **Sedentary client.** Health benefits may be seen at as low as 40% of $\dot{V}O_2$ (60% HRmax) (ACSM 2009).

When the intensity level causes a sharp increase in lactic acid production and in fatigue, your client has reached the *anaerobic threshold*. The duration of the training session will be shortened dramatically if she exercises above this intensity level. The greatest benefits without early fatigue are provided with intensities just below the anaerobic threshold. Anaerobic threshold can be measured accurately in a laboratory. With some guidance, however, your client can learn to recognize the abrupt increase in ventilation and rating of perceived exertion (RPE) that occur when she exceeds her threshold.

If you have not determined an anaerobic threshold through aerobic assessment or a submaximal test, you can calculate a crude but generally effective target heart rate (THR) from the equation

$$THR = RHR + 75\% \ (HRmax - RHR)$$

where RHR = the resting heart rate and HRmax = the maximum heart rate (estimated as 220 − age). The percentage is based on the client and outcome guidelines listed earlier in this chapter. Use the target heart rate initially as an approximate guide. Then, by trial and error, adjust the intensity to keep your client just below the anaerobic threshold. Your client can maintain or adjust the intensity level for CT by monitoring her peak training heart rate and her perceived exertion level.

Interval Training

In interval training (IT), periods of low-intensity exercise (which use the body's aerobic energy system) are alternated with periods of higher-intensity exercise (which use anaerobic energy systems). Interval training is a high-intensity effort designed to enhance performance, usually in a competitive sport. Because one energy system can recover while the other is being used, your client is able to exercise for long periods of time with a greater total amount of work performed.

Interval training improves the body's ability to adapt and recover. Like CT, it improves cardiorespiratory fitness (Heyward 2010). It also provides paced training that athletes can monitor and modify to suit their training phase and purpose. These and many other advantages make IT attractive for many people:

- When you know which energy systems you want to emphasize, IT allows for great variations. You can regulate it to develop mainly aerobic, anaerobic, or muscular systems. You can target specific energy systems for improvement.

- Interval training often stimulates the aerobic system without producing the high levels of lactic acid that occur with continuous higher-intensity exercise. During the recovery phase of IT, heart rate declines at a proportionately greater rate than the return of blood to the heart, resulting in brief increases in stroke volume many times during a workout. This process increases myocardial strength and enables the muscles to be quickly cleared of waste products (lactic acid) (Wilmore and Costill 2004).

- Interval training achieves the greatest amount of work possible with the least fatigue (although longer workout times are usually necessary).

- This form of training offers several ways to provide a training overload: intensity of work interval, work-to-relief ratio, and total number of intervals (reps).

- High-intensity intervals are more effective in improving lactate threshold, perhaps because of the recruitment of fast-twitch fibers (Powers and Howley 2009).

- By examining the requirements of a particular event and the energy systems used, you can design an IT program that provides specificity of training.

- If used late preseason and selectively during the season, IT can peak an athlete's performance.

- For clients in poor condition who have trouble maintaining their training intensity, the work relief intervals of IT allow them to complete more total work.

- The ACSM (2009) recommends IT for symptomatic individuals who can tolerate only low-intensity exercise for short periods of time (1-2 min).
- The frequent breaks in activity allow you to monitor your client and make appropriate adjustments.
- The possibility of greater variety is a motivating factor.

To prescribe IT, you will need to know the following terms (Karp 2000):

- **Work interval:** That portion of the IT program consisting of the work effort (e.g., a 220 yd [about 200 m] run performed within a prescribed time).
- **Relief interval:** The time between work intervals in a set. The relief interval may consist of light activity such as walking (rest relief) or mild to moderate exercise such as jogging (work relief).
- **Work–relief ratio:** The ratio of the work and relief intervals. A work–relief ratio of 1:2 means that the work interval is half as long as the relief interval.
- **Set:** A group of work and relief intervals (e.g., six 220 yd runs, each performed within a prescribed time, separated by designated relief intervals).

- **Repetition:** The number of work intervals per set. Six 220 yd runs would constitute six repetitions.
- **Training time:** The rate of work during the work interval (e.g., each 220 yd run might be performed in 28 s).
- **Training distance:** Distance of the work interval (e.g., 220 yd).
- **IT prescription:** Specifications for the routines to be performed in an IT workout. For sample prescriptions, see the case studies in this chapter.

Table 6.3 shows which energy system athletes should develop according to their sport (Fox 1979). For example, because a basketball player relies heavily on anaerobic systems for ATP energy, his IT program should focus on anaerobic systems.

Match your IT prescription to your client's outside activities. For a specific sport, for example, find out the typical length of time during which your client puts in continuous, strenuous effort. Consider ice hockey, which typically has players on the ice for about a 45 to 90 s shift. Use tables 6.3 and 6.4 together. According to table 6.3, ice hockey predominantly uses the ATP–PC–LA energy system. Therefore your hockey-playing client's prescription should emphasize this same system. Now go to table 6.4, find ATP–PC–LA

Table 6.3 Various Sports and Their Predominant Energy Systems

Sport or activity	% Emphasis of energy system		
	ATP–PC–LA	LA and O$_2$	O$_2$
Basketball	85	15	—
Ice hockey	80	20	—
Recreational sports	—	5	95
Skiing, downhill	80	20	—
Skiing, cross-country	—	5	95
Soccer, wings/strikers	80	20	—
Soccer, halfbacks	60	20	20
Swimming, 100 m	80	15	5
Swimming, 1500 m	10	20	70
Tennis	70	20	10
Track and field, field events	90	10	—
Track and field, 400 m	40	55	5
Volleyball	90	10	—

Note: ATP = adenosine triphosphate; PC = phosphocreatine; LA = lactic acid.

Adapted from Fox and Mathews 1974.

in the top row, and note the training time that is closest to the range of a hockey shift (i.e., 30-80 s). According to table 6.4, the prescription for your client should include 4 or 5 repetitions starting with 3 sets, with a work–relief ratio of 1:3 or perhaps 1:2.

Table 6.4 assumes that a high-intensity effort, proportionate to the length of time, is given for the work interval. There is evidence to show that if short-duration, high-intensity intervals interspersed with relatively short relief periods are performed (15 s work:15 s relief; i.e., 1:1 ratio), peak oxygen consumption can also be improved (Helgerud et al. 2007).

These IT prescription factors may need fine-tuning if

- the work is not difficult or is too difficult,
- your client is in poor or very good condition,
- your client is fresh or near the end of the workout, or
- the training signs (e.g., recovery heart rates) do not seem appropriate.

Two of the most important considerations with an IT prescription are sufficient work rate and sufficient relief and recovery. For short, highly intensive performance, the relief interval may be three times as long as the work interval. For longer, less intensive work periods, the relief interval may be equal to or less than the work interval. When the work interval has produced lactic acid, the most rapid removal rate occurs during continuous aerobic activity.

The intermittent nature of IT allows you to monitor the client's heart rate at the end of work intervals and relief intervals. Therefore, relief interval lengths may be determined initially by an appropriate work–relief ratio and then adjusted based on your client's work and relief heart rates. Table 6.5 provides some guidelines for suitable target heart rates for different ages at the conclusion of different intervals.

Cardiovascular function benefits have been reported to be similar between 50 min continuous moderate-intensity cycling and 2 to 3 min all-out cycling(4-6 bouts of 30 s) at a supramaximal workload (Gillen 2012). Along with a considerable number of other scientific findings, low-volume HIIT (high-intensity interval training) may be a highly potent and time-efficient exercise strategy that can provide a range of health benefits in a variety of populations. Gillen (2012) has suggested some step-by-step tips for practitioners and individuals about low-volume HIIT workouts:

- Using a stationary bicycle, warm up for 2 to 3 min at a comfortable pace.
- Increase the resistance on the bicycle to a workload that feels to be about a 9 out of 10 (1 = nothing at all; 10 = maximal effort); then pedal hard for 1 min.

Table 6.4   Guidelines for Interval Training Program Prescription

Energy system	ATP-PC	ATP-PC-LA	LA-O$_2$	O$_2$
Training time*	10-30 s	30-80 s	80 s-3 min	3-5 min
Work–relief ratio	1:3	1:3	1:2 or 1:1	1:1 or 1:1/2
Volume	4-5 sets 8-10 reps	3-5 sets 4-5 reps	1-2 sets 4-6 reps	1 set 3-4 reps

*All-out effort for training time.

Note: ATP = adenosine triphosphate; PC = phosphocreatine; LA = lactic acid.

Steps for Constructing the Interval Training Prescription

Review the steps for constructing an appropriate IT prescription:

1. Using table 6.3, determine which energy system is to be improved.
2. Select the type of exercise to be used during the work interval (e.g., running, cycling, stair climbing, a sport).
3. From table 6.4, select the training times (per work interval), the number of repetitions and sets, the work–relief ratio, and the type of relief interval.
4. Fine-tune the prescription based on your observations of your client's first few workouts.

Table 6.5 Monitoring Target Heart Rates in Interval Training Prescription

Age (years)	Work HR (beats/min)	Relief HR (between reps)	Relief HR (between sets)
Under 20	190	150	125
20-29	180	140	120
30-39	170	130	110
40-49	160	120	105
50-59	150	115	100
60-69	140	105	90

Note: HR = heart rate. Heart rates are for both men and women.

From Fox and Mathews 1974.

- Follow this with 1 min of light cycling that feels like a 4 out of 10. (If needed, this minute can be used for complete rest.)
- Repeat this 1 min on, 1 min off protocol 10 times, for a total of 19 min.
- Cool down at a low intensity for 2 to 3 min.

You can also apply these steps to other modes of exercise, such as swimming, running, or stair climbing. The key is to repeatedly push "hard" for 1 min at a time, with periods of low-intensity exercise or rest interspersed.

Case Studies

Case Study 1: Moderately Fit 34-Year-Old Female

This client wants to follow her favorite aerobic video while interval training for cardiovascular conditioning. The prescription is as follows:

4 × 4:30 (4:00)

where 4 = number of repetitions, 4:30 = training time in minutes and seconds, and (4:00) = time of relief interval in minutes and seconds.

Each work interval consists of following the video for 4 1/2 min, then a relief interval of walking on the spot and stretching while the video is on pause for 4 min. Four repetitions of this sequence constitute a set. The prescription works the oxygen system, with a work-to-rest relief interval of 1:1. For most moderately fit clients, exercise intensities should fall within 70% to 85% of $\dot{V}O_2$ (80-90% of HRmax), starting at the lower end. Create the initial overload by progressively increasing the length of the work period; later, you can decrease the length of the rest relief interval.

Case Study 2: Competitive Squash Player

This client complains of fatiguing too early. The ATP–PC and LA systems are predominant (table 6.3). It is preseason, so you decide to start by working his LA–O$_2$ system. You design a series of carefully timed, on-the-court drills:

- **Set 1:** 6 × 2:30 (3:45) in which each of six drills lasts 2 1/2 min (high intensity) with a 3 min 45 s light exercise (jogging, or using a nearby bike or treadmill)
- **Set 2:** 8 × 1:30 (3:00) in which the drills are slightly shorter but use the same format, intensity, and energy system

Because the recovery intervals will be incomplete, the client will increase his tolerance to lactic acid as well as his anaerobic capacity—important for a squash player. As the season approaches, you progress to a more intense workout of his ATP–PC–LA system. According to the guidelines in table 6.4, this progression will mean shorter (more intense) training intervals and more repetitions per workout, so you will need to prescribe a slightly longer work–relief ratio.

Case Study 3: General Fitness Beginner

This client has had some trouble motivating himself with a CT approach, so his personal fitness trainer has designed two general fitness IT sessions to be alternated on the 2 days in the week they are together. One is a low-intensity IT program, and the second is a high-intensity IT program, both geared to his beginner level.

- Low-intensity IT:
  - 5 min warm-up
  - 4 × 4:00 (4:00) @ 60% to 65% HRmax and walk relief periods
  - 5 min cool-down
- High-intensity IT:
  - 5 min warm-up
  - 2 sets: 4 × 1:00 (2:00) @ 70% to 75% HRmax and light exercise relief periods
  - 5 min cool-down

Circuit Training

Circuit training usually consists of 10 to 15 different exercise stations with the circuit repeated two or three times.

The following advantages of circuit training make it particularly suitable to certain clients:

- Makes efficient use of time for the benefits obtained
- Provides moderate gains in aerobic fitness, muscular strength, and endurance
- Can be adapted for beginners or athletes
- Provides a focus and a challenge to the training
- Can maintain fitness levels when client is recovering from an injury

The stations are either calisthenics (such as stride jumps, stepping, sit-ups, high knee hops, push-ups, pull-ups, skipping), resistance equipment (such as machines, free weights, bands), or a combination. Stations are near one another to facilitate efficient movement. The exercises are selected to avoid repeated use of the same muscle group and early fatigue.

When you prescribe weights, select a moderate intensity (40-60% of maximum capacity) with either a repetition limit such as 15 reps or a timed limit around 30 s. The relief periods between the stations are an important part of the design. For example, with lighter-intensity exercises (or lighter weights), rest periods between stations need be only 15 s—or about the time to move to and get set up at the next station. Circuit weight training typically has an exercise-to-rest ratio of 1:1 (Baechle and Earle 2008). Greater aerobic gains are achieved when relief times involve aerobic activities such as jogging or use of aerobic machines (space and facilities permitting). A client training at home can use the stairs, a skipping rope, an aerobic video, or any number of aerobic calisthenics such as stride jumps, high knee hops, or leg exchange lunges between the weight stations.

Circuit weight training is a compromise between muscular conditioning and aerobic conditioning. Monitoring target heart rate is important. The metabolic requirements of circuit weight training usually meet minimum requirements for the development of aerobic capacity with an aerobic cost of 40% to 60% $\dot{V}O_2$ or 60% to 75% HRmax (ACSM 2009). Some research showed that compared to traditional forms of endurance exercise, circuit training programs were just as beneficial for improving fitness levels and resulted in higher postexercise metabolic rates and strength levels (Kaikkonen et al. 2000). Others reported that the degree of improvement in aerobic capacity using circuit training alone was modest (about 8%), although work capacity in the specific activities increased to a greater degree (ACSM 2010).

Circuit training does not need weights or machinery. A circuit of 8 to 10 aerobic calisthenics will elevate and maintain a heart rate more effectively than weights. For the sample circuit presented in figure 6.1, a 4 to 6 ft (1.2 to 1.8 m) piece of surgical tubing or exercise band can provide added resistance but is not necessary.

In the first or second workout, and then about every 10th workout, you should assess each exercise. Establish the client's starting level by noting, with ample time for recovery between each exercise test, the maximum number of perfectly executed exercises done at each station during 30 s. Watch for excessive momentum, incomplete ranges of motion, and poor alignment. Allot your client 1 min at each station to do the number of repetitions performed on the assessment. With 15 s between each station, one full circuit should take 10 min. After the first circuit trial, you can fine-tune the number of reps. Start with two sets or circuits per session and progress by adding reps to selected stations; you can also progress by including the surgical tubing or exercise band

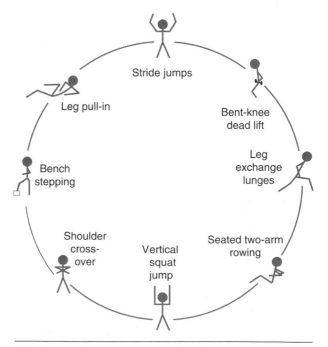

Figure 6.1 The compact versatility of this circuit is a major advantage for clients working in their home with little space or equipment.

or by adding a third circuit. The calisthenics in figure 6.1 involve large muscle groups, including most of the major groups, and should minimize local muscle fatigue.

Cross-Training

Cross-training involves a variety of fitness activities. It provides the flexibility of mixing activities, allowing joints and soft tissues to rest without stopping workouts. Appropriate for the beginner as well as the athlete, cross-training can expand the training benefits of a single-sport exerciser.

Yacenda (1995) explained how runners can use aerobics and swimming to shorten the duration of fatigue in their legs. Runners typically have a high incidence of lower leg overuse problems, but missing workouts means losing an acquired level of aerobic conditioning. Their chronic knee and shin problems may also be mediated with complementary cycling or circuit weight training workouts. Swimmers can gain endurance and joint stability from low-impact aerobic classes. The contrasting stresses are a positive challenge. Cross-training is often selected at a time of injury recovery, because most aerobic training gains are maintained if another mode of activity is substituted for several weeks while an injury is allowed to heal. If your client maintains the cross-training after the injury recovery, it will protect against other single-activity overuse injuries.

The four primary prescription factors for cardiovascular fitness (FITT: frequency, intensity, time, type) can be approximately duplicated regardless of the activity selected. Table 6.6 will help you select aerobic activities based on intensity levels. You can calculate the intensity of exercise as a percentage of your client's maximum metabolic equivalent (MET) value (see "Metabolic Calculations"). If you don't know the appropriate MET training level, start by identifying the activity level that your client can consistently maintain

Table 6.6   Intensity Levels of Aerobic Activity

Activity		Intensity level						
	METs	3-4	4-5	5-6	6-7	7-8	8-9	10+
	kcal/min	4-5	5-6	6-7	7-8	8-10	10-11	11+
Walking	mph	3.0	3.5	4.0	5.0	—	—	—
	min/mile	20	17	15	12	—	—	—
Running	mph	—	—	—	—	5	5.5	6-8
	min/mile	—				12	11	10-7.5
Stationary bicycle (tension kp)	130 lb (59 kg)	1/2	1	1 1/4	1 3/4	2	2 1/4	3+
	175 lb (79 kg)	3/4	1 1/4	1 3/4	2 1/4	2 3/4	3 1/4	4+
Outdoor cycling	mph	6	8	10	11	12	13	15
	min/mile	10	7:30	6	5:30	5	4:40	4
Swimming	mph	—	0.85	1.0	1.25	1.5	1.7	2.0
	s/25 yd (23 m)	—	60	50	43	35	30	25
Bench stepping	154 lb (70 kg)	8 in. × 12/min	8 in. × 18/min	8 in. × 24/min 11 in. × 18/min	11 in. × 24/min 12-6 in. × 18/min	8 in. × 30/min 12-6 in. × 24/min	11 in. × 30/min 15-8 in. × 24/min	(11 mets) 15 in. × 30/min

Note: MET = metabolic equivalent; kp = kiloponds, a measure of brake resistance.

and move across the row to the workload. Any other activity in this column should be close to what your client can perform. Powers and Howley (2009) and the ACSM (2009) have published extensive lists of activity energy expenditures.

Fartlek Training

Fartlek (translation of Swedish term that means "speed play") is a form of training developed in Sweden. It combines elements of CT with IT. Although fartlek is timed and formalized by athletes as a serious mode of training, you can adapt it as an interesting change to a fitness program that can be a lot of fun alone or in a small group.

Fun is the main goal, and distance and time are secondary. People are relatively free to run whatever course and speed they prefer, although the speed should periodically reach high intensity levels. Fartlek involves fast-paced accelerations interspersed with endurance running. The accelerations vary in distance, and the "form" may be a sport-specific action, straight running, or simply playful activity. Fartlek training is often performed in the countryside where there are a variety of hills and terrain. Warm-up is important for this type of training. More than 10 min of jogging and long static stretches of the running muscles are necessary. Runs may last for 40 min or longer.

Here are the advantages of fartlek training that can help you match it to appropriate clients at appropriate stages in their programs:

- The break in monotony from changing speeds and scenery makes it psychologically stimulating.
- It improves both anaerobic and aerobic capacity.
- It is an enjoyable means of achieving cardiovascular fitness and to a lesser extent other health-related aspects of fitness.
- It is a good training break for a small group of athletes and a welcome addition to a serious training program.
- If your client lives in a rural area, the match is a natural one.

Many city parks have fitness trails with exercise stations spread along the pathway. Whereas the true cross-country speed play of fartlek may prove to be too intense for many exercisers, a customized park fitness trail is well suited for many clients.

To simulate a Swedish fartlek, the athlete can start in the country by a lake. After a walk–jog warm-up and some lower body static stretching, the athlete begins with a moderately paced 1 km (0.62 miles) run on flat paths. Coming to a hill, she should attack it at near top speed, walk back down the hill, and repeat this four or five times. She should follow this with a level run at about 75% speed for 3 to 4 min and repeat this sequence two or three times. A few short sprints over local obstacles and an easy jog will bring her back to the lake. Follow with a social sauna, fluid replacement, some stretching, and a plunge in the lake!

Active Living

Gord Stewart (1995) described active living as an enhancement of the simple activities in a daily routine, like walking to the corner store instead of taking the car, or climbing stairs instead of riding the elevator. At first sight, this may not seem like a method of training; but for a majority of adults, the leap into an aerobic class, weight room, or running track is too large a step (see discussion of stages of change in chapter 1).

Recent research has shown that regular, moderately intense activity can provide impressive health benefits (Bouchard et al. 2007; Kesaniemi 2001). Active living is particularly well suited for a previously sedentary or older client concerned about blood pressure, blood lipids, heart health, and preventive medicine. Active living can relieve stress, improve energy, inject enjoyment, and provide feelings of well-being.

In a study with adolescents, Horswill and colleagues (1995) demonstrated how the choice of a leisure activity such as playing a musical instrument rather than watching television can increase energy expenditure by 41%. Even these small changes in lifestyle habits can have a substantial, cumulative effect on long-term energy balance and weight management. For your older clients, the benefits of active living translate to greater independence and the prevention of disabilities (chapter 13).

If your client is inactive, initially prescribe an expenditure of 1000 kcal/week, striving eventually for 2000. Any one of the following will burn about 1000 kcal over the week:

- 4 to 5 h of housework
- 4 to 5 h of active child care and play
- 4 to 5 h of shopping and putting groceries away
- 3.5 to 4.5 h of gardening or yard work
- 3 to 4 h of painting

- 2.5 to 3 h of dancing
- 3 h of walking
- 2.5 h of ice skating
- 2 to 2.5 h of manual labor
- 2 h of tennis

The variety is limited only by your ingenuity. Help your clients see their opportunities: stationary cycling while watching television, finding alternatives to the car for transportation, using more manual tools for daily chores, playing with the kids, taking an active vacation, playing cartless golf, or walking at lunchtime.

Active living extends beyond the physical and has the potential of becoming a way of life. Your clients may need some initial guidance, but active living is about making choices—it is truly client centered.

We have examined six different cardiovascular training methods: continuous, interval, circuit, cross, fartlek, and active living. The next two steps (steps 4 and 5) of the Cardiovascular Exercise Prescription Model (table 6.1) are critical as they select a personalized FIT (frequency, intensity, and time/duration) for the client.

Step 4:
Set Intensity and Workload

Now we are ready to discuss setting the intensity and the corresponding workload on a specific exercise mode for your client. Intensity is probably the most important and complex determinant of the cardiovascular exercise prescription. If it is set too high, our clients will be discouraged and will risk injury. If it is set too low, results may be deferred and objectives not met. Before we can prescribe a client's exercise intensity, we must know how to calculate intensity. After you have learned how to calculate exercise intensity, we will discuss how to set the target intensity for given segments of your prescription, for example, the warm-up, the cool-down, the plateau to be reached in constant training, and the peaks and valleys in IT.

Calculating Exercise Intensity

The most direct way of calculating intensity is to use a percentage of the measured functional capacity (e.g., percent of maximum oxygen consumption). If, however, a graded exercise test was not performed, there are several indirect methods to estimate a training zone. The method selected will depend not only on your access to test data but also on your experience as an exercise professional, the availability of monitoring equipment, and the client's exercise program and level of fitness.

The following are the primary methods of calculating and prescribing exercise intensity:

- Methods with assessment:
  - MET level method ($\dot{V}O_2$ reserve)
  - Graph method
  - Percentage of maximum heart rate
- Methods without assessment:
  - Percentage of maximum heart rate (estimated)
  - Heart rate reserve (HRR)

MET Level Method

The MET level method uses a percentage of the client's measured $\dot{V}O_2$ reserve ($\dot{V}O_2R$; i.e., functional reserve) converted to MET equivalents (1 MET = $3.5 \; ml \cdot kg^{-1} \cdot min^{-1}$). Although exercise intensity has traditionally been expressed as a percentage of a client's maximum oxygen consumption ($\dot{V}O_2$), ACSM now recommends using the percent $\dot{V}O_2R$ instead. $\dot{V}O_2R$ is the difference between $\dot{V}O_2$ and resting $\dot{V}O_2$. Therefore,

$$\dot{V}O_2R = \dot{V}O_2 - \dot{V}O_2 \; rest \; (ACSM \; 2009).$$

With this change, %$\dot{V}O_2R$ and %HRR methods for prescribing intensity are much closer. As an example, to calculate a target intensity of 50% to 85% of functional reserve, given a $\dot{V}O_2 = 35 \; ml \cdot kg^{-1} \cdot min^{-1}$:

$$\dot{V}O_2 = 35 \; ml \cdot kg^{-1} \cdot min^{-1}$$
$$\text{Therefore, } \dot{V}O_2R = \dot{V}O_2 - \dot{V}O_2 \; rest$$
$$\dot{V}O_2R = 35 \; ml \cdot kg^{-1} \cdot min^{-1} - 3.5 \; ml \cdot kg^{-1} \cdot min^{-1}$$
$$= 31.5 \; ml \cdot kg^{-1} \cdot min^{-1}$$
$$\text{or METs} = 10 - 1$$
$$= 9 \; \text{METs, or functional reserve}$$

If the intensity prescription is set at 50% to 85% of functional reserve:

$$[50\% \; of \; (10 - 1 \; METs)] + 1 \; MET = 5.5 \; METs$$
$$[85\% \; of \; (10 - 1 \; METs)] + 1 \; MET = 8.6 \; METs$$

Therefore, the client should select activities with similar energy expenditures that require 5.5 to 8.6 METs. Table 6.7 (ACSM 2009) indicates that possible activities include aerobic dance, badminton, conditioning exercise, downhill skiing, hiking, or tennis. Wilmore and Costill (2004) and Powers and Howley (2009) provided a more exhaustive list of physical activities and their respective MET values.

The highlight box "Metabolic Calculations" will allow you to progress from a target MET level to a corresponding workload on a specific exercise mode.

When you are deciding whether to use the MET level method, consider the following points:

- The MET level method is useful for clients selecting activities like racket sports or horseback riding who want approximate energy costs.
- This method can be used for weight loss programs (e.g., 1 MET is 1 kcal $\cdot$ kg^{-1} $\cdot$ h^{-1}).

Therefore, an 80 kg (176 lb) client in average condition, working at 6 METs, would expend 480 kcal/h or 8 kcal/min.

- MET is a commonly used measure with referrals.
- The MET level method can be used when the test mode is different from the training mode.

Table 6.7 Leisure Activities in METs

Activity	MET range
Aerobic exercise class	6-9
Badminton	4-9+
Basketball	7-12+
Bowling	3-4
Canoeing, rowing	3-8
Calisthenics	3-8+
Child care, active play	3-4
Chores • Cleaning and indoor • Yard work and manual labor	 3-5 4-6
Competitive sports (continuous)	10+
Cycling (recreation)	3-8+
Dance • Moderate • Vigorous	 5-6 7-8
Golf • Pulling a cart • Carrying clubs	 3-4 4-7
Hiking	3-7
Painting	3-4
Rope skipping • <75 rpm • >75 rpm	 8-9 10+
Skating	5-8
Skiing • Cross-country • Downhill • Water	 6-12+ 5-8 6-7
Squash or racquetball	8-12+
Table tennis	4-5
Tennis • Doubles • Singles	4-9+ 4-5 6-8
Volleyball	3-6+

Note: MET = metabolic equivalent.

- Assessment in other modes may be difficult and costly.
- The actual energy cost of activity may be affected by environment, weather, clothing, diet, mechanical efficiency, or fatigue.
- When used in conjunction with perceived exertion, "talk test," or heart rate, the MET level method allows fine adjustments to be made.

Graph Method

Plot your client's steady-state heart rate response to each stage of a graded maximal or submaximal exercise test. Heart rate is linearly related to metabolic load (energy cost) and therefore can be plotted on a graph against oxygen consumption equivalents (or METs). Do this for each stage of the test, and then draw a "best fit" line between the points. Now at any oxygen consumption or MET level, a corresponding heart rate can be read from the graph. Determine the training zone range by taking appropriate percentages of the functional reserve (e.g., $\%\dot{V}O_2R$) and finding the heart rate responses at those points (Golding 2000).

Figure 6.2 provides an example of using the graph method. The five plots on the graph represent the five steady states obtained during the assessment. The final stage elicited a heart rate of 170 beats/min, which corresponded to an energy cost of 10 METs. Remember, the functional reserve

Metabolic Calculations

You can use ACSM equations (2009) to calculate the speed or workloads corresponding to a specific MET intensity for walking, jogging, running, cycling, and bench stepping activities.

Example 1

How fast should a client jog on a level route to be exercising at an intensity of 8 METs?

$$\dot{V}O_2 = 8 \text{ METs} \times (3.5 \text{ ml} \cdot \text{kg}^{-1} \cdot \text{min}^{-1})$$
$$\dot{V}O_2 = 28 \text{ ml} \cdot \text{kg}^{-1} \cdot \text{min}^{-1}$$

ACSM Running Equation

$$\dot{V}O_2 = 0.2 \text{ (Speed)} + 3.5 \text{ ml} \cdot \text{kg}^{-1} \cdot \text{min}^{-1} = [\text{Speed (m/min)} \times 0.2 \text{ ml} \cdot \text{kg}^{-1} \cdot \text{min}^{-1}] + 3.5 \text{ ml} \cdot \text{kg}^{-1} \cdot \text{min}^{-1}$$
$$28 \text{ ml} \cdot \text{kg}^{-1} \cdot \text{min}^{-1} - 3.5 \text{ ml} \cdot \text{kg}^{-1} \cdot \text{min}^{-1} = \text{Speed (m/min)} \times 0.2 \text{ ml} \cdot \text{kg}^{-1} \cdot \text{min}^{-1}$$
$$24.5 \text{ ml} \cdot \text{kg}^{-1} \cdot \text{min}^{-1} = \text{Speed (m/min)} \times 0.2$$
$$122.5 \text{ m/min} = \text{Speed}$$
If 1 mph = 26.8 m/min, 122.5 m/min ÷ 26.8 m/min = 4.57 mph.
If pace = 60 min/h ÷ mph, pace = 60 min/h ÷ 4.57 mph, pace = 13.1 min/mile.

Note: The ACSM walking equation should be used for normal level walking speeds:

$$\dot{V}O_2 = 0.1 \text{ (Speed)} + 3.5$$

Example 2

What workload should be set for an 80 kg (176 lb) client on a bicycle ergometer, exercising at an intensity of 4.3 METs?

$$\dot{V}O_2 = 4.3 \text{ METs} \times (3.5 \text{ ml} \cdot \text{kg}^{-1} \cdot \text{min}^{-1})$$
$$\dot{V}O_2 \text{ (ml/min)} = 15 \text{ ml/kg} \cdot \text{min} \times 80 \text{ kg}$$
$$\dot{V}O_2 \text{ (ml/min)} = 1200 \text{ ml/kg}$$

ACSM Leg Ergometer Equation

$$\dot{V}O_2 = 1.8 \text{ (Work rate)/(Body mass)} + 7$$
$$15 = 1.8 \text{ (Work rate)/80} + 7$$
$$8 = 1.8 \text{ (Work rate)/80}$$
$$640 = 1.8 \text{ (Work rate)}$$
$$355 \text{ kg} \cdot \text{m/min} = \text{Work rate}$$

is the level from rest to functional capacity (1 MET up to 10 METs), so the reserve is that area above 1 MET. Once the percentage of the functional reserve has been calculated, the actual energy cost includes the resting MET, so it is added back on.

If the intensity prescription is set at 60% to 80% of functional reserve:

[60% of (10 − 1 METs)] + 1 MET = 6.4 METs
[80% of (10 − 1 METs)] + 1 MET = 8.2 METs

The broken lines on the graph show that these levels correspond to heart rates of 132 and 152 beats/min, respectively.

Consider the following client issues as you decide whether to use the graph method of calculating intensity:

- If test mode is the same as training mode, the relationship of the prescribed workload and heart rate should be very close.

- Assessment may be difficult and costly, but this method is the most reliable for prescription.

- There may be a loss of accuracy if the test mode differs from training mode (modulate the intensity with RPEs and monitor more often).

- Exercise can be prescribed at a training heart rate range that is below the point of adverse signs or symptoms experienced by the client during the test.

Percentage of Maximum Heart Rate

Maximum heart rate can be determined by an appropriate health care practitioner directly through a maximal functional capacity test using

a treadmill or bicycle ergometer and going to a point of fatigue or a limiting symptom. Determine the training zone by taking a percentage of the measured HRmax. This method is based on the fact that the %HRmax is related to %$\dot{V}O_2R$ and %HRR (ACSM 2009) (figure 6.3 and table 6.8).

The ACSM (2009) recommends an exercise intensity of 50% to 85% $\dot{V}O_2R$. Based on table 6.8, the target heart rates would be set at 70% to 92% of maximum. If the measured maximum heart rate is 180 beats/min, then

70% of 180 = 126 beats/min.
92% of 180 = 166 beats/min.

Consider the following issues as you decide whether to use the HRmax method of calculating intensity:

- This method has been validated across many populations.

- If the test mode is the same as the training mode, the relationship of the prescribed workload and heart rate should be very close.

- Assessment may be difficult and costly, but it is accurate with use of an electrocardiogram.

- Discomfort and some risk during this test are possible with the average client (ensure that the certification you have allows maximal assessments).

Estimated Percentage of Maximum Heart Rate

Traditionally, maximum heart rate has been estimated as 220 − age. Although the traditional formula is still widely used, a new formula has been proposed to estimate maximum heart rate

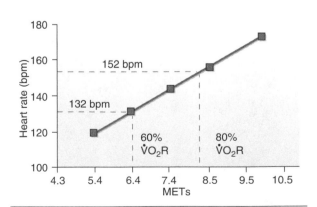

Figure 6.2 Direct method of determining the target heart rate zone. MET = metabolic equivalent; $\dot{V}O_2R$ = functional reserve.

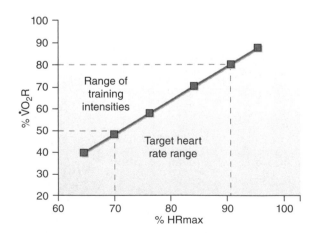

Figure 6.3 Relationship of percentage of maximum heart rate (%HRmax) and percentage of maximum aerobic power.

Table 6.8   Methods of Classification of Exercise Intensity

Sample MET	%HRmax	%$\dot{V}O_2R$	%HRR	RPE	Perceived intensity
3.0	55	30	30	11	Light
4.0	64	40	40	12	
5.0	70	50	50	13	Somewhat hard
6.0	77	60	60	14	
7.0	85	70	70	15	Hard (heavy)
8.0	90	80	80	16	
8.5	93	85	85	17	Very hard
9.0	95	90	90	18	

The sample MET data are for a client with a $\dot{V}O_2$max of 35 ml · kg^{-1} · min^{-1}; %HRmax = percentage of maximum heart rate; %$\dot{V}O_2R$ = percentage of $\dot{V}O_2$ reserve; %HRR = percentage of heart rate reserve.

based on broad age and fitness level ranges of healthy subjects:

$$HRmax = 208 - 0.7 \times Age \text{ (Tanaka et al. 2001)}$$

The old formula underestimated HRmax in those older than 40 years, a group in higher need of exercise prescription (Schnirring 2001). The training zone is determined by taking a percentage of the estimated HRmax.

$$\text{Heart rate training zone}$$
$$= [(208 - 0.7 \times Age) \times \text{Training zone \%}]$$

For example, for a 50-year-old client training between 60% and 70% HRmax,

$$[(208 - 0.7 \times 50) \times 60\%] = (208 - 21) \times .6$$
$$= 173 \times .6 = 104 \text{ beats/min.}$$
$$[(208 - 0.7 \times 50) \times 70\%] = 173 \times .7$$
$$= 121 \text{ beats/min.}$$

Consider the following client issues in deciding whether to use the %HRmax method:

- The formula (HRmax = 208 − 0.7 × Age) is conservative and variable (±10 beats/min) (Tanaka et al. 2001).

- You should use RPE and subjective exercise comments to guide this method.

Heart Rate Reserve

As already noted, heart rate reserve (HRR) is the difference between the maximum heart rate and the resting heart rate. To use the HRR method, determine at what intensity you want the client to exercise. Take that percentage of the "reserve" and add it to the resting HR to determine the heart rate training zone. The percentage of HRR is approximately equal to the percentage of $\dot{V}O_2$ reserve (Swain and Leutholtz 2007) (figure 6.4).

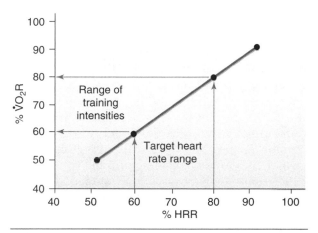

Figure 6.4 Relationship of percentage of heart rate reserve and percentage of maximal aerobic power.

$$\text{Heart rate training zone} = [(HRmax - HRrest)$$
$$\times (50-85\%)] + \text{Resting HR (ACSM 2009)}$$

For example, for a 40-year-old client with a resting heart rate of 70 beats/min at an intensity of 60%,

$$[(180 - 70) \times 60\%] + 70 = 66 + 70$$
$$= 136 \text{ beats/min.}$$

Consider the following client issues in deciding whether to use the HRR method:

- This method is very popular. A well-informed client may be familiar with or already using this method.

- True resting HR is not always available, but this does not seem to introduce a serious error.

- HRmax estimates may be inaccurate.

- This method physiologically represents reserve of the heart for increasing cardiac output.

Client-Centered Guidelines for Setting Cardiovascular Intensity

You can vary the prescribed intensity level for your clients, depending on their fitness level, exercise history, objectives, and risk factors. Chapter 3 discusses health gains possible at lower levels of intensity (Haskell 1995; Kesaniemi et al. 2001; Bouchard et al. 2007). Intensities that provide adequate cardiovascular improvement for most of the population are in the following ranges:

- 60% to 80% of $\dot{V}O_2R$ (ml · kg^{-1} · min^{-1} or METs)
- 60% to 80% of HRR
- 75% to 90% of HRmax

These ranges are narrower than, but still within, the ACSM guidelines (2009). Intensity guidelines can be further personalized when they are based on client descriptions (table 6.9).

Rating of perceived exertion is a subjective measure of exercise intensity that takes into account the client's feelings of exercise fatigue, including musculoskeletal, psychological, and environmental factors. The Borg scale of RPE assigns a numerical value between 6 and 20. You can use RPEs from a graded exercise test independently or in combination with heart rate to prescribe exercise training intensities. For example, a client had reported an RPE of 13 (somewhat hard) at a stage of the assessment that you selected as the target intensity for his prescription. Then, regardless of the mode of activity, whenever he perceives an intensity level of "somewhat hard" (13), he is at the correct level of exertion. Using Borg's verbal descriptors seems more client-friendly and perhaps more client centered for some client types. To extend the prescriptive and monitoring value of RPEs, Heyward (2010) showed the relationship of perceived exertion and relative intensity (table 6.9).

Here are some practical considerations to help you set the correct intensity for a client. Following these principles will put you well on the way to successful prescription.

Information Gained From the Cardiovascular Assessment

Graded exercise tests provide general categorizations of fitness status to help you select the training zone. For example, table 6.9 shows an intensity of 50% to 65% HRR for a client in a low fitness category and 65% to 80% for an average fitness category. The following "flags" identify the point just *above* which you should set the intensity:

- A sudden jump in heart rate, blood pressure, or physical effort during a test (or supervised change in workload if a test was not done)
- Systolic blood pressure rising significantly or rapidly
- A long time to steady state
- A slow recovery

Often it is helpful to start at a lower intensity and increase the volume of work gradually. Also consider using intervals to encourage adaptation in smaller increments. Set relief times based on recovery heart rates (table 6.5). The final cooldown should be gradual.

Table 6.9 Client-Centered Intensity Prescription

Zone	Client description	Intensity (%HRR/%$\dot{V}O_2R$)	Beats ± AT	RPE
1 Aerobic base	Low fitness status, inactive, several risk factors, wants lower intensity, longer duration	50-65%	30-20 beats below AT	13-14
2 Steady-state tempo	Average fitness status, normal activity, few risk factors	65-80%	20-10 beats below AT	14-16
3 Threshold	Excellent fitness status, very active, low risk, an athlete, interval training	80-90%	10 beats ± AT	16-18

Note: %HRR = percentage of heart rate reserve; %$\dot{V}O_2R$ = percentage of $\dot{V}O_2$ reserve; AT = anaerobic threshold; RPE = rating of perceived exertion.

Relationship of Intensity to the Other Prescription Factors

Duration, frequency, and mode interact with intensity in terms of total work and the stage of progression. Duration and frequency are often chosen to accommodate the selected intensity: Intensity may be dangerously high if selected to accommodate low duration or low frequency. Extending the duration of the work (or the work interval) provides the safest initial progression. Wider intensity ranges may be appropriate for some IT programs. For example, you may prescribe an upper heart rate limit slightly beyond the standard aerobic training zone because the work interval is short, or you may prescribe a lower heart rate limit below the standard zone because it represents an interval recovery rate (see discussion of interval training earlier in this chapter). The aerobic warm-up intensity at the beginning of a workout should approach the lower end of the heart rate training zone.

Personal Goals of Your Clients

What your clients want must be balanced against your physiological objectives. Although the most rapid improvements usually occur when intensity is increased, the type of improvement your clients want (e.g., sport specific) should influence intensity selection. High-intensity intervals will produce aerobic and anaerobic benefits; moderate, steady intensities improve stamina and aerobic endurance. Listen to your clients and their perceptions of the intensity. The Borg scale (RPE) is an excellent tool for tracking your clients' adjustments to their workloads, whether you are present or the ratings are logged.

Before continuing on to the next step, review the choices presented in step 4 of the Cardiovascular Exercise Prescription Model (table 6.1).

Step 5: Set Volume

We have considered the first four steps in the client-centered model for cardiovascular exercise prescription, and now we are ready to discuss setting the desired duration and frequency of exercise, referred to as the weekly *volume* of activity and often measured in calories per week.

The optimal duration of an exercise session for a particular client depends on her prescribed intensity. Generally, the higher the intensity, the shorter the duration. You must know your clients well enough to prescribe an appropriate mix of intensity and duration to challenge their

cardiovascular systems without overexertion. The frequency of exercise depends on the duration and intensity of the session. If the intensity is kept low and duration is short, plan more sessions per week.

Frequency may be the most difficult factor in the fitness formula. The number of sessions per week is limited by your clients' lifestyle—but it also depends on how motivated the client is. Your key role in motivation, then, may be one reason for the growth of the personal fitness training field.

The American College of Sports Medicine (2009) recommends 3 to 5 days a week for most aerobic programs.

Very low fitness: 1 or 2 days/week (if intensity and duration low)

Low fitness: 3 days/week

Average fitness: 3 to 5 days/week

Maintenance: 2 to 4 days/week

Figure 6.5 shows that improvements in oxygen uptake (cardiovascular endurance) increase with the frequency of the exercise sessions. These benefits begin to level off after 4 days/week. In fact, if a client has been previously sedentary, exercising more than 4 days per week seems to be too much, and the incidence of injuries and dropouts increases (Powers and Howley 2009). If sessions are shorter and less intense, frequency can safely increase.

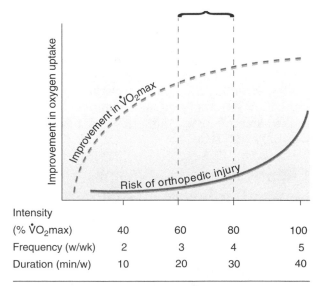

Optimal training
intensity, frequency, and duration

Intensity (% $\dot{V}O_2$max)	40	60	80	100
Frequency (w/wk)	2	3	4	5
Duration (min/w)	10	20	30	40

Figure 6.5 The effects of intensity, duration, and frequency on cardiovascular improvements. w = workout.

Total Work Done

The most important variable for cardiovascular gains is the total work done. Although other health gains are possible at quite low intensities, cardiovascular improvements appear to require a minimum threshold for the total work done in an exercise session. So if your client is working at a low intensity, the duration must be longer to achieve the same amount of total work as that of another client who is working at a higher intensity.

The body responds well to workouts lasting 20 to 30 min, with benefits leveling off after this time. Figure 6.5 shows that improvements in oxygen uptake increase with the duration of the exercise session. But figure 6.5 also shows that, with moderate intensity, workouts much longer than 40 min increase the risk of orthopedic injury. This being the case, you must adjust your client's workout duration to accommodate his fitness level. Here are ranges of duration that generally work well:

- Low fitness: 10 to 20 min (100-200 kcal/workout)
- Average fitness: 15 to 40 min (200-400 kcal/workout)
- High fitness: 30 to 60 min (>400 kcal/workout)

Total work may be expressed in terms of the caloric cost of an activity. The caloric equivalent of 1 MET is $1 \text{ kcal} \cdot \text{kg}^{-1} \cdot \text{h}^{-1}$. For example:

An 80 kg client in average
condition works at 6 METs.

He expends 6 METs $\times$ 80 kg $\times$ 1 kcal $\cdot$ kg^{-1} $\cdot$ h^{-1}, or 480 kcal/h, or 480 kcal/h / 60 min = 8 kcal/min.

If this same 80 kg client's initial recommended workout load includes expending 200 kcal, working at an intensity of 6 METs he would need to work out for 25 min (200 kcal/workout at 8 kcal/min). If the duration gradually increased to 40 min at the same intensity, the total work per session would be 320 kcal.

Client-Centered Guidelines for Setting Cardiovascular Duration

If your client's objective is cardiovascular improvement, *duration* should refer to the time within the training zone. Activity below the training zone still may positively affect body composition or decrease risk factors. Longer durations can help your client tolerate submaximal challenges, but they are less effective in changing maximum oxygen uptake.

Determine the duration of higher-intensity "spurts" of activity in those sports that demand cardiovascular endurance; then design IT programs with similar durations.

Duration is an important prescription factor for clients who have symptoms that limit their level of intensity. Because such people have less chance of intensity-related injury, you can progressively increase the duration of their activities. If recovery is incomplete within 1 h, or heart rate is still more than 20 beats/min above the preexercise level after 10 min of recovery, then either total work or duration may be too high.

Client-Centered Guidelines for Setting Cardiovascular Frequency

Frequency is a key prescription factor in building a habit. Daily walking routines appear to have lower attrition than less frequent programs, because walking becomes part of your clients' lifestyles. Daily doses of lower-intensity activity for those with a lower functional capacity will minimize fatigue and help build muscular endurance.

The work-a-day, then rest-a-day routine will improve cardiovascular health, lower the incidence of injury, and achieve weight loss goals (ACSM 2009). If aerobic improvement is a primary objective, there should be no more than 2 days between workouts.

Although exercising only twice a week may cause some cardiovascular improvements, the higher intensity necessary to bring about the improvements can be hazardous. If your client is just beginning a weight-bearing activity such as jogging or aerobic classes, suggest 36 to 48 h of relative rest between aerobic workouts to prevent overuse injuries. The rest is even more important for overweight people or those who have lower leg alignment problems (see chapter 8). Lower body stretching before and after the aerobic workout will improve safety and performance, but you must instruct your client about the dangers of overstretching and how to avoid this.

Before continuing on to the next step, review the choices presented in step 5 of the Cardiovascular Exercise Prescription Model (table 6.1).

Step 6: Design Progression and Monitoring

The previous steps have led us to the ongoing process of progression and monitoring, the sixth step in the Client-Centered Model for Cardiovascular Exercise Prescription.

The perpetual challenge for fitness professionals is to find a rate of progression that builds aerobic capacity without overtraining or reducing compliance. Monitoring progress at follow-up sessions should begin by reviewing the steps taken toward goals. If the goals were specific and measurable, it is easy to focus on the projected outcomes. Feedback should go beyond recognition and encouragement. Involve clients in taking ownership of their program and in strategizing for change. Follow-up and monitoring provide

- regular feedback for clients,
- a basis to judge the effectiveness of your prescriptions, and
- trends that are invaluable for planning changes or progressions.

The rate of improvement depends on an individual's age, functional capacity, health status, and objectives. Clients who are more fit or closer to their genetic potential and some older individuals will not improve as much as those who are less fit (Heyward 2010). The fastest rate of progression is during the first 6 to 8 weeks, when physiological changes enable clients to significantly increase the total work performed. According to Sharkey (1984), aerobic endurance may improve as much as 3% a week during the first month, 2% a week during the second month, and 1% a week or less thereafter. Your clients can achieve safety and comfort by building a level of endurance before initiating higher-intensity workouts or engaging in competitions.

Stages of Progression

The three stages of progression for cardiovascular exercise programs are

- initial conditioning,
- improvement conditioning, and
- maintenance conditioning (ACSM 2009).

The *initial conditioning stage* usually lasts 4 to 6 weeks and is characterized by longer warm-ups and cool-downs, intensities of 40% to 60% of HRR, durations of 12 to 15 min progressing up to 20 min, and frequencies of three times per week on nonconsecutive days. Active clients with better than average fitness may skip this stage.

The *improvement conditioning stage* usually lasts 16 to 20 weeks and is characterized by more rapid progressions, intensities moving from 50% to 85% of HRR, durations increasing every 2 to 3 weeks up to 30 continuous minutes, and frequencies of three to five times per week.

The *maintenance conditioning stage* usually begins after 6 months of training. It is characterized by maintenance of an energy cost comparable to that of the conditioning stage. However, the workout is altered to include some cross-training activities, more group 2 or 3 activities (see section "Endurance Activities by Intensity") involving skill and variety, a change of training method for some of the workouts, or a change of goals.

Client-Centered Guidelines for Setting Cardiovascular Progression

Progression should occur gradually and should be tailored to your client's responsiveness to the training program. A prudent goal for many clients would be to increase the total volume of exercise by 10% per week (Swain and Leutholtz 2007). Table 6.10 will help you establish prescription factors appropriate to your clients' stages of cardiovascular progression. During the first few weeks, move your clients through gradual increases in duration, holding intensity nearly constant until they have achieved 20 to 30 min of endurance in the training zone. Building frequency and duration will increase workout volume, with resulting beneficial changes in body composition, reduction of risk factors such as blood lipids, and physiological changes at the submaximal levels (McArdle et al. 1991).

Table 6.10 Cardiovascular Progressions

Stage	Week	Frequency (workouts/week)	Intensity (%HRR)	Duration (min)
Initial stage	1	3	40-50	12
	2-5	3	50-70	15-20
Improvement stage	6-10	3-4	70-80	20
	11-24	3-5	70-80	20-30
Maintenance stage	25+	3	70-85	30-45

With an IT program, you can maintain the total duration of the workout but prescribe progression by changing the ratio of work time and relief time. Base your progressions on data from regular monitoring. For example, monitoring resting (morning) heart rate over a 4- to 5-week period of aerobic endurance training should reveal a decrease of about 5 to 10 beats/min. An increase in resting heart rate over several days, however, may indicate physical or mental fatigue. Suspect overtraining or possible illness in such a case, and adjust the workouts accordingly.

Small alterations to the prescription factors (intensity, mode, duration, frequency, and progression) can favor different aerobic objectives in different clients. Table 6.11 illustrates how you can manipulate the prescription factors to highlight the potential gains for specific aerobic objectives.

Monitoring Heart Rate

Heart rate has long been a key physiological parameter. It is reliably used to estimate the relative intensity of an exercise and to quantify training loads. Following are guidelines for heart rate monitoring and advantages of using a heart rate monitor rather than relying on manually taking a pulse.

• Training intensities should be determined on an individual basis. Time spent at a specific heart rate can vary considerably among clients exercising at the same workload.

• Training zones should be established from the results of graded exercise tests. The tests should use the same modes of exercise as you will be prescribing for the clients.

• At a given submaximal workload, heart rate will tend to be higher in children and females than in adult males (on whose data most heart rate norms are based!).

• Because of dehydration and increased core temperature, heart rate tends to be higher toward the end of a prolonged exercise even though the intensity remains constant (Marion et al. 1994).

Table 6.11 Prescription Factors for Specific Aerobic Objectives

Aerobic objective	Selection of prescription factor
1. Ability to do prolonged work (>30 min); development of aerobic capacity and lactic acid tolerance	• Alternate increasing intensity and then duration. • Apply these progressions regularly (approximately every 2 weeks during improvement stage). • Encourage supplemental activity and cross-training.
2. Ability to resist fatigue and maintain high energy	• Use interval training (e.g., upper to lower levels of training zone). • Gradually decrease time of relief. • Use active recovery.
3. Ability to rapidly recover from higher rates of work; preparation for sports	• Include very hard work for short intervals (<2 min) of work. • Allow quite a lengthy and yet active recovery.
4. Ability to adapt to psychological stress and gain a feeling of well-being	• Incorporate low to moderate intensity of a longer, continuous nature (no fatigue). • Use a lengthy, gradual recovery. • Provide positive mood and climate (e.g., music, voice, lighting, smile).
5. Weight loss	• Avoid lactic acid buildup by keeping client below the anaerobic threshold. • Use nonfatiguing, longer activity to better mobilize fats and continue to burn calories.

Recording Data

Some data, such as heart rates, times, perceived exertions, training loads, and other fitness measures, are best collected during the workout on a monitoring form or program card. This may involve keeping a multipurpose exercise log or plotting recovery heart rates after a standardized work segment. Forms 6.2 and 6.3 at the end of this chapter may be copied for your clients' use.

• Overdressing or protective equipment (e.g., while hiking or engaging in sports such as lacrosse) will cause higher heart rates at submaximal exercise and recovery.

• Day-to-day variations can account for up to ±5 beats/min for the same individual at identical submaximal workloads (Åstrand and Rodahl 2003).

• During IT, a pulse rate check at the end of the relief period can verify if the client is ready to repeat the work interval.

• Your client's heart rate can tell you when it is time to apply the progressive overload principle. Record the heart rate at the end of a standardized workload on a daily basis (use form 6.3). As the heart rate decreases (figure 6.6), increase the intensity of the workout.

Although it is helpful for clients to take their own heart rate, using a heart rate monitor has a number of quantifiable advantages. Heart rate during exercise can fluctuate, and manual heart rate readings may be inaccurate by as much as ±15 beats/min (Black 2001). Other muscle movements and heavy breathing can make a pulse difficult to count. Howard (2003) listed some of the benefits associated with the industry's most widely used portable exercise devices:

• Provide immediate, individual feedback
• Are relatively inexpensive (lower-end models)
• Provide precise measure of intensity
• Can be used to monitor and measure progress
• Regulate quantity and intensity of workouts
• Add motivation by indicating improvements
• May boost exercise adherence

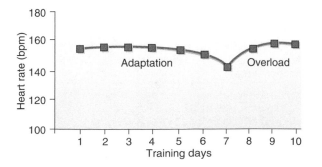

Figure 6.6 Progression based on heart rate adaptation.

Other Effective Means of Monitoring

Unfortunately, many adults—particularly those just starting an exercise program—find it difficult or inconvenient to monitor their heart rate. Ratings of perceived exertion and the talk test are remarkably effective in keeping clients within safe yet productive intensity levels. Pedometers help monitor volume with the incentive of continuous feedback.

• **Ratings of perceived exertion.** We saw earlier how RPEs could be used for exercise prescription. You can also use RPEs to monitor exercise intensity. This approach is very client centered; it sensitizes people to judge local cues (such as muscular discomfort) as well as central cues (such as breathing and heart rates). Table 6.12 uses heart rate and RPE to provide guidelines for either the adjustment of an exercise session or the progression of the prescription after a training effect has taken place. There is a bit of a learning curve with RPE because it is subjective. You will need to help your clients understand how to match their body feelings with the RPE scale.

• **The talk test.** When using the talk test, clients should exercise at an intensity where they can still carry on a normal conversation and maintain a steady state. When this point is exceeded, the body cannot supply enough energy and must supplement the energy needs through anaerobic mechanisms. This is called the anaerobic threshold (AT). A convenient way to estimate AT is to assess ventilatory (breathing) patterns during exercise, because they are affected by lactic acid buildup. The increase in respiration often coincides with the AT (Porcari et al. 2000), making the talk test a simple, noninvasive way to individualize exercise intensity.

• **Pedometers.** America on the Move, a national program launched in 2003, is a pedometer-based walking program designed to get Americans to walk an additional 2000 steps per day. Pedometers measure distance traveled and can also provide motivation—particularly for beginning clients who prefer to be exact. Positive cardiovascular and health benefits have been seen in pedometer-based programs for sedentary adults, those with type 2 diabetes or osteoarthritis, moderately hypertensive people, and obese children (Gaesser 2003).

Before continuing on to the next step, review the choices presented in step 6 of the Cardiovascular Exercise Prescription Model (table 6.1).

Step 7: Design Warm-Up and Cool-Down

The prescription model reaches full circle with this final, seventh step. Within the client's needs and goals (step 1), we have selected the activity and equipment (step 2), determined a training method and mode (step 3), and specifically set intensity and workload (step 4) and volume through duration and frequency (step 5), while putting in place methods for progression and monitoring (step 6).

The cardiovascular prescription model suggests that the warm-up and cool-down should be designed last. These components must be pre-scription specific and client centered. You need to understand the purpose as well as the methods of both warming up and cooling down.

Warm-Up

The warm-up should increase heart rate, blood pressure, and oxygen consumption; dilate the blood vessels; and increase elasticity of muscle and connective tissue in a gradual fashion. Warm-up also increases the mental readiness of your client for exercise or the motor specifics of the activity. Duration of the warm-up should be longer if the intensity of the aerobic segment is high or your client's fitness level is low. As seen in table 6.13, range of motion exercises, stretches,

Table 6.12   Interpretation of Intensity Monitoring

Intensity monitoring method		
%HRR	RPE	Exercise prescription
85	>16	• Decrease intensity, duration, or both. • Continue to monitor at the reduced intensity.
80-85	15-16	• Use caution, and monitor heart rate. Make sure client is working at the prescribed workload. • Use for a client with good fitness status.
60-80	12-15	• Use for clients with average fitness status and few risk factors. Increase duration when RPE remains lower for consecutive workouts. • Increase intensity instead of duration every third and fourth progression.
<60	<12	• Use for clients with low fitness status or several risk factors. Progress with longer durations. Usually means intensity or duration needs to increase.

Note: %HRR = percentage of heart rate reserve; RPE = rating of perceived exertion.

Table 6.13   Warm-Up Segment Design

Prescription	Design issues
Range of motion (moving major joints through their range of motion)	• Use warm-up to increase joint lubrication and synovial fluid (protect joints). • Have client check on how body feels before work. • Use warm-up to provide some flexibility gains.
Circulatory warm-up (light aerobic; same mode as cardiovascular work)	• Continue warm-up to increase tissue temperature and synovial fluid in preparation for stretching. • Use segment to gradually prepare heart and circulatory system (this segment should be a minimum of 5 min). • Simulate joint mechanics with low trauma.
Stretching and self-myofascial release	• Promote flexibility gains (static and dynamic). • Target muscles used, especially if used eccentrically. • Include dynamic stretches for sport preparation. • Foam rolling (myofascial release) for tight or imbalanced muscles.
Transition (easing into next segment)	• Add a light overload in the activity to follow (start of progressive overload). • Look for opportunities to do a mini warm-up and skill practice (especially in intermittent sports such as baseball).

and gradual low-level aerobic exercise are essential for safety, delay of fatigue, and economy of movement.

Your client's warm-up activities should provide a graduated level of activity mechanically similar to that within the aerobic segment. This will improve mechanical efficiency and facilitate the transmission of neural impulses that augment coordination and power (Nieman 2010).

- Participants in racket sports should begin with a light jog or brisk walk, followed by a gradually increased tempo of volleying.
- Swimmers should begin with a slow crawl (perhaps in intervals) and gradually increase stroke pace.
- Outdoor cyclists should begin on flat terrain in lower gears.
- Stationary cyclists should begin at half the intended work setting and a slower speed.
- Joggers should warm up with a walk–jog interval or a slower-paced jog.

A warm-up for a sporting event or a highly eccentric workout should be a more active, dynamic-style warm-up. Dynamic warm-up has been shown to be a more effective method for power performance enhancement, including jump performance, agility, and sprint performance. Recent studies have suggested that 10 min of dynamic stretching and 1 or 2 sets of 20 m of dynamic stretches can enhance jump and sprint performance, respectively (Turki et al. 2011). These 20 m shuttles can include skips (with strong arm actions), laterals (side-to-side stepping with a crouch), crossovers (like laterals but crossing trail leg front, then back), verticals (high knees), lunges, lunges with trunk twist, or other sport-specific

movements. Take time and care to demonstrate and teach the warm-up to new clients. Only once a client has demonstrated a complete understanding of the techniques necessary to operate the cardiovascular equipment, perform the stretches, and use any equipment such as foam rollers, can he begin performing the warm-up on his own. This will then allow for increased training time in which to focus on other aspects of the training program.

Cool-Down

The cool-down should gradually decrease the cardiac work and metabolism with low-level aerobic activity similar to that in the preceding aerobic segment. For clients with higher cardiovascular risk, the cool-down is crucial. Lower extremity blood pooling and high concentrations of exercise hormones can significantly strain the heart. An effective cool-down should also gradually cool body temperature, returning muscles to their optimal length–tension relationships. Table 6.14 shows that the circulatory cool-down should be followed by stretching—particularly of the active muscles.

The length of the cool-down segment is proportional to the intensity, mode, and duration of the aerobic activity and to your client's level of fitness. Additionally, a cool-down should occur after any hard bout of exercise or at any point within the workout between the aerobic segment and a subsequent segment (e.g., resistance training). After a moderate-intensity workout, most people should allot for their cool-down a period equal to about 15% of the time they spent exercising. Ensure that heart rate is below 100 beats/min or within 20 beats/min of the original HR and that your client looks and feels recovered.

Table 6.14 Cool-Down Segment Design

Prescription	Design issues
Circulatory cool-down and transition	• Make sure cardiovascular indicators (e.g., heart rate, depth of breathing, blood pressure) are reduced. • Ensure that muscles feel worked but not sore or tight. • Ice any "hot spots" or minor injuries. • Tier down gradually; avoid final sprints or sudden stops (better cardiovascular adaptations permitted).
Stretching (emphasizing static stretching)	• Use this segment for greatest flexibility gains—tissue is warm. • Have client hold stretch for up to 30 s. • Use target muscles, especially if used eccentrically. • Consider self-myofascial release (e.g., foam rolling) if muscle imbalance or tightness is a priority. • Consider proprioceptive neuromuscular facilitation if flexibility is a priority.

Before continuing on to the case studies, review the steps and choices presented in the Cardiovascular Exercise Prescription Model (table 6.1).

Case Studies

The following case studies deal with specific client situations and demonstrate the application of many of the cardiovascular prescription tools. A reproducible blank cardiovascular card is provided for your use (see form 6.4). It follows the seven-step prescription process and will guide you through recording the decisions that you have made when designing the cardiovascular prescription. Complete prescription samples using the template are provided for case 4 (Ingrid) and case 6 (Rory). An abbreviated version of Client-Centered Cardiovascular Exercise Prescription Worksheet is provided for case 5 (Josh).

Case Study 4: Well-Conditioned Woman

Ingrid was a 37-year-old woman in good condition, interested in cycling. She was at a maintenance stage, having cycled 3 days per week for the last 2 months. Although Ingrid had been cycling for a while, she remained at a comfortable lower intensity. Recent monitoring showed that her peak heart rate rarely went over 130 beats/min. She was interested in a progressive prescription that would get her over her fitness plateau and help her meet some goals.

Assessment

Ingrid had set a goal of cycling 50 km (31 miles) in a single day, and although training results were leveling off, I could sense her determination. During our counseling, I learned that when Ingrid had been single, she had played some racquetball and participated for a couple of years in aerobic dance classes. We decided to stick with just cycling as long as no overuse patterns emerged. As the weather got warmer, we could move outside with some street cycling. But the big challenge was to work around her busy schedule. We agreed that a very specific prescription based on the cardiovascular assessment would yield the best results.

I assessed Ingrid on a bicycle ergometer using a multistage graded exercise protocol. Her blood pressure, perceived exertion, and other signs were within normal ranges. Figure 6.2 plots heart rate against MET levels. Ingrid's final heart rate was 170 beats/min. Using the plotted curve, the point on the horizontal axis that corresponds to 170 beats/min is 10 METs.

Prescription

With her needs and goals well established from the counseling and assessment, we selected a bicycle ergometer to easily measure the workload and found a comfortable gel seat and her favorite music to lessen the load. A CT method suited her goal of amassing 50 km. The following calculations demonstrate how we established a starting intensity and workload. The duration (20 min) and frequency (3 days/week) reflected the time she had on lunch break.

Calculation of Exercise Intensity

Given Ingrid's "good" rating (Howley and Franks 1997), I selected a training zone of 60% to 80% of max METs. With the intensity, prescription is set at 60% to 80% of functional reserve:

$$[60\% \text{ of } (10 - 1 \text{ METs})] + 1 \text{ MET} = 6.4 \text{ METs}$$
$$[80\% \text{ of } (10 - 1 \text{ METs})] + 1 \text{ MET} = 8.2 \text{ METs}$$

The graph in figure 6.2 shows that these levels correspond to heart rates of 132 beats/min and 152 beats/min, respectively.

At an initial intensity of 60% of the functional capacity:

$$\dot{V}O_2 = 6.4 \text{ METs} \times (3.5 \text{ ml} \cdot \text{kg}^{-1} \cdot \text{min}^{-1})$$
$$\dot{V}O_2 = 22.4 \text{ ml} \cdot \text{kg}^{-1} \cdot \text{min}^{-1}$$
$$\dot{V}O_2 \text{ (ml/min)} = 22.4 \text{ ml} \cdot \text{kg}^{-1} \cdot \text{min}^{-1} \times 70 \text{ kg}$$
$$\dot{V}O_2 \text{ (ml/min)} = 1568 \text{ ml/min}$$

The American College of Sports Medicine (2009) provides an equation for calculating work rate on the bicycle ergometer.

$$\dot{V}O_2 \text{ (in ml/min)}$$
$$= 1.8 \times \text{Work rate} + 3.5 \text{ [Body weight (in kg)]}$$

where work rate (WR) is in kg · m/min. Substituting the measurements for Ingrid:

$$1568 = 1.8 \text{ WR} + 3.5(70)$$
$$1.8 \text{ WR} = 1568 - 245$$
$$\text{WR} = 735 \text{ kg} \cdot \text{m}^{-1} \cdot \text{min}^{-1}$$

It is most practical to assign a 720 kg · m^{-1} · min^{-1} workload (i.e., 2 kg at 60 rpm). Although Ingrid was not primarily concerned with burning calories, it may be useful to remember that the caloric equivalent of 1 MET is 1 kcal · kg^{-1} · h^{-1}. For example, if our 70 kg (154 lb) client worked at 6.4 METs, she would expend 6.4 × 70 = 448 kcal/h, or 7.5 kcal/min.

General Prescription

The general prescription is summarized next (see figure 6.7), with Ingrid starting at the lower levels for each of the prescription factors. The essential segments of a cardiovascular exercise program include warm-up and cool-down, aerobic segment prescription factors (intensity, mode and training method, duration, frequency), and a progression plan.

Client name _Ingrid_	Trainer name _JG_
Client goals	**Special considerations**
Progress beyond her earlier fitness plateau _50 km (31 miles) cycling in 1 day_ _Maintenance_	_Variety to maintain interest_

Circulatory Warm-Up			
Equipment and mode	**Workload**	**Time**	**HR/PE objective**
Stationary cycling (walking and calisthenics)	_1 kg at 60 rev/min (brisk walk, light exercise)_	_3-5 min_	_HR >90, <120 beats/min_

Stretching Warm-Up	
Name and brief description	**Guidelines**
• _Range of motion (lower-body joints moved through their ROM)_ • _Stretch (emphasis on static stretching legs and trunk)_	

Cardiovascular Workout
Intensity training range

Lower limit: _60%_ HRR ($\dot{V}O_2R$) _132_ beats/min _12_ RPE _6.4_ (METs)

Upper limit: _80%_ HRR ($\dot{V}O_2R$) _156_ beats/min _15_ RPE _8.2_ (METs)

	Equipment	Training method	Frequency	kcal/session
1	_Bicycle ergometer_	_Continuous_	_3_	_150_
2				

Figure 6.7 Ingrid's cardiovascular prescription card. _(continued)_

Phase	Workload	Time	Phase	Workload	Time
Warm-up	*Ease into peak work with 1 kg at 60 rev/min*	*3-5*	Warm-up		
Peak	*720 kg · m−1 · min−1 work-load (i.e., 2 kg at 60 rev/min)*	*20*	Peak		
Cool-down	*Taper to 1 kg then 1/2 kg, ensure HR <90 beats/min*	*3-5*	Cool-down		

Interval Training Prescription					
Set	Reps	Work time	(Relief time)	Ratio	Intensity

Progression and Monitoring
Phase (weeks):

See Summary of Progressions

Cool-Down	
Name and brief description	**Guidelines**
• *Circulatory cool-down (light cycling)* • *Transition (reverse of warm-up parts)* • *Stretch (legs)*	*Emphasis on static stretching of the legs—good opportunity to work on whole-body flexibility*

Figure 6.7 *(continued)*

			Summary of Progressions		
Phase (weeks)	Intensity (% $\dot{V}O_2R$)	Intensity (METs)	Workload (kg · m⁻¹ · min⁻¹)	Duration (min)	Frequency
Initial					
1	60	6.4	720	20	3
2	60	6.4	720	25	3
3	60	6.4	720	30	3
4	60-65	6.4-7.0	720-780	30	3
Improvement					
5-6	65-70	7.0-7.5	780-830	30	3
7-8	70-75	7.5-8.0	830-880	30	3
9-10	70-75	7.5-8.0	830-880	35	4
11-12	75-80	8.0-8.5	880-930	35	4
13-14	75-80	8.0-8.5	880-930	40	5
15-16	80	8.5	930	40	5
Maintenance					
17	+80	8.5	930	40-45	3
	80-85	8.5-9.0	Squash	40-50	1
	80-85	8.5-9.0	Aerobics	40-50	1

Note. HR = heart rate; PE = perceived exertion; ROM = range of motion; HRR = heart rate reserve; $\dot{V}O_2R$ = $\dot{V}O_2$ reserve; RPE = rating of perceived exertion; MET = metabolic equivalent.

Figure 6.7 *(continued)*

The warm-up I prescribed was standard: range of motion (lower body joints moved through their range of motion), circulatory (light aerobic activity, such as stationary cycling, walking, or calisthenics), stretch (emphasis on static stretching of legs and trunk), and transition (easing into the aerobic segment with easy cycling).

The prescribed cool-down also was rather standard: circulatory cool-down (light cycling), transition (reverse of warm-up parts), and stretch (emphasis on static stretching of the legs to work on whole-body flexibility).

During the initial stage of the exercise program, I assigned Ingrid a workload corresponding to 60% of $\dot{V}O_2$ (6.4 METs or 720 kg · m⁻¹ · min⁻¹) for 3 weeks. The workload is calculated using the ACSM formula for leg ergometry (see "Metabolic Calculations" in the earlier section "MET Level Method"). Her heart rate was near or slightly above 132 beats/min, duration was 20 min, and frequency was three times per week.

Results

Ingrid was very keen, worked out regularly, and recorded her heart rates and RPEs when I was not there. After a few weeks, Ingrid's heart rates were regularly below 132 beats/min, even with slight increases

in duration. I increased the workload about 10% in the fourth week. With gradual increases in duration during this initial stage, her energy expenditure progressed from 150 to 250 kcal per workout (7.5 kcal/min), excluding warm-up and cool-down.

As the summary of progressions segment of the cardiovascular prescription card indicates, I progressively increased intensity, duration, and frequency during the improvement stage. Although I varied the prescription factors to suit Ingrid's schedule, the total work per week remained the same. In this stage, the caloric expenditures ranged from 250 to 400 kcal per workout. Within 8 to 10 weeks, she reached her objective of progressing beyond her earlier fitness plateau and was doing some extra mileage outdoors. Ingrid eventually did a total of 50 km (31 miles), 25 km in the morning and 25 km later that same summer day. To add variety and keep Ingrid's interest high in the maintenance stage, after about 4 months I had her supplement the cycling with racquetball and aerobic dancing.

Justification of Cardiovascular Prescription

Each personal fitness trainer would have a slightly different approach to the case study prescription. However, as you make choices, be sure you have a strong rationale for each one. The following list provides physiological justifications and client-centered (behavioral) justifications for each choice made.

1. **Review Client Needs and Confirm Goals**
   - The client was willing to increase work even at her maintenance stage.
   - Intensities based on assessment results should use limited time optimally.
   - The client's highest priority was to get over a fitness plateau in cycling.
   - Racquetball or aerobic dance could be considered later as alternatives.
   - The client was motivated to cycle 50 km (31 miles) in a day.

2. **Select Activities and Equipment**
   - Ingrid found cycling fun.
   - She had access to a bicycle ergometer and a road bike.
   - Cycling could serve as transportation, making it time efficient.
   - The gel seat will add comfort and might increase exercise time.

3. **Select Training Method**
   - Cycling is continuous, and the client had sufficient fitness and exercise tolerance.
   - Cycling suits the objective of 50 km in a day.
   - Cycling is safe, well tolerated, and convenient.

4. **Set Intensity and Workload**
   - Workload was calculated using the ACSM formula and assessment results.
   - Heart rate was easily maintained in appropriate range for objectives.
   - RPEs were helpful.

5. **Set Volume (Duration and Frequency)**
   - A schedule of 20 min three times/week suited her lunch hour availability.
   - Cycling is an active lifestyle integration.
   - Volume progression was needed to reach her 50 km goal.

6. **Design Progression and Monitoring**
   - Progressive overload would improve cardiovascular conditioning at a given RPE.
   - The chart provided was quite detailed and easy to self-administer.
   - Increasing time and pace would rapidly increase cardiovascular improvements.
   - Monitoring would guide time and extent of cardiovascular overload.
   - Cycling was easy to monitor.
   - A 10% increase in workload was based on monitoring and was reasonable.

7. **Design Warm-Up and Cool-Down**
   - Range of motion and stretching focused on joints and muscles used in cycling.
   - Circulatory warm-up was used to increase muscle temperature.
   - Transitions would allow her to ease into aerobic workout intensities and clear metabolic wastes in cool-down.
   - Stretches targeted previously active muscles.
   - The cool-down provided a gradual return to the preexercise state.

Case Study 5: Prescribing Without Cardiovascular Assessment

I met Josh while I was working with a fitness center that did not offer cardiovascular fitness assessments, maintaining that they were too expensive—an unfortunate but not uncommon situation. When hard data are in short supply, we have to be creative in obtaining information that will guide us in our prescription designs.

Assessment

Josh wanted to improve his cardiovascular fitness significantly. More extensive questioning during the counseling stage revealed the following:

- This 27-year-old had been active in several aerobic sports but in the last 4 months had been using only a home exercise bicycle once or twice a week.
- He did not mind the cycling but found it hard to motivate himself.
- After only 10 to 12 min on his bike, his legs were tired—and he believed it took him a long time to recover.
- On the rare occasions when he did a warm-up, it consisted of two or three stretches that were completed in less than a minute; he never did a cool-down.
- He was interested in improving his squash game and in beginning to compete.
- He had no injuries or other health problems, and his weight was controlled.
- Most days he had an hour to work out and was confident he could work out four times per week.

I had to use an indirect method to estimate a training zone. Heart rate reserve (HRR) physiologically represents the reserve of the heart for increasing cardiac output. I had Josh monitor his resting heart rate on 3 consecutive days before he got up in the morning, and I found a consistent 62 beats/min.

Josh was young and healthy and was still somewhat active. Some of his early fatigue appeared to be caused by an inappropriate intensity (workload setting) and the lack of proper warm-ups or cooldowns. His history of involvement in multiple sports suggested that he would enjoy the squash competition, and I considered the intensity level and interval nature of squash in the program design.

Prescription

Josh's goals were split between aerobic fitness and squash. Some of his needs involved getting assistance on the use of equipment and better guidance with a minimum of information about his physical condition. Although Josh had access to an exercise bicycle at home and at the fitness center, the method of establishing intensity and workload differed at each location. We started with 25 min of continuous cycling but eventually moved to an IT program more representative of a game of squash. He was quite open to change and trying new exercises. Warm-up and cool-down were important to add to Josh's activity, especially at the higher intensities.

Calculation of Exercise Intensity

$$HRmax = [208 - (0.7 \times Age)]$$
$$= (208 - 19) = 189 \text{ beats/min}$$

I used the HRR method and a moderate to high training zone of 70% to 80% HRR:

$$\text{Heart rate reserve}$$
$$= [(HRmax - HRrest) \times \text{Training zone \%}] + HRrest$$
$$= [(189 - 62) \times (70 \text{ to } 80\%)] + 62$$
$$= [127 \times (70 \text{ to } 80\%)] + 62$$
$$= (89 \text{ to } 102) + 62$$
$$= 151 \text{ to } 164 \text{ beats/min}$$

General Prescription

One of the difficulties of prescription without assessment is allocation of a workload. Sometimes Josh used his home exercise bicycle, sometimes the bicycle ergometer at the fitness center. At home I had him cycle at a load and speed about half of what he had been using and then check his heart rate after 3 min of steady cycling. If his heart rate was less than 151 beats/min, he increased the workload for another 3 min and monitored heart rate again. He continued this process until his heart rate was between 151 and 164 beats/min, at which point he recorded the tension setting and speed for the next session. The ergometer at the center gave a more precise measure of work. I informed him that his perceived exertion should be "somewhat hard" (about 13-14 on the Borg scale).

Josh's warm-up included light cycling for 5 min followed by static stretches for his quadriceps, hamstrings, calves, shins, and low back. The first 3 min of the cycling were at one-half to two-thirds of the training zone. For the cool-down, he tapered the cycling for the final 3 to 5 min and redid the warm-up stretches—holding them longer, because tissue temperature was high, for added flexibility gains.

Results

Once Josh began to tolerate intensity levels closer to his upper limit for 25 to 30 min, I introduced him on alternate days to some IT. He started with 3 min periods of cycling at his upper limit load but at a faster speed, and then did 3 min of cycling at his warm-up level. He repeated this cycle six to eight times. Squash eventually became his primary focus, and I adjusted the intervals accordingly. To more intensely work the ATP–PC–LA system, I designed an IT program with 3 sets of 5 repetitions, each 2 min in length. Exercise heart rates started around 160 beats/min but crept up to 170 beats/min by the fifth repetition. During the 3 min relief period between repetitions, heart rates came down to 120 to 130 beats/min. This IT program for Josh successfully prepared him to be in better condition for squash.

Justification of Cardiovascular Prescription

1. **Review Client Needs and Confirm Goals**
   - Goal: improving aerobic fitness and squash
   - Needs and preferences: tired legs, poor recovery, motivation
   - Assessment interpretation: no tests done
   - Limitations: an hour to work out; four times/week

2. **Select Activities and Equipment**
   - Equipment: cycle ergometer at club and home stationary bike
   - Activity: cycling and squash
   - Specific exercises: stretches for warm-up and cool-down

3. **Select Training Method**
   - Continuous: initial method
   - Interval: interval training program (ITP) added every second workout once 30 min of continuous work was easily tolerated

4. **Set Intensity and Workload**

- Training zone: continuous: 25 min @ 70% to 80% HRR
- Corresponding workload: continuous, 151 to 164 beats/min, perceived exertion 13 or 14 (adjust tension and speed accordingly)

5. **Set Volume**

- Duration: continuous, 25 min
- Frequency: four times/week
- Intervals: 6 to 8 × 3:00 @ 160 to 164 beats/ min (3:00 @ warm-up load)

6. **Design Progression and Monitoring**

- Methods of progression—FITT, continuous, increase to 30 min, then up intensity to 80% HRR
- Rate of progression: ITP, 3 sets of 5 × 2:00 @ 164 to 170 beats/min (3:00 @ 120 to 130 beats/min)
- Monitoring: Fine-tune progression on ITP to address needs for squash fitness
- Primary safety precautions: ensure adequate recovery during ITP

7. **Design Warm-Up and Cool-Down**

- Warm-up: Light cycling for 5 min (50-60% HRR) followed by static stretches for his quadriceps, hamstrings, calves, shins, and low back. Add dynamic stretches before squash competitions and substitute easy stroke executions for cycling.
- Cool-down: Taper cycling for the final 3 to 5 min and redo warm-up stretches—holding them longer.

Case Study 6: 23-Year-Old Male Sprinter

A serious 23-year-old male sprinter, Rory specialized in the 200 m event. He wanted to train all year long and was looking for a safe, progressive program.

Assessment

I used the treadmill for Rory's aerobic assessment because I wanted him to achieve his highest measurable oxygen uptake, because he was familiar with the device, and because he wanted a prescription for running. Not surprisingly, his results ($\dot{V}O_2 = 60$ ml · kg^{-1} · min^{-1}) were in the "excellent" category. His maximum measured heart rate was 196 beats/min. And when the assessment was redone in 3 months, we had a benchmark for comparison. Perhaps most valuable for a client-centered prescription was Rory's personal best in the 200 m (219 yd) at 24 s. This time was used as a basis for building times for the IT programs. Percentage of HRmax and adequate heart rate recovery helped monitor and fine-tune the prescription.

Prescription

Rory's program would span three phases: preparation, competition, and transition (figure 6.8). Rory's goal was performance based, and although he was motivated, he needed to work smarter and more systematically. Running was the activity, but the venue varied from cross-country to treadmill to track. Continuous and fartlek training would strengthen his aerobic base followed by various interval prescriptions with some plyometrics (see chapter 7). Intensities are discussed farther on. However, in combination with duration and frequency of the workouts, the volume increased during the preparation phase and then tapered into the competition phase. Warm-ups were progressive and cool-downs were long, and both had lots of lower body stretching.

Phases of Training

Periodization is the process of dividing the annual training plan into shorter, more manageable phases. Each phase can be further subdivided to allow the planning of specialized training with each phase and cycle, ordered to ensure proper peaking for competition.

- **Preparation phase.** The early portion of Rory's preseason effort emphasized aerobic training, a balance between flexibility and strength, and muscular endurance. The volume of training was high and the intensity low. As the preseason progressed, however, I had him ease up on volume and increase intensity. The technical skill preparation involved drilling fundamental techniques such as running the turn. The progression was from simple to complex skills as the preseason advanced. For example, he practiced with basic acceleration form before proceeding to block form.

- **Competition phase.** Rory's next phase included high intensity and a decline in volume. The training was specific, concentrating on fitness and motor components that simulated sprinting. Adequate recovery from workouts was important. As is true in many sports at this stage, Rory needed increased emphasis on speed of movement, reactive training (e.g., plyometrics), and technique work.

- **Transition phase.** The off-season provided an opportunity for Rory to recover physiologically and psychologically, through a period of active rest that involved lower-intensity activities requiring motor skills similar to those needed for sprinting.

Calculation of Exercise Intensity

During the continuous work of the preparation phase, we aimed for heart rates of 156 to 175 beats/ min (80-90% HRmax). During the interval work of the late preparation and competitive phases, heart rates would routinely reach the 180 to 190 beats/min

Client name Rory	Trainer name JG
Client goals	**Special considerations**
• Safe, progressive annual program for 200 m sprint • Early portion of preseason, emphasize aerobic training, flexibility and strength balance, muscular endurance, and technical skill preparation	Personal best in the 200 m = 24 s

Circulatory Warm-Up			
Equipment and mode	**Workload**	**Time**	**HR/PE objective**
Track and park (treadmill in bad weather)	Light cross country pace (60-70% HRmax)	7-10 min + stretching (longer in competitive phase)	117-136 beats/min

Stretching Warm-Up	
Name and brief description	**Guidelines**
• Combination of static and PNF stretching • Emphasis on hips and lower leg	Vary with the current workout emphasis or injury

Cardiovascular Workout
Intensity/training range

Lower limit: 80% HRmax 156 beats/min _____ RPE _____ (METs)

Upper limit: 90% HRmax 175 beats/min _____ RPE _____ (METs)

	Equipment	Training method	Frequency	kcal/session
1	Track and park	Preparation phase (P): (a) continuous runs, Fartlek, or cross country runs; (b) ITP—higher volume	5×/week	NA
2	Track	Competitive phase (C): ITP—higher-intensity sprints including plyometrics	4×/week	NA

Figure 6.8 Rory's cardiovascular prescription card. *(continued)*

Phase	Workload	Time	Phase	Workload	Time
Warm-up			Warm-up		
Peak	(P) Continuous 75-80% HRmax, 150 beats/min	30-40 min	Peak		
Cool-down			Cool-down		

Interval Training Prescription					
Set	Reps	Work time	(Relief time)	Ratio	Intensity
(P)1 (P)2	6 3	200 m at 40 s 400 m			60% of PB
(C)1	3	200 m at 26.6 s	1½ to 2 min walk (120-130 beats/ min)	1:3 or 1:4 work-to-relief ratio	90% (PB) intensity

Progression and Monitoring
Three phases (weeks):   • (P) Preparation: work up to 70% of PB (34-35 s) in 5 to 6 weeks   • (C) Competition: increase intensity by 5% and decrease the volume by 10% (20 m for every 200 m) every 2 to 4 weeks   • (T) Transition: jog at family's cottage and play some recreational soccer

Cool-Down	
Name and brief description	Guidelines
• Light jog • Combination of static and PNF stretching • Emphasis on hips and lower leg	Vary with the current workout emphasis or injury

Note. HR = heart rate; PE = perceived exertion; HRR = heart rate reserve; $\dot{V}O_2R = \dot{V}O_2$ reserve; PNF = proprioceptive neuromuscular facilitation; RPE = rating of perceived exertion; MET = metabolic equivalent; ITP = interval training program; NA = not applicable; PB = personal best.

Figure 6.8 *(continued)*

range, with relief heart rates dropping to at least 140 to 150 beats/min.

General Prescription

In the early preseason, the preparation was general: continuous runs, fartlek, or cross-country runs. I prescribed specific times, not distances, such as starting with 20 min and building up to 45 min. In the late preseason, the volume or total work was double that of the competitive phase. For Rory, this was a mixture of continuous and interval work. A 400 m runner typically may be given a volume of 2400 m (4 × 600 m) (or 2624 yd, 4 × 656 yd). Because Rory ran 200 m (219 yd), I gave him a volume of 1200 m (6 × 200 m or 4 × 300 m). The intensity at the start was 60% of his personal best. Since his personal best was 24 s for 200 m, I calculated 60% to be 24 s × (100/60) = 40 s for 200 m. He worked up to 70% (34-35 s) in 5 to 6 weeks. After this time, I increased the intensity by 5% and decreased the volume by 10% (20 m for every 200 m) every 2 to 4 weeks.

In the competitive phase, IT was at a 1:3 or 1:4 work–relief ratio. The volume was about half that of the late preseason or about three to four times the racing distance. For example, I prescribed a volume of 600 m (3 × 200 m) (or 656 yd, 3 × 218 yd) at 90% intensity. Because his personal best in the 200 m was 24 s, 24 × (100/90) = 26.6 s was the workout time. Therefore, the prescription was 3 × 200 m at 26.6 s with a walking recovery lasting 1 1/2 to 2 min or until his heart rate returned to 120 to 130 beats/min.

Results

Initially, Rory needed a longer recovery time near the end of a workout than I expected. As the volume decreased and his condition improved, he no longer needed to extend his recoveries. In the competitive season, Rory ran better than his personal best in all but one competition. He never sustained a serious injury the whole year, and his personal best dropped to 22.6 s. In the off-season, Rory jogs at his family's cottage and plays some recreational soccer.

Summary

The client-centered cardiovascular exercise prescription model allows you to design a tailored aerobic-based program by following clear steps that prompt the critical decisions. The benefits and observed results will be shaped by your client's goals and sound physiological principles.

Based on access to test data, past experience, availability of monitoring equipment, and your client's exercise needs and level of fitness, the seven-step model will help you chose the appropriate exercise intensity, volume, and progression.

Cardiovascular improvements are comparable for most modes of aerobic exercise as long as intensity, frequency, and duration of exercise are prescribed in accordance with sound scientific principles. Select a training method or exercise mode by drawing on your conversations with your client about preferences and interests, goals and objectives, availability and convenience (facility, equipment, time), skills and background, suitability (e.g., level of fitness and risk), and other desired benefits (e.g., skills, social opportunities, targeted energy system). The two broad categories of aerobic training methods are CT and interval training. Benefits to the oxygen transport system from CT are more easily transferred from one mode of training to another. Interval training improves the body's ability to adapt and recover. Match your interval training prescription to the reality of your client's outside activities or specific sport. Circuit training usually consists of 10 to 15 different exercise stations with the circuit repeated two or three times. Cross-training, fartlek, and active living are training methods also examined in the chapter.

Calculating and prescribing exercise intensity should be based on one of the following: the graph method and percentage of maximum heart rate (with assessment), the percentage of maximum heart rate (estimated), or heart rate reserve (without assessment). You can vary the prescribed intensity level for your clients depending on their fitness level, exercise history, objectives, and risk factors. The weekly volume of activity involves setting the desired duration and frequency of exercise. Although health gains are possible at quite low intensities, cardiovascular improvements appear to require a minimum threshold for the total work done in an exercise session. Your perpetual challenge is to find a rate of progression that builds the aerobic capacity without overtraining or reducing compliance. Follow-up and monitoring allow you to give your clients regular feedback, judge the effectiveness of your prescriptions, and track trends that are invaluable for planning changes or progressions.

The warm-up should increase heart rate, blood pressure, and oxygen consumption; dilate the blood vessels; and increase elasticity of muscle and connective tissue in a gradual fashion. The cool-down is essentially the reverse, with stretching focused on the most active muscles.

FORM 6.1   Client-Centered Cardiovascular Exercise Prescription Worksheet

Decisions	Key Points
1. Consider client needs and goals.	Goal: Needs and preferences: Assessment interpretation (e.g., functional): Limitations:
2. Select activities and equipment.	Equipment: Activity: Specific exercises:
3. Select training method and mode.	Continuous: Interval: Circuit: Other:
4. Set intensity and workload.	Training zone (e.g., % $\dot{V}O_2$ reserve, % max METs, % HRR, %HRmax, RPE): Corresponding workload:
5. Set volume (duration and frequency).	Duration: Frequency: Intervals (duration of work and rest):
6. Address progression and monitoring.	Methods of progression—FITT: Rate of progression: Monitoring to suit client's objectives: Primary safety precautions:
7. Design warm-up and cool-down.	Warm-up: Cool-down:

From J.C. Griffin, 2015, *Client-centered exercise prescription*, 3rd ed. (Champaign, IL: Human Kinetics).

FORM 6.2 Exercise Log: Multipurpose

Date	Type of exercise	Distance (km/miles)	Duration (min)	Pulse and RPE before/after	Observations and comments

Note: RPE = rating of perceived exertion.

From J.C. Griffin, 2015, *Client-centered exercise prescription*, 3rd ed. (Champaign, IL: Human Kinetics).

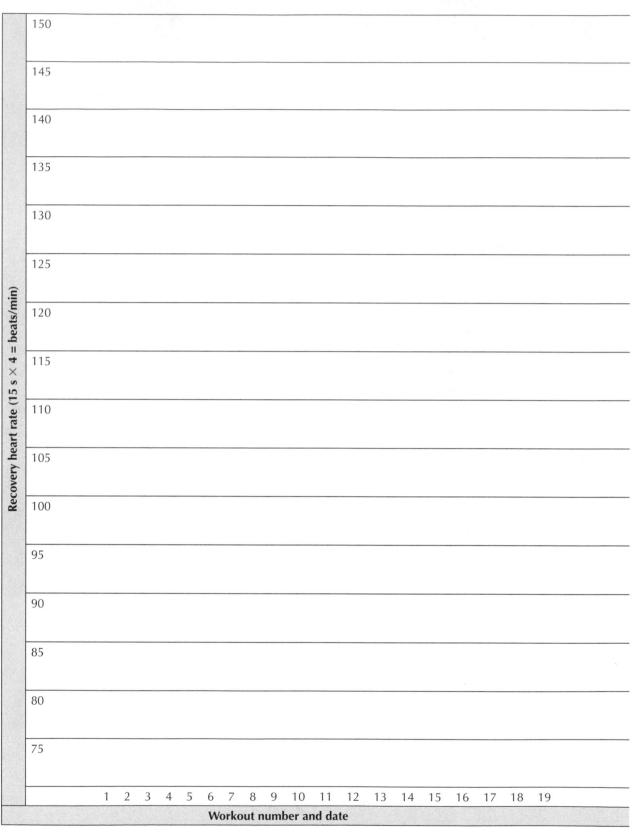

At a standardized time (e.g., 1 min or 3 min) of recovery, mark your heart rate for each workout in the table.

From J.C. Griffin, 2015, *Client-centered exercise prescription,* 3rd ed. (Champaign, IL: Human Kinetics).

FORM 6.4 Cardiovascular Prescription Card

Client name	Trainer name
Client goals	Special considerations

Circulatory Warm-Up

Equipment and mode	Workload	Time	HR/PE objective

Stretching Warm-Up

Name and brief description	Guidelines

Cardiovascular Workout

Intensity training range

Lower limit: _____%HRR ($\dot{V}O_2R$) _____ beats/min _____ RPE _____ (METs)
Upper limit: _____%HRR ($\dot{V}O_2R$) _____ beats/min _____ RPE _____ (METs)

	Equipment	Training method	Frequency	kcal/session
1				
2				

(continued)

(continued)

Phase	Workload	Time	Phase	Workload	Time
Warm-up			Warm-up		
Peak			Peak		
Cool-down			Cool-down		

Interval Training Prescription						
Set	Reps	Work time	(Relief time)	Ratio	Intensity	

Progression and Monitoring
Phase (weeks):

Cool-Down	
Name and brief description	**Guidelines**

Note: HR = heart rate; PE = perceived exertion; HRR = heart rate reserve; $\dot{V}O_2R$ = $\dot{V}O_2$ reserve; MET = metabolic equivalent; RPE = rating of perceived exertion.

From J.C. Griffin, 2015, *Client-centered exercise prescription,* 3rd ed. (Champaign, IL: Human Kinetics).

Client-Centered Resistance Training Prescription Model

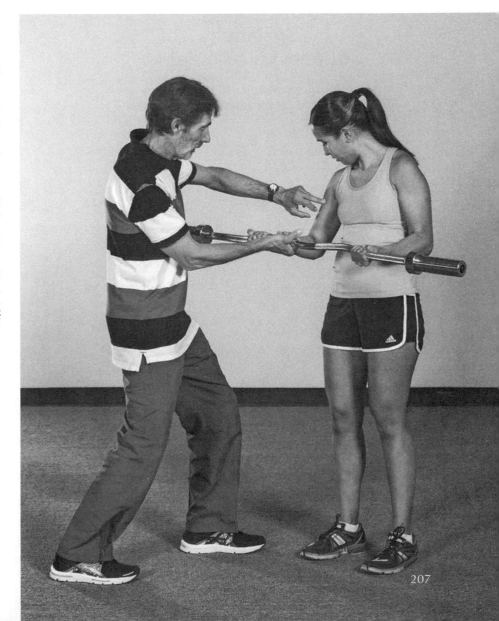

Chapter Competencies

After completing this chapter, you will be able to demonstrate the following competencies:

1. Shape the resistance training overload to suit your client's objectives and training level.
2. Decide on the best type of resistance and equipment and the interface of equipment with the client.
3. Select the resistance training methods that will meet your client's needs, time constraints, experience, motivation, and level of condition.
4. Design a physiologically sound and client-centered exercise prescription for resistance training using the eight-step model of sequenced decisions.
   - Step 1. Review client needs and confirm goals.
   - Step 2. Select resistance equipment.
   - Step 3. Select resistance training method.
   - Step 4. Select exercises and order of performance.
   - Step 5. Set resistance intensity and weight.
   - Step 6. Set resistance volume.
   - Step 7. Design progression and monitoring.
   - Step 8. Design warm-up and cool-down.

This chapter outlines an eight-step model for the design of a physiologically sound and client-centered exercise prescription for resistance training. Each step presents you with several choices. The correct amount of overload depends on your client's objectives and training level. The challenge is to shape the overload to suit your client by manipulating the prescription factors according to the principle of specificity—namely, that gains in muscular fitness are specific to the muscle group, training method, and exercise volume. After the client-centered prescription model is introduced, a case study illustrating its application is presented.

Muscular strength is required for fitness, performance, health, and a good quality of life. Resistance training not only increases muscular strength but can also enhance muscle endurance, power, hypertrophy, and muscle balance. A number of principles will allow you to effectively design and implement a prescription for resistance training.

will respond in a fashion that reflects the demands themselves. Knowing this in advance of our prescription design is a powerful tool. The desire to seek an adaptation, whether it is fitness related (muscle strength or endurance), health related (bone density or back care), or performance related (speed or power), is the primary motivation of most clients. The type of adaptation resulting from resistance training is related to the type of resistance, the metabolic demands, and the neuromuscular nature of the recruitment. These factors can be manipulated through prudent selection of appropriate exercises, prescription factors, machines, and training methods. The training benefit is directly related to the nature of the training. Your clients may desire enhanced muscle size, strength, power, balance, recoverability, movement pattern, rate of force production, energy system, tension through range of motion, or posture, and all of these can be enhanced with an appropriate prescription.

Specificity of Resistance Training

At the core of resistance training is the body's ability to adapt to the demands placed on it. The kinetic chain on which we place these demands

Matching Prescription to Client Needs

To be genuinely client centered, you must control each prescription factor to meet specific client needs. Table 7.1, although only a guideline, shows

Facts About Strength Training

- Strength is the maximum force generated during muscle contractions.
- Strength can be exerted without joint movement (isometric) or with joint movement (isotonic).
- Power is the ability to exert strength quickly.
- Muscular endurance is the ability to apply force repeatedly or sustain a contraction for a period of time.
- Muscle hypertrophy refers to an increase in muscle size.
- A repetition is the completion of a designated movement through a full range of motion. A set is a specified number of repetitions attempted consecutively. Intensity is the power output of an exercise and is dependent on the resistance and the speed of the movement.
- Low-repetition, high-resistance weight training favors strength and hypertrophy gains.
- Low-resistance, high-repetition training favors muscular endurance gains and possibly some aerobic gains if rest periods are brief.
- High-speed specific tasks can enhance power outputs.
- With a concentric contraction, the muscle shortens as it exerts a force to overcome a resistance. With an eccentric contraction, the muscle lengthens as it exerts a force.
- A closed kinetic chain exercise involves the foot or hand being in contact with the ground or some other surface. The ankle, knee, and hip joints form the kinetic chain for the lower extremity. Here the forces begin at the ground and work their way up through each joint.

Table 7.1   Prescription Factors for Resistance Training

Component factor	Preparation	Hypertrophy	Strength-hypertrophy	Strength	Strength-endurance
Intensity and load	Low 60-69% of one-repetition maximum (1RM)	Moderate 70-76% of 1RM	Moderate-high 77-84% of 1RM	High 85-100% of 1RM	Low-moderate 60-69% of 1RM
Reps	13-20	9-12	6-8	1-6	13-20
Sets	1-4	3-5	3-5	2-4	1-3
Rest between sets	60-120 s	30-60 s	30-120 s	1.5-3 min	10-60 s
Frequency	2-3	5-6 (split)	5-6 (split)	5-6 (split)	3
Volume	Medium	High	Medium	Low	Medium-high

Adapted from Fleck and Kraemer 2004; Heyward 2010.

how manipulation of prescription factors can affect the specificity of training effects.

For example, a client interested in general conditioning may have a prescription outline as follows:

- **Goal and component need:** Fitness, general conditioning, strength-endurance
- **Equipment:** Stack weights and free weights
- **Training method:** Standard sets (i.e., set–rest–set)
- **Selection of exercises:** 10 to 12 basic exercises for all major muscle groups, plus selected exercises for areas of weakness or imbalance
- **Order:** Large-muscle, multijoint exercises (all sets) before small-muscle, single-joint exercises; lighter warm-up set for each large-muscle exercise
- **Resistance intensity or loads:** 70% percent of maximum
- **Resistance volume (sets, reps, frequency):** Two sets; 12 to 15 repetitions; 60 s rest between sets; slow–moderate speed; 3 days/week
- **Resistance progression and monitoring:** Increase repetitions up to 20; then increase load by 10% while reducing reps to 12; log workouts and reassess after 6 to 8 weeks.

The American College of Sports Medicine (ACSM 2010) has guidelines for the development of muscular fitness in healthy adults. These include strength training of a moderate intensity, sufficient to develop and maintain a healthy level of fat-free weight (FFW). As a minimum, ACSM recommends 1 set of 8 to 12 repetitions of 8 to 10 exercises that condition the major muscle groups, at least 2 or 3 days per week. Muscular strength and endurance are the most common component goals for fitness and health programs.

Resistance Training Prescription Model

A resistance prescription can stand alone or can be incorporated into a cardiovascular or weight loss prescription for a number of supportive health, fitness, and performance benefits. Table 7.2 outlines an eight-step model for the design of a physiologically sound and client-centered exercise prescription for resistance training. Each step involves choices that you must make, and the table lists many of these choices. Following a brief background to each of the steps, a sample case study is presented including the choices that were made for the client.

Step 1: Review Client Needs and Confirm Goals

Client needs may be related to health (low bone density or low back pain), fitness (strength and endurance), performance (sport-specific power or occupational fitness), or education (e.g., regarding diet and supplements). Your client's motivation could also be appearance (hypertrophy, weight loss or gain), rehabilitation (injury and posture), or functional (muscle balance, stability, and mobility in daily activities). Client needs can also be defined by results of fitness assessments such as those described in chapter 4 (sit-ups/% one-repetition maximum [1RM]), by lack of self-esteem, or by special designs necessitated by physical limitations or high performance demands.

As discussed in chapter 1, goal setting is the process of specifying what needs to be done, when and how to do it, and what the anticipated outcomes will be. It is often easier to begin with long-term goals that are more global and then

Table 7.2 Resistance Training Prescription Model

Decisions	Choices
1. Review needs and confirm goals.	• Limitation (e.g., risk, injury) • Design (e.g., time, facility, equipment) • Health, fitness, appearance • Motivational strategy and personality—learning style • Strength, hypertrophy, muscular endurance, power • Functional needs (muscular balance, posture, occupation) • Rehabilitation • Weight loss or gain • Preferences and expectations (e.g., equipment, venue, outcomes)
2. Select resistance equipment.	• Equipment (and brand) pros and cons • Constant, variable, accommodating resistance • Free weights, machines • Bands, tubes, balls, boards • Equipment features (e.g., range of motion limits, pivot locations)
3. Select resistance training method.	• Standard (simple) sets • Circuit • Supersets • Compound sets or tri-sets • Pyramids (ascending or descending) • Split routine • Negatives (forced repetition) • Plyometrics
4. Select exercises and order of performance.	• Large to small muscle groups • Multijoint to single joint • Agonist-antagonist (alternating push and pull) • Upper body–lower body (alternating) • Stabilizers (e.g., trunk) later in order • Complex or sport-specific exercises • Open or closed chain, functional • Exercises in more than one plane • Overdevelopment of unnecessary areas • Balanced, unbalanced (e.g., more front than back exercises) • Weak, high-need areas first • Coordinated with training method
5. Set resistance intensity and weight (load).	• Based on goal (e.g., strength, hypertrophy) • Established from assessment or during demo (e.g., percent of 1RM [relative intensity] or trial and error [5- to 10RM]) • Interdependent with volume (sets × reps × load) • Match reps to load (based on goals) • Momentary failure for trained clients (greater neural activity) • Large muscle groups may require higher percent 1RM
6. Set resistance volume (reps, sets).	• Sets × reps × load = volume • See table 7.9, Hypertrophy Versus Strength–Endurance • Rest between sets reflects objective, size of muscle group, and reps × load • Time under tension (e.g., slower movements) • Time under tension for workout affected by rest time • Minimum 2-3 days/week

Decisions	Choices
7. Design progression and monitoring.	• Volume first, intensity second • One volume factor modified at a time. (Example 1: increase reps: 2 × 12-15, then 3 × 10; example 2 (strength): 2 × 12 at 100 lb; then 3 × 8 at 110 lb; then 4 × 6 at 120 lb) • 5% increase in load tolerable (when upper limit of reps met) • Minimum length of program 6 weeks • Periodization stages used when program duration is longer • Monitoring used to cue progression timing • Related to client's objectives (motivation) • Follow-up checks established (objective, subjective) • Primary safety precautions and execution mechanics listed and demonstrated
8. Design warm-up and cool-down.	• Cardiovascular warm-up and cool-down transitions • Specific joint and muscle stretching • Suits nature of the prescription and special client considerations

formulate several shorter-term goals that could be accomplished before major changes in assessment measures such as maximal lifts, change in body contours, or target weight gain. You can play a vital role by helping your client set realistic, measurable goals and then recording outcomes. Physical goals may need to be preceded by activity integration goals relating to flexibility in the program design, purchase of home equipment, or time management. As well, be sensitive to your client's preferences and expectations regarding outcomes, style of assistance, venue selection, and choice of equipment or training method.

Step 2: Select Resistance Equipment

When you prescribe resistance training, you must make some important decisions—in consultation with the client—about the best type of resistance and equipment and the interface of equipment with the client (ergonomics).

Most fitness centers have several types of machines along with free weights and benches. Moreover, resistance equipment is increasingly popular in the home market. Any type of resistance will affect muscle conditioning. Table 7.3 summarizes the advantages and disadvantages of free weights and machines, but there are many other decisions you must make about the type of resistance. This section examines the advantages and client suitability of specific types of resistance: body weight, free weight, constant resistance, variable resistance, hydraulics and pneumatics, electronics, isokinetics, and others. The best workout for your client will include the equipment that meets his needs.

Your choices for type of resistance and equipment may be limited by various venues in which you train. It is often helpful to think in terms of selecting the equipment to cover the following body areas. For example:

- Chest (e.g., bench press, supine fly, pec deck)
- Upper back (e.g., lat pull-down, rowing, cable crossover)
- Shoulders (e.g., lateral arm raise, shoulder press)
- Arms (e.g., curl, extension)
- Front thigh (e.g., leg press, knee extension)
- Back thigh (e.g., knee curl, deadlift)
- Calf (e.g., toe raise)

If you are setting up a training area in your own home or advising your client, your equipment list should include the following:

- Dumbbells (with at least a flat and incline bench)—good for isolation and smaller muscle groups
- Barbells (benches should have spotting racks)
- Olympic bar lifting—for more serious bodybuilders

Sometimes rather simple equipment can provide great benefit in return for very low cost:

- Pulley systems (high and low, fixed and swivel base), which allow versatile movements; good for rehab
- Bands and tubing—benefits similar to those of pulleys
- Body weight apparatus (e.g., chin-up bar, dips, stall bars, mats)
- Other small equipment (e.g., medicine or plyo balls, body bars, kettlebells, wobble

Table 7.3   Advantages and Disadvantages of Free Weights and Machines

Advantages	Disadvantages
Free weights	
• Weights can be tailored to specific demands of individual clients and permit unlimited variety of exercises. • Supporting muscles are also used, which should assist with muscle balance. • Free weights may be more effective in increasing muscle mass (O'Hagan et al. 1995).	• Safety is a consideration for the novice (i.e., proper execution and slippage). • A spotter is needed with heavier weights. • There is a learning curve whereby technique may initially impair performance.
Machines	
• Machines can isolate a single large muscle group. • Machines provide greater safety because they guide the movement, remove the concern for balance, and make it more difficult to use bad form. • Machines are easier to use than free weights, are appropriate for beginners, and guide clients through a full range of motion. • It's easy to change loads (e.g., pin placement). • The lifter can move quickly from one exercise to another; machines are well suited for circuit training. • Certain machines may be able to adjust resistance to suit the force output, control resistance to suit the force output, control speed of movement, dictate type of muscle contraction, simulate a sport skill, or provide electronic feedback.	• Exercise is restricted to predetermined movement patterns (i.e., less versatility). • Exercise is restricted to predetermined joint angles. • Cost and space restrict home use. • Machines do not train balance of movement or supportive muscle action. • Machines do not teach coordinated power movements that are often needed for sports. • Many machines (especially home models) have insufficient adjustments to comfortably and safely fit a small or large client.

boards, exercise balls, balance discs, BOSU trainer, wrist and ankle weights, boxing gloves and shields)

Body Weight

Body weight is the most versatile source of overload and is truly client centered! It provides a load that often reflects the real demands placed on the body. Body weight resistance is well suited to clients recovering from an injury (chapter 11). Lifting your body weight or a segment of your body against gravity demands a concentric contraction of the muscles (i.e., shortening of the muscle under tension). The lowering action involves an eccentric contraction of the same muscles (i.e., lengthening of the muscle under tension). Examples include chin-ups, dips, curl-ups, aerobic floor exercises, and calisthenics. The Gravitron is a specialized piece of equipment that uses a percentage of your body weight to do exercises such as chin-ups and dips. Body weight can be functionally increased with weighted vests, wind-resisted chutes, and harnesses linked to weighted sleds. Plyometrics, also known as "jump training" or "plyos," comprises exercises based around having muscles exert maximum force to move body weight in as short a time as possible,

with the goal of increasing both speed and power. Plyometrics often employs small equipment such as hurdles, plyo boxes, or cones. Suspension training (e.g., TRX) is another form of resistance training that includes body weight exercises in which a variety of multiplanar, compound exercise movements can be performed. Intensity is varied by modifying body angle, changing the base of support, or raising or lowering the center of gravity.

Free Weight

Dumbbells and barbells are probably the oldest and most easily understood forms of resistance. Bars come in 5, 6, and 7 ft (1.5, 1.8, and 2.1 m) (Olympic) lengths and are straight, cambered, or angled for arm curl work (e.g., EZ Curl). A stable adjustable-incline bench allows a large range of exercises and joint angles. Free weights may be the obvious choice for the client who has no access to a larger facility, has a limited budget, and has limited space at home. Free weights are also the method of choice for many bodybuilders interested in muscle isolation and hypertrophy. Free weights lend themselves to single-joint exercises such as the biceps curl and to multijoint exercises such as a squat. Free weights are categorized as constant resistance (i.e., weight does not change through the range of motion). Although the load remains the same, the perception of effort changes as the biomechanical leverage changes through the range of motion. As with calisthenics, the muscles work concentrically when lifting and eccentrically when lowering. Safety is a consideration for the novice, such as when the client hits a sticking point with no spotter. Proper instruction and supervision are critical. A number of other free weight tools have emerged as popular pieces of equipment for both gym and home. Medicine, plyo, and stability balls have expanded movement options and allowed the application of speed with training.

Strength bars (soft covered weighted bars) are excellent introductory devices for teaching technique without excessive weight or balance issues and come in weights of 10 to 16 lb (4.5 to 7.3 kg). Kettlebells have become a very popular free weight tool. McGill and Marshall (2012) demonstrated that selected kettlebell movements offer the opportunity to train both rapid muscle contraction–relaxation cycles emphasizing posterior chain hip power and core muscle activation. However, some swing exercises create large ratios of shear to compression load on the lumbar spine, leading to greater risk of injury if not countered by active stabilization.

Machine Resistance

Beyond the debate between free weights and machines, you must understand the use, applications, and benefits of various machine resistance modalities. Generally, machines are safer to use and easier to learn and, if available, should be used to complement training programs at all levels.

Constant-resistance machines generally duplicate free weight exercises and offer both concentric and eccentric contractions. Although the machine may alter the direction of motion required, the resistance is still the movement of weight against gravity. Popular machines include selectorized, multigym, plate loaded, and pulleys. The cable system used simply redirects gravity, and with some cable crossover alignments a person can cut in half the stack resistance, permitting the exercise of smaller muscle groups in more gradual increments.

Variable-resistance equipment is designed around the principle that the force a muscle produces during contraction is not constant. In fact, muscles produce the greatest force in the middle of the range of motion and the least force at either extreme (Baechle and Earle 2008). Most often a cam-shaped pulley alters the effective resistance of the weight stack to match the strength curve of the muscle. Some believe that such equipment provides particularly high training efficiency: With optimal resistance through a full range of motion, the client can get an intense workout quickly. One of the difficulties with cam equipment is that no two people are alike in their muscle strength curves, so the machines are built for an average force curve. Nonetheless, many clients prefer the comfortable lift provided by variable-resistance equipment. Devices such as springs, rubber bands, or sliding fulcrums increase the resistance through the range of motion, which is not how most muscles actually work. Through hands-on experience, you should get acquainted with the feel of different brands of variable-resistance equipment. Also look for devices that limit range of motion and that allow users of different size to fit comfortably and safely. Equipment examples include Nautilus, David, Polaris, Cybex, Atlantis, and Eagle.

Hydraulics and Pneumatics

Alternatives to weight stacks include hydraulics and pneumatics. **Hydraulics** use a cylinder of compressed water or oil to vary the resistance. They offer concentric–concentric work in which the muscles on one side of the joint raise the weight and the antagonist muscles on the other side of the joint pull it down. With both the agonist and antagonist working, these machines are efficient, because only half the number of machines is needed. One advantage is reduced muscle soreness for the novice exerciser; a disadvantage, however, is that many daily activities and sport skills involve eccentric contractions. **Pneumatics** use compressed air and make the muscle work eccentrically (i.e., the muscle is developing tension while it is being elongated). Hydraulic and pneumatic machines differ from weight stacks in that the client does not have to deal with overcoming the inertia of the weight or the momentum created once the machines are moving. These machines are quite safe, are good for higher-speed training, and can be adapted for clients interested in sport training. Hydra-Gym is a manufacturer of hydraulic equipment, and Keiser is an example of pneumatic equipment.

Isokinetics

Computerized equipment can offer a number of different exercise modes: isometrics, isotonics, or isokinetics. Such equipment usually has an integrated display panel, and the detail and immediacy of the feedback are very motivating. Isokinetic machines mechanically control the speed of movement. The resistance is accommodating and matches the force produced by the muscle group throughout the entire range of motion. Although some hydraulic and pneumatic machines simulate isokinetics, they allow some acceleration through the initial range of motion (O'Hagan et al. 1995). In contrast, electronic resistance machines, particularly dynamometers, provide true isokinetic conditions. Some electronic machines provide resistance only during concentric contractions, whereas others offer resistance during both concentric and eccentric phases. Advantages of isokinetic devices include accommodating forces; reduced muscle soreness (concentric only); display feedback; collection of data; high- or low-speed training; and development of muscular power, strength, and endurance (Heyward 2010). These devices also offer a great deal of safety, because resistance dissipates with the onset of pain, injury, or fatigue. Machines with high-speed settings are appropriate for clients training for sports with high-speed skills (e.g., football or track). Disadvantages include cost, accessibility, need for motivation, and a constant-speed action that is not natural to most activities. Equipment examples include Cybex, Orthotron, Omni-tron, and Kin-Com. On the low-tech, high-touch side, as a personal fitness trainer you can offer manual accommodating resistance. However, this resistance cannot be precisely controlled.

Other Devices

Other types of devices or mediums used in resistance training are possible: elastic bands and tubing, water, instability devices, and manual resistance.

• **Elastic.** Some home multigyms use various thicknesses of tubing as a basis of resistance. Surgical tubing or commercial bands (e.g., Thera-Band) are popular and come in a variety of thicknesses that offer a range of resistance. The effective resistance increases as the device is elongated. By carefully positioning both your client and the secured end of the tubing, you can obtain a variety of movements and joint angles. For about $2.00 to $4.00, you can supply your client with a personal home gym or a hotel workout! Elastic has a short life, however—beware of breakage or release while bands are under tension. To extend their longevity, the bands need to be dusted with talcum powder after each use; place the bands in a bag, sprinkle with powder, and stir with your hand. Avoid exposing the bands to extended periods of sunlight, and store them in a cool, dry location.

• **Water.** In water, gravity and impact are not issues. Water controls speed and offers a natural, accommodating resistance. Your client can vary the resistance by trying different body segments, body positions, or specialty devices. The enveloping resistance allows for an endless combination of joint angles and simple and complex movements. The multiplane movements possible with water exercise are particularly appropriate for older clients and those with arthritis or joint problems. Community pools usually have an assortment of aquafit classes and other water activities with specialized instructors. However, you can also provide aquatic exercises using the resistance of the water. These may include calisthenic-type exercises or simulated weight training movements like squats, lunges, or arm raises. Aquatic resistance equipment such as webbed gloves, water fan paddles, aqua dumbbells, and ankle or wrist weights can increase intensity and resistance.

• **Instability devices.** The use of unstable surfaces has been shown to increase the muscular activity in lieu of increasing mechanical load (Norwood et al. 2007). This is well suited to young athletes in training, aging recreationalists, people rehabilitating injuries, and in-season elite athletes who cannot train with high loads. The use of stability or exercise balls, BOSU balls, and disc pods or pillows can increase the activation of core stabilizers and make better connections with the limb kinetic chains during dynamic multijoint movements. Instability devices appear to be more beneficial for the activation of stabilizing muscles compared to the prime movers. Other devices such as balance pads and wobble or rocker boards are effective in joint stabilization, balance, and proprioceptive training.

• **Manual resistance.** You can simulate many of the principles of exercise machines by working as a training partner. Knowing what muscles cause specific joint movements, you can position yourself to provide manual resistance. If the resistance is greater than your client's force, the contraction will be eccentric; if the resistance equals that of the client, the contraction will be isometric; if the resistance is less than the client's force, the contraction will be concentric. You can also control the speed of movement to simulate isokinetic training. With creativity, you can mold the nature of the resistance to the direct needs of the client. Many of the trainer–client positions for manual resistance are similar to those used for proprioceptive neuromuscular facilitation stretching (chapter 8).

Step 3: Select Resistance Training Method

Your selection of resistance training method is important in shaping the prescription to meet your client's needs, time constraints, experience, motivation, and level of condition. Your design can become quite distinctive when you manipulate prescription factors within a given system. Training methods such as standard sets, pyramid, circuit, supersets, compound or tri-sets, plyometrics, and others are discussed next.

Standard Set System

The standard set system consists of one (single set) or more sets (multiple set) of each exercise. This system usually demands 8 to 12 repetitions with a weight that elicits a point of momentary failure. A standard set system can be performed at any resistance, for any number of repetitions or sets, to match the client's goals. This system is very versatile, allowing the beginner and advanced client enough variation to suit their needs. Novice exercisers can use either single- or multiple-set programs for the first 3 to 4 months, but data indicate that for continued progress, multiple-set programs should be used (ACSM 2002).

Pyramid System

The pyramid system begins by working a specific muscle group using a relatively light weight so that about 10 to 12 repetitions can be performed. After each set the weight is increased so that fewer and fewer repetitions can be done, until only 1 or 2 repetitions can be performed. The resistance is then progressively decreased each set, and the session ends with a set of 10 to 12 repetitions (e.g., table 7.4). The system can be modified to include any number of reps for the desired number of sets and is favored by many bodybuilders for its potential hypertrophy gains. The first half of the pyramid is called the **light-to-heavy system**. The reverse **heavy-to-light system** is preferred over the former in producing strength gains (Fleck and Kraemer 2004). For an example, see table 7.4.

Superset System

The superset system uses several sets of two exercises performed one after the other with little or

Table 7.4   Pyramid System

Sets	Reps	Weight
1	10	
1	8	
1	6	
1	4	
1	1-2	
1	4	
1	6	
1	8	
1	10	

no rest. The two exercises are for the same body part but for antagonistic muscles. For this reason, the method is sometimes called *agonist–antagonist paired set* (APS). For example, you might follow a bench press with rowing exercise, arm curls with triceps extensions, or leg curls with leg extensions. Have your client rest for 1 or 2 min after both exercises are complete and then complete the remaining 2 to 5 sets. The repetitions are usually limited to 8 to 10. Supersets can lead to significant increases in strength (Robbins et al. 2010), and, if your client is fit and motivated, he can reduce his workout time by including more exercises in a given training session.

A variation of the superset system uses 1 set of several exercises for the same muscle group performed one after another with little rest. For example, this may include bench press, military press, and incline flys, or one set of lat (latissimus dorsi) pull-down, seated rowing, and bent-over rowing. This variation is also effective in improving muscular strength and hypertrophy.

Table 7.5 prescribes a sample superset program. Your client should do the first set of exercise 1(a), followed immediately by the first set of exercise 1(b). Have him rest 1 to 2 min and then go on to second sets of 1(a) and 1(b). Follow this format for the prescribed number of sets and reps.

Compound or Tri-Set System

A compound set involves two exercises, and a tri-set is a group of three exercises for the same body part, one done after another with little or no rest between exercises or sets. Use tri-sets to work three different muscle groups, to work the same muscle from three different angles, or to work the same area of the muscle (from the same angle). Three sets of each exercise are usually performed. Fleck and Kraemer (2004) reported that tri-sets are good systems to increase local muscular

Table 7.5   Superset Program

Exercises	Reps (sets)	Exercises	Reps (sets)
1(a) Leg extension (quadriceps)	10-8-6 (3)	4(a) Bench press (pectoralis major)	10-8-6 (3)
1(b) Leg flexion (hamstrings)	10-8-6 (3)	4(b) Lat pull-down (latissimus dorsi)	10-8-6 (3)
2(a) Resisted hip abduction (hip abductors)	10-8/leg (2)	5(a) Dumbbell fly (anterior deltoid and pectoralis major)	10-8 (2)
2(b) Resisted hip adduction (hip adductors)	10-8/leg (2)	5(b) Reverse fly (posterior deltoid and latissimus dorsi)	15-15 (2)
3(a) Standing toe raise—calf machine (gastrocnemius)	8 to 12 (1)	6(a) Standing barbell curl (biceps)	10-8 (2)
3(b) Seated barbell toe raise (soleus)	15 to 20 (1)	6(b) Dips (triceps)	Up to 15 (2)

endurance. A tri-set might include lateral raises, arm curls, and triceps extensions all working the upper arms and shoulder area but distinctly different muscles. A tri-set for the same muscle group (different angles) may comprise decline flys, bench presses, and incline flys. This can be a useful change of pace for a client who has hit a training plateau.

Plyometrics

Although weight training can produce gains in strength, the speed of movement is limited. Because power combines strength and speed, many athletes need to decrease the amount of time it takes to produce muscular force. A form of training that combines speed of movement with strength is plyometrics.

Plyometric training involves rapid eccentric lengthening of a muscle followed immediately by rapid concentric contraction of that muscle to produce a forceful explosive movement. The increase in explosive power comes in part from the storage of elastic energy within the prestretched connective tissue tendon. The concentric contraction can be magnified only if the preceding eccentric contraction is of a short range and is performed quickly and without delay (Voight and Tippett 1994). Plyometrics emphasizes this speed of the eccentric phase and control in dynamic movements.

Examples of plyometric exercises for the lower extremity include hops, bounds, and depth jumping. In depth jumping, your client jumps to the ground from a specified height and then quickly jumps again as soon as she makes ground contact. For the upper extremity, you can prescribe medicine balls or other weighted equipment.

One benefit of plyometric training is that it can be organized into circuits. The program shown in figure 7.1 involves a high-volume circuit designed to improve both vertical and linear power patterns (Chu 1992).

Plyometrics is a very valuable tool, but you must use it judiciously according to your client's tolerance. Demonstrate all movements, provide adequate recovery, avoid overtraining, and match the activity to your client's abilities. The following guidelines will help you avoid injuries and maximize your client's improvement:

• Precede each workout with an extended warm-up and gradual buildup. Plyometrics involves a lot of eccentric (i.e., ballistic) actions, and the muscles must be stretched and exposed to light eccentric movements in the warm-up.

• Remember that the greater the intensity, the longer the recovery. This guideline applies both between sets during the workout and between workouts.

• Emphasize proper technique and explosive intensity. Stop the exercise if your client's form begins to fail.

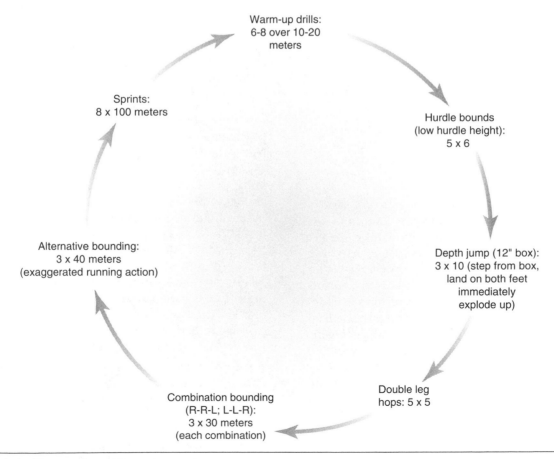

Figure 7.1 Plyometrics program.

Plyometrics + Resistance Training = Complex Training

Complex training involves pairing two exercises that are similar in movement pattern—one high-intensity resistance exercise and one plyometric exercise (speed and rebound ability). These are examples of complexes of absolute and elastic strength:

- Squatting, then jumping
- Pressing, then passing
- Lunging, then bounding or skipping
- Pulling, then tossing or throwing

Complex training is well suited for an athlete working in the strength–power continuum.

- Train specific movement patterns for specific activities.

- Modify prescription factors for progressive overloads by increasing the number of exercises, increasing the number of repetitions or sets, or decreasing the rest periods between sets. Discourage use of ankle or wrist weights because they may cause excessive momentum.

- Carefully observe, monitor, and test your client to gain important feedback for motivation and progression.

- Assign a frequency of no more than three times per week in the preseason (higher volume) and less during the season (higher intensity).

- At the end of a workout, use a plyometrics segment that is shorter and less stressful than that at the beginning, because your client is partially fatigued.

Circuit Weight Training System

Circuit resistance training consists of a series of resistance exercises in a multiple-station system: approximately 10 to 15 repetitions of each exercise, at a resistance of 40% to 60% of maximum (RM), with 15 to 30 s rest between exercises (Fleck and Kraemer 2004). Design the circuit to meet specific goals or use available equipment. This is a very efficient method of developing strength and endurance (with some aerobic and calorie-burning benefits). It can be a good way to add variety to traditional cardiovascular training and resistance training. Alcaraz and colleagues (2011) compared the effects of 8 weeks (3-6 sets of six exercises at 6RM) of high-resistance circuit training (35 s interset recovery) and traditional strength training (3 min interset recovery). Both training methods produced substantial strength, power, and

muscle mass gains. However, the circuit group showed significant decreases in percent body fat and accomplished this in less time, an important training feature for those with limited time to train. Heyward (2010) presented a sample circuit resistance training program, shown in figure 7.2.

Systems That Are Extended Forms of Other Systems

Some systems of resistance training are extensions of other systems or can be used within an existing system. They enable further manipulation of the prescription factors that allow individual needs to be addressed. The following are examples of such extensions.

- **Split routine system.** Developing hypertrophy is a time-consuming process for bodybuilders. Not all body parts can be covered in one training session. The split routine system trains various body parts on alternate days—arms, legs, and abdomen on 3 days per week, for example, and chest, shoulders, and back on alternate days. Variations in this example may allow a reduction of training days. Calder and colleagues (1994) found that split routines (four sessions/week) produced results that were similar to those for whole routines (two sessions/week) over 5 months of training. The increased time for recovery helps reduce overuse injuries and overtraining and allows for a more intense training level.

- **Forced repetition system.** The forced repetition system allows you to work very closely with your client. After a set to exhaustion, help your client determine just the amount of weight that will permit her to do 3 or 4 additional repetitions. By demanding stimulation from a partially fatigued muscle, this approach is well suited to clients who want increased strength and muscular endurance.

• **Periodization.** Periodization is characterized by systematic cycles of alternating prescription variables such as intensity and volume during different phases of a resistance training program. This provides the necessary recovery time for certain muscle fibers while other fibers are overloaded, leading to greater increases in muscle characteristics and performance and reduced risk of overtraining. In general, there are two basic approaches to periodizing a resistance training program: linear and nonlinear. Linear periodization methods use a progressive increase

in intensity with small variations in each 1- to 4-week microcycle. An example of a 4-week-cycle linear periodized program is presented in table 7.6 (Thompson 2010).

Nonlinear (undulating) periodization creates different exercise stimuli to provide variation and challenge. This concept of periodization allows you to vary intensity and volume within each 14-day training cycle by rotating different exercise protocols (Kraemer 2003). Compared with use of the same repetition maximum for every workout or a lower-volume circuit design, the nonlinear periodization program has shown significant superiority during a 6-month training

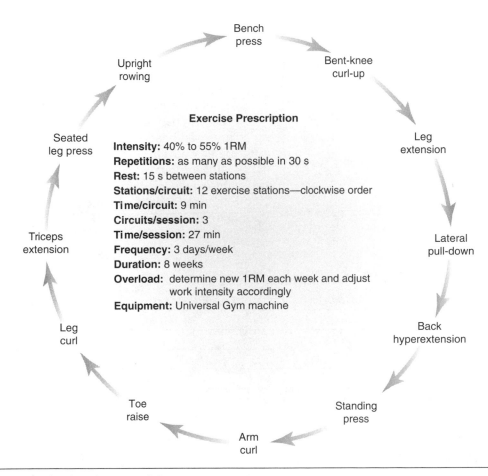

Figure 7.2 Sample circuit resistance training program.

Table 7.6 **Linear Periodization Program**

Microcyle 1	Microcyle 2	Microcyle 3	Microcyle 4	Microcyle 5 (2 weeks)
3-5 sets of 12- to 15RM	4-5 sets of 8- to 10RM	3-4 sets of 4- to 6RM	3-5 sets of 1- to 3RM	Active rest/recovery

This protocol uses 4 week cycles.

period (Marx et al. 2001). Sorace and LaFontaine (2005) suggested using an undulating periodization program to train strength, hypertrophy, and endurance within the same cycle (table 7.7).

• **Exhaustion set system.** Momentary failure is the point at which another full repetition is not possible—that is, the set has been done to exhaustion. You can incorporate sets to exhaustion into almost any training system. This system appears to recruit a large number of motor units and to produce significant strength gains (Baechle and Earle 2008). An added burn can be achieved by performing 5 or 6 partial repetitions after exhaustion.

The weight used to reach momentary failure is called a repetition maximum (RM). If eight repetitions of 150 lb (68 kg) are done to exhaustion, the 8RM is 150 lb. If you have assessed your client's 1RM (chapter 4), the following chart can estimate a prescription for intensity (% of 1RM) and number of repetitions that will elicit momentary failure (Fleck and Kraemer 2004; Heyward 2010):

60% 1RM = 15- to 20RM

65% 1RM = 14RM

70% 1RM = 12RM

75% 1RM = 10RM

80% 1RM = 8RM

85% 1RM = 6RM

90% 1RM = 4RM

95% 1RM = 2RM

100% 1RM = 1RM

For example, the prescription in the first line would be a set of 15 to 20 repetitions to exhaustion at 60% 1RM.

Step 4: Select Exercises and Order of Performance

Chapter 5 outlines an exercise design model that identifies a component, targets the muscles, and identifies the appropriate joint movements for effective design or selection of exercise. Exercises should be selected so that they stress the muscles, joints, and movements specified by the client's needs analysis. Exercises can be classified as multijoint or single-joint exercises. Multijoint exercises require the coordinated action of two or more muscle groups and joints, such as squat, deadlift, bench press, lat pull-down, and military press. Isolated single-joint exercises may include biceps curls, knee extensions, and knee curls. Multijoint exercises require neural coordination among muscles and are important for whole-body strength movements, most sports, and functional activities in everyday life (e.g., climbing stairs). Multijoint exercises have greater metabolic

Table 7.7   Undulating Periodization Program

	Monday	Wednesday	Friday
Sets	3-5	3-4	5-6
Reps	6-12	12-20	2-5
Intensity/load (% of 1RM)	70-80	60-70	80-100
Rest and recovery (min)	1-2	<1	2-5

This protocol uses a 3-day rotation with 1-day rest between workouts.

Flexible Periodization Method

Jensen (2010) describes a flexible periodization method that is well suited to fitness enthusiasts as well as athletes. He emphasizes different periodized program variables for each macrocycle. For example, goal periodizations include the following:

• First improve the weak link, and then improve the function of the entire kinetic chain.
• First improve the endurance of stabilizing muscles, then improve the strength of prime movers.
• First improve structural strength, then improve functional strength.

Therefore within the specific training block, periodization of volume and intensity would naturally follow the goal periodizations.

demands and are time efficient because several different muscle groups are activated at the same time. Knowing the purpose and benefit of each exercise can help maintain muscle balance and avoid overworking a particular body area. Keep in mind physical limitations, past injuries, and conditions such as hypertension.

The order in which the selected exercises are performed affects the quality and focus of the workout. For example, if multijoint exercises are performed early in the workout, more resistance can be used because of a limited amount of fatigue in the smaller muscle groups. It is believed that this stimulates a greater neural, metabolic, and circulatory response, which potentially may augment the training with subsequent muscles or exercises later in the workout (Thompson 2010). In most cases, and certainly with novice clients, order your selection of specific exercises (muscle groups) to meet the following criteria:

- Choose successive exercises that do not involve the same muscle group.

- Prescribe large-muscle, multiple-joint exercises (e.g., bench press, squat) to precede small-muscle, single-joint, isolation exercises (e.g., biceps curl, crunch). This will avoid early fatigue and poor performance later in the workout.

- Work areas of weakness or imbalance while your client is still fresh.

- Prioritize sport-specific movements for athletes.

- Choose exercises that are functional for the demands on the client; these often include exercises in more than one plane.

- For the large-muscle exercises, have the client perform a warm-up set with less weight.

- Prescribe one exercise for each muscle group that maintains agonist–antagonist and bilateral symmetry, which promotes a balanced development and helps prevent overuse injuries. For example, a frequent cause of shoulder rotator cuff injury is overtraining of the upper chest muscles and undertraining of the upper back and posterior shoulder muscles.

- Alternating upper and lower body exercises, pushing and pulling exercises, or both allows more time to recover between exercises.

- Include stabilizers (e.g., lower spine muscles) later in the session.

- Choose exercises that complement the training method (which may be counter to some of these guidelines).

Step 5: Set Resistance Intensity and Weight

Specific neuromuscular adaptations to resistance training depend in large part on the resistance or loads used. Generally, as the intensity or load (weight) is increased, there is an increase in the motor unit activation. This results, over a period of training, in an increased force production as measured by strength or power. Encouraging trained clients to reach the muscle's threshold (momentary failure) increases the neural activity and speeds the training results. Resistance can be expressed as either RMs (the maximum load that can be lifted the specified number of repetitions) or the absolute resistance (actual poundage). Throughout the training program, the absolute resistance is then adjusted to match the changes in strength so a true RM target (e.g., 10RM) continues to be used. Determining resistance with a percentage of 1RM (e.g., 70% of the 1RM) requires that the maximum strength in all exercises be evaluated regularly. This method has good theoretical value but obvious shortcomings in practical application. Without knowledge of 1RMs for each exercise, you can use educated trial and error to determine the training zone intensity. Choose a weight that your client can do for 6 repetitions to failure. This will give you a 6RM and a weight to begin strength training with. For review, chapter 4 (table 4.5) provides the relationship between %1RM and repetitions accomplished in a trial set.

Training intensity is a critical prescription factor providing the stimulus needed for improvement in specific muscular components (table 7.8).

Step 6: Set Resistance Volume

Exercise volume is one of the most important prescription factors. The intensity or load must be heavy enough to cause temporary discomfort and momentary muscle fatigue. For combined strength and endurance improvements, the resistance should be about 75% of the maximum load your client is able to lift. Baechle and Earle (2008) indicated that most people can complete 8 to 12 repetitions with about 75% load. If your client is a beginner or is training at high intensity, 1 or 2 sets are sufficient to produce excellent benefits. The greater training stimulus associated with the higher volume from multiple sets is needed to create further improvement and progression, but 1-set programs are effective for developing and maintaining a certain basic level of muscle strength and endurance.

Table 7.8   Intensity and Load

Component factor	Intensity	Load
Preparation	Low	60-69% of 1RM (11-20 reps)*
Hypertrophy	Moderate	70-76% of 1RM (9-11 reps)*
Strength-hypertrophy	Moderate-high	77-84% of 1RM (6-9 reps)*
Strength	High	85-100% of 1RM (1-6 reps)*
Strength-endurance	Low-moderate	60-69% of 1RM (11-20 reps)*

*Momentary failure

Do Bigger Weights Produce Bigger Muscles?

Loading the muscle with an intensity >70% to 80% of 1RM is thought to be fundamental to the development of muscle hypertrophy and a stimulus for strength. Recent research has challenged this assumption that high loading intensities are needed for increasing skeletal muscle mass. A recent Canadian study demonstrated that 80% to 90% of 1RM to fatigue for 5 to 8 repetitions was similar to 30% of 1RM to fatigue for 20 to 25 repetitions with respect to increases in the synthesis of new muscle proteins. The authors concluded that the amount of weight lifted is not the major concern; emphasis should be placed on exerting a hard effort with good form to reach voluntary fatigue, with the degree of muscle fiber recruitment as the primary stimulus (Burd et al. 2012). This idea is valuable for the design of resistance training programs aimed at maintaining a healthy independent lifestyle across the life span.

In another study challenging the dogmatic view, researchers compared high load–low velocity (70% of 1RM, 3 sets of 12 reps) and low load–high velocity (35% of 1RM, 6 sets of 12 reps), equated by volume, and found that the low-load–high-velocity protocol offered similar hypertrophic benefits because of the greater time under tension, power, force, and work output. They suggested that the real benefit to this training may be due to the greater eccentric velocities and subsequent protein synthetic response (Mohamad et al. 2012). To maximize the anabolic effect of resistance exercise, there appears to be a need to activate the highly trainable type II muscle fibers. This type of loading better simulates the velocities associated with athletic movement and therefore may optimize transference from the gym-based gains to on-field performance.

Prescribe a frequency of 3 days per week for strength development. At least 2 days per week are necessary for maintenance. Detraining will occur when frequency is less than 1 day per week.

Volume is often described as sets × reps × load. The length of time you are actually working with the resistance is the "time under tension." However, the rest between the sets and the speed of the movements both contribute to the total training effects of time under tension. Longer rests (>3 min) may be needed to replace creatine kinase during high-intensity strength training with larger muscle groups (Thompson 2010). If the goal is to optimize both strength and muscle mass, both long rest with heavy loading and short rest with moder-

ate loading types of workout protocols could be used. However short-rest resistance programs (i.e., 1 min or less) can cause greater fatigue and discomfort. Watch for symptoms such as loss of force production in the beginning of the workout, nausea, or dizziness. It is interesting to compare volume between a prescription for hypertrophy with one for a more traditional strength–endurance component (table 7.9). Although the load is only 10% higher for hypertrophy and the rest between sets is comparable, the total lifts per workout are quite a bit greater and the lifts per week are substantially more.

In a full component workout, time is needed for a warm-up, aerobic activity, resistance work, and a cool-down. Depending on the type and availability of equipment, the time devoted to resistance training will limit the number of reps and sets and the number of exercises selected. For example, in a 30 min lunchtime workout, your client may only have 10 min for resistance work compared to a 60 min session allowing perhaps 25 min for resistance work (table 7.10).

For more serious athletes, periodization is used in their long-term training plans (see earlier in the chapter). Periodization systematically varies the volume and intensity of training over units of training called mesocycles that last for a few weeks to several months (Bompa 1999). Most often, training volume progressively decreases as the intensity increases. This changes the training stimulus through each of the mesocycles and has been shown to provide peak strength and power performances at times appropriate for the competitions (Stone et al. 1999).

Step 7: Design Progression and Monitoring

The universal principle of conditioning is progressive overload, that is, a periodic increase in workload that increasingly overloads the muscle group. The correct amount of overload depends on your client's objectives and training level. The challenge is to shape the overload to suit your client by manipulating the prescription factors according to the principle of specificity—namely, that gains in muscular fitness are specific to the muscle group, training method, and exercise volume.

At the beginning of the training program, correct technique with the exercises is critical, and the resistance and volume should be kept low. As the skill and experience of the client improve, consider the following progressions:

- **Unloaded to loaded.** Teach the movement patterns with unloaded or low intensity to develop basic skills.

- **Simple to complex.** Set the groundwork with basic skills for more complex movement patterns in later training phases (e.g., increase the use of multijoint movements involving the body's kinetic chains, recruiting many muscle groups to mimic functional movements).

- **Stable to unstable.** Begin with stable positions with the client balanced. As abilities improve, change the base of support to a more unstable position or surface to create a greater proprioceptive challenge.

If your client is doing resistance work at least twice a week, you need to change (increase) the overload each week when possible. For example, table 7.11 shows a progressive overload at a given weight appropriate for strength and endurance gains (e.g., 70% 1RM). This represents an increase in volume of about 20% over the 4 weeks.

To ensure safe and effective progression, modify only one volume factor at a time. For example:

Table 7.9 Hypertrophy Versus Strength–Endurance

Component factor	Hypertrophy	Strength–endurance
Intensity and load	Moderate 70-76% of 1RM	Low-moderate 60-69% of 1RM
Reps	9-12	13-20
Sets	3-5	1-3
Rest between sets	30-60 s	10-60 s
Frequency	5-6 (split)	3
Volume	High	Medium-high

Table 7.10 Length of Resistance Workout

30 min workout	45 min workout	60 min workout
10 min resistance	15-20 min resistance	25 min resistance
4-5 exercises (1 set)	4-5 exercises (2 sets) or 6-8 exercises (1 set)	6-8 exercises (2 sets)

Hints for Helping Your Novice Clients Set Training Volume

With a specific focus on training volume, recent research can help us be more client centered for our novice and untrained participants:

- Exercises with a larger muscle mass (to increase energy expenditure) and longer between-set rest intervals (to avoid early fatigue) allow greater training volume (Farinatti and Neto 2011).

- Single-set programs for an initial short training in untrained individuals result in strength gains similar to those of multiset programs. As progression occurs, multiset programs are more effective.

- When the training goal is maximal strength, 3 min of rest should be taken between sets to avoid significant declines in repetition and training volume. Rest intervals of 3 min versus 1 min between sets of biceps curls at 40% of 1RM to voluntary fatigue resulted in greater workout volume but no differences in muscle soreness in untrained subjects (Evangelista et al. 2011).

- With older clients, more gradual progression may be needed when rest period lengths between sets are cut.

- An upper body agonist–antagonist (paired set) protocol allowed greater volume in a time-efficient manner (Robbins et al. 2010).

- In a group of untrained, middle-aged women, there was no difference in initial short-term gains in lean mass and strength between 3 nonconsecutive days and 4 consecutive days of the week when both groups completed 72 sets per week of 8 to 12 repetitions at 50% to 80% of 1RM (Benton et al. 2011).

- Strength recovery over a 4-day period of time demonstrated that women require longer rest periods between sessions than men, although they develop and dissipate muscle soreness in a similar manner.

Table 7.11   Progressive Overload

Week	Set 1	Set 2
1	12 reps	12 reps
2	13 reps	12 reps
3	14 reps	13 reps
4	15 reps	14 reps

1. Increase reps: 2 × 12 to 15; then 3 × 10 to 15.
2. Increase intensity: 2 × 12 at 100 lb; then 3 × 8 at 110 lb; then 4 × 6 at 120 lb.

The following guidelines will assist you in monitoring progress:

- Clients interested in strength gains will continually want to increase their load.

- Monitoring girth measures will track gains in hypertrophy.

- Clients working on strength-endurance should increase their reps up to about 15 and then increase the load and drop the reps back down. As their condition improves, they may decrease the rest between sets.

- A 5% to 10% increase in load is very tolerable (when upper limit of reps is met).

- Use a perceived exertion scale to measure the intensity of a training segment or session.

- Clients working on muscular endurance should use repetitions or sets (volume) as a method of progression. Decreasing rest time between sets can further challenge this component.

- Monitoring total poundage per workout will easily demonstrate improved work capacity.

- Program cards that allow quick recording of these factors can save time and encourage regular recording.

- A minimum length of program is usually 6 weeks.

- You should visually (and at times, physically) monitor primary safety precautions and execution mechanics (see tables 7.12 and 7.13).

Table 7.12 Common Design and Execution Faults for Selected Resistance Exercises

Exercise	What's wrong?	Why? Key points
Lat pull-down	Pulling down behind the head	• Muscle imbalances such as rounded shoulders can compromise the position of the scapula and shoulder joint at the start of the movement. • At times a restricted lateral rotation of the shoulder can force the lumbar spine into increased lordosis.[a] • Wide grip with bar and a pull to anterior chest require more work from lats.[b]
Seated row	Leaning forward to start and backward to finish	• Rounded low back may create compression in a flexed position. • Rounded shoulders create a loosely packed, unstable position. • Leaning back activates the erector spinae, not the desired lats, posterior deltoids, and midtraps. More weight may be lifted but not by the intended muscles.
Dumbbell press	Lowering the weights too far	• The problem can be caused by excessive microtrauma of the chest musculature. • The client may be in a position of lumbar lordosis as the chest rises. • Also, subacromial space diminishes (potential impingement) when the elbows are brought down.[c]
Fly cable crossover	Failing to lock elbows throughout range of motion	• Bringing elbows from a bent to a straightened position will use the triceps. • Keeping elbows stable in a slight flex will focus horizontal movements on the pectoralis.
Squat	Squatting to a depth at which the thighs are parallel to the ground	• Most lifters bend forward excessively at the hips, which rotates the pelvis forward and increases lumbar lordosis in an attempt to stay upright. • Some may round the back (flex at the spine), creating a shear force with the compression on the intervertebral disc. • Spine should be stable in a neutral position.
Leg press or hack squat	Bringing the weight too low Turning the feet inward or outward to isolate parts of the quads	• When the knee tracks beyond the toes, excessive forces are placed on the posterior cruciate ligament.[d] • There is no consensus that foot position can alter quad muscle recruitment.[e] • Select the most comfortable foot position that poses the least stress.
Hamstring curl	Allowing buttocks to rise from the bench and the hips to flex	This may be one of three things: • The weight is too high. • The rectus femoris is too tight, pulling to rotate the pelvis. • The abdominal muscles are too weak to hold a neutral spine position.
Triceps kickback	Positioning elbow below the body	• The ROM in which the triceps have to lift against gravity is reduced. However, a raised elbow puts the long head of the triceps in a shortened position, so this head has less involvement. • A modification of a triceps exercise in which the upper arm is raised (shoulder flexion) will involve the long head as well as the medial and lateral heads.
Barbell curl	Moving the torso or shoulder joint	• Extending the torso in the up phase creates momentum. • Flexing the shoulder joint draws assistance from the anterior deltoid and upper pectoralis major. • These actions do not allow the elbows to move through a full ROM and decrease the muscle fiber recruitment of the biceps.

(continued)

(continued)

Exercise	What's wrong?	Why? Key points
Exercise ball crunch	Using a position on the ball that does not allow for a ROM suited to the client's strength	• A position of support in the middle and upper back will decrease the ROM and reduce the lever arm length, creating an easier modification. • A lower starting position allowing the spine to slightly hyperextend will prestretch the abdominal muscles, change the fulcrum, and increase the lever arm, therefore increasing the contractile ROM.

Note: ROM = range of motion.

[a]Hagan 2000; [b]Signorile et al. 2002; [c]Lyons and Orwin 1998; [d]Escamilla et al. 1998; [e]Lockwood 1999.

Table 7.13 Spotting Guidelines for Monitoring Lifting Techniques

Area	Spotting guidelines
Upper body	• Position yourself close to the client where you have the most effective position for assistance. • Assist the client with heavier weights to bring the weight to the starting position. • Position your hands on the barbell. • During dumbbell exercises, position your hands at the joint that is immediately below the weight. • Assist the client at the end point of a movement during the final reps.
Lower body	• Position yourself close to the client where you have the most effective position for assistance. • Assist the client to bring the weight to the starting position for squats and lunges. • Position your hands just above the waist for squats and lunges. • Position your hands on the machine or the involved limb for pulley, machine, or hand exercises. • Assist the client at the end of a movement or if the speed decreases because of fatigue.
Trunk	• Use the assistance of gravity by using incline or decline positions of the bench. • Teach a pelvic stabilization to minimize low back curvature and strain. • Manually assist when client has difficulty with correct movements. • Manually assist at the ends of normal range of motion once fatigue has occurred.

Table 7.12 identifies a number of common faults in the design or execution of popular resistance exercises. Monitoring good form through effective spotting can significantly reduce execution faults. Table 7.13 lists the major spotting guidelines for monitoring technically sound mechanics.

Step 8: Design Warm-Up and Cool-Down

The warm-up and cool-down should reflect the type and magnitude of the work done in the resistance training portion. In the warm-up, introduce and progress low-impact movements to raise temperature and heart rate. Increasing the temperature of a muscle increases the elastic properties and the ability to stretch. After some warming, stretch the muscle groups to be used in the workout. Add supplemental static stretches if muscles are tight or sore or if you expect higher intensity than usual.

If workout is to be highly eccentric, build eccentric overloading gradually with a more active, dynamic-style warm-up. Although some studies have shown no difference between the effects of dynamic and static warm-up before physical activity or sport, dynamic warm-up has been shown to be a more effective method for high strength and power performance enhancement including jump performance, agility, and sprint performance (Pacheco et al. 2011; Van Gelder and Bartz 2011). For the serious athlete, the inclusion of near-maximal muscular actions may acutely improve neuromuscular performance by inducing postactivation potentiation (PAP). Recent studies have suggested that 10 min of dynamic stretching or 1 or 2 sets of 20 m of dynamic stretches can enhance jump and sprint performance, respectively (Turki et al. 2011).

In the cool-down, relieve muscle tightness that may result from eccentric work (e.g., in quadriceps, calves, chest, and erector spinae). Stretch tight postural muscles (e.g., anterior chest, hip flexors, hamstrings). Light aerobic work will prevent blood pooling (dizziness) and help remove blood lactate to aid in recovery.

Case Studies

Form 7.1, Resistance Training Prescription Worksheet, addresses the essential prescription factors and is a quick reference for basic exercise selections. Add your own exercises for each body area based on available equipment or preferences. This should prove quick and useful for direct client program design. Initially, form 7.2, Resistance Training Prescription Card, may seem detailed and time-consuming to fill out. Like a lesson plan for a teacher, it has great value as a learning tool, guiding critical choices so as not to leave any gaping holes or allow oversights in the design.

Case Study 1: Off-Season Athlete

Ranjeev is a 16-year-old lacrosse athlete who has requested an off-season training program to develop his lower body power. He wants to be able to accelerate past or through his opponents, change directions quickly, and maintain this power into the third period. The worksheet reflects his trainer's focus on reactive ability, which is critical for power output and separates elite athletes from the average. It means faster, more precise directional changes and better agility, speed, and joint stability, as well as a decreased risk of injury. Figure 7.3 outlines Ranjeev's off-season program.

Case Study 2: 38-Year-Old Beginner

Michael was a 38-year-old male with little experience in resistance training. He was interested in feeling better and gaining general conditioning for the whole body but was particularly concerned with his upper body posture and poor abdominal tone.

Assessment

The assessment provided me with the following data:

- Weight: 85 kg (187 lb)
- Height: 180 cm (5 ft 11 in.)
- Body mass index: 26.2
- Resistance exercises: 10RM established for each exercise and 1RM estimated
- Circuit time: Initial time recorded for two circuits (10 reps) including 2 min rest between cycles

Counseling revealed that Michael was at a preparation stage. He had purchased a membership at the local YMCA and although his time was tight, he thought that he could spend 40 to 45 min there two or three times per week. There were no overt health or musculoskeletal limitations; however, his technique during the 10RM assessments was consistent with a novice motor knowledge level. We agreed to use some equipment that seemed appealing to Michael and complement those pieces with others that could form a circuit centered on his goals.

Resistance Training Prescription

Most of the equipment selected was variable resistance, and Michael found it quite smooth. There was a minimum of weight stack adjustment from station to station in the circuit. The equipment that Michael had chosen fit easily into the circuit. Most of the exercises were multijoint with some isolations for posture and trunk. They alternated lower body and upper body with a balance of agonist and antagonist. Precautions were listed on the program card. The abdominal and core work on the stability ball was done after the circuit and was one of Michael's favorites. The intensity (weight) and volume (sets and reps) were based on the preparation stage and his 10RM assessment. A training log was kept, reflecting these primary prescription factors and Michael's subjective feelings. The progression was volume based, building reps from 13 up to 20 (momentary failure), then going to 3 sets of 15 (up to 20). Because of a lack of time, the stretches within the warm-up and cool-down included specific postural stretches. Details of the prescription are on the resistance training prescription card (figure 7.4).

Justification of Resistance Prescription

When we design an exercise prescription, we must integrate principles of exercise science and training with the psychosocial factors of our clients and the circumstances affecting their exercise prescription. Every decision made should be based on a sound physiological justification and a rationale that is client centered. The following list provides the critical thinking that was involved in Michael's resistance training prescription.

1. **Review Client Needs and Confirm Goals**
   - Client has no overt limitations.
   - Modified circuit will allow efficient use of time and cover whole body.
   - Major muscles are included.
   - Weaker phasic muscles (e.g., rhomboids, lower traps, abdominal muscles) need to be strengthened.
   - Length and difficulty of program suit exercise and time.
   - Rounded shoulders and lumbar lordosis stated as concern (exercises 6 and 7).

COMPONENT OBJECTIVE:
POWER PROGRAM (FUNCTIONAL REACTIVE ABILITY—LOWER BODY)

Client name   Trainer name

Exercise (brief description)	Body area/ muscles	Intensity and weight	Reps	Sets	Rest between sets	Precautions
Scissor jumps • *From a lunge position, spring up and switch legs (use your arms)* • *Land in a lunge position with opposite leg in front*	Extensors	Body weight (BW)	8-10 each side	1		Adjust to pre-fatigue with good form
Hurdle – 2 leg bounds (5 @ 3 ft each), with 1/2 squat • *Set up 5 small hurdles (hockey sticks) – 3 ft apart* • *Using a double leg jump & tuck, land and immediately continue hurdling*	Extensors	(BW)		2	(1 min rest)	Adjust to pre-fatigue with good form
X-country ski-alternating single leg bound • *Alternate single leg bounds (keep alignment and work knee-hip flexion)* • *Co-ordinate straight arm rhythmic swing (as in X-country skiing)*	Extensors	(BW)	5-8 each side	1		Adjust to pre-fatigue with good form
Side hops with sprint 5 steps • *Start in a squat position with a cone beside you* • *Hop sideways over the cone with both feet* • *Progress by adding a 5-step spring in various directions on landing*	Extensors and abductors	(BW)	3-4 each	1		Adjust to pre-fatigue with good form
Lateral line hops (alternating legs) • *Start in a squat position about 2 feet from a line* • *Push off laterally and upward from outside foot* • *Land on the opposite foot and push back in opposite direction*	Extensors and abductors	(BW)	8-10 each side	1		Adjust to pre-fatigue with good form
Depth jumps (12-18 inches), down and up (optional) • *From the edge of a sturdy box, step off to land on both feet* • *Spring up into vertical jump right away (ground contact in short)*	Extensors	(BW)	10-12	1		Adjust to pre-fatigue with good form
Method of Progression: *Increase reps to upper limit, then go back to lower limit and add another set (1 min rest)*						

Figure 7.3 Ranjeev's resistance training prescription worksheet.

Exercise Selection Examples (by body area)			
Chest	**Shoulders**	**Upper back**	**Arms**
Bench press	Shoulder press	Lat pull-down	Chin-up
Supine/Incline fly	Lateral fly	Bent-over fly	Biceps curl
Supine bent-arm pullover	Upright row	Bent-over row	Triceps extension
Pec deck		Cable crossover	Push-up
Cable crossover			
_____	_____	_____	_____
_____	_____	_____	_____
Legs	**Inside/Outside legs**	**Abdominal muscles**	**Lower back**
Leg press	Hip adduction (e.g., cable)	Crunch/Curl-up	Superman
X Lunge (modif.)	Hip abduction	Reverse sit-down	Deadlift
X Squat (modif.)	*X Lateral line hop*	Plank (front/side)	All-fours alternate arm and
Knee extension	*X Side hop*	Oblique crossover	leg lift
Knee flexion			Prone leg/arm lift
Calf raise			
X Hurdle			
X Single leg bound			

Figure 7.3   *(continued)*

2. **Select Resistance Equipment**
   - Multijoint exercise is more functional and efficient for only six exercises.
   - Choice is suitable for client's comfort and motor knowledge.
   - Choice provides variable resistance and smooth strength curve.
   - Equipment provides stabilization for novice.
   - Exercises are suited to goals and time.
   - Equipment is readily available at YMCA.
   - Station switch is quick and easy.

3. **Select Resistance Training Method**
   - Standard sets are provided in a circuit format.
   - Choice is good for prep stage.
   - Time under tension is maximized with circuit.
   - Program is fast moving, should keep interest.

4. **Select Exercises and Order of Performance**
   - Lower body and upper body are worked alternately.
   - Exercises suit circuit and there is ample recovery time.
   - Feedback on execution mechanics ensures personal safety and benefits.
   - Agonist–antagonist muscles are worked (exercises 1 and 3, 2 and 4).

   - Exercise 1: Hip and knee extensors, balances with exercise 3.
   - Exercise 2: Anterior shoulder and chest (horizontal adduction of shoulder and extension of elbow), balances with exercise 4.
   - Exercise 3: Knee flexors, balances with exercise 1.
   - Exercise 4: Posterior and anterior shoulders (adduction of shoulder and flexion of elbow), balances with exercise 2.
   - Exercise 5: Outer and inner thigh (concentric in and out); exercises 1 to 5 involve the whole body.
   - Exercise 6: Posterior shoulders (horizontal abduction of shoulders and retraction of scapula), strengthens weaker muscles to address rounded shoulders.
   - Exercise 7: Trunk flexors and rotators, suits client goals of abdominal tone, core stability, and mobility.

5. **Set Resistance Intensity and Weight**
   - Resistance intensity and weight are established from assessment (i.e., 10RM is close to starting load).
   - Load is fine-tuned in the demonstration.
   - Resistance intensity and weight are interdependent with volume (sets × reps × load).

| Client name | *Michael* | Trainer name | *John* |

Client goals	Special considerations
Preparation stage—concerned with upper-body posture, abdominal tone, and feeling better.	*General fitness needs—whole body* • *local YMCA 2-3 x per week* • *40-45 min—time efficient*

Circulatory Warm-Up

Equipment and mode	Workload	Time	HR/PE objective
Treadmill	*Moderate to brisk walk; gradually increase speed*	*5-7 min*	*HR: 100-110 beats/min* *RPE: 11-12*

Stretching Warm-Up

Name and brief description	Guidelines
• *Four to six stretches for lower body after treadmill, including low back, hip flexors, hip extensors, and calf and shin muscles* • *One stretch each for the chest, upper back and shoulders, triceps, biceps, and hip adductors and abductors in preparation for the circuit* • *Stretches for pectoralis minor and shoulder medial rotators to maintain or improve posture*	*Static stretches after treadmill* *Hold for 15-20 s* *Between the two circuit sets, redo any of the warm-up stretches of muscles that feel tight*

Resistance Workout

Equipment type (e.g., free weights)	Training method
• *Selectorized equipment (variable resistance)* • *Exercise ball*	*Modified circuit with standard (simple) sets* *Mainly multijoint exercises, some isolations for posture and trunk*

Guidelines

• *Circuit fashion (i.e., perform all exercises once and then do second set)*
• *Rest 2 min between circuits*
• *10RM established in each exercise*

Exercise (brief description)	Muscles	Intensity/ weight	Reps	Sets	Rest between sets	Precautions
1. Leg press (seated) 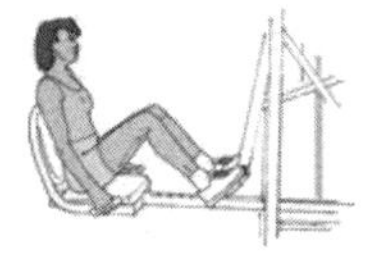 	*Quadriceps, hamstrings, gluteus maximus*	*65-70% of 1RM*	*10-13*	*2*	*30 s*	• *Maintain alignment* • *Avoid full knee extension*

Figure 7.4 Michael's resistance training prescription card.

Exercise (brief description)	Muscles	Intensity/ weight	Reps	Sets	Rest between sets	Precautions
2. Bench press 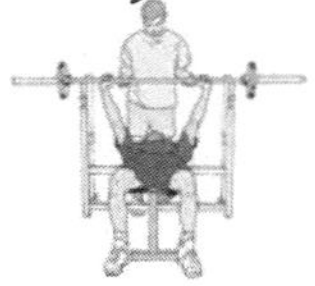	Pectoralis major, anterior deltoid, triceps	65-70% of 1RM	10-13	2	30 s	• Use soft elbows • Avoid bounce at bottom of ROM
3. Hamstrings curl 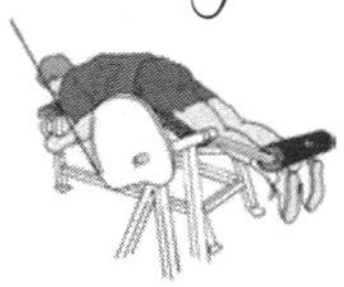	Hamstrings	65-70% of 1RM	10-13	2	30 s	• Stabilize low back • Maintain form even with low ROM
4. Lat pull-down 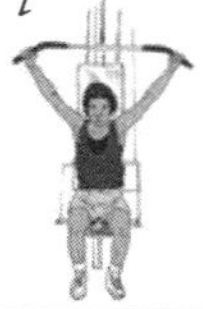	Latissimus dorsi, pectoralis major	65-70% of 1RM	10-13	2	30 s	• Lower to top of sternum and squeeze scapulae
5. Leg abductor–adductor 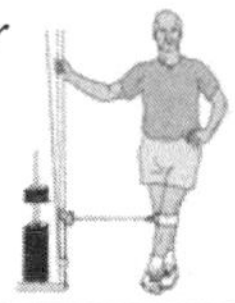	Hip abductors and adductors	65-70% of 1RM	10-13	2	30 s	• Use slow and controlled movements
6. Seated row 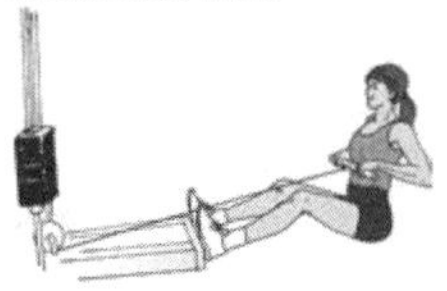	Posterior deltoid, trapezius, biceps	65-70% of 1RM	10-13	2	30 s	• Squeeze scapulae together
7. Abdominal curls and twists on ball 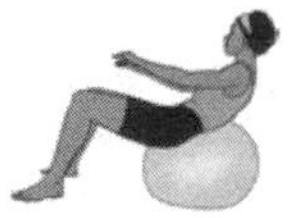	Rectus abdominis, obliques, spinal stabilizers	Body weight	3 3 7 (left, front, right)	2	30 s	• Maintain stable core and breathing • Keep ball on low back

Progression
• Build reps from 13 up to 20 (momentary failure) then go to 3 sets of 15 (up to 20)—"volume overload." • Use log provided to record load, reps, sets, volume, and subjective feelings. • Retest 1ORM in 4 weeks.

Cool-Down	
Name and brief description	**Guidelines**
Repeat warm-up stretches.	Hold static stretches for 15-20 s.

Note. HR = heart rate; PE = perceived exertion; RPE = rating of perceived exertion; ROM = range of motion.

Figure 7.4 *(continued)*

- Segment is based on preparation stage and goals (i.e., posture and abdominal tone).

6. **Set Resistance Volume**
   - Initial overload is focused on volume.
   - Momentary failure peaks neural stimulation.
   - Choice supports load setting.
   - Volume is best for a beginner.
   - Circuit allows recovery (rest between sets).
   - Minimum frequency of two times/week is possible.

7. **Design Progression and Monitoring**
   - Reps and sets (volume) adjust one factor at a time.
   - Training log reflects primary prescription factors.
   - Program provides for retesting load and readiness for next stage.
   - Program is steady but reasonable and allows self-administration.
   - Review of subjective feeling is a good predictor of compliance.
   - Program is related to client's motivation type.

8. **Design Warm-Up and Cool-Down**
   - Cardiovascular warm-up raises muscle temperature.
   - Specific joint and muscle stretching is provided for resistance exercises.
   - Segment suits special client considerations (e.g., postural stretches).

Summary

The client-centered exercise prescription model for resistance training allows you to shape the overload to suit your client by manipulating the prescription factors according to the principle of specificity—namely, that gains in muscular fitness are specific to the muscle group, training method, and exercise volume. Whether your client's needs are related to health, fitness, performance, appearance, or rehabilitation, the eight-step model guides your design decisions for a tailored program.

Specific types of resistance include body weight, free weights, constant resistance, variable resistance, hydraulics and pneumatics, electronics, isokinetics, and others such as elastic bands and tubing, water, and manual resistance.

Many resistance training programs use the standard set system of training consisting of 1 (single set) or more sets (multiple sets) of each exercise. This resistance training method can be performed at any resistance, for any number of repetitions or sets, to match the goals of the client. With the pyramid system, the client begins by using a relatively light weight and after each set increases the weight so that fewer repetitions can be done. Specific needs may be met with other systems of training such as superset, compound set, circuit, and a split-routine system. For speed and force, plyometric training—rapid eccentric lengthening of a muscle followed immediately by rapid concentric contraction of that muscle to produce a forceful explosive movement—is effective. Periodization is a method that can be applied to resistance training and is characterized by systematic cycles of alternating prescription variables such as intensity and volume.

Knowing the purpose and benefit of each exercise can help maintain muscle balance and avoid overworking a particular body area. Training intensity is a critical prescription factor providing the stimulus needed for improvement in specific muscular components. Volume is often described as sets × reps × load. However, the rest between the sets and the speed of the movements all contribute to the total training effects of "time under tension." The correct amount of progressive overload depends on your client's objectives and training level and should be monitored carefully along with his technique. The warm-up and cool-down should reflect the type and magnitude of the work done in the resistance training portion.

Client name   Trainer name

Exercise (brief description)	Body area, muscles	Intensity and weight	Reps	Sets	Rest between sets	Precautions

(continued)

(continued)

Exercise (brief description)	Body area, muscles	Intensity and weight	Reps	Sets	Rest between sets	Precautions

Method of Progression:

_____

Exercise Selection Examples (by Body Area)

Use the prescription model guidelines and add prescription exercises to the list of examples as needed.

Chest	**Shoulders**	**Upper back**	**Arms**
Bench press	Shoulder press	Lat pull-down	Chin-up
Supine/incline fly	Lateral fly	Bent-over fly	Biceps curl
Supine bent-arm pullover	Upright row	Bent-over row	Triceps extension
Pec deck		Cable crossover	Push-up
Cable crossover			
_____	_____	_____	_____
_____	_____	_____	_____

Legs	**Inside and outside legs**	**Abdominal muscles**	**Lower back**
Leg press	Hip adduction (e.g., cable)	Crunch/curl-up	Superman
Lunge	Hip abduction	Reverse sit-downs	Deadlift
Squat		Plank (front/side)	All-fours alternate arm and leg lift
Knee extension	_____	Oblique crossover	Prone leg/arm lift
Knee flexion			
Calf raise	_____	_____	_____
_____		_____	_____
_____			

FORM 7.2   Resistance Training Prescription Card

Client name	Trainer name
Client goals	**Special considerations**

Circulatory Warm-Up			
Equipment and mode	**Workload**	**Time**	**HR/PE objective**

Stretching Warm-Up	
Name and brief description	**Guidelines**

Resistance Workout	
Equipment type (e.g., free weights)	**Training method**

Guidelines

Exercise (brief description)	Muscles	Intensity and weight	Reps	Sets	Rest between sets	Precautions

(continued)

(continued)

Exercise (brief description)	Muscles	Intensity and weight	Reps	Sets	Rest between sets	Precautions

Progression

Cool-Down

Name and brief description	Guidelines

Note: HR = heart rate; PE = perceived exertion.

From J.C. Griffin, 2015, *Client-centered exercise prescription,* 3rd ed. (Champaign, IL: Human Kinetics).

Client-Centered Functionally Integrated Exercise

Chapter Competencies

After completing this chapter, you will be able to demonstrate the following competencies:

1. Describe the factors affecting muscle balance.
2. Describe the causes and results of muscle imbalance.
3. Select and describe assessment items for muscle balance.
4. Describe the factors affecting the quality of a stretch.
5. Describe the advantages and client suitability of various stretching techniques.
6. Select appropriate exercises (stretching or resistance) that target designated muscle groups to improve range of motion or muscle balance.
7. Design a physiologically sound and client-centered exercise prescription for muscle balance and flexibility using the six-step model of sequenced decisions.

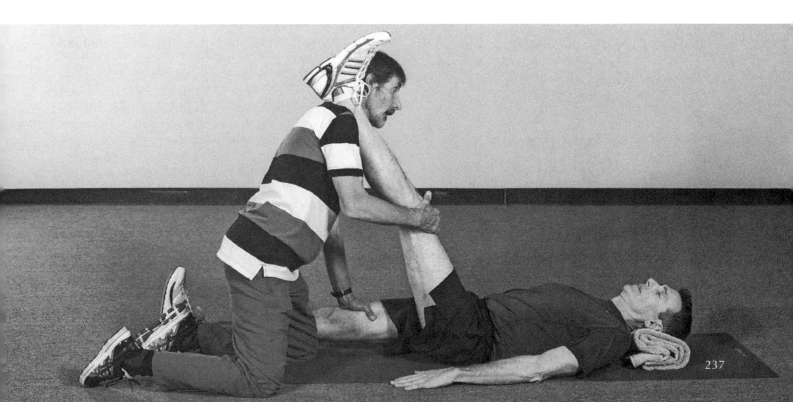

The buzzword in the fitness industry nowadays is *functional*. A functional program can be defined simply as a program that simulates actions similar to the desired activity or that mimic the demands and skills of a sport or daily activity. Functional integration is often the process of changing previously learned motor programs in the body. It is not something that can be cognitively controlled on a consistent basis. The body must be reeducated to function as it was designed to function.

Clients who have muscle imbalances or postural alignment problems can be helped with functionally integrated exercise. Muscle balance is affected by muscle tightness, flexibility, strength, and endurance, because these factors work together to provide support and movement. Thus, looking at muscle balance is a necessary part of a holistic approach to muscular fitness. Although not a new concept, muscle balance is a new approach to solving problems. It gets right to the heart of your clients' needs, whether they are athletes or fitness enthusiasts or are recovering from injuries.

A muscle must be long enough to allow a normal range of motion and short and strong enough to provide joint stability. Thus, only after assessing a client's muscle tightness and flexibility, and weakness versus strength and endurance, can we adequately personalize the training program. Setting objectives for muscle balance usually centers around stretching tight muscles, strengthening weak muscles, reducing spasms or inefficient firing, building muscular endurance, or improving posture.

In addition to discussing the preceding issues, this chapter presents guidelines for functional exercise design, causes and detection of muscle imbalance, client-centered flexibility prescription, the steps involved in the model for muscle balance prescription, and two case studies with personalized prescriptions.

Functionally Integrated Exercise

Functional, integrated training is "lifelike" and free moving, involving multiplane and multijoint movements that overcome the force of gravity and require stabilization, changes of direction, and acceleration and deceleration. To actually live up to the meaning of the term "functional," the prescription for functional exercise must follow some important guidelines:

• Integrate kinetic chain movements. The brain thinks in terms of whole motions, not individual muscles. For example, a baseball batter thinks about hitting the ball. To achieve this action, he swings in one fluid action, not by consciously trying to activate individual muscle groups. The brain initiates a series of impulses to attain a synchronized movement pattern. We should respond by training movements, not muscles. Combining movements of the upper and lower extremities can often fulfill this principle and expand the kinetic chain movements.

• Use multiplane motion. A tennis player rushing the net or a senior citizen climbing stairs is combining motion patterns in the sagittal, frontal, and transverse planes. Reaching, rotating, climbing, lifting, and pushing are activities that involve a free-flowing, nonrigid movement in the functional spectrum of these three planes. Resistance machines often prevent the body from moving in the most functional manner within the three planes.

• Involve a loading and unloading cycle. Dynamic activity that requires the client to slow, stop, or change direction creates the need to reduce force (eccentric contraction) in one direction, stabilize, and then produce force (concentric contraction) in another direction. When performed quickly, this is referred to as agility and efficiently incorporates the use of stored energy during the eccentric or loading phase. Even at slower rates, changes in acceleration and stabilization are part of functional training that requires the body to absorb gravitational forces when moving downward and reacting with concentric forces to move back up.

• Incorporate actions that require balance, stabilization, and proprioceptive stimulation. For example, a side-to-side hop requires clients to preload before unloading to achieve efficient movement. The client must be balanced as she moves from one phase to the next. Ways to add challenge to functional movements include changing body angles, adjusting body weight, changing vision direction, or providing unstable surfaces. These modifications require skill development and the ability to know where the limbs are in space and in relationship to other body parts.

A functional, integrated training program can dramatically enhance your clients' results. When creating the training program, consider your client's objectives and design a functional prescription based on the goal of the program. Many

Functional Exercise for Muscle Imbalance

Functional exercises can help clients work on issues such as muscle imbalances or postural alignment problems. On the other hand, structural problems and muscle imbalances can predispose your client to injury or exacerbate an existing injury or symptom. These postural and structural changes occur over time. Certain muscles can become shorter and tighter; others can become longer and weaker. These changes can alter the muscles' mechanical lines of pull, causing other muscles and muscle groups to compensate. The postural changes then begin to directly alter joint mechanics. This alteration or compensation leads to a decrease in performance. Functionally integrated exercises need to be designed to address interdependency of the structural weakness. Although the exercise design may initially be focused and targeted (e.g., rehabilitation), optimal performance of the task at hand and incorporating function into the training process are our ultimate goal. These exercises can be an adjunct to your strength training or your flexibility program.

To effectively conduct a postural evaluation or an evaluation of muscle imbalance and apply it to your prescription, you will need a thorough knowledge of kinesiology and a working knowledge of biomechanics. Clients who have significant or chronic postural deviations or pain, a history of spinal problems, or radiating nerve pain to the upper or lower extremities should be referred to a qualified health professional. It is important that you not diagnose and that you recognize when the client's situation is beyond your capabilities.

activities occur from positions such as sitting, lying, and kneeling, but try originating your exercises from a standing position. Standing affects the hip, knee, and torso, which are also affected by motion of the trunk and arms—all typical of functional movement.

For example, traditional abdominal exercises are often done from the ground in the sagittal plane only. Although this activates the abdominal muscles, they are isolated and do not work to decelerate the trunk during rotation or help stabilize the spine when it is extending. A functional alternative would be to use a medicine ball and perform rotational movements, perform overhead two-handed throws, or balance on one foot while holding the medicine ball overhead. Now the abdominal muscles are recruited for stabilization, rotation, and deceleration, and they work in tandem with the hips to maintain a strong core when one is in an upright posture. This functional or integrated approach begins with linking and stabilizing the muscles that work together to achieve a neutral spine. It is upon this foundation of a neutral spine that all power of movement by the arms and legs can be successfully generated.

We need to treat the human body as a highly integrated structure instead of a series of independent parts. Functionally integrated exercise improves any performance, reduces the risk of overuse injuries, and allows you as the trainer to be more creative in your exercise design. Functional training exercises enhance clients' overall function and at the same time let them have some fun.

Muscle Balance

Muscle balance is vital to optimal bodily functioning. A loss of muscle balance may be reported as a pain or a general feeling of fatigue or tightness. During screening, you may recognize muscle imbalance from poor posture or poor alignment (chapter 4), and postural deviations will become more common and more exaggerated with aging. The client's posture is the "snapshot" of his muscle imbalances. Repetitive activity can overuse certain muscles and underuse opposing muscles. This overuse creates a weakness of one group that is overpowered by the strength of the opposing group. A client's job may demand a prolonged position or repeated movements that create an imbalance.

Imbalance may be the underlying cause of headaches, low back discomfort or other joint abnormalities, apparently random aches and pains, or an old injury that keeps emerging. Most clients will approach you with relatively vague initial concerns. Careful questioning about signs, symptoms, or concerns can reveal a potential cause of the muscle imbalance. Such problems are usually multifaceted: They are not limited to strength, flexibility, or endurance but may involve strength of one muscle group and flexibility of an opposing muscle group. Muscle balance also

Baseball-Related Muscle Imbalance

Your client plays recreational baseball and complains of some discomfort when raising his arm to throw. Because his shoulder felt weak, he had initiated a strengthening program for his shoulders and chest, with no apparent improvement. Your initial observations include a rounded shoulder posture and well-developed chest muscles. This is a classic example of muscle imbalance that needs an integrated approach to prescription. Many of the major upper body muscles internally (medially) rotate the shoulder. Throwing the ball powerfully uses these muscles. The external (lateral) rotators, however, are relatively small. The stronger and tighter internal rotators involved in throwing are overpowering the weaker external rotators. In baseball, the magnitude and speed of this force are significant. The rounded shoulders are the result of this imbalance and a contributing cause of the shoulder pain. The single-component approach used by the client to strengthen the shoulder actually increased the imbalance. The anterior muscles (internal rotators) need to be lengthened, and the external rotators (posterior) need improved strength and muscular endurance. This is the muscle balance approach.

depends on neuromuscular efficiency or the ability of the neuromuscular system to properly recruit movers (agonists), stabilizers, and synergists to produce force or reduce force (antagonists). By considering all these factors, you can best serve your clients.

A key to structural balance and posture is equal pull by opposing muscles. A joint is a pivot point or a fulcrum whose alignment is constantly affected by the pull of the muscles around it. Figure 8.1 shows a loss of structural alignment when a short muscle overpowers a longer muscle. If the muscle is short, it will restrict normal range of motion. Muscles that are too short are usually strong and hold the opposite muscle in a lengthened position. Excessively long muscles are usually weak and allow adaptive shortening of antagonists (Kendall et al. 2005).

To better understand how these imbalances happen, consider the specialized roles played by different sorts of muscles. Muscles can be categorized into two groups (Norris 2000):

1. **Postural stabilizers.** These muscles have a static postural function and primarily stabilize a joint. Their function is more slow twitch or tonic than that of other muscles. They are often tight and short because of long work periods. Examples include upper trapezius, levator scapulae, transversus abdominis, pelvic floor, quadratus lumborum, iliopsoas, multifidus, erector spinae, and hip adductors.

2. **Phasic mobilizers.** These muscles are primarily responsible for movement. They tend to be more superficial and are often biarticular. They may be weak and fatigue early. Examples include rectus abdominis, gluteus maximus, rectus femoris, peroneals, deltoid, and biceps.

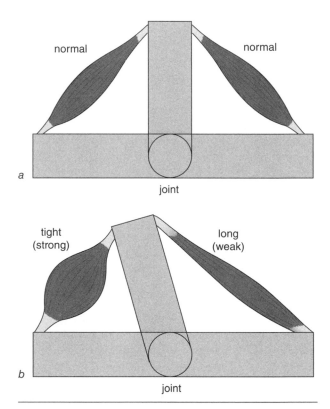

Figure 8.1 Muscle balance: *(a)* joint in structural balance and *(b)* joint misaligned—muscle imbalance.

With insufficient variety in muscle use, postural muscles can be activated disproportionately, which inhibits and weakens phasic muscles (Nordin and Frankel 2001). This process can lead to muscle imbalance, poor posture, loss of mobility, and an increase in joint load. Stabilizers and mobilizers react differently to reduced or excessive usage. Most often, we will see tightness in the postural stabilizers and weakness in the phasic mobilizers (table 8.1).

Table 8.1   Postural Stabilizers and Phasic Mobilizers

Tight postural stabilizers	Weak phasic mobilizers
Upper trapezius, levator scapulae	Lower trapezius, rhomboids
Iliopsoas	Rectus abdominis
Erector spinae, multifidus	Gluteus maximus
Hip adductors	Gluteus medius

Let's look more closely at the specific causes of imbalance. Muscles can be unbalanced in several ways. They can have unmatched levels of flexibility, strength, or contracture, or a combination of these factors, all of which are discussed subsequently. In addition, muscles can be neurally imbalanced (Blievernicht 2000).

Imbalance Resulting From Tight Muscles

Flexibility is the range of joint motion; **muscle tightness** is the range of muscle length. For muscles that pass over one joint, these two measures are very similar. For muscles that pass over two or more joints (e.g., gastrocnemius, hamstrings, rectus femoris, erector spinae), the range of muscle length will be less than the total range of motion of the joints over which the muscle passes. For example, the knee must be flexed to permit a full range of hip flexion because the hamstrings are too tight if the knee is straight.

Often there is tightness in the most active muscle group, which overpowers the more passive, longer, opposing muscle group. For example, you should always examine the lower leg balance of clients who are runners. Without proper stretching, constant use of the calf muscles will cause tightness. Calf stretching will help prevent alterations in the running mechanics and subsequent injuries.

Imbalance Resulting From Weak Muscles

Muscle strength testing not only can determine muscles of compromised strength but may also isolate the position of weakness. Muscle weakness has many causes. Even in active people, certain muscles are seldom overloaded. If weakness is attributable to lack of use, prescribe specific exercises for those muscles. With the runner in the previous example, strengthening the anterior shin would prevent problems resulting from unmatched levels of calf strength. If weakness is caused by overwork, fatigue, or strain, prescribe rest—at least in the short term. Relieve the stress before prescribing additional muscular work. Weakness often means an altered proprioceptive input to that muscle, and to improve joint stability, normal proprioception must be restored (Roskopf 2001).

Imbalance Resulting From Muscle Contracture

Commonly known as muscle spasms, muscle contracture also can cause imbalance. Contracture may result from injury, prolonged shortening, or weakness in the opposing muscle. These continued involuntary contractions usually respond to application of heat or cold, progressive static stretching, and, at times, isometric contractions.

A forward-bent position of the trunk and head (spinal flexion), often seen in office workers, requires continuous, prolonged muscle contractions—often at 20% of maximum voluntary contraction (Nordin and Frankel 2001). The pain that results from a lack of oxygen and an accumulation of metabolites can lead to a vicious circle of muscle spasm. In addition, prolonged isometric contractions can cause inflammation and passive shortening of the muscle.

Clients who have chronic low back pain are often diagnosed as having "back spasms." Traditional treatments include rest, ultrasound, various forms of heat, and massage. Although these treatments may relieve symptoms, they do not address the cause of the underlying muscle imbalance.

Imbalance Resulting From Combined Factors

You need to prescribe both strengthening and stretching for total body balance. A reduction of tightness is often needed before certain strength exercises can be properly performed. Therapeutic exercises to strengthen weak muscles, stretch tight muscles, and retrain postural awareness and movement patterns are the most effective and lasting means by which muscle balance is restored and maintained.

Low back spasms are often caused by weakness of opposing muscles. In the earlier example of the office worker, the weakness would be in the abdominal muscles around the trunk and the gluteus maximus and hamstrings around the posterior pelvis. Because traditional treatment is passive, it would actually leave the client with *two* weak muscles: the abdominal muscles and the low back muscles! When pain subsides and the traditional treatment has relieved some inflammation and spasm, you would start your client on abdominal strengthening exercises (with precautions for the back—see chapter 11). As in one of the case studies later this chapter, tight hip flexors can place added pressure on the low back. Neuromuscular awareness of postural alignments while standing, sitting, lying, and performing any of the prescribed movement patterns is a critical part of this integrated approach.

Neural Imbalance

Muscles that are strong and shortened are also neurally facilitated, whereas muscles that are weak and lengthened are neurally inhibited. Neurally facilitated muscles contract early and with excessive force during movements. Neurally inhibited muscles respond later and with less force than they would otherwise.

Results of Muscle Imbalance

One common imbalance involves shortened back extensors and hip flexors versus weakened abdominal and buttocks muscles. This imbalance results in an anterior pelvic tilt and excessive lumbar lordosis. In the upper body, there often is tightness of the pectoralis major, upper trapezius, and levator scapulae versus weakness of the rhomboids, lower trapezius, serratus anterior, and the deep flexor muscles of the neck. This is manifested in rounded shoulders, shoulder girdle elevation and abduction, forward head position, and possible cervical lordosis (Nordin and Frankel 2001).

Muscle imbalance may also lead to faulty movements through muscle groups firing in an uncoordinated way. For example, clients with tight rectus femoris and weak abdominal muscles may alter their body mechanics when they perform a hamstring curl. The hips may flex and the back hyperextend near the end of the range of motion.

The rectus femoris is stretched under tension as the knee bends, but if the rectus femoris is tight, it will pull on its origin, the anterior superior iliac spine, causing hip flexion. If the abdominal muscles are not strong, they cannot counter the anterior pull on the pelvis, and an anterior tilt results along with a low back hyperextension.

Imbalances may also exist within synergists, that is, a group of muscles that work together to produce a movement. For example, when clients with rounded shoulders perform lateral raises with dumbbells or reach overhead as in lifting a box to a top shelf, substitution patterns may occur. Normally the scapula rotates laterally (upwardly) to allow the shoulder joint to abduct. Clients with rounded shoulders often have an imbalance between the synergists responsible for this movement. They have a tight upper trapezius and weaker lower trapezius and serratus anterior. What results is excessive elevation of the shoulder girdle because of the dominant upper trapezius.

Faulty mechanics usually results when some stabilizers are more passive than others during certain movements. For example, during a strenuous biceps curl, the shoulder girdle may elevate. The middle and lower trapezius should stabilize the shoulder girdle in an adducted and depressed position during elbow flexion. Because the long head of the biceps brachii attaches to the scapula above the shoulder, the levator scapula and upper trapezius overpower their lower antagonists to place the biceps in a stronger prestretched position when fatigue sets in. This also occurs during activities such as shoveling or lifting, when the anterior deltoid or pectoralis major (clavicular) is prestretched by the shoulder girdle elevators. This substitution pattern will often result in a tense neck and upper back.

The human kinetic chain is made up of the muscular, fascial, skeletal, and neural systems. If one segment of the kinetic chain is misaligned or not functioning properly, predictable patterns of dysfunction develop, leading to neuromuscular inefficiency and tissue overload (Ninos 2001a). For example, tightness of the gastrocnemius can cause a runner to alter the support phase of her gait. The reduced dorsiflexion and slight turnout may result in increased stress on the plantar fascia and longitudinal arch. As a result, some excess pronation may occur in midstance when the foot is rolling forward but runs out of dorsiflexion range of motion. Further up the chain, this may cause an increased external rotation of the tibia, which in turn adds to the stress being placed on the patellofemoral joint (Ninos 2001b). Tightness of the calf can also affect the mechanics of doing a squat. Without adequate dorsiflexion, lifters will widen their stance and externally (laterally) rotate their feet to compensate for the tight calf. Essentially, the body's kinetic chain seeks the path of least resistance by placing an excessive torque load on the knees, resulting in ever-increasing disability.

The ultimate goal of the kinetic chain is to maintain dynamic postural equilibrium. To accomplish this, it must have adaptive potential. Limited flexibility, muscle weakness, and inappropriate neural firing decrease this adaptive potential. It is your job to look for signs of any existing muscle imbalance and begin the process of working with your client to restore balance.

Joint Stress Cycle

As should be clear by now, loss of muscle balance may lead to acute injury or can be the underlying cause of chronic overuse injury. Figure 8.2 is a model of how muscle imbalance can induce injury.

The **joint stress cycle** works like this: If your client has a muscle imbalance, such as tight anterior chest muscles (including shoulder internal rotators), there is often a misalignment (e.g., rounded shoulders). These muscles lose flexibility, and the joint becomes progressively more stiff until the muscle is in constant partial contracture; it has progressively less endurance

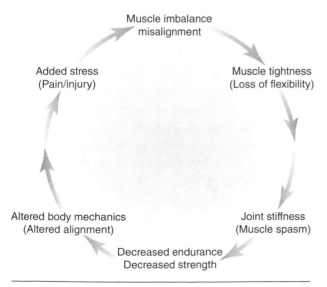

Figure 8.2   The joint stress cycle.

and strength. At this point, a person will alter his mechanics—for example, he may throw a ball with a distinct sidearm style. But the adjustments themselves cause additional problems, creating a vicious circle of pain and misalignment.

How do you know if your client is within this joint stress cycle? Most clients, whether active or inactive, are somewhere on the cycle, and you must decide where your client is on the cycle.

Start by obtaining a client history of musculoskeletal problems. Use form 8.1, Joint Stress Questionnaire and Observations, to gather the client's answers and to record your own observations. This information will tell you where your client is on the joint stress cycle and how to get her out of it. As seen in the joint stress cycle, problems most often begin with muscle tightness and loss of flexibility. In a functionally integrated approach to musculoskeletal training, our first concern should be with this component.

Mechanisms of Stretch and Flexibility

Flexibility is an often neglected component of physical fitness. Enhancing flexibility improves not only joint range of motion (ROM) but also muscle relaxation, muscle balance, and preparation for activity. Flexibility should integrate multiplanar soft tissue extensibility with neuromuscular efficiency throughout the full ROM. Lack of flexibility is often the cause of musculoskeletal injuries, low back pain, and headaches.

The effectiveness of a stretch is related to the behavior of the connective tissue and muscle when under stress. Limitation to ROM is attributable 47% to joint structure, 41% to muscle fascia, and 10% to tendons (Brooks 1993). The mechanism of stretch explains why this is so.

The myosin filaments within the sarcomere of the muscle fiber have a strand of very elastic protein called titin extending out to be anchored at the Z line. When a relaxed muscle is stretched passively, its muscle fibers elongate and the actin and myosin filaments slide past each other so that the sarcomeres also lengthen. When the stretch force is removed, the muscle fibers and the sarcomeres spring back to their original resting lengths because of the actions of titin pulling the Z lines closer together (Germann and Stanfield 2002). This elastic mechanism is not dependent on time.

However, muscles are not purely elastic; rather, they are viscoelastic, having both viscous (resistant to flow) and elastic properties. Lengthening of a muscle under force is called **creep.** When a muscle is stretched to a constant length, over time the force (tension) will decrease, and this is called **stress-relaxation.** If the muscle returns to its original length when the force is removed, this is **elastic deformation** (figure 8.3). When connective tissue is stretched, some of the elongation is elastic and some may be more permanent when the force is removed **(plastic deformation)** (Hendrick 2000). Connective tissue is the major structure limiting joint ROM (i.e., sheathing around muscle, tendons, ligaments, and joint capsules).

New evidence suggests that the stretch mechanism has both a direct and an indirect process of decreasing a muscle's "stiffness," which is defined as the force required to change its length. The direct process is via passive viscoelastic changes or deformations. The indirect process is attributable to reflex inhibition and consequent changes in the viscoelasticity from decreased actin–myosin cross-bridging (Shrier and Gossal 2000). There is also evidence that we get an increase in ROM not only because of a decrease in muscle stiffness but also because of an increase in our stretch tolerance (i.e., more force can be applied before we feel pain).

Role of Fascia

The common method of defining muscle action by determining what would happen if the two ends came closer together is useful but not definitive. When one part of the body moves, the body as a whole responds. Functionally, the only tissue that can mediate such responsiveness is the connective tissue. Muscle has an effect on its neighbors by tightening its fascia and pushing against those adjacent muscles. As well, fascia has an effect of pulling on proximal or distal structures beyond the muscle.

The word "myofascia" connotes the bundled-together, inseparable nature of muscle tissue *(myo)* and its accompanying web of connective tissue *(fascia)*. Critical to understanding movement, the term *myofascial continuity* refers to the connection between adjacent structures within a fascial webbing. Myers (2009) refers to myofascial meridian lines as lines of pull, which transmit strain and movement through the body's myofascia around the skeleton. One such line is the superficial back line, which is a collection of muscles and their accompanying fascia running from the plantar fascia continuously to the cranial fascia (see figure 8.4). Myofascial lines must show a continuity of fascial fibers in which these lines of pull or lines of transmission through the myofascia go fairly straight. Many have a direct connection that is purely fascial. For example, the iliotibial tract ties directly into the tibialis anterior; the external and internal obliques have a clear direct connection across the abdominal aponeurosis and the linea alba. Other myofascial lines have mechanical connections passing through intervening bone. For example, the rectus abdominis and the rectus femoris have an indirect mechanical connection through the pelvic bone in sagittal motions such as anterior and posterior tilt of the pelvis (Myers 2009).

The mechanical role of fascia or connective tissue is to meet the combined need of flexibility and stability in our structure. Stretch fascia quickly and it will tear. However, if the stretch is

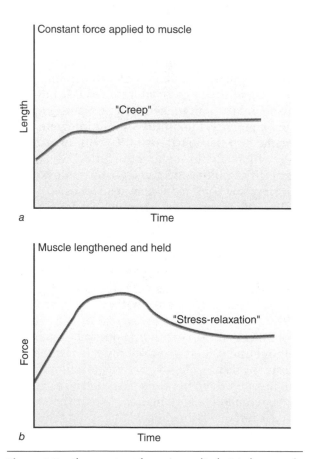

Figure 8.3 If a constant force is applied, *(a)* the muscle will stretch immediately and then slowly increase in length. If a muscle is stretched to a certain length and held, *(b)* the force on the muscle gradually reduces.

applied slowly, the fascia will deform plastically: It will change its length and retain that change. It has been generally assumed that fascia is solely a passive contributor, transmitting tension that is created by the muscles or other forces. However, fascia may be able to contract autonomously and thereby play a more active role. It can integrate proprioceptive signals and assist in load bearing (e.g., lumbar fascia). Fascia myofibroblasts are cells that are capable of exerting continuous force over long periods of time, which may influence structural stability of the tissue. Myofibroblasts may represent an intermediate cell type between a smooth muscle cell and a fibroblast (Myers 2009). The sustained contractile ability of myofibroblasts may play a role in chronic contractures. The contraction produced by the cells can generate stiffening or shortening of large areas in the sheets of fascia where they often reside. This responsiveness of fascia can prepare the body for greater loads or facilitate transfer of loads from one fascia to another. The fact that myofibroblasts do not respond to neural stimulation may have implications for therapeutic fascia loading and unloading techniques that may be used for pain management (O'Sullivan and Bird 2011).

Long-duration contraction of the connective tissue may play a role in acute or chronic musculoskeletal pain. Fascia contraction occurs very slowly over a period of 20 to 30 min and may be sustained for more than an hour before slowly subsiding (O'Sullivan and Bird 2011). The contraction develops in response to a sustained load. Connective tissue can be remodeled by the positioning and movements of the body segments. Repetitive movement of a specific muscle group can produce a thickening or shortening of the fascia surrounding the activated muscle, which may provide more stability and allow the muscle to generate more power. During the process of fascia remodeling, inadequate lengthening (regular stretching) may produce a dysfunctional state that could increase risk for fascia tearing. Unlike muscle fibers, fascia is extremely susceptible to microtears when stretched quickly (e.g., high-intensity eccentric loading). If the fascia stretch is applied slowly over a long period of time, however, it may undergo plastic deformation. In the repair process, activation of fibroblasts results in the deposition of collagen at the location of the injury, which is assembled into fibers that become aligned with mechanical tension in the tissue. If the tissue is immobilized, dense connective tissue forms. Pain can be alleviated through a reduction in the mechanical stress on the tissue (i.e., fascia unloading), which reduces load on free nerve endings within the fascia (O'Sullivan and Bird 2011).

Lunge With Knee-Height Reach

Train the superficial back myofascial line with this exercise (figure 8.4).

1. Take a step forward, and while driving pelvis toward the floor, reach arms down in front of knees (look downward).
2. Reach from scapula and allow thoracic spine to flex while hips and knees flex (flex with rhythm).
3. Return to start position and repeat with opposite leg.

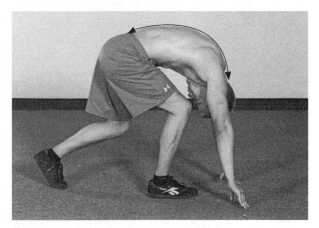

Figure 8.4 Lunge with rounded reach.

✅ Application

Training the myofascial lines dissipates force through the entire system, minimizing excessive isolated joint tension while giving the joints freedom to move and improving total body awareness and coordination. To place force through a line, the line (of muscle and fascia) must first load then unload, or stretch then shorten. This allows us to take advantage of the viscoelastic properties of fascia, helping us generate and transmit force through the entire body system while minimizing energy expenditure.

Flexibility Training Methods

You must have thorough knowledge of your clients before you can determine the best training method approach. A client who participates in competitive sport once or twice a week probably has tight muscle–tendon–fascia structures, whereas a previously inactive client may lack the strength of opposing muscles to pull the joint through a larger ROM. If your client's objective is to attain a ROM that allows ease of daily function or improved posture, static stretching may be the best training method.

Most types of flexibility training fall into one of three categories: static, dynamic, and proprioceptive neuromuscular facilitation (PNF). Regardless of the method of flexibility selected, always be aware of safety during the demonstration, supervision, and modification (see chapter 5).

Active Loosening

Relaxation, or the minimization of muscular tension, must exist before a stretch is attempted. Reduced tension can assist in stretching out connective tissues. Active loosening can relieve muscle tension and promote relaxation (Kuprian 1982). Active loosening exercises include rhythmic swinging of the limbs, active shaking of the limbs, or rotating the torso or limbs.

Many athletes know the effects of shaking the extremities to loosen particular muscles. A sprinter never gets into the starting blocks without thoroughly loosening her legs and arms. She shakes her legs one at a time while in a slight straddle position, and she shakes her arms while standing with the upper body slightly inclined and the arms hanging loosely. Loosening exercises facilitate more rapid recovery from stress through

a facilitated blood flow. Failure to loosen up leads to an early loss of strength, slowing of movements, and fatigue (Eitner 1982).

Other examples of effective loosening exercises include these:

- Lifting the shoulders and allowing them to fall
- Lying on the upper back, supporting the waist with the hands, and shaking the legs in the air
- Standing, twisting the trunk to the left and right (avoid excessive momentum, and avoid if any history of back problems)
- Standing, leaning against wall with outstretched arms, swinging each leg back and forth
- Lying supine with knees bent, shaking the legs (especially calves and hamstrings)
- Standing, one arm leaning on a table, letting other arm swing in a circle by rocking body weight in a circular pattern (figure 8.5)

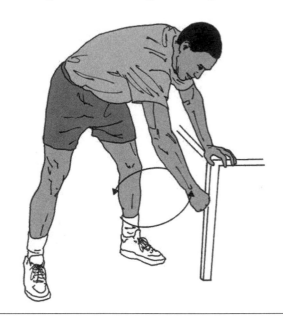

Figure 8.5   Active loosening.

Static Stretching

Static stretching involves controlled elongation of an antagonistic muscle by placing it in a maximal position of stretch and holding it. The Golgi tendon organs (GTOs) in the muscle's tendon are sensitive to the tension of a static stretch. The GTOs' signal to relax overrides the muscle spindles' signal to contract. The muscle spindles need a few seconds to adapt to the lengthened position before they decrease their discharge. The reflex contraction of the muscle to be stretched decreases, and the muscle is more relaxed and prepared to stretch. Recommendations for the optimal time for holding the stretch range from as short as 10 s to as long as 60 s (Heyward 2010). Thirty seconds duration is often suggested assuming that muscle temperature is elevated. If the stretch time is reduced to 15 s, 2 or 3 repetitions should be completed (Sapega et al. 1991). Static stretching can be either active or passive. Covert and colleagues (2010) found that 30 s of static stretching and ballistic stretching of the hamstrings three times per week both produced increased muscle length; however, static stretching was superior.

Active static stretching is accomplished by moving the agonist muscle to the end of its ROM and holding it in that position with an isometric contraction of the agonist muscles—without other aid. For example, to stretch the anterior chest and pectoralis minor muscles (figure 8.6), a client would contract the posterior shoulder girdle and shoulder joint muscles. This type of stretch is especially useful for people whose ROM is limited by the strength of the agonist muscles. You will recognize these clients by noting a large difference between their active ROM and assisted (passive) ROM. Active static stretching may also be effective after strength training or heavy eccentric work when a forced stretch may elongate the fibers excessively.

Active isolated stretching (A-I) is similar to active static stretching in that it uses the same principle: As one muscle in a pair is innervated to contract, the opposing muscle is inhibited (reciprocal inhibition). The client contracts the opposite muscle to be stretched through a full ROM. The unique feature of the A-I technique is the assistance provided by the trainer to gently increase the ROM. The client repeats the movement about 10 times, with the assist lasting no longer than 1 1/2 to 2 s. Good positioning and constant communication are important. Read your client's face and make sure she lets you know if she is feeling any irritation. To perform an active isolation stretch, one could do the stretch in figure 8.6 while sitting on a chair. The trainer would stand behind the client with his hands on the inside of the elbows. When the client reaches the stretch point, the trainer provides gentle assistance at the end of the ROM.

In **passive static stretching,** an outside agent applies the force. This form of stretching is effective when the ROM is limited by soft tissue extendibility. Its effect on warmed muscle is to lengthen the connective tissues passively. Pressure or held traction, external leverage, or support of a partner may provide the outside force.

- **Pressure or held traction.** This technique is demonstrated in figure 8.7, a side-lying quadriceps stretch in which the heel is pulled toward the buttock. The stretch should be gently and gradually increased.

- **External leverage.** This can be seen in figure 8.8, in which the shoulder internal rotators are elongated by the position of leverage in the doorway.

- **Support of a partner.** The partner assists the stretch beyond an active ROM but must remain in close communication with the client and carefully control the stretch intensity. Figure 8.9 shows a partner hamstring stretch.

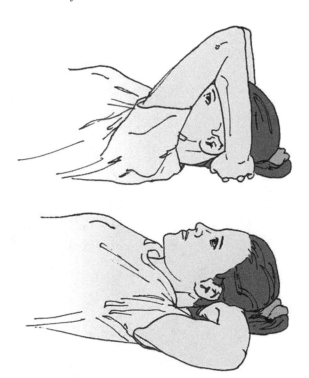

Figure 8.6   Active static stretch.

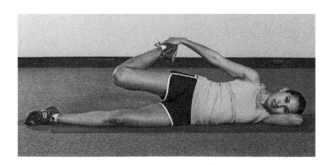

Figure 8.7   Passive static stretch with pressure and traction.

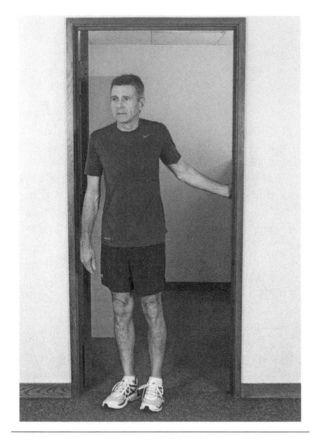

Figure 8.8   Passive static stretch with external leverage.

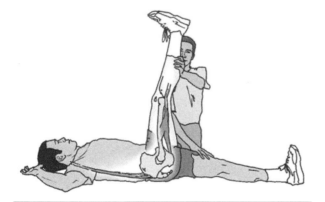

Figure 8.9   Passive static stretch with support of a partner.
Reprinted by permission from Howley and Franks 1997.

Dynamic Stretching

Active, bouncing movements initiated by contraction of the agonist muscle produce a quick stretch of the antagonist muscle. If uncontrolled momentum becomes a factor in the stretch, it is referred to as a ballistic stretch. Ballistic stretching can cause overstretching, resulting in microtears within the musculotendinous unit. Connective tissue has a safe elastic range, but if stress exceeds a yield point, small tears will occur. Repetition of such microtrauma can cause inflammation (chapter 11). The tearing can also lead to formation of scar tissue, with a gradual loss of elasticity. The risk of injury is higher with this type of stretching than with others and is dependent on the intensity and velocity of the stretch and the temperature of the muscle (Alter 2004).

However, many sports require dynamic or ballistic movements. Because ballistic stretching is functional and does increase ROM (Hendrick 2000), it is reasonable to integrate it into athletic training programs as long as the ballistic stretches correspond to actions required by the sport. If you prescribe this type of stretching for a client, target the specific muscle to be stretched, establish safe alignment, and avoid excessive momentum. Dynamic stretching should follow static stretching and only after the body temperature is sufficiently warm. Dynamic stretching should consist of rhythmic actions similar to those in the client's sport. Start with small movements and gradually increase the ROM. The exercises can be performed while the client walks 10 to 20 m (11-23 yd). Depending on the sport, common dynamic flexibility exercises include lunge walk (figure 8.10), lunge with a twist, walking knee tuck, high–low walks, and grapevines (with a twist).

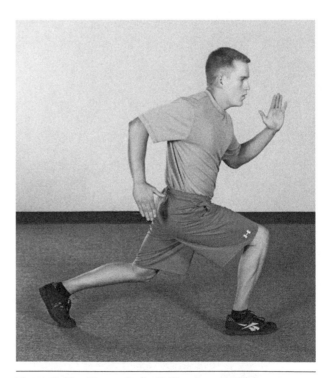

Figure 8.10   Dynamic flexibility: lunge walk.

Proprioceptive Neuromuscular Facilitation

Proprioceptive neuromuscular facilitation (PNF) invokes neurological responses that facilitate stretching. It works by generating a force or tension (generally an isometric muscle contraction) in the muscle that stimulates the GTOs, which then inhibit the muscle spindles and relax the muscle (autogenic inhibition) (Holcomb 2000). Before the stretch, have your client hold a submaximal isometric contraction against a resistance at the end of the limb's ROM for about 6 s. The static stretch that follows (approximately 15-30 s) also stimulates the GTOs to further relax the muscle to be stretched. Your client should repeat the sequence several times to allow for a greater reflex inhibition and thus a greater stretch.

McAtee and Charland (2007) summarized the common PNF variations as follows:

- **Hold-relax** uses an isometric contraction of the antagonist at the limit of the initial ROM, followed by a period of relaxation. Then the limb actively moves farther in the same direction against minimal resistance through the new ROM to the new point of limitation. The strong isometric contraction is thought to recruit more muscle fibers and then fire the inverse stretch reflex, relaxing the target muscle and permitting further stretch (Osternig et al. 1990). Hold-relax is effective when ROM has decreased because of muscle tightness on one side of a joint.

- **Contract-relax** (CR) is similar to hold-relax. You provide resistance as the client attempts to move the limb to the initial limit of the ROM of the target muscle. Because your resistance prevents the limb from moving, his muscles contract isometrically. Then your client relaxes, and you again move the limb passively beyond the initial limit. Contract-relax is preferred to hold-relax when ROM is good and when motion is pain free.

- **Contract-relax, antagonist-contract** (CRAC) is similar to contract-relax, except that after the isometric contraction, the client actively moves his limb into the new ROM (figure 8.11). This active contraction of the agonist is thought to relax the target muscle (called reciprocal inhibition), thereby allowing a better stretch (McAtee and Charland 2007).

- **Manual isometric stretch** is a modification of PNF, using the relaxed state of the muscle immediately following an isometric contraction (figure 8.12). Have your client manually resist the

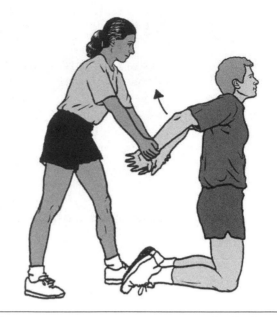

Figure 8.11   Proprioceptive neuromuscular facilitation stretch: pectoralis major (sternal).

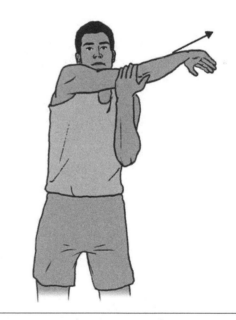

Figure 8.12   Manual isometric stretch.

contraction of a muscle in the midrange of movement for 6 to 10 s and then move the muscle into a passive static stretch, allowing enough time for connective tissue elongation and neuromuscular relaxation. Figure 8.11 may be performed as a manual isometric stretch of the shoulder.

Proprioceptive neuromuscular facilitation is considered an advanced method of stretching, both for the client and for personal fitness trainers, who have varying levels of skill in its application.

It has a number of advantages and is well suited for certain clients:

- Specific benefits are associated with the PNF method used (see McAtee and Charland 2007).
- Range of motion gains, especially passive mobility, have been equal to or greater than gains with other stretching methods.
- Proprioceptive neuromuscular facilitation produces strength, muscle balance, and joint stability.
- It increases relaxation of the muscle, which allows greater stretch of the connective tissue.
- Because PNF generally requires a partner, it gives you an opportunity to increase rapport with your client.
- It can be used to stretch any muscle in the body.
- It provides an excellent opportunity to motivate your client.
- It is popular with therapists because it approximates "natural" movements.
- It can be adapted to be done without a partner.

Despite all these pluses, use PNF with caution. Because it may produce excessive tissue stretch, PNF stretching should be performed only with the supervision of a knowledgeable and experienced personal fitness trainer.

In prescribing any flexibility exercise for your client, in addition to the training method, consider the following factors that directly affect the quality of stretch:

- Duration of the applied force (how long to hold a stretch)
- Intensity of the applied force (how hard to push a stretch)
- Temperature of the tissue (related to pre-stretch warm-up)
- Degree of relaxation of the muscle (amount of tension in a muscle)
- Type of applied force (e.g., ballistic, static, PNF)
- Alignment of muscle fibers to be stretched (direction of pull on the muscle)

Other prescription factors you should consider in your client's program design include these:

- Number of exercises (within the flexibility program)
- Number of repetitions (number of times the same stretch is performed)
- Other activities within the workout (aerobic, strengthening, sports)
- Frequency of workouts (how often the flexibility program is done per week)
- Impact of a stretch on an injury

Muscle Balance Prescription Model

Muscles that are too short are often strong and hold antagonists in a lengthened and weakened position. These muscles need to be lengthened and made more flexible through stretching. Muscles identified as weak and long need to be strengthened. This is best done through simple

Muscle Relaxation

Attempting to stretch muscles in spasm may cause injury. Connective tissue can be stretched effectively only if the muscle is relaxed. Strain is most often felt around the tendon of a tense muscle. Heat, light aerobics, loosening (see "Active Loosening"), massage, or ROM exercises can provide some relaxation, particularly if your client has come directly from an environment of repeated movements or static posture, such as sitting at a computer terminal. The mode of training can also affect the state of relaxation. For example, PNF involves a phase of isometrically contracting the muscle to be stretched. The proprioceptor is sensitive to the isometric tension, producing a reflex inhibition of the muscle, less resistance to stretch, less discomfort, a possible analgesic effect, and a greater ROM. But remember—if the muscle–tendon structure is inflamed, rest may be the best prescription.

If the alignment of the muscle–tendon structure is directly in the line of the stretch (or movement), the tensile stretch (or force application) is optimized. Pay special attention to alignment detail when you demonstrate the program to your client.

exercises that isolate and use the muscles in question. For muscle balance to be restored and maintained, therefore, therapeutic exercises to strengthen weak muscles should be combined with stretches for tight muscles.

The steps involved in the model for muscle balance prescription follow this approach. Client goals are established based on counseling concerns and assessment of posture, muscle tightness or joint ROM, and muscle weakness (see table 8.2). For each goal, a series of exercises is designed for flexibility of the tight muscles and strength of the weak side. Use form 8.2, Muscle Balance Prescription Worksheet, to record program recommendations and guidelines for safety and monitoring for each patient. The worksheet is a useful template to guide this program design process, ensuring that it is client centered and goal oriented. The two case studies at the end of the chapter demonstrate the use of the model and prescription worksheet.

For a client dealing with a weakness underlying muscular imbalance, refer to the detailed resistance training guidelines in chapter 7.

Table 8.2 Muscle Balance Prescription Model

Decisions	Choices
1. Review needs and confirm goals.	• Health, injury, fitness, or performance improvement • Fitness assessments (posture, tightness, ROM, weakness) • Observed movement compensation
2. Select the training method.	• Client's needs, time constraints, experience, and level of conditioning • Manipulate prescription factors within a given system • Standard sets or a specific circuit for strengthening • Static stretching or PNF for tightness or ROM

3. Select exercises, equipment, and order of performance.	• Combine therapeutic exercises to strengthen weak muscles with stretches for tight muscles
	• Choose exercise and equipment that retrain muscles that have been over- or underworked
	• Choose exercises that are functional for the demands on the client
	• Modify for physical limitations and current or past injuries
	• Simple equipment includes bands and tubing, pulleys, medicine balls and plyo balls, body bars, dumbbells, wobble boards, exercise balls, balance discs, BOSU trainers, and mats
	• Exercise order guidelines:
	  • Deal with each identified goal sequentially
	  • Work areas of imbalance while client is fresh
	  • Do a light warm-up and then stretch, followed by strengthening exercises and then functional neuromuscular exercises
	  • Maintain agonist–antagonist and bilateral symmetry
	  • Include stabilizers (e.g., lower spine muscles) later in the session

4. Set intensity and volume.	• Volume is often described as sets × reps × load • Intensity or load must be heavy enough to cause temporary fatigue • Strength and endurance improvements will come with 8 to 12 repetitions and a 75% load • Two sets are usually sufficient • Frequency may be >3 days per week when retraining an imbalance
5. Design progression and monitoring.	• Manipulate prescription factors to suit client according to specificity—gains in muscular fitness are specific to the muscle group, training method, and exercise volume • Modify only one volume factor at a time (e.g., increase reps up to about 15, then increase the load and reduce the reps) • Use program cards to record these factors • Visually monitor execution mechanics and precautions
6. Design warm-up and cool-down.	• Should reflect type and magnitude of the work (to be) done • After some warming, statically stretch the muscle groups to be used • In the cool-down, relieve anticipated muscle tightness and stretch tight postural muscles (e.g., anterior chest, hip flexors, hamstrings)

Step 1: Review Client Needs and Confirm Goals

Clients' needs may be related to health or injury, fitness, or performance improvement. Their needs can also be identified by fitness assessments (posture, tightness, ROM, weakness) or an observed compensation in some movement patterns.

Clients are not going to say that they have muscle imbalance. But you can find out if they do by asking the right questions. Faulty body mechanics, as determined by postural screening, should be confirmed by the muscle tests. Select assessment items only after you and your client together have decided on priorities. Chapter 4 describes and interprets the following assessments:

- Postural assessments (including static and dynamic)
- Muscle length and flexibility assessments
  - **Upper body:** pectoralis minor, pectoralis major (sternal), shoulder internal rotators, shoulder external rotators, shoulder abduction ROM
  - **Lower body:** hip flexors (one and two joint), tensor fascia latae, hamstrings, hip internal rotators, hip external rotators, gastrocnemius, tibialis posterior, and soleus (ankle ROM)
  - **Trunk:** lumbar and cervical rotation ROM, sit-and-reach
- Strength assessments
  - **Upper body:** Push-ups (pectorals, serratus anterior), weightlifting 5RM (repetitions maximum) to 10RM (selected muscles)
  - **Lower body:** Weightlifting 5RM to 10RM (selected muscles)

- **Trunk:** Biering–Sorenson (erector spinae), five-level sit-up (abdominal muscles), leg lowers (lower abdominal muscles), lateral lift (quadratus lumborum)

Postural analysis will indicate which muscle length and flexibility tests and strength assessments to perform. Interpretation of these tests will tell you what muscles need to be strengthened and which ones need to be lengthened.

Step 2: Select the Training Method

You must select the training method that best meets your client's needs, time constraints, experience, and level of condition. Your design can become quite distinctive when you manipulate prescription factors within a given system. Training methods such as standard sets or a specific circuit may be appropriate for strengthening, whereas static stretching or PNF may be selected for tightness or ROM (presented in the earlier "Flexibility Training Methods" section).

There are two approaches to improving flexibility: decreasing the resistance to the stretch and increasing the strength of the opposing muscle. Decreasing resistance to the stretch can be accomplished by either increasing the connective tissue length or attaining a greater degree of relaxation or analgesic effect in the target muscle. Table 8.3 describes the appropriate stretching techniques for each approach.

Step 3: Select Exercises, Equipment, and Order of Performance

To restore and maintain muscle balance, combine therapeutic exercises to strengthen weak muscles with stretches for tight muscles. You must know the purpose and benefit of each exercise (and

Table 8.3   Stretching Techniques

Approach	Technique
1. Decrease resistance to the stretch	
• Lengthen connective tissue. • Relax stretch reflex of targeted muscle. • Use analgesia.	• Warm-up (including light aerobics), massage, loosening, dynamic stretching • Static stretch with brief intermittent isometric contractions, relaxation techniques • Ice or heat applied during a static stretch
2. Increase strength of opposing muscles	
• Resistance train opposing muscles (muscle balance).	• Isolation of specific muscles and isometric or concentric contractions
3. Combine approaches	
• Train for stretch and strength (facilitation).	• Proprioceptive neuromuscular facilitation

equipment, if used) and choose those that maintain muscle balance and retrain muscles that have been over- or underworked. Modifications may be necessary because of physical limitations and current or past injuries. Often there is no need for specialized equipment. Simple equipment that can be useful may include bands and tubing, pulleys, or other small equipment such as medicine balls and plyo balls, body bars, dumbbells, wobble boards, exercise balls, balance discs, BOSU trainers, and mats.

Order your selection of specific exercises using the following guidelines:

- Deal with each identified goal sequentially, as a unit of exercises.
- Work areas of weakness or imbalance while your client is still fresh.
- Have the client do a light warm-up and then stretch, followed by strengthening exercises and then any functional neuromuscular exercises.
- Select exercises for each related muscle group maintaining agonist–antagonist and bilateral symmetry, which promotes a balanced development.
- Choose exercises that are functional for the demands on the client; these often include exercises in more than one plane (see guidelines for functional exercise earlier in the chapter).
- Include stabilizers (e.g., lower spine muscles) later in the session.

A well-rounded flexibility or conditioning program should include at least one exercise for each major muscle group. Your prescription should include the stretch specific to the area of tightness, the proper positioning and execution of the stretch, and the method of stretching best suited to your client. Postural screening and muscle length testing may suggest greater emphasis on, or avoidance of, certain muscle groups.

Step 4: Set Intensity and Volume

Program strengthening recommendations may involve exercise load and volume. Exercise volume is one of the most important prescription factors. Volume is often described as sets × reps × load. The intensity or load must be heavy enough to cause temporary fatigue. If your client is using weights, strength and endurance improvements will come with 8 to 12 repetitions and a 75% load. Two sets are usually sufficient to produce

excellent benefits. Frequency is sometimes more than 3 days per week for retraining an imbalance.

You can provide the appropriate overload for flexibility in the form of additional isolation stretches, more repetitions, longer duration, more frequent sessions, or a change of stretching technique. Heyward (2010) suggested 2 to 6 repetitions of each exercise for a minimum of 3 days a week, with the duration of stretch from 10 to 60 s. Covert and colleagues (2010) suggested one 30 s stretch per muscle group, but it is likely that longer periods or more repetitions are required in some people, for some muscle groups, or in the presence of injuries.

A stretch of relatively long duration and low force at elevated tissue temperatures will provide an effective permanent stretch **(plastic deformation)** (Sapega et al. 1991). If the duration of stretch is short, the intensity of force is high, and the tissue temperature is normal or cold, the muscle–tendon structure will return quickly to its original length **(elastic deformation)** and much of the benefit of the stretch will be lost.

Teach your clients to read their body's feedback and make their prescription client centered:

1. Stretch until you feel tension or slight pulling, but no pain.
2. Hold that length of the muscle until there is a noticeable decrease in the tension (stress relaxation).
3. Increase the muscle length until you feel the original tension level.
4. Take a deeper breath and slowly exhale. Repeat steps 2 and 3 until no further increase.

Step 5: Design Progression and Monitoring

The universal principle of conditioning is progressive overload, that is, periodically raising the workload to increasingly challenge the muscle group. The object is to shape the overload to suit your client by manipulating the prescription factors according to the principle of specificity—namely, that gains in muscular fitness are specific to the muscle group, training method, and exercise volume.

To ensure safe and effective progression, modify only one volume factor at a time (e.g., increase reps up to about 15, then increase the load and drop the reps back down). Program cards that allow quick recording of these factors can save time and encourage regular recording.

Visually monitor primary safety precautions and execution mechanics.

After constantly repeating a particular faulty movement pattern, clients need to be reprogrammed to perform the movement correctly. This can be difficult, because the faulty movement is by now ingrained in the central nervous system and has contributed to the muscle imbalance and poor posture. To address this condition, put your client's kinesthetic and postural awareness to use. Have clients perform the exercises with little or no load initially. Once they can do the unloaded movement properly, add a TheraBand or tubing and continue to monitor the movement mechanics. There are several good examples of situations in which this has proven to be very effective:

- Clients with weak lower trapezius and overactive upper trapezius: Excessive scapular elevation can occur with dumbbell lateral raises. Start with light tubing and teach the client to pull outward, not upward, avoiding any shoulder shrugging.

- Clients who need to be aware of a neutral spine position: Promote postural awareness in a seated position on a stability ball. Establish awareness of what muscles are contracting to stabilize and then begin small movements in all directions while maintaining a good kinesthetic sense of the lumbar–pelvic position.

- Clients with winged scapulae that need to be stabilized against the rib cage: Teach clients to "set" their scapulae in proper alignment with your tactile feedback. Progress to a modified push-up and emphasize the involvement of the serratus anterior with fully protracted scapulae at the top of the exercise. Similarly, emphasize the rhomboids by pinching the scapulae in the lowered position.

Check your clients for alignment and compliment good form during their resistance exercises. Balance the number of push–pull movements in the maintenance prescription. Progress to more functional total-body exercises and identify the things clients do in everyday life that need the same degree of attention as their workout. Few of us are immune from these daily risks: the new mother who undergoes repeated spinal flexion with caring for her child, the career driver with a poor seat or poor core stability who has constant intervertebral compression, the office worker with his telephone wedged between his ear and shoulder, and the personal trainer who constantly stoops to pick up weights and leans over to spot clients.

Step 6: Design Warm-Up and Cool-Down

The warm-up and cool-down should reflect the type and magnitude of the work done in the training portion. After some warming, have the client statically stretch the muscle groups to be used in the workout. In the cool-down, relieve anticipated muscle tightness and have the client stretch tight postural muscles (e.g., anterior chest, hip flexors, hamstrings).

There has been some controversy about the merits of stretching, particularly as an element of the warm-up, and you must give your clients accurate information in this area. Warming up for stretching has replaced the notion of stretching to warm up. Besides simply raising tissue temperature, warm-up activity stimulates muscle calcium release and motor unit recruitment. However, warm-up without stretching does not increase ROM (Shrier and Gossal 2000). There is evidence that high strength and power outputs are negatively affected after a static stretching session. It is possible that long-lasting changes in the ability of a muscle to store elastic energy when stretched, as well as muscle excitability, can be negatively influenced by static stretching (LaRoche et al. 2008). This may suggest the avoidance of passive stretching before activities requiring high muscle force and power, with preference given to dynamic sport-specific muscle preparation. However, most clients who have tightness will benefit from a prewarmed, long, static stretch routine done frequently and without the ballistic effect of other activities.

Table 8.4 shows (for the lower body) the progression from postural assessment to the identification of probable areas of muscle imbalance, and it provides guidelines for exercise design. Depending on the exercise movement, every muscle, at some time, is a prime mover (agonist) in a specific action, and each muscle has an opposing muscle (antagonist). Refer to table 8.5 to determine muscle pairs and to aid you in designing exercises based on muscle testing.

When designing isolated corrective exercises, ensure that the resistance is light enough to prevent the client from compensating by using other muscles. As muscle balance improves, start to replace isolated exercises with more complex, functional movements. However, if the isolated weakness is not corrected, multijoint strengthening exercises will also tend to cause compensation and reinforce the imbalance or create new ones.

When a muscle has excessive tension, the stress should be relieved before you prescribe additional

Table 8.4 Exercise Design From Muscle Testing: Lower Body

Postural fault	Muscles in shortened position	Muscles in lengthened position	Exercise implication
Flexed knee	Popliteus Hamstrings at knee	Quadriceps Sartorius	• Stretch knee flexors • Stretch hip flexors if tight; may contribute
Medially rotated femur (often associated with pronation of foot or toeing in)	Hip medial rotators	Hip lateral flexors	• Stretch hip medial rotators • Strengthen hip lateral rotators
Knock-knee	Tensor fascia latae Lateral knee joint structures	Medial knee joint structures	• Stretch tensor fascia latae
Postural bowlegs	Hip lateral rotators Quadriceps Foot everters	Hip medial rotators, popliteus, tibialis posterior, and long toe flexors	• Strengthen hip medial rotators
Ankle pronation	Peroneals and toe extensors	Tibialis posterior and long toe flexors	• Strengthen inverters and muscles supporting the arch
Ankle supination	Tibialis (especially posterior)	Peroneals	• Strengthen peroneals

Table 8.5 Opposing Muscles

Movement direction	Agonists	Antagonists
Foot and ankle		
Anteroposterior	Dorsiflexors (tibialis anterior, peroneus tertius)	Plantar flexors (gastrocnemius, soleus)
Lateral and rotary	Tibials (tibialis anterior and posterior)	Peroneals (peroneus longus and brevis)
Knee		
Anteroposterior	Flexors (hamstrings, gastrocnemius)	Extensors (quadriceps)
Hip		
Anteroposterior	Flexors (iliopsoas, rectus femoris, pectineus, tensor fascia latae, sartorius)	Extensors (gluteus maximus, hamstrings)
Lateral	Abductors (gluteus medius, tensor fascia latae)	Adductors (adductor longus, brevis, magnus, gracilis, pectineus)
Rotary	Internal rotators (gluteus minimus, tensor fascia latae)	External rotators (gluteus maximus, six external rotators)
Trunk		
Anteroposterior	Flexors (rectus abdominis, external oblique)	Extensors (erector spinae, deep posterior spinal group)
Lateral	Lateral flexors—left oppose right (quadratus lumborum, external and internal obliques, erector spinae group)	Same
Rotary	Rotators to the same side (internal oblique, erector spinae group)	Rotators to the opposite side (external oblique, deep posterior group)
Pelvis		
Anteroposterior	Forward tilt (hip flexors, trunk extensors)	Backward tilt (trunk flexors, hip extensors)
Lateral	(Gluteus medius and minimus)	(Quadratus lumborum, external oblique)

(continued)

(continued)

Movement direction	Agonists	Antagonists
Shoulder joint		
Anteroposterior	Flexors and horizontal adductors (anterior deltoid, pectoralis major)	Extensors and horizontal abductors (posterior deltoid, latissimus dorsi, teres major)
Lateral	Abductors (deltoids, supraspinatus)	Adductors (latissimus dorsi, teres major, pectoralis major)
Rotary	Internal rotators (subscapularis, teres major)	External rotators (infraspinatus, teres minor)
Shoulder girdle		
Vertical	Elevators (trapezius 1 and 2, levator scapula, rhomboids)	Depressors (trapezius 4, pectoralis minor)
Lateral	Abductors (serratus anterior, pectoralis minor)	Adductors (trapezius 2, 3, and 4, rhomboids)
Rotary	Lateral rotators (trapezius 2 and 4, serratus anterior)	Medial rotators (pectoralis minor, rhomboids)
Elbow		
Anteroposterior	Flexors (biceps brachii, brachialis, brachioradialis)	Extensors (triceps brachii, anconeus)
Radioulnar		
Rotary	Pronators (pronator quadratus, pronator teres, brachioradialis)	Supinators (supinator, brachioradialis, biceps brachii)
Wrist		
Anteroposterior	Wrist flexors	Wrist extensors
Lateral	Abductors (radial side)	Adductors (ulnar side)

muscular work. There is often reduced neuromuscular input in these muscles. Roskopf (2001) suggested using isometric contractions to restimulate the muscle by increasing sensory input to the brain. Corrective isometrics can act as precursors to designing exercises to strengthen concentric contractions. Roskopf suggested a protocol using 6 repetitions of 6 s contractions progressing from 50% intensity to 70%, 100%, and maximal force on the last three contractions.

Case Studies

This chapter presents guidelines for the design of functional exercise: Integrate kinetic chain movements; use multiplanar motion; involve a loading and unloading cycle; and incorporate actions that require balance, stabilization, and proprioceptive stimulation. Although applicable to resistance exercises and those for muscle imbalance, these guidelines should also be integrated into flexibility exercise design given the continuity of the body's myofascial lines. Case study 1 illustrates this point.

Inherent in musculoskeletal fitness are alignment and muscle balance. Screening for common postural faults provides a direction for follow-up muscle testing. The goals of training for performance, rehabilitation, or fitness may differ, but the need to maintain muscle balance is important for all. Setting objectives for muscle balance usually centers around stretching tight muscles, strengthening weak muscles, reducing spasm, building muscular endurance, or improving posture. Remain vigilant for those clients whose postural assessment or other screening indicates that they should be referred to another health care professional.

Case studies 2 and 3 illustrate the progression from postural analysis to selection of muscle length test items and on to a personalized prescription. These case studies detail a number of muscle tests presented in chapter 4.

Case Study 1:
Functional Stretching for a Track Club

A local track club has arranged to use your fitness center for training and to have your staff assist with warm-up, cool-down, and flexibility training. The members include runners of various distances and some recreational runners. Traditionally, the active muscles needing to be stretched would be the calf, hamstrings, and quadriceps–hip flexors. Rather than doing isolated stretches, you appreciate that efficient locomotion depends on integrated kinetic chain movements and therefore design an approach that is more functional. In addition to the guidelines for functional exercise design, you want to keep things simple to promote habit and keep the program progressive to suit individual needs.

After a moderate aerobic warm-up sufficient to increase local muscle blood flow and tissue temperature, the runners will perform two stretches (or progressive movement patterns), one focusing on leg extensors and the superficial back myofascial line and the other on leg flexors and the superficial front myofascial line, as well as four multiplanar dynamic stretch exercises.

Leg Extensor Stretch Along the Superficial Back Myofascial Line

1. Stand in front of a chair or bench with one leg (straight) on the chair (neutral position).

2. Hinge or flex at the hip (not the back) and hold for 20 to 30 s (passive static stretch) (see figure 8.13a).

3. While holding a flexed hip position, bend the knee, then contract the quadriceps to straighten the knee; pulse gently for 2 s and repeat five times (active isolation stretching).

4. Slightly bend the knee, dorsiflex the ankle (may be assisted, e.g., towel), and flex at the hip and hold for 15 to 20 s (see figure 8.13b).

5. While in that position, slowly rotate–oscillate the trunk, leading with the pelvis, in both directions (fascial mobilization of the hip joint structures—multiplanar) (see figure 8.13c).

6. Soften the flex of the ankle and knee and allow the knee and toes to face outward; flex at the hip, which changes the plane to include the gluteals and iliotibial band (lateral myofascial line); hold for 20 s or pulse as with the A-I stretch technique (see figure 8.13d).

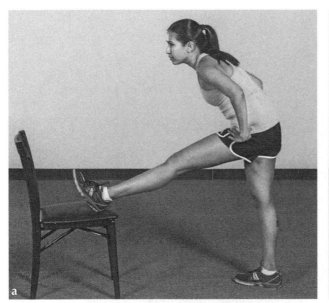
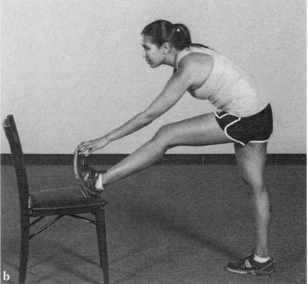
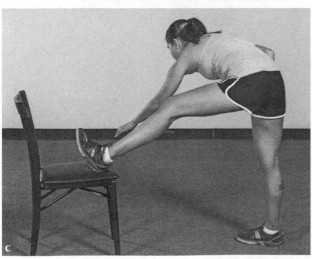
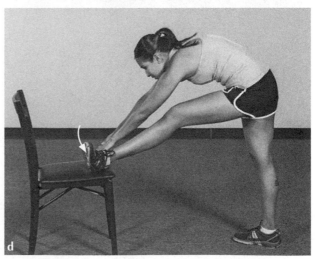

Figure 8.13 Leg extensor stretch.

7. Return to a neutral position (straight leg) with a slightly bent knee; curl the spine and reach forward for 10 to 15 s (gentle stretch pressure only).

8. Repeat the last movement pattern, turning the trunk, and reach up and over your head on the side of the stretch; hold for 20 s (lateral myofascial line).

9. Repeat with the opposite leg.

Leg Flexor Stretch Along the Superficial Front Myofascial Line

1. Stand in front of a chair or bench with one leg (bent) on the chair.

2. Lower gently into a lunge position with the back knee straight and hold for 20 to 30 s (passive static stretch).

3. Roll–tilt the pelvis under by contracting the gluteals and abdominal muscles; pulse gently for 2 s and repeat five times (active isolation stretching) (see figure 8.14a).

4. From the lunge stretch, pivot slowly on your rear toe outward and hold, then inward and hold (fascial mobilization of the hip joint structures—multiplanar) (see figure 8.14b).

5. Realign; bend the back knee and lower your body; hold for 20 s or pulse as with the A-I stretch technique.

6. Reach up and across with the active-side arm; hold for 20 s (lateral myofascial line) (see figure 8.14c).

7. Repeat, reaching with a trunk twist across to the far knee, and give a gentle pull; hold for 20 s (see figure 8.14d).

8. Repeat with the opposite leg.

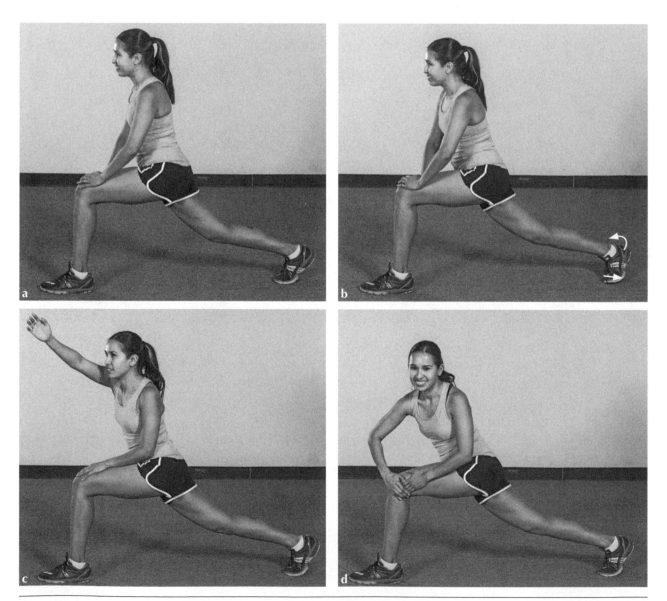

Figure 8.14 Leg flexor stretch.

Dynamic Stretch Exercises (Multiplanar)

These exercises can be performed while the clients walk 10 to 20 m (11-23 yd).

- Short lunge while reaching down and across body; alternate legs (see figure 8.15)
- Step and lift knee up and across body; alternate legs (see figure 8.16)
- Long lunge while reaching up and across body; alternate legs (see figure 8.17)
- High-knee steps while leg rotates outward; alternate legs (see figure 8.18)

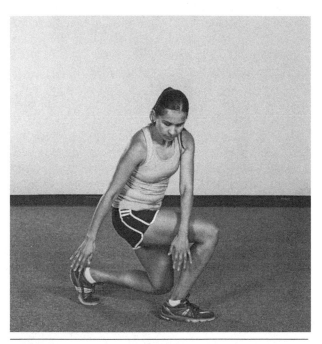

Figures 8.15 Short lunge reach across.

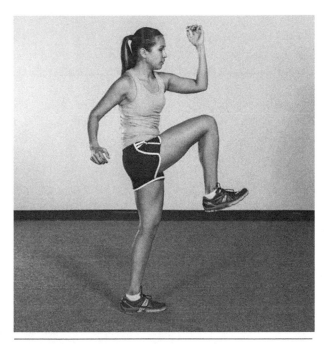

Figures 8.16 Step and lift.

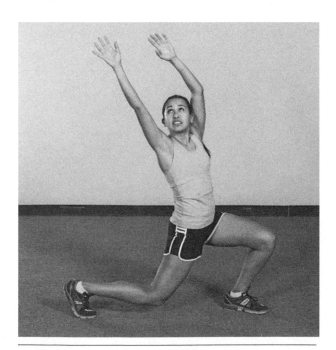

Figures 8.17 Long lunge reach above.

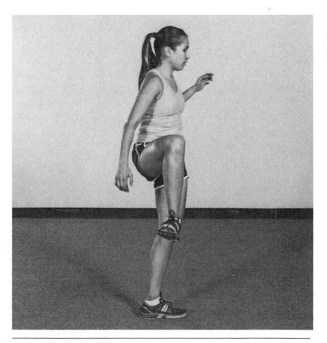

Figures 8.18 High-knee step outs.

Case Study 2:
37-Year-Old Working Mother

Rose was a 37-year-old bank teller with two children, ages 3 years and 18 months. She did not exercise regularly. Rose had headaches caused by neck tension and pain. She wanted to exercise at home and could devote 25 to 30 min, 4 or 5 days per week, to her program. Her primary objectives were to improve upper body endurance and eliminate neck pain.

Assessment

A cursory check of Rose's posture, with particular attention to upper torso alignment, revealed some areas that warranted further examination. I believed that an apparent lack of balance could be confirmed with some muscle tightness assessment.

The postural assessment helped to fine-tune the priorities. I observed no significant problems with Rose's feet, knees, or pelvis, but I did note the following misalignments: depressed chest, increased cervical curve, forward shoulders, palms rotated medially, scapulae abducted, and a forward head (tables 8.6 and 8.7).

Interpretation

The combination of postural faults just described often creates neck and shoulder tension and discomfort, because the weight of the head is supported by the posterior muscles rather than the skeletal system. Strengthening of the anterior neck muscles (deep neck flexors and sternocleidomastoid) can help restore balance.

The shoulder girdle and neck musculature are linked. It was clear to me that muscle length testing could help determine the underlying cause of Rose's rounded shoulder posture. This condition is referred to as the upper crossed syndrome (Page et al. 2010), a muscle imbalance characterized by tightness in the cervical extensors or anterior shoulder muscles or both. In particular, the upper fibers of the trapezius, levator scapula, and pectoralis major and minor are the muscles prone to becoming short and tight. Specifically, the deep cervical flexors, the middle and lower fibers of the trapezius, the rhomboids, serratus anterior, and latissimus dorsi run the risk of weakness and inhibition. The pectoralis minor exerts a forward and downward pull on the front of the scapula and

Table 8.6   Assessment of Segmental Posture: Upper Body

Alignment scale:	5 (Good)	4		3 (Faulty)	2	1 (Very faulty)
Joint	View	Good alignment	Faulty alignment	Score	Left (L)/ Right (R)	Comments
Head	L P	Erect and balanced	Protruding, chin forward Tilted and rotated	3		*Head and chin forward*
Arms and shoulders	A	Arms relaxed; palms facing body	Arms stiff, away from body Palms facing backward	3		*Palms rotated medially*
	L	Shoulders back	Shoulders rounded and forward	2		*Shoulders rounded*
	A/P	Shoulders level	One or both shoulders up, down, or rotated	5		
	P	Scapulae: flat on rib cage; 4-6 in. (10-15 cm) apart	Scapulae: prominently winged, far apart	3		*Scapulae abducted: 6 in. (15 cm) apart*
Score:				*16/25*		

Note: A = anterior; P = posterior; L = lateral.

Table 8.7   Assessment of Segmental Posture: Spine

Alignment scale:	5 (Good)		4		3 (Faulty)	2	1 (Very faulty)
Joint	**View**	**Good alignment**	**Faulty alignment**	**Score**	**Left (L)/ Right (R)**	**Comments**	
Spine and pelvis	A/P	Hips level, weight even on both feet	One hip higher (lateral tilt), hips rotated (forward one side)	5			
	P	No lateral curve to spine (posterior view)	C- or S-curve scoliosis Ribs prominent one side	5			
	L	Natural lumbar curve	Lordosis: forward tilt of pelvis and flat back: pelvis tilts backward	5			
	L	Natural thoracic curve	Kyphosis: thoracic rounding	4		*Some thoracic rounding*	
	L	Natural cervical curve	Cervical lordosis: forward head	3		*Increased cervical curve and forward head*	
Trunk	L	Flat or slightly rounded abdomen	Protruding lower or entire abdomen	5			
	L	Chest slightly raised	Hollow chest and rounded back	3		*Depressed chest*	
Head	L P	Erect and balanced	Protruding, chin forward Tilted and rotated	3		*As noted in table 8.6*	
Score:				***33/40***			

Note: A = anterior; P = posterior; L = lateral.

may alone cause the roundness. Tightness of the pectoralis major will contribute to the forward pull of the shoulders and may cause an internal rotation of the shoulder, as seen in the palms facing backward. Because Rose was relatively untrained, I suspected weak and overstretched posterior scapular adductors (trapezius and rhomboids) and a depressed chest (which often accompanies rounded shoulders).

Chapter 4 describes procedures for muscle length assessments for the pectoralis minor, pectoralis major (sternal), shoulder internal rotators, and shoulder external rotators. The "normal" values quoted for the tests are conservative: Any deviation from them

deserves attention. Here is what I found for Rose (table 8.8):

- Pectoralis minor: moderate tightness, left and right
- Pectoralis major (sternal): left and right arms 5° off table
- Shoulder internal rotators: left and right forearms 10° off table
- Shoulder external rotators: normal ROM
- Early and excessive elevation of scapulae when shoulder joint abducted

Table 8.8   Assessment of Shoulder and Chest Tightness

Assessment	Results (observations)	Normal range of motion	Pain
Shoulder internal (medial) rotation: tightness of infra-spinatus, teres minor	L: *70°* R: *70°*	70°	*No*
Shoulder external (lateral) rotation: tightness of sub-scapularis	L: *80°* R: *80°*	90°	*No*
Pectoralis major (sternal) length	*5° off table*	Table level	*No*
Pectoralis minor length	L: *Moderately tight* R: *Moderately tight*		*No*
Shoulder joint abduction (dynamic shoulder align-ment)	*Early and excessive eleva-tion of scapulae*	180°	*Neck tightness*

Prescription

It seemed clear that Rose's forward chin, cervical lordosis, and tight neck would benefit from exercises designed to stretch the neck extensors and strengthen the neck flexors. Her rounded shoulders should respond to stretches for tight pectoralis minor and major and to strengthening exercises for shoulder extensors, external rotators, and scapular adductors (see table 8.6).

Several exercises are beneficial for both areas, with simple training methods appropriate for the home environment. Static stretching is the suggested method for lengthening the tight muscles. Isometric exercises, tubing, and calisthenics are the appropriate strength training techniques. I prescribed these exercises for Rose as shown in figure 8.19.

Follow-Up

Weekly phone conversations with Rose seemed very promising. She managed to devote nearly an hour every day to her prescription. She liked the convenience of working out at home and the easy-to-follow program. I joined her for a workout in the third week and was amazed at her rapid increase in muscular endurance, especially in the posterior shoulder area. However, the dull ache in her neck had not disappeared. My concern at this point was that Rose might be overtraining and perpetuating the symptoms.

I didn't want to discourage Rose from her exercise habit, but some modifications were necessary. We designed a workout log to track the volume of work and any symptoms. She agreed to exercise only 3 days per week for 30 min. To maintain an adequate overload, I moved her up to heavier tubing and substituted bent-over flys with some newly acquired dumbbells for the supine scapular retraction exercise. We selected a starting weight that brought Rose to fatigue by the 8th to 10th repetition on the first set.

I scheduled a reassessment in 5 weeks to judge the effectiveness of the prescription for Rose's posture and muscle balance. Continued weekly phone calls confirmed a reduction in neck pain and tension headaches.

Prescriptions are rarely a straight highway to success. But with regular monitoring and follow-up modifications, the journey can resume in the right direction.

Note: If your clients are seeking gains in strength and endurance, select a starting weight that brings them to fatigue by the 8th to 10th repetition on the first set. Adjust the weight, if necessary, and have them do as many repetitions as possible on the second set. Refer to figure 8.19 for progressions and other guidelines.

Case Study 3: 45-Year-Old Weekend Warrior

Kevin was a divorced 45-year-old broker who worked long hours. He played old timers hockey once a week for 6 months of the year. He had moderate low back discomfort. He had just joined a local fitness club and was willing to commit to three 50 min workouts per week. He wanted to lose fat from the trunk area and improve the condition of his back.

Assessment

Kevin was concerned about his back and trunk region. An overview of his posture revealed some areas to examine further. His prolonged stress and sitting posture at work were obvious concerns. To confirm an apparent lack of balance, I assessed the strength and tightness of the muscles that attach to the spine and pelvis. The postural assessment (table 8.9) helped to fine-tune the priorities.

Client name: Rose	Trainer name: John
Client goals: 1. Relieve neck pain by stretching neck extensors and strengthen neck flexors 2. Correct rounded shoulders by stretching chest and front shoulder and strengthen back shoulder and scapular muscles	Assessment rationale: 1. Forward chin and head lean—cervical lordosis, tension in neck 2. Rounded shoulders, internal rotation of shoulder, abducted scapulae, tight anterior muscles
Flexibility prescription for Goal 1: **Chin tuck** Pull head straight back, keeping jaw and eyes level. 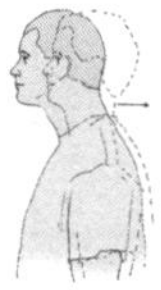	Strengthening prescription for Goal 1: **Resisted neck flexion** Facing forward with finger tips on forehead, bend head forward through a full range. Give moderate resistance. (20 s × 2) 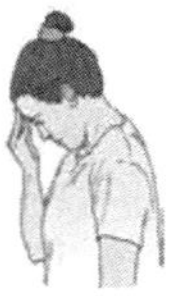
Lateral neck stretch Grasp arm and pull downward and across body while gently tilting head. 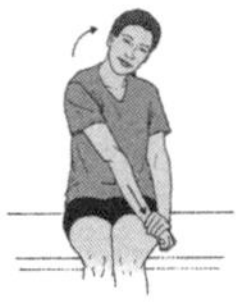	
Flexibility prescription for Goal 2: **Shoulder internal rotator stretch** Keep palm of hand against door frame, elbow bent at 90°. Turn body from fixed hand until stretch is felt. 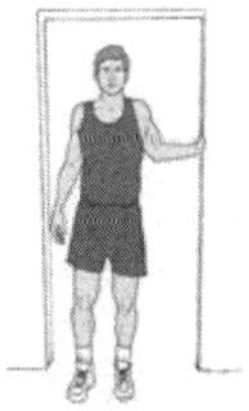	Strengthening prescription for Goal 2: **Resisted diagonal shoulder extension** Grasp tubing with arm reaching above shoulder and across body. Gently pull downward and away from your body. Return slowly to starting position. 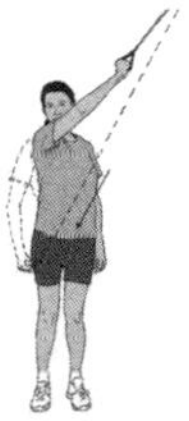
Supine wand thrust Hold wand with involved side palm up, push with uninvolved side (palm down) out from body, keeping elbow at side until you feel a stretch. Then pull back across body, leading with uninvolved side. 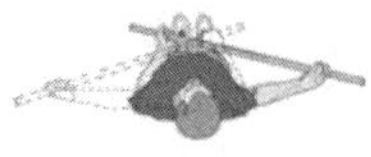	**Resisted shoulder external rotation** Using tubing, and keeping elbow in at side, rotate arm outward away from body. Keep forearm parallel to floor. 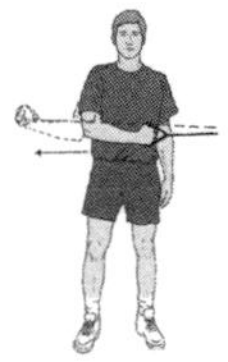
Door frame pec stretch Keep palm of outstretched horizontal arm against door frame. Turn body until a stretch is felt. Vary the level of the arm. 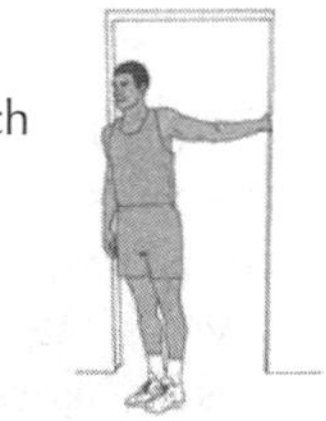	**Supine scapular retraction** With fingers clasped behind head, pull elbows back while pinching shoulder blades together. 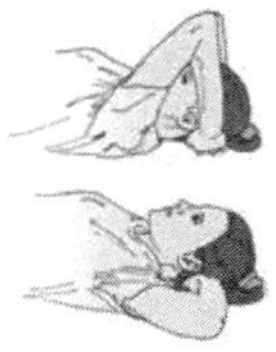
Program recommendations: • For clients who prefer dumbbells, upper back strengthening exercises may be replaced with bent-over flys or reverse flys. • For stack-weight users, rowing and pull-downs could be substituted. • For clients seeking gains in strength endurance, select a starting weight that brings them to fatigue by the eighth to tenth repetition on the first set.	Safety and monitoring guidelines: • Hold stretches for 15-30 s, longer but not harder if tension is more significant. • Repeat stretches 2 or 3 times. • Do a circulatory warm-up before muscle balance workout.

Figure 8.19 Rose's muscle balance prescription card.

Table 8.9 Assessment of Segmental Posture: Spine

Alignment scale:	5 (Good)		4	3 (Faulty)		2	1 (Very faulty)
Joint	View	Good alignment	Faulty alignment	Score	Left (L)/ Right (R)	Comments	
Spine and pelvis	A/P	Hips level—weight even on both feet	One hip higher (lateral tilt); hips rotated (forward one side)	5			
	P	No lateral curve to spine (posterior view)	C- or S-curve scoliosis Ribs prominent one side	5			
	L	Natural lumbar curve	Lordosis: forward tilt of pelvis and flat back: pelvis tilts backward	3		*Increased curve in low back—anterior pelvic tilt*	
	L	Natural thoracic curve	Kyphosis: thoracic rounding	5			
	L	Natural cervical curve	Cervical lordosis: forward head	5			
Trunk	L	Flat and slightly rounded abdomen	Lower or entire abdomen protrudes	3		*Protruding abdomen (entire trunk)*	
	L	Chest slightly raised	Hollow chest and rounded back	5			
Head	L P	Erect and balanced	Protruding, chin forward Tilted and rotated	5			
Score:				36/40			

Note: A = anterior; P = posterior; L = lateral.

Kevin's postural chart showed nothing significant at the feet, knees, shoulder, scapulae, or head. I did note the following misalignments: an anterior tilt to the pelvis, a protruding abdomen, and an increased curvature to the low back with accompanying discomfort.

Muscle testing showed tightness in the one-joint hip flexors (the iliopsoas crosses only the hip) and two-joint hip flexors (the rectus femoris crosses both hip and knee). Further assessment revealed some tightness of the hamstrings; five-level sit-up test (chapter 4) revealed weak abdominal muscles, and a modified trunk forward flexion assessment disclosed low back tightness (tables 8.10 and 8.11).

Chapter 4 describes procedures for muscle length assessments for hip flexors, hamstrings, and forward trunk flexion. As was true with the previous example, any deviation from the "normal" values given for these tests should lead to further investigation. The observations I made for Kevin were as follows:

- Hip flexors: one-joint and two-joint hip flexors tight, tensor fascia latae also tight
- Hamstrings: 75° to 80° (low normal)
- Forward trunk flexion: hamstrings normal, short muscles in low back (no roundness)
- Lumbar rotation: 40° to 45° (low normal)

Table 8.10   Assessment of Hip, Knee, and Back Tightness

Hip/knee assessment	Results (observations)	Normal ROM	Pain Y/N
Hamstring length	L: **80°** R: **75°**	80° (males) 90° (females)	**N**
Hip flexors: 1 joint (tightness of iliopsoas)	L: **10° off table** R: **10° off table**	Thigh table level	**N**
Hip flexors: 2 joint (tightness of rectus femoris)	L: **60°** R: **60°**	Knee: 80°	**N**
Tensor fascia latae tightness	L: **abduction and rotation** R: **abduction and rotation**		**N**
Hip internal (medial) rotation (tightness of gluteus maximus, piriformis)	L: _____ R: _____	35°	
Hip external (lateral) rotation (tightness of gluteus minimus, anterior gluteus medius)	L: _____ R: _____	45°	
Back assessment	**Results (observations)**	**Normal ROM**	**Pain Y/N**
Spinal rotation: Lumbar Cervical	L: **40°**; R: **45°** L: _____; R: _____	45° 65°-70°	**N**
Sit-and-reach test: Actual Visual	**24 cm** **Short muscles in low back—no roundness in low back**	"Good": 28-33 cm (males), 32-37 cm (females)	**Felt tight**

Interpretation

The increased lumbar lordosis had caused the weight of the upper body to settle on the low back, aggravating any low back problems. Although it is common in such cases to see exaggerated curves in the thoracic and cervical regions (to compensate for the lumbar curve), Kevin did not exhibit such symptoms. The anterior tilt to his pelvis, in conjunction with the lumbar lordosis, is very common and likely resulted from one or several muscle imbalances. The condition is referred to as the lower crossed syndrome (Page et al. 2010) and is an imbalance characterized by tightness in the lumbar extensors and the hip flexors. The tightness can manifest itself in the erector spinae and quadratus lumborum in the lower back and the iliopsoas and rectus femoris in the anterior hip. Weakness is generally seen in the hip extensors and abdominal muscles. Specifically, the gluteus maximus and medius, the hamstrings, and the rectus abdominis tend to be elongated and inhibited. Tight hip flexors pulled his pelvis forward and down—a condition often associated with short spinal extensors, which also contribute to anterior pelvic tilt. Weak and perhaps overstretched abdominal muscles are not sufficient to withstand such forces. I decided that strengthening the hip extensors (gluteus maximus and hamstrings) would resist the pull of the very strong hip flexors.

Prescription

Because Kevin had lumbar lordosis and anterior pelvic tilt and tested positive for tight erector spinae and hip flexors, he could alleviate his low back stress with exercises that stretched the back extensors and hip flexors and that strengthened the abdominal muscles and hip extensors. Table 8.5 is a useful reference for muscle pairs.

Table 8.11   **Strength and Endurance Testing**

Muscle	Test	Rating system	Comments
1. 2. 3. 4.	Weightlifting	1. Exercise: _____ 5- to 10RM _____ ; 1RM _____ 2. Exercise: _____ 5- to 10RM _____ ; 1RM _____ 3. Exercise: _____ 5- to 10RM _____ ; 1RM _____ 4. Exercise: _____ 5- to 10RM _____ ; 1RM _____	
Erector spinae	Biering–Soren-son	For example, ages 20-29 male and female (s) Needs improvement · fair · good · very good · excellent Male: 85 · 86-98 · 99-132 · 133-175 · 176-180 Female: 65 · 66-101 · 102-135 · 136-179 · 179-180	
Rectus abdominis	Five-level sit-ups	(1) (2) *3* (3) (4) (5) **No. of reps: 8 at level 1**	*Terminated because of loss of form and partial fatigue*
Lower abdominal muscles	Leg lowers	75° = poor, 60° = fair, 30° = good, 5° = excellent ° = degrees when back arches while lowering legs	
Quadratus lumborum	Lateral lift	**Right shoulder** Grade 1: Shoulder 12 in. off floor without difficulty Grade 2: Shoulder 12 in. off floor with difficulty Grade 3: Shoulder 2-6 in. off floor Grade 4: Unable to raise shoulder off floor **Left shoulder** Grade 1: Shoulder 12 in. off floor without difficulty Grade 2: Shoulder 12 in. off floor with difficulty Grade 3: Shoulder 2-6 in. off floor Grade 4: Unable to raise shoulder off floor	
Serratus anterior	Push-up	Strong = scapula flat in down phase Weak = scapular "winging" in down phase	

The exercise design began with therapeutic exercises for the lumbar lordosis, followed by exercises for the related anterior pelvic tilt (see figure 8.20). The methods of training included static stretching for muscle tightness. To strengthen the abdominal muscles, Kevin started with only the resistance of gravity and body weight. For the hip extensors, I suggested that he add resistance from tubing or from the appropriate machines at the fitness club.

Follow-Up

I had an opportunity to talk with Kevin during most of his club visits. The first 4 weeks of his program preceded the start of his hockey season. After a guided demonstration and three workouts on his own, I introduced some aerobic intervals that simulated the shift changes for his hockey. I explained that the aerobic activity would have an added benefit for his back.

Because he enjoyed the aerobic intervals, we continued them throughout the hockey season using different equipment for a cross-training effect (see chapter 6). A month into the season, Kevin began coming in only twice a week as opposed to three times as prescribed. This would not have been a concern had not Kevin indicated that his home workouts had pretty much dropped off.

Kevin was in an "action stage" (see chapter 1), and his risk of relapse was high. I could tell he felt guilty about the transgression, but I reassured him that this was a normal state of affairs and our job now was to deal with the lapse. With his two club aerobic workouts and weekly hockey, he was pleased with the cardiovascular improvements he was feeling. However, he was taking 2 days of rest after his hockey because his back felt tight and fatigued. Although he agreed that he needed to do the muscle balance exercises

Client name: Kevin	Trainer name: John
Client goals: 1. Alleviate low back discomfort and reduce lumbar lordosis by stretching back extensor muscles and strengthening abdominals 2. Relieve back discomfort symptoms and pelvic tilt by stretching hip flexors and rotators and strengthen hip extensors	Assessment rationale: 1. Increased curve in low back; tight low back during sit-and-reach; protruding abdomen; only 8 reps at level 1 2. Anterior pelvic tilt, tight one- and two-joint hip flexors, tight tensor fascia latae, deep buttock ache
Flexibility prescription for Goal 1: **Supine knees to chest** Pull both knees in to chest until a comfortable stretch is felt in low back. Keep back relaxed. Illustration by Michael Richardson. Reprinted by permission from Alter 2004. 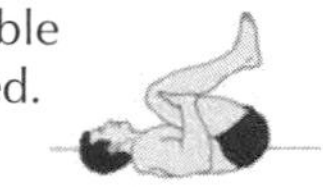	**Strengthening prescription for Goal 1:** **Curl-up—Level 1** With arms at side, tilt pelvis to flatten back. Raise shoulders and head from floor. Return in a controlled fashion. 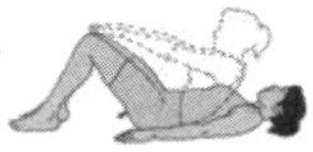
Seated back stretch Sit on the edge of a chair with legs spread apart. Tuck your chin and slowly bend downward. Relax in a comfortable stretch. Return slowly. Illustration by Michael Richardson. Reprinted by permission from Alter 2004. 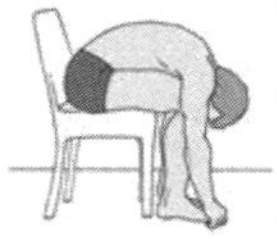	**Abdominal crunch** With legs over footstool or chair and arms positioned at side of head, tilt pelvis to flatten back. Raise head and shoulders from the floor. 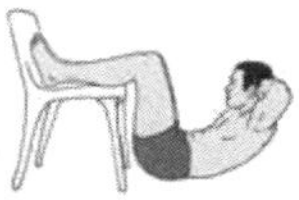
Flexibility prescription for Goal 2: **One-joint hip flexor lunge** Slowly push pelvis downward from a front lunge until stretch felt in front of hip. Illustration by Michael Richardson. Reprinted by permission from Alter 2004. 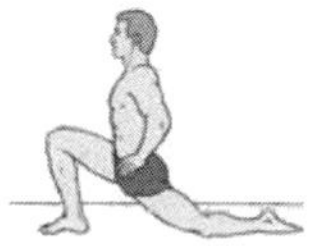	**Strengthening prescription for Goal 2:** **Supine hip thrusts** Start in a supine position with lower legs vertical and pillow under head. Slowly raise buttocks, keeping stomach tight. 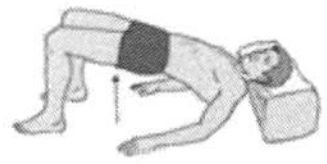
Side-lying quad stretch Pull heel toward buttocks until comfortable stretch in front thigh. Tilt pelvis backward. Illustration by Michael Richardson. Reprinted by permission from Alter 2004. 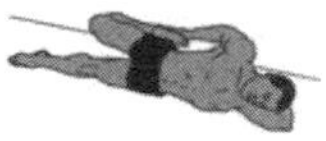	**Resisted hip extension** With tubing around involved ankle and opposite end secured, bring leg backward, keeping knee secure. 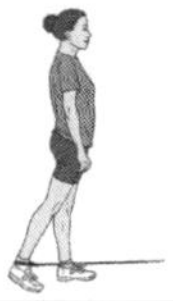
Wall lean stretch With arm against wall, slowly lean hips toward wall. Cross inside leg behind for increased stretch. 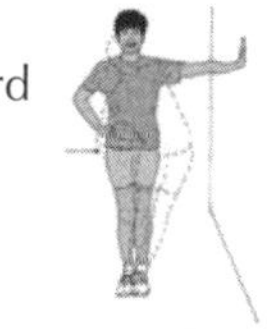	
Supine piriformis stretch Cross legs with involved leg on top. Gently pull opposite knee toward chest. Stretch should be felt in buttock and hip area. 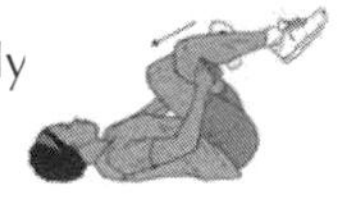	
Program recommendations: • Stack weight leg extensions or other machines may be substituted to strengthen hip extensors. • For clients seeking gains in strength endurance, select a starting weight that brings them to fatigue by the eighth to tenth repetition on the first set.	**Safety and monitoring guidelines:** • Hold stretches for 15-30 s, longer but not harder if tension is more significant. • Repeat stretches 2 or 3 times. • Do a circulatory warm-up before muscle balance workout. • Monitor discomfort in buttocks and low back; if symptoms worsen, seek medical attention.

Figure 8.20   Kevin's muscle balance prescription card.

more frequently, Kevin admitted that he had little motivation to follow his home program. We came up with two modifications. First, I linked Kevin up with one of our apprenticing personal trainers for an additional 15 min per visit of guided strengthening and stretching similar to his prescribed exercises. To deal with the tightness created by the hockey, I gave him five stretches—specifically adapted to the bench in his locker room—that he agreed to do before and after each game.

Client-centered prescription involves carefully listening to your client's feedback and modifying the path as necessary in response. It often involves side trips and doubling back, but it always moves in the direction of better health for your client.

Summary

A functional program can be defined as a program that simulates actions similar to the desired activity or that mimics the demands and skills of a sport or daily activity. To actually live up to the meaning of the term "functional," the prescription for functional exercise must follow some important guidelines: Integrate kinetic chain movements, use multiplanar movements, involve a loading and unloading cycle, and incorporate actions that require balance, stabilization, and proprioceptive stimulation. Muscle balance is affected by muscle tightness, flexibility, strength, and endurance, as these factors work together to provide support and movement. A joint is a pivot point or a fulcrum whose position is constantly affected by the pull of the muscles around it. Joint alignment and posture are affected by these forces. If the muscle is short, it will restrict normal ROM. Excessively long muscles are usually weak and allow adaptive shortening of antagonists. Muscle imbalance may also lead to faulty movements as muscle groups fire in an uncoordinated way. Faulty body mechanics, as determined by postural screening, should be confirmed by the muscle tests for tightness, ROM, and weakness.

Critical to understanding movement, the term *myofascial continuity* describes the connection between adjacent structures within a fascial webbing. The mechanical role of fascia or connective tissue is to meet the combined need for flexibility and stability in our structure. Stretch fascia quickly and it will tear. However, if the stretch is applied slowly it will deform plastically: It will change its length and retain that change.

Most types of flexibility training fall into three categories: static, dynamic (ballistic), and PNF. Each of these stretching techniques has individual advantages and client suitability factors. A number of factors that affect the quality of a stretch are discussed in the chapter and then applied in a sample functional stretch program.

Clients who have muscle imbalances or postural alignment problems can be helped with functionally integrated exercise. Muscle balance is affected by muscle tightness, flexibility, strength, and endurance, because these factors work together to provide support and movement. Appropriate exercises (stretching or resistance) must be selected that target designated muscle groups to improve ROM or muscle balance. Objectives for muscle balance should be centered on stretching tight muscles, strengthening weak muscles, reducing spasms or inefficient firing, building muscular endurance, or improving posture. Whatever your client's needs, this six-step model of sequenced decisions will provide a physiologically sound and client-centered exercise prescription for muscle balance and flexibility.

FORM 8.1   Joint Stress Questionnaire and Observations

1. Do you currently have any pain? _____

2. If so, in what joint or area do you feel the pain? _____

3. In what positions do you feel the pain? _____

4. During what movement do you feel the pain? _____

5. Does your occupation or fitness activity overuse one body segment? _____

6. Do you feel you are currently overtraining? _____

7. Do you feel tight anywhere? _____

8. Do you feel this tightness during or after activity? _____

9. Do you get tired (muscularly) more easily than you used to? _____

10. Have you experienced a loss of strength? _____

11. Are you compensating in your movements to avoid pain or loss of strength? _____

12. Are things getting worse? _____

13. What do you think is causing this problem? _____

14. How could it be alleviated? _____

Watch your client during a workout. Look for altered body mechanics, stiffness, or postural faults, and then answer these questions:

Did you notice any altered body mechanics, stiffness, or postural faults when your client walked in?

_____

_____

_____

Did you notice any altered body mechanics, stiffness, or postural faults when your client was active?

_____

_____

_____

Can any altered body mechanics, stiffness, or postural faults be accounted for because of acute symptoms from current or chronic injuries?

_____

_____

_____

According to these questions and initial observations, where is your client on the joint stress cycle?

_____

_____

_____

Assessment (chapter 4): Perform a postural screening particularly on the area of greatest concern. Perform muscle length testing to determine whether the muscle length is limited or excessive.
Objectives: Establish specific objectives and a plan for exercise design and monitoring.

From J.C. Griffin, 2015, *Client-centered exercise prescription*, 3rd ed. (Champaign, IL: Human Kinetics).

FORM 8.2   Muscle Balance Prescription Worksheet

Objective: _____

Exercise (brief description); alternate stretch and resistance	Body area, muscles	Intensity and weight	Reps	Precautions

Method of Progression:

_____

From J.C. Griffin, 2015, *Client-centered exercise prescription,* 3rd ed. (Champaign, IL: Human Kinetics).

FORM 8.3 Muscle Balance Prescription Card

Client name:	Trainer name:
Client goals:	**Assessment rationale:**
1.	1.
2.	2.
3.	3.
Flexibility prescription for goal 1:	**Strengthening prescription for goal 1:**
Exercise name and description	Exercise name and description
Exercise name and description	Exercise name and description
Exercise name and description	Exercise name and description
Flexibility prescription for goal 2:	**Strengthening prescription for goal 2:**
Exercise name and description	Exercise name and description
Exercise name and description	Exercise name and description
Exercise name and description	Exercise name and description
Flexibility prescription for goal 3:	**Strengthening prescription for goal 3:**
Exercise name and description	Exercise name and description
Exercise name and description	Exercise name and description
Exercise name and description	Exercise name and description
Program recommendations:	**Safety and monitoring guidelines:**

From J.C. Griffin, 2015, *Client-centered exercise prescription*, 3rd ed. (Champaign, IL: Human Kinetics).

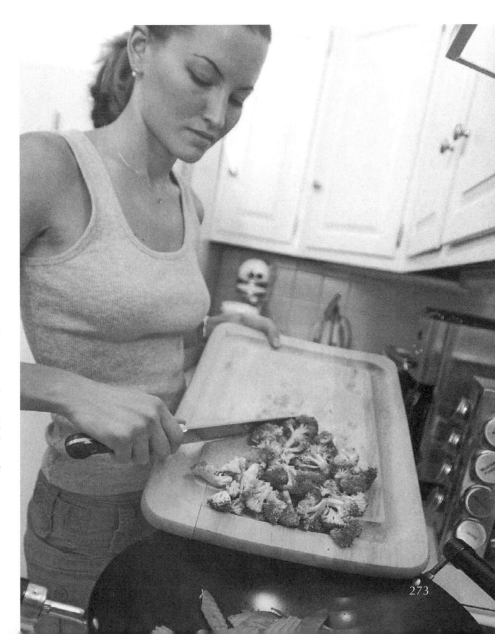

Client-Centered Weight Management Prescription Model

Chapter Competencies

After completing this chapter, you will be able to demonstrate the following competencies:

1. Take a two-pronged approach to improving a client's "shape" and helping him lose weight by (a) modifying eating behaviors and (b) integrating activity (not merely fitness prescription).

2. Identify behaviors most often identified as the reasons for a client's weight problem, that is, what is eaten (e.g., overeating or eating the wrong foods) and why it is eaten (e.g., emotional eating).

3. Describe several ways to expend energy: resting metabolism, metabolizing food (thermic effect of food), and physical activity (thermic effect of exercise).

4. Provide information to clients about counting calories and the merits of diet versus exercise.

5. Use the Energy Deficit Point System to encourage clients to become more active and to estimate the weight loss value of these lifestyle changes.

6. Use a 10-step model to design a physiologically sound and client-centered exercise prescription for weight management.

Together, overweight and obesity are exhibited by approximately 66.3% of adults in the United States (Donnelly et al. 2009). Statistics Canada (2011) reported the rates of overweight and obese females and males as 44.2% and 60.1%, respectively. We must help our clients accept a large range of healthy weights and variations in body size, and we also need to educate them about the merits of diet versus exercise and the issue of counting calories. The Energy Deficit Point System is presented in this chapter to encourage clients to become more active and to estimate the weight loss value of these lifestyle changes. We must recognize the importance of integrating a resistance training segment into a weight management prescription that will prevent loss of lean body mass while increasing resting energy expenditure, and often increasing energy expenditure per pound. The 2010 USDA Dietary Guidelines and the 2009 position stand "Appropriate Physical Activity Intervention Strategies for Weight Loss and Prevention of Weight Regain for Adults" are integrated into this chapter.

A large and growing number of clients ask for assistance to "get into shape." By "getting into shape," most clients mean that they want to shed extra pounds. It is a formidable task to create behavioral change in the midst of overwhelming cultural pressures to succumb to the junk food diets and sedentary living that have led to epidemic weight gain and ill health. So how can we most effectively help those who wish to transform their physical shape?

A great deal of confusion seems to exist among health–fitness professionals about where to draw the line when it comes to assisting participants with nutrition-related questions and goals. The American Council of Sports Medicine believes that health–fitness professionals should have a general understanding of basic nutrition and weight management information that they can share with participants in a "general" sense. This does not include "individual" nutrition assessments, dietary advice, meal plans, or recommendations for supplements or nutrient intakes (Sass et al. 2007). These professionals should refrain from calculating, outlining and counseling on, or prescribing an individualized weight management plan, but can explain the basic principles of weight loss. For more detailed questions or personal information, especially as it relates to disease, it is important to refer to a registered dietitian. Depending on the training of the health–fitness professional, this may include:

Healthy Eating Resources

One of the best nutrition resources for active people is Nancy Clark's 5th edition (2014) of *Sports Nutrition Guidebook*. The following websites and journals are excellent sources of information.

U.S. Websites and Publications

- Academy of Nutrition and Dietetics: www.eatright.org
- Food and Nutrition Information Center: www.nal.usda.gov/fnic
- American Journal of Clinical Nutrition: www.ajcn.org
- Nutritional Reviews: www.ilsi.org/Pages/NutritionReviews.aspx
- USDA Center for Nutrition Policy and Promotion: www.choosemyplate.gov
- Make Your Calories Count: www.accessdata.fda.gov/videos/cfsan/hwm/hwmintro.cfm

Canadian Websites and Publications

- Dietitians of Canada: www.dietitians.ca
- Canada's Food Guide for Healthy Living: www.has.uwo.ca/hospitality/nutrition/pdf/foodguide.pdf
- Canadian Institute of Food Science and Technology: www.cifst.ca
- Dairy Farmers of Canada: dairynutrition.ca/fitness
- Fact Sheets for Canadian Fitness Professionals: csep.ca/partners
- Sport Nutrition Advisory Committee: coach.ca
- Applied Physiology Nutrition and Metabolism: www.nrcresearchpress.com/journal/apnm

- Providing information about food guidance systems (e.g., MyPyramid, USDA Dietary Guidelines, or Canada's Food Guide)
- Providing examples of healthy snacks
- Talking about carbohydrates, proteins, fats, vitamins, minerals, and water
- Demonstrating how to prepare and cook food
- Giving statistical information about relationships between chronic disease and the excess or deficiencies of certain nutrients
- Providing information about nutrients contained in foods or supplements (Sass et al. 2007)

Improving a client's shape and helping him lose weight require a two-pronged approach: (a) modifying eating behaviors and (b) integrating activity (not merely fitness prescription). Many of the techniques discussed in chapter 1, "Activity Counseling Model," will be helpful in the encouragement of behavioral change for weight management. The most effective weight loss programs focus on these two components. Inadequate attention to either one of these decreases the likelihood of long-term, healthy weight management. The combined roles of nutrition and energy balance serve as the foundation of this approach.

In the case study in this chapter, you will learn how to apply the model for weight management prescription with physiological justifications and client-centered behavioral justifications for each choice made.

Nutrition Essentials

A number of nutrition essentials and resources should be among your tools of the trade, although you cannot replace the services of a qualified nutritionist.

The USDA's ChooseMyPlate and Harvard Health Publications' Healthy Eating Plate models help with daily food choices with four colorful quadrants on the plate. Half the plate is filled with fruits and vegetables—the more color and variety, the better. One-quarter of the plate is grains, preferably whole grains. Consumers are encouraged to pick a healthy source of protein to fill another quarter of the plate. Milk and dairy products are limited to 1 or 2 servings per day. The Dietary Guidelines for Americans (2010) recommends consuming a variety of nutrient-dense foods within the basic food groups while limiting the intake of saturated and trans fats, cholesterol, added sugars, salt, and alcohol. Canada's Food Guide encourages selecting a variety of foods from each of four food groups. The number of servings depends on age, body size, activity level, sex, and pregnancy or breast-feeding status. Canada's Food Guide suggests 5 to 12 servings of grain products, 5 to 10 servings of vegetables and fruit, 2 or 3 servings of meat and alternatives, and 2 to 4 servings of dairy products.

Portion sizes and servings may not be as large as most clients think. With the emphasis on getting more for your money, many people have lost sight of standard portion sizes. Eating large portion sizes can lead to overeating, resulting in overweight. To help keep your eye on portion size, use the visual images presented in table 9.1 (Dietitians of Canada 2005). A recent study found that most clients inaccurately estimated the total number of servings they ate per day ("A Lot on Their Plate" 2013). The article noted that the Canada Food Guide defines a meat serving as 2 1/2 oz. (70 g) or 1/2 cup of cooked fish, poultry, or lean meat; if you normally think of an 8 oz. (225

Table 9.1 Visualizing Portion Sizes

Food group	Specific foods	Portion size	Looks like
Grain products 5-12 servings	Pasta, rice Bagel	125 ml (1/2 cup) 1/2 small	1/2 baseball 1 hockey puck
Vegetables and fruits 5-10 servings	Fresh (e.g., apple, orange) Dried fruit Baked potato	1 medium piece 60 ml (1/4 cup) 1 medium	1 baseball 1 golf ball Computer mouse
Meats and alternatives 2-3 servings	Meat, poultry, fish Cooked kidney beans Nuts (e.g., peanuts, almonds)	50-100 g cooked 125-250 ml (1/2-1 cup) 75 ml (1/3 cup)	Deck of cards 1/2-1 baseball Cupped palm of hand
Milk products 2-4 servings	Yogurt Cheese	175 ml (3/4 cup) 50 g (2 oz.)	Yogurt container (6 oz.) 3 dominoes

Data from Fleck and Kraemer 2004, Heyward 2002.

g) steak as a reasonable single serving, that alone exceeds the guide's maximum daily allowance for a woman by more than 50%.

Being food label savvy is important, and a good place to start to keep track of the foods you eat is the grocery store. Nutritional labeling posts the nutritional values on most packaged foods. The marketing claims often placed on the front of the package can be misleading. Claims of fat free, low sodium, or high fiber are recorded accurately on the nutrition label. Nancy Clark (2014) shows how to use the nutritional facts on the label to evaluate the value of a cereal (figure 9.1).

Packaged programs, self-inflicted diets, and gym gurus are often unsuccessful because one approach does not fit everyone. Clients seeking professional advice on weight loss programs that are individually tailored to their lifestyle and food needs are best referred to a registered dietitian. Use the information in "Healthy Eating Resources" to locate a local registered dietitian or to find reliable information.

Energy Expenditure

There are three ways to expend energy: resting metabolism, metabolizing food (thermic effect of food), and physical activity (thermic effect of exercise).

Resting Metabolic Rate

The resting metabolic rate (RMR) is the energy expended to maintain normal body functions if we are simply lying in bed. It is usually the primary source of energy expenditure (60-75%) and would be about 1600 kcal/day for someone

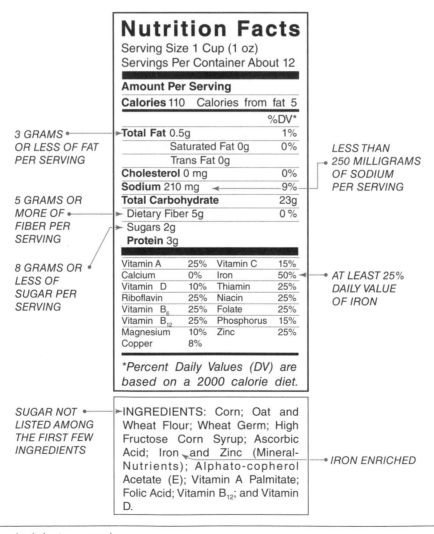

Figure 9.1   What to look for in a cereal.

Reprinted by permission from Clark 2014.

weighing 70 kg (154 lb)—the equivalent of jogging 16 miles (26 km)!

Obese people have daily RMRs approximately 500 kcal higher than nonobese people. This may seem like good news. However, when an obese person loses excess weight, the RMR may drop to 15% to 20% below that of a normal-weight person of similar height and weight (Nieman 1990). This is because fat is less metabolically active than muscle, and dramatic dieting can decrease lean body tissue so that the proportion of fat to lean tissue actually increases, slowing the "internal furnace"! This makes it even more difficult to lose weight at the same levels of energy expenditure than before the dieting. You can estimate RMR by multiplying the body weight in pounds by a factor of 10 for women and 11 for men (Heyward 2010). For example, if our 70 kg client was a female, her RMR would be approximately 1540 kcal (154 lb × 10 kcal/lb or 70 kg × 22 kcal/kg). Given the higher energy expenditure of muscle, of course, individuals with more muscle have a higher RMR than those of the same weight with less muscle.

Thermic Effect of Food

The thermic effect of food (TEF) is the increase in energy expenditure above the RMR that can be measured for several hours after a meal. The average client's TEF is 7% to 10% of the total ingested calories and may last more than 3 h. The TEF is higher after carbohydrate and protein meals than after fat meals (Miller 1991). With appropriate adjustments in meal plans, you could eat more and still lose weight.

Thermic Effect of Exercise

Any physical activity raises the baseline rate of metabolism (RMR). The energy expended for physical activity is the thermic effect of exercise (TEE). The most significant factor affecting this TEE is the intensity of the exercise. For example, a briskly walking average-sized adult male may expend 5 kcal/min (compared with 1 kcal/min while lying down). The same man jogging easily may burn 10 kcal/min. And if the intensity is up to a level barely sustainable by the best athletes for a full workout (10-12 mph, or 16-19 kph), the rate of caloric expenditure may be more than 20 kcal/min (Williams 1995). On the other hand, Klesges and colleagues (1993) indicated that the resting energy expenditure decreases during watching television in approximately inverse proportion to the temptation to consume high-calorie snacks.

Energy expenditure is affected not only by the intensity but also by the efficiency of movement. A more awkward swimmer or runner will burn more calories going the same distance at the same speed as an expert swimmer. Heavier people also burn more calories for any given amount of work, because it takes more energy to move a heavier load.

In young male subjects, vigorous exercise for 45 min resulted in a significant elevation in postexercise energy expenditure that persisted for 14 h. The 190 kcal expended after exercise above resting levels represented an additional 37% to the net energy expended during the 45 min cycling bout. The magnitude and duration of increased energy expenditure after a 45 min bout of vigorous exercise may have implications for weight loss and management (Knab 2011). Present this bonus to your clients as their physical condition improves and their enjoyment of activity increases.

Energy Sources and Metabolism

The two major sources of energy during exercise are fats (in the form of fatty acids) and carbohydrates (in the form of muscle glycogen).

A mixture of fats and carbohydrates is usually used during exercise, the ratio depending on the intensity and duration of the exercise and on the diet and physical condition of the individual. Fat cells are specialized for the synthesis and storage of triglycerides. Before energy release from fat, triglycerides are broken down into free fatty acids (FFAs). Although some fat is stored in all cells (some in the muscle cells and a small amount in the blood), the most active sources of FFAs are the fat cells within adipose tissue. Once FFAs diffuse into the bloodstream, they are delivered to active tissues where they can be used for energy (figure 9.2). As blood flow increases with exercise, more FFAs are removed from fat cells and delivered to active muscle. During exercise, the muscle cells first use fatty acids from the blood and from the muscles' own stores of triglycerides. As exercise continues or increases in intensity, the blood FFAs begin to be in short supply and must be replenished by the vast stores of triglycerides in the adipose tissue.

During rest, the body metabolizes only about 30% of the FFAs that are released from adipose tissue. The other 70% are converted back into fat (i.e., triglycerides). During exercise, only about 25% of these FFAs are reconverted into triglycerides, providing much more FFA to the muscle cells.

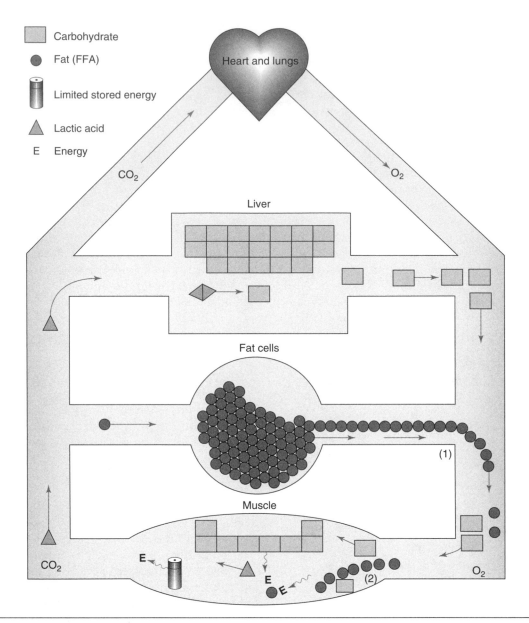

Figure 9.2   Schematic of energy production during light exercise. 1: Free fatty acids move from the fat cells to the muscle during exercise. 2: Free fatty acids reconvert into triglycerides.

During light exercise (25-50% of $\dot{V}O_2$max), about 30% to 50% of the total energy cost is derived from carbohydrate whereas the other 50% to 70% comes from FFAs. As the exercise intensity increases toward 60% to 65% $\dot{V}O_2$max, the muscle triglycerides become increasingly important as the source of fatty acids (Romijn et al. 1993) (figure 9.3).

Carbohydrate is the preferred energy source during high-intensity exercise, such as 65% to 70% of $\dot{V}O_2$max and above. Free fatty acids alone cannot sustain exercise at this intensity, and their contribution diminishes. Hodgetts and colleagues (1991) suggested that an increase in blood lactic acid levels may block release of FFAs from the adipose tissue.

Although carbohydrate becomes more important as an energy source during high-intensity exercise, trained endurance athletes may be able to use fats more efficiently at higher exercise intensities. Even regular exercisers who increase their anaerobic thresholds will be able to burn more fat during intensity levels of 65% to 70% of their $\dot{V}O_2$max.

Energy Balance

American and European surveys (Bartlett 2003; McArdle et al. 2010; Statistics Canada 2006) showed that approximately 35% to 40% of adult women and 25% to 30% of adult men were

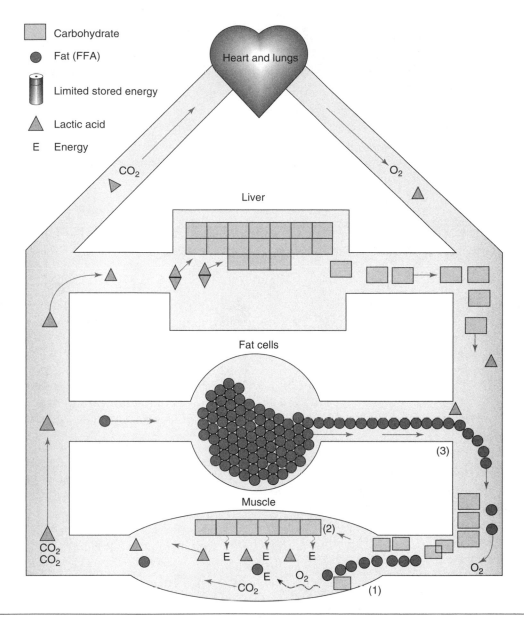

Figure 9.3   Schematic of energy production during high-intensity exercise. 1: Free fatty acids alone cannot sustain exercise at this intensity. 2: Carbohydrate is the preferred energy source during high-intensity exercise. 3: Release of FFAs blocked.

currently attempting to lose weight. What all of these people must understand is that every calorie they eat must be expended or conserved in the body, so weight gain has usually resulted from a long period in which energy intake has exceeded energy expenditure. Calorie intake and calorie outgo must be balanced if clients are to maintain weight and "unbalanced" in the appropriate direction if clients are to gain or lose weight (Jakicic 2009).

Physical activity (PA) is recommended as a component of weight management for prevention of weight gain, for weight loss, and for prevention of weight regain after weight loss. Evidence supports moderate-intensity (3.0-5.9 METs) PA between 150 and 250 min per week as effective to

prevent weight gain. This same prescription will provide only modest weight loss. Greater amounts of PA (>250 min/week) have been associated with clinically significant weight loss. After weight loss, weight maintenance is improved with PA >250 min/week (Donnelly et al. 2009).

We have at our disposal a positive and powerful tool for manipulating this energy balance: physical activity. We have seen the unique role that this tool has on fat metabolism, metabolic rate, heart health, and energy expenditure. In this section we examine how to integrate everyday activity and exercise into our prescriptions and ensure that each combination is suited both to the goals of weight control and to the individual client.

Aerobic Training and Body Composition

Heyward (2010) described four changes relating to fat loss and the conservation of lean body tissues that results from aerobic training:

- The percentage of the energy used during submaximal exercise that is derived from the metabolism of FFA is larger than the percentage used during rest or intense exercise.

- Endurance training raises the point at which lactic acid levels sharply increase (called the anaerobic threshold). Because lactic acid inhibits fatty acid metabolism, conditioned people burn more fat during exercise than do unconditioned people.

- Resting energy expenditure (REE) may not decrease during calorie-restricted diets if regular exercise is maintained.

- Increased levels of epinephrine and norepinephrine released during exercise stimulate the mobilization of fat from storage and activate the enzyme lipase, which breaks down triglycerides into FFAs.

Creating the Deficit

To manage their weight, clients need to understand the following principles:

- Weight loss should not exceed 1 kg (2 lb) per week.
- Caloric deficit should not exceed 1000 kcal/ day.
- Aerobic activity should be performed daily, in one or several sessions.
- Aerobic activity, if sustained for at least 10 min, may include home or occupational activities in addition to fitness, recreation, and sport activities (see table 9.2 later in the chapter).
- Total energy expenditure is higher with longer-duration, lower-intensity exercise; however, RMR can remain elevated for 30 min or longer after high-intensity exercise (Heyward 2010).
- Resistance training effectively maintains FFM, which uses more calories at rest.

Inactive, sedentary individuals may expend only 15% additional energy beyond their RMR. At the other extreme, laborers and very active athletes may expend double their RMR. For most clients, our goal is to help them move into light activity, which may provide 35% to 40% of additional expenditure beyond their RMR. Larger deficits will come by encouraging moderate activity, adding 50% or more to their total daily caloric expenditure.

If at rest the average-sized adult burns 60 to 70 kcal/h, with even light activity this can be tripled. As conditioning increases to allow a moderate level of activity such as tennis, brisk power walking, or moderate aerobics, the furnace can be stoked to about eight times its normal burning capacity, increasing our potential to burn more calories in the same period of time.

Many resources (including table 9.2) list the energy costs of a wide variety of physical activities. When using these lists, remember that

- they refer only to the time that your client is actually moving, which may be only 35 to 40 min of an hour-long basketball game; and
- actual energy expenditure may vary because of skill level, air resistance, and terrain, and body weight and sex can affect the data (body weight adjustment is listed below the table).

Energy Deficit Point System

Table 9.2 provides the energy requirements for many home, occupational, and fitness activities. You can calculate the total caloric expenditure for each activity by multiplying the $kcal \cdot kg^{-1} \cdot min^{-1}$ by the client's body weight (kg). By multiplying this by the number of minutes of that activity, you have the client's energy expenditure for the session. Doing the detailed calculations and keeping a physical activity log can be very helpful for some clients; however, it is time-consuming and, of course, is still an estimate. To simplify the use of this information, the first column lists energy points associated with each group of activities. These points are a conservative estimate of the number of calories burned per minute of activity.

The Energy Deficit Point System is based on the calculations and the accumulated research represented in table 9.2, yet it is as easy as 1–2–3. Simply perform the following steps:

Table 9.2 Point System for Energy Requirements

Energy points	Energy range	Home or occupational activity	Fitness or recreational activity
2	1.5-2.0 METs 2.0-2.5 kcal/min $0.013\text{-}0.016 \text{ kcal} \cdot \text{lb}^{-1} \cdot \text{min}^{-1}$ $0.029\text{-}0.035 \text{ kcal} \cdot \text{kg}^{-1} \cdot \text{min}^{-1}$	Desk work Word processing Playing cards	Strolling (1 mph)
4	2.0-3.0 METs 2.5-4.0 kcal/min $0.016\text{-}0.026 \text{ kcal} \cdot \text{lb}^{-1} \cdot \text{min}^{-1}$ $0.035\text{-}0.057 \text{ kcal} \cdot \text{kg}^{-1} \cdot \text{min}^{-1}$	Dressing Driving a car Riding a lawn mower Making a bed Washing Playing a musical instrument	Walking (2.0 mph) Cycling (5 mph) Stretching Hatha yoga Bird watching Bowling Playing catch, baseball, Frisbee
5	3.0-4.0 METs 4.0-5.0 kcal/min $0.026\text{-}0.032 \text{ kcal} \cdot \text{lb}^{-1} \cdot \text{min}^{-1}$ $0.057\text{-}0.070 \text{ kcal} \cdot \text{kg}^{-1} \cdot \text{min}^{-1}$	Showering House painting Sweeping floors Cleaning windows Pushing light power mower Vacuuming Active child care and play	Walking (3.0 mph) Golf, using power cart Cycling (6 mph) Bicycle ergometer (300 kg $\cdot$ m^{-1} $\cdot$ min^{-1}) Light calisthenics Tai chi Curling Volleyball, noncompetitive
6	4.0-5.0 METs 5.0-6.0 kcal/min $0.032\text{-}0.039 \text{ kcal} \cdot \text{lb}^{-1} \cdot \text{min}^{-1}$ $0.070\text{-}0.086 \text{ kcal} \cdot \text{kg}^{-1} \cdot \text{min}^{-1}$	Gardening, weeding, raking Mopping floors Light carpentry Washing and waxing the car	Walking (3.5 mph) Golfing: walking and carrying clubs Cycling (8 mph) Bicycle ergometer (450 kg $\cdot$ m^{-1} $\cdot$ min^{-1}) Stepping: stair height (rate: 18/min) Jogging on mini-trampoline Water aerobics and calisthenics Weightlifting (moderate) Many calisthenics Baseball, general Basketball, shooting baskets Badminton, social singles or doubles Dancing: line, polka, fast pace Skiing, downhill, light effort
7	5.0-6.0 METs 6.0-7.0 kcal/min $0.039\text{-}0.045 \text{ kcal} \cdot \text{lb}^{-1} \cdot \text{min}^{-1}$ $0.086\text{-}0.099 \text{ kcal} \cdot \text{kg}^{-1} \cdot \text{min}^{-1}$	Gardening, digging Walking downstairs Scrubbing floors Carrying objects (15-30 lb, 7-14 kg) Manual labor (moderate)	Walking (4.0 mph) Walk and jog combination Jogging in place (60-70 steps/min) Hiking, cross-country Cycling (10 mph) Bicycle ergometer (600 kg $\cdot$ m^{-1} $\cdot$ min^{-1}) Aerobic dance (low impact) Stepping: stair height (rate: 24/min) Softball, fast or slow pitch Skiing, downhill, moderate effort Tennis, doubles
8	6.0-7.0 METs 7.0-8.0 kcal/min $0.045\text{-}0.052 \text{ kcal} \cdot \text{lb}^{-1} \cdot \text{min}^{-1}$ $0.099\text{-}0.114 \text{ kcal} \cdot \text{kg}^{-1} \cdot \text{min}^{-1}$	Chopping wood Climbing stairs (slowly)	Walking (5.0 mph) Cycling (11 mph) Stepping: stair height (rate: 30/min) Aerobic dance (moderate) Water aerobics (vigorous) Rowing machine (moderate) Weightlifting (vigorous) Racquetball, casual, general Soccer, casual, general Skiing, cross-country, light effort

(continued)

(continued)

Energy points	Energy range	Home or occupational activity	Fitness or recreational activity
10	7.0-8.0 METs 8.0-10.0 kcal/min 0.052-0.065 kcal · lb^{-1} · min^{-1} 0.114-0.143 kcal · kg^{-1} · min^{-1}	Sawing hardwood Snow shoveling	Jogging (5.0 mph) Jogging in place (120 steps/min) Cycling (12 mph) Bicycle ergometer (750 kg · m^{-1} · min^{-1}) Swimming laps (slow to moderate) Circuit resistance training Heavy calisthenics (e.g., push-ups, sit-ups, jumping jacks) Skating, roller or ice Skiing, cross-country, moderate effort Tennis, singles
11	8.0-9.0 METs 10.0-11.0 kcal/min 0.065-0.071 kcal · lb^{-1} · min^{-1} 0.143-0.156 kcal · kg^{-1} · min^{-1}	Climbing stairs (moderate speed) Shoveling, 10 shovels/min (30 lb or 14 kg load)	Running (5.5 mph) Cycling (13 mph) Bicycle ergometer (900 kg · m^{-1} · min^{-1}) Rowing machine (vigorous) Aerobic dance (vigorous/step: 6-8 in.) Water jogging Rope skipping (<75 rpm) Hockey, recreational
11+	≥10.0 METs ≥11.0 kcal/min ≥0.071 kcal · lb^{-1} · min^{-1} ≥0.156 kcal · kg^{-1} · min^{-1}	Climbing stairs (quickly)	Running (6.0 mph = 10 METs, 7.0 mph = 11.5 METs, 8.0 mph = 13.5 METs, 9.0 mph = 15 METs) Deep-water running Cycling (>13 mph) Bicycle ergometer (1050 kg · m^{-1} · min^{-1}) Swimming, laps (vigorous) Rope jumping (120-140 beats/min = 11-12 METs) Martial arts

Note: 1 MET = energy expenditure at rest; approximately 3.5 ml · kg^{-1} · min^{-1}.

Energy range depends on efficiency, rest pauses, and body size. Values are based on client of 154 lb or 70 kg. Add 10% for each 15 lb or 7 kg above 154 lb or 70 kg.

Data from Ainsworth et al. 2000; Heyward 2010; Hoeger, Hoeger, Locke, and Lauzon 2009; and Powers and Howley 2009.

1. **Prescribe and record the fitness activity of your client's choice.** In addition, identify or credit home or occupational activities that are performed during the week. Record the energy points associated with the activities. For example,

Activity A: ___ Energy points

Activity B: ___ Energy points

2. **Prescribe and record the length of time in minutes that your client will devote to those activities** (minimum continuous time is 10 min). This provides the energy points for that session of activity. For example,

Activity A: ___ Energy points × ___ min = ___

Activity B: ___ Energy points × ___ min = ___

3. **Prescribe and record the number of times in a week that this will be repeated.** This provides the energy points for that activity for the week. For example,

Activity A: ___ Energy points × ___ min × ___ /week = ___

Activity B: ___ Energy points × ___ min × ___ /week = ___

Total weekly energy points: ___

Let's apply this technique to a plausible situation you might encounter with a client. You recommend that your client take her dog for a 20 min brisk walk every day. To create an additional energy deficit, you design a 30 min calisthenic circuit including TheraBands that she will do three times a week. She also recognizes that if she helps with the weekly Saturday cleaning of the apartment, she deserves some credit. To apply the Energy Deficit Point System:

Step 1: Prescribe the Activities

Activity A: Walking the dog (3.0 mph or 4.8 kph) = 5 energy points

Activity B: Calisthenic circuit = 6 energy points

Activity C: Cleaning = 5 energy points

Step 2: Prescribe the Durations

Activity A: 5 energy points 3 20 min = 100

Activity B: 6 energy points 3 30 min = 180

Activity C: 5 energy points 3 100 min = 500

Step 3: Prescribe Frequency

Activity A: 5 energy points 3 20 min 3 7/week = 700

Activity B: 6 energy points 3 30 min 3 3/week = 540

Activity C: 5 energy points 3 100 min 3 1/week = 500

Total weekly energy points: 1740

This represents a conservative estimate of 1740 kcal/week and should represent 1 lb (0.45 kg) of weight lost every 2 weeks.

Eating Behaviors

The human body is a remarkable machine. It can consume nearly a ton of food in a year and not change its weight. However, overeating, eating the wrong foods, and emotional eating are the behaviors most often identified as the reasons for weight problems.

What You Eat

It is unfair, and for the most part unproven, to suggest that all people with weight problems overeat. Even if the cause of increased fat deposit is not overeating, treatment for overweight clients usually involves a reduction in daily energy intake. Yet dieting can reduce the RMR, shift the energy balance back in the direction of energy storage, and counteract caloric reduction. Repeated diets may have decreased your client's ability to lose weight and increased his ability to gain weight (Williams 1995).

The average American consumes nearly 40% of calories from fat (25-30% is recommended). This amount of dietary fat can itself be a cause of obesity. It has been shown that naturally lean people have a difficult time gaining weight on a low-fat diet but gain easily on high-fat diets (Tremblay et al. 1989). Eating a high-fat diet promotes body fat formation. The body uses one-fourth to one-third less energy to process dietary fat than it does to convert protein or carbohydrate to body fat (McArdle et al. 2010). In other words, a given caloric quantity of excess dietary fat is more fattening than a calorically similar quantity of excess carbohydrate. This means that what you eat (diet composition) may be as important as total calories in the promotion of obesity.

Miller (1991) demonstrated that middle-aged obesity is characterized by reduced carbohydrate intake. His data suggested that consumption of natural or complex carbohydrates (such as whole grains) assists in weight loss, whereas obesity correlates with excess consumption of "added" or refined sugars. He also found that a high fiber intake assists in weight loss because of the increased consumption of natural carbohydrates (vegetables, fruits, grains).

The Dietary Guidelines for Americans (2010) highlighted three major goals:

1. Balance energy intake with PA (energy expenditure) to manage body weight.
2. Consume more fruits, vegetables, whole grains, fat-free and low-fat dairy products, and seafood.
3. Consume fewer foods with sodium, saturated fats, trans fats, cholesterol, added sugars, and refined grains.

Similarly, the Canadian Community Health Survey (Statistics Canada 2006) showed that Canadians still eat too many nutrient-poor foods, such as chips, commercial muffins and Danish pastries, soft drinks, sugary beverages, and fried foods. As well, we don't get enough milk products or fruits and vegetables.

Clients are more likely to follow eating recommendations if you can integrate their food preferences, assuming moderation, and include all food groups. Even the most knowledgeable clients need encouragement to make the best choices on a daily basis. The National Heart, Lung, and Blood Institute (2000) provided recommended elements of a basic low-calorie diet for healthy adults (table 9.3). Recommended daily intake or allowances (RDAs) are one part of a broader set of dietary guidelines called the Dietary Reference Intake used by both the United States and Canada.

Nutrient-dense foods and beverages provide the greatest number of nutrients with the least number of calories. That is, the nutrients have not been diluted by adding calories from solid fats, refined starches, or added sugars. Nutrient-dense foods include whole grains, vegetables, fruits, seafood, eggs, beans and peas, unsalted nuts and seeds, fat-free and low-fat milk and milk products, and lean meats and poultry. Nutrient density is beneficial when weight loss is a goal. Compare the following caloric content of similar food forms (Bushman 2011):

Extra lean ground beef patty (184 kcal)   versus   Regular beef (52 extra fat calories)

Baked chicken breast (138 kcal)   versus   Breaded and fried (108 extra calories)

Corn flakes (90 kcal)   versus   Added sugars (57 calories)

Baked potato (117 kcal)   versus   French fries (141 extra fat calories)

Unsweetened applesauce (105 kcal)   versus   Added sugars (68 calories)

Fat-free milk (83 kcal)   versus   Whole milk (66 extra milk fat calories)

Why You Eat

Helping clients discover why they eat is as important as knowing what they eat. Clients who were rewarded with food as children may confuse being fed with being loved. Some people eat when they are bored. With the boom in television watching, many are not aware of the amount they consume each night after their "last" meal!

These clients need extra help to become more aware of when and why they eat. A daily log of the food, quantity, time, place, and emotional state may provide insights for you and your client and help you devise strategies to counteract her personal triggers for overeating or for eating the wrong things. Many clients may need guidance in preparing food, packing a nutritious lunch, or judging food serving sizes. To avoid temptations to give in to excuses, instruct your clients to do the following:

- Plan alternatives ahead of time. Have some prepared meals in the freezer that can be thawed faster than a pizza delivery.

- Use stick-on notes to post inspirational messages on the refrigerator, for example, "Contrary to popular belief, chocolate is not one of the food groups."

- Share goals and temptations with a friend or spouse and ask for the person's help when the going gets tough.

- Use smaller plates and bowls so food portions seem larger.

Research indicates that tracking food choices can help with healthy weight management

Table 9.3   Recommended Daily Intake

Component	Recommended daily intake
Calories	500-1000 kcal/day reduction
Protein	About 15% of total calories
Carbohydrate	>55% of total calories
Fat (saturated and unsaturated)	<30% of total calories
Cholesterol	<300 mg/day
Sodium chloride	<2400 mg/day
Calcium	1000-15,000 mg/day
Fiber	20-30 g/day

From the National Heart, Lung, and Blood Institute 2000.

Fast Food Fat

I have a friend who often found himself on the road at mealtime. He usually picked up a cinnamon bun with butter in the late afternoon to hold him till dinner. His wife prepared wonderful nutritious dinners, for example, chicken breast, baked potato, salad, and juice. What changed his habit was his shock in learning that the afternoon snack had more calories than his dinner! He was also surprised that not all hamburgers are created equal. For example, McDonald's Big Mac has almost 600 kcal with its high-fat sauce, whereas a regular hamburger contains only 150 kcal (from carbohydrate, fat, and protein). Fast food snacks may be high-fat meals—choose carefully!

(Thomas et al. 2011). Completing a journal or mini-assessment such as the one in form 9.1, Assess Your Energy Profile, can provide such assistance (Dairy Farmers of Canada [DFC]/Canadian Society for Exercise Physiology [CSEP] 2012a).

Common Client Concerns About Diet and Exercise

Clients usually come to you with a mix of information and misinformation about weight management. Some of the common issues or areas of confusion are (1) counting calories, (2) the relationship of diet and exercise, (3) special nutritional concerns for active clients, and (4) the role of resistance training in weight management.

Should Clients Count Calories?

If a person routinely consumes more calories than he expends, he will gain weight regardless of the composition of his diet. Conversely, if your client uses more calories than he ingests, he will lose weight. A 3500 kcal deficit will result in a loss of 1 lb (0.45 kg); a 3500 kcal excess will result in the gain of 1 lb of body tissue. If your client needs to count the calories he expends and the calories he consumes to ensure the balance (for weight maintenance) or deficit (for weight loss) between them, counting calories is important. A recent study compared menu labels displaying the amount of exercise (brisk walking) needed to burn the calories in the food item. The results indicated that this new angle to calorie counting was more effective than menus with calorie-only labels and menus without calorie labels in terms of fewer calories ordered and consumed (Shah and James 2013). Clients often need to start out counting calories but will eventually reach the point where they develop a feel for their caloric balance.

When making food choices, they should keep in mind that protein and carbohydrate contain only 4 kcal/g, whereas fat contains 9 kcal/g and water contains no calories (McArdle et al. 2010).

Because the body has different components (water, fat, fat-free mass), changes in these components may bring about weight fluctuations that appear to contradict the caloric balance concept. For instance, early weight loss may be primarily loss of water. Also, exercise increases the fat-free mass (which is heavier, although more compact than fat) while it is decreasing fat, so weight loss on the scales may be slower than might be expected (figure 9.4).

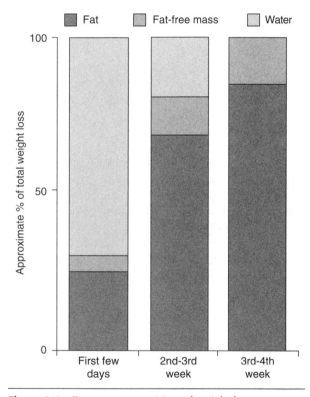

Figure 9.4   Percent composition of weight loss.

Counting Calories for the Blue Jeans

Gwen is a good example of someone who benefited from counting calories. Gwen entered our employee fitness program weighing 150 lb (68 kg) and set realistic goals of losing 10 lb (4.5 kg) and fitting into her blue jeans. She had been maintaining her weight for the last year and believed that she could achieve a daily 500 kcal deficit (3500 kcal/week) by reducing her diet by 250 kcal and increasing her activity by 250 kcal, on average. Gwen joined our noon aerobics class 3 days a week (3 × 300 kcal) and started walking to work 5 days a week (5 × 150). A weekend golf game or tennis match burned an extra 500 kcal. At the end of each day, Gwen recorded food deficit calories and the caloric worth of her activities. Each day did not add up to 500 kcal, but the week's total gave her a 3500 kcal deficit. After a greater than 1 lb (0.45 kg) loss in the first 2 weeks (probably water loss), it looked as though things were starting to plateau. However, by the end of 10 weeks, she had lost the 10 lb. More important for Gwen, she arrived at work that Friday casually dressed in blue jeans.

Which Is More Effective: Diet or Exercise?

There are pros and cons to using exercise alone or dieting alone, but either can be effective in reducing weight. You must consider each client individually when establishing an appropriate treatment strategy. Overweight clients are somewhat less likely to stay with an exercise program. Inactivity may be the cause of the problem, or it may be the result of the excess weight. Clients should include exercise because if they only follow a calorie-restricted diet, they risk losing lean body tissue. Walberg (1989) showed that diet-only programs led to decreased REE and ongoing weight management difficulties. The slower metabolism helps conserve a dwindling energy reserve from lack of food. But the restrictive dieting also makes it progressively harder to lose weight. It may be only a matter of time before the weight is gained back and another crash diet starts a "yo-yo" cycle. Many clients have already tried diet restriction alone for some time and are among the 95% of all people who lose weight only to gain it back within 2 years.

Compared with exercise alone, dieting alone can produce more rapid weight reduction early in a program. Although exercise may provide slower results, it can help maintain lean body mass and prevent any decrease in REE. Weight lost by dieting is about 75% fat and 25% protein. Combining exercise and diet can reduce that protein loss to only 5% (Garfinkel and Coscina 1990). Exercise counterbalances the disadvantages of dieting alone; and once excess body fat has been lost, continued exercise is important to maintaining a stable, healthy body weight. Marks and colleagues (1995) showed that aerobic cycle exercise and resistance training are equally effective in maintaining fat-free mass while encouraging weight loss. Evidence has shown that weight loss and additional healthful outcomes are more likely with exercise in combination with diet than with diet alone (Volpe 2011; Bond Brill et al. 2002).

Every client is different in terms of her degree of motivation to change diet or exercise. Keeping in mind that a 3500 kcal deficit will result in a loss of 1 lb (0.45 kg) of body tissue, table 9.4 identifies four "routes" that a client may take, each resulting in the loss of about 1 lb/week.

Are There Special Nutritional Concerns for Active Clients?

Nutrition plays a critical role in athletic performance, but many active people do not eat a diet that helps them to do their best. Active clients need to consume enough energy for the demands of their workout. By consuming adequate calories from a variety of foods, they should satisfy their need for macronutrients (carbohydrate, protein, fat) and micronutrients (vitamins, minerals). To keep the body energized and to manage hunger, refuel every 3 to 4 h with either a meal or a snack. Preworkout consumption fuels muscles with water and carbohydrates, provides energy for the activity, and can assist in a more rapid recovery. The best fuels are carbohydrates without too much fiber (e.g., rice, pasta, bagels, boiled potatoes). Moderate amounts of protein and fat can be tolerated up to 1 to 2 h before the work. For a preworkout breakfast, you may suggest orange juice, whole-grain cereal or bread, partly skim milk cheese, applesauce, or a banana. A larger meal 1 to 2 h preworkout may include a pasta salad, tuna on a whole wheat tortilla or chicken breast, and vegetable or fruit juice. Preworkout snack ideas may include a fruit smoothie, whole-grain granola bar, small oatmeal muffin with raisins, fruit yogurt, or a whole wheat bagel with sliced banana. Try to avoid fatty foods and high-protein foods that take longer to digest and sugary foods that can cause energy to spike and then plummet (DFC/CSEP 2012a).

After a workout, clients need to recover quickly and reenergize. Within 30 min after exercising, muscles need carbohydrates with a little pro-

Table 9.4 Diet and Exercise Plans to Lose 1 lb (0.45 kg) per Week

Exercise	Intensity	Duration	Frequency	Required kcal exercise expenditure per week	Required diet kcal deficit per week	Required diet kcal deficit per day	Total kcal deficit per week
None	—	—	—	—	3500	500	3500
Yes	Moderate	30 min	3 times/week	1050	2400	350	3500
Yes	Moderate	30 min	5 times/week	1750	1700	250	3500
Yes	Moderate	60 min	5 times/week	3500	None	None	3500

tein and water. All liquids count: water, milk, juice, drinkable yogurt, sports drinks, and so on. Spaccarotella and Andzel (2011) found low-fat chocolate milk to be as good as carbohydrate–electrolyte beverages at promoting recovery between training sessions. Postworkout snack ideas may include trail mix, cottage cheese with fruit, tuna and cheddar on whole-grain bread, ham and cheese sandwich, almond butter and banana wrap, yogurt and fruit, or an energy bar. Eating high-protein meals soon after strength training workouts promotes muscle growth and can help repair muscle damage. While very active athletes, such as those who train intensely every day or for several hours per day, may need extra protein, there is no need to overload. Most strength training clients naturally meet higher energy and protein needs through their increased appetite, and excess protein may be stored as fat (American College of Sports Medicine [ACSM], American Dietetic Association, Dietitians of Canada 2009). A 70 kg (154 lb) person needs 0.8 g/kg a day or about 56 g protein. Endurance or strength training athletes may require 1.2 to 1.7 g/kg per day (DFC/CSEP 2012a). Besides beef, poultry, and fish, try yogurt with berries and granola, hard-boiled egg and orange juice, trail mix with nuts and seeds, grilled cheese with tomato, or vegetarian chili with cheese.

We need to make sure that our clients are drinking enough fluid to support their PA. Dehydration can make your clients' workouts seem harder and less effective. Fluid is lost in sweat, urine, digestive processes, and breathing and through the skin. Watch for symptoms such as thirst, fatigue, weakness, headache, dizziness, and reduced mental alertness and muscle control (Institute of Medicine 2006). The simplest way to determine whether your clients are getting enough fluid is to have them monitor their urine color and amount. A large volume of light-colored urine indicates that hydration is sufficient. A small volume of dark-colored urine may indicate the need to drink more fluid. Physically active people need to drink enough fluid to balance out these losses and avoid dehydration. Although plain water is sufficient for most workouts, diluted juice or a sports drink may be better during exercise if it's very hot, when clients are wearing protective sports equipment, or if they are sweating a lot (DFC/CSEP 2012b).

Active people need specific nutrients. They have to take care that their diet delivers the nutrients that meet their energy requirements. An inadequate diet (e.g., strict dieting) can lead to deficiencies, especially in calcium and iron. In addition to helping build and maintain bone mass, calcium plays a role in muscle contraction and relaxation. Adequate calcium intake is therefore essential for ensuring that muscles work properly and for minimizing the risk of muscle cramps. The body responds to a calcium shortage by drawing from its reserves in the bones. Bones can become more fragile and brittle, increasing the risk of fractures (McArdle et al. 2010). To ensure your clients meet their calcium needs, have them choose good dietary sources of calcium-rich foods every day: milk, yogurt, and cheese. Remember, supplements don't replace food. Iron plays a critical role for active clients. Iron in the blood carries oxygen to the muscles that help produce the energy needed for activity. Inadequate levels of iron use up reserves, causing a deficiency, and symptoms of anemia may appear: paleness, fatigue, lack of energy, irritability, and infections. Although many foods contain iron, vegetable sources are not absorbed as well as animal-source foods like meat, poultry, and fish.

Is Resistance Training for Weight Loss or Weight Gain?

Most clients want resistance training programs to build muscle strength, endurance, power, or size. However, resistance training can also be a valuable adjunct to a weight management prescription. Here are some facts about weight management and resistance training that will encourage your clients who are interested in weight loss or maintenance:

• A weight reduction program can cause loss of protein tissue (primarily muscle) along with body fat. Weight training can prevent significant loss of lean body mass.

• Weight training can also prevent decreases in REE, keeping the furnace stoked. In fact, each additional pound of muscle tissue can raise the RMR by 35 kcal/day (Campbell et al. 1994). If your client adds 2 lb (0.90 kg) of muscle tissue as the result of resistance training, it could raise her RMR by 70 kcal/day (35 × 2), which equals 25,550 kcal/year (70 × 365) or the equivalent of 7.3 lb (3.3 kg) of fat (25,550/3500).

• Andersen and Jakicic (2003) reported that acute strenuous resistance exercise is associated with modest but prolonged elevations in postexercise metabolic rate and possibly fat oxidation.

• Lifting lighter weights for more repetitions (e.g., 15-25) and 1 or 2 sets can maintain muscle endurance and tone with little chance of significantly altering muscle size.

- Clients need not worry that new muscle cells will turn into fat in the future: It is physiologically impossible.

- Although resistance training does burn calories, the effect is relatively small compared with that of aerobic exercise. Thus, the optimal prescription for many is a combination of aerobic exercise and moderate resistance training.

The ACSM position stand (Donnelly et al. 2009) states that resistance training alone does not seem to be effective for weight reduction. It increases fat-free mass when used alone or in combination with weight loss from diet restriction. Resistance training may increase loss of fat mass when combined with aerobic exercise.

Can Abdominal Exercises Trim the Waistline?

Abdominal obesity tends to increase with weight gain and is strongly associated with increased levels of visceral fat and various diseases such as heart disease, type 2 diabetes, and the metabolic syndrome (McArdle et al. 2010). Is resistance training effective in decreasing abdominal subcutaneous and visceral fat and keeping the waistline trim? Abdominal exercises, such as core conditioning exercises, are often promoted as effective means to reduce abdominal fat and waistline measures. Support for "spot reduction" in body fat is mixed and often based on subcutaneous skinfolds. Vispute and colleagues (2011) used dual-energy X-ray absorptiometry (DXA) to assess whole and regional percent body fat. In addition, the group of 14 men and 10 women, 18 to 40 years, were assessed for body composition, anthropometrics, and abdominal endurance. All participants maintained an isocaloric diet, and the exercise group performed seven abdominal exercises, for 2 sets of 10 repetitions, on 5 days/week for 6 weeks. There was no significant effect of abdominal exercises on body weight, body fat percentage, android (trunk and abdomen) fat percentage, abdominal circumference, abdominal skinfold, and suprailiac skinfold. However, this group did perform significantly better on abdominal endurance. Other researchers have shown a loss of abdominal subcutaneous and visceral fat after combined aerobic and resistance exercise (McArdle et al. 2010).

Integrating Activity Into Lifestyle

The late Jean Mayer, an international authority on weight control, reported that no single factor is more frequently responsible for obesity than lack of PA. If inactivity is not a major cause for obesity in some cases, it is the consequence of obesity and plays a definite role in maintaining obesity.

We live busy lives, and lack of time is the most frequently quoted barrier to becoming more active. Combine this with a dislike for strenuous exercise and often a sense of physical embarrassment and you have the formula for sedentary living. We need a new strategy to help overweight clients. Recent public health guidelines (ACSM 2009; Donnelly et al. 2009; Volpe 2011; Warburton et al. 2006) and research (Andersen and Jakicic 2003) suggest that sedentary individuals can derive significant health benefits from accumulating 30 min or more of moderately intense activity on most days.

Although some clients will follow a structured aerobic-based exercise prescription for weight loss, many will not. With these clients, your challenge is to help them buy in to the concept and practice of activity "integration." We need to direct these clients toward activities that could be part of their current lifestyle. Thoughtful counseling should identify daily opportunities to walk, such as delivering a message in person three floors up, or to perform manual tasks, such as washing the car, gardening, or doing repair jobs around the house. Andersen and Jakicic (2003) compared the effects of performing several 10 min bouts of home exercise throughout the day with a single, longer bout. Overweight patients were more likely to adhere to the shorter prescription than those who exercised in longer bouts.

A compelling argument against exercise as a means of weight loss is that it expends so few calories: "One piece of cake and I've blown my whole aerobics class!" In the short term this is true. But compare mild exercise with the return we expect when we invest money at interest. The immediate payback usually is not large; but if we are patient and stay with the investment, it will grow substantially over time. For example, if you walked briskly for about 2 miles (3.2 km) a day, you would expend enough calories in a month to 6 weeks to account for a loss of nearly 2 lb (0.90 kg). When we combine mild diet reduction with increased activity, it is reasonable to expect a 10% reduction in body weight in 6 months (Bartlett 2003).

In modern society, most adults spend most of their time sitting, whether at work, at home, or during leisure time. This leads to low levels of energy expenditure and is likely to be a significant cause of obesity. This inactivity physiology is a strong argument for increasing lifestyle PA

Body Image

Fitness professionals often take a purely physiological approach to weight management, examining weight and health in terms of metabolic normality, body composition (leanness and fat), and functional capacity. This approach tends to focus on health enhancement, on an acceptable standard, on performance, or on aesthetics. Such a focus, however, may not connect with your client's needs.

Our eyes see what our brains tell them to see. Body image is the mental image we have of our own physical appearance. More than 50% of adult women are dissatisfied with their weight. The concern with weight often starts in high school, but the handicap is felt long afterward in terms of personal and professional fulfillment. For such clients, the mental image of the ideal weight is often distorted. You need to help them realize that an acceptable and realistic standard may be a "tolerable" weight that is within a healthy standard (chapter 4).

Once your clients realize that you are considering the psychological and social pressures they face, and that you don't simply see their weight as a risk factor, the doors will be open to talk about weight in relation to well-being, body image, and social acceptance. De-emphasize any absolute measure of weight or body composition in the counseling, and encourage your client to find her own desirable and healthy weight. Ask her if she is happy with her weight. To really enjoy a high quality of life, she needs to be happy with herself. Then ask her if she wants to change enough to implement exercise and dietary changes. These simple questions will help establish a degree of commitment to define a "tolerable" weight for her.

For clients with a body image goal, I like to use a "mirror" analogy: I challenge them to change the reflection they see. It becomes an attitude challenge. Our goal is to promote personal acceptance of a large range of healthy weights and variations in body size. Searching through magazines to find appropriate images of body shape can be helpful. Less frequent use of scales and a few new pieces of clothing can also help toward a more positive self-attitude. Be realistic about your "reflection" but recognize the continuing benefits of appropriate eating and PA habits.

and should be taken into account in weight management efforts (Donnelly et al. 2009). Other examples of strategies to integrate PA into a client's lifestyle include work around the home, commuting, personal care, occupational activity, and leisure-time activities. These usually include problem solving, goal setting, self-monitoring, and so on.

Weight Management Prescription Model

The model for weight management prescription is similar to that used in chapter 6 for cardiovascular prescription. Resistance exercise is incorporated into this weight loss prescription to minimize the reduction of lean body mass and to increase the RMR, so you will need to consult chapter 7 for the model recommended for the design of resistance training programs.

Table 9.5 outlines a 10-step model for the design of a physiologically sound and client-centered exercise prescription for weight management. Each step involves a sequenced decision that you must make. Many of the choices available for each decision are listed for each step. Following a brief

background on each of the steps, a sample case study is presented, including the choices made for the client and a justification for those choices.

Step 1: Review Client Needs and Confirm Goals

Client needs may be related to medical or high-risk (elevated blood lipids, hypertension), educational (eating habits), or motivational factors. Client needs also can be defined by results of fitness assessments (skinfolds), by lack of self-esteem, or by special designs necessitated by physical limitations owing to weight or orthopedics. Careful screening procedures can identify when medical intervention is warranted. Often the client is unaware of emerging needs such as borderline hypertension or lack of core strength. Recording an activity profile can establish current levels of energy expenditure (see table 9.2).

As discussed in chapter 2, goal setting is the process of specifying what needs to be done, when and how to do it, and what the anticipated outcomes will be. Integrating needs, wants, and lifestyle (chapter 1) will increase the probability of compliance with any prescription. It is often easier to begin with long-term goals that are more

Table 9.5 Exercise Prescription Model for Weight Management

Decisions	Choices
1. Review needs and confirm goals.	• Screening: medical history, intervention needed (e.g., meds) • Limitations (e.g., CV risk, orthopedic, injury, test results) • Activity profile and history (review current energy expenditure) • Design considerations (e.g., time and equipment availability) • Priorities: health, fitness, appearance • Motivational strategy, personality, learning style • Stress management issues • Food management habits and strategies (review current diet) • Weight loss goal (kcal deficit goal)
2. Select aerobic activities and equipment.	• Treadmill, run, walk • Bicycle, ergometer • Elliptical trainer • Rower • Stepper • Swim • In-line skating • ACSM groups 1 and 2—aerobic (less weight bearing)
3. Select aerobic training method.	• Continuous • Interval • Circuit • Cross-training, sports • Active living
4. Set aerobic intensity and workload.	Recommended training zone: • % $\dot{V}O_2$ reserve, % maximum METs, %HRR, perceived exertion (e.g., 50-70% $\dot{V}O_2$ reserve or HRR; moderate-intensity activity of 3.0 to 5.9 METs; sufficient to complete duration and tolerate the exercise without risk) • Calculate corresponding workload (e.g., ACSM metabolic formulas), or client selects a workload that elicits an appropriate HR (e.g., 50-70% HRR); verify selection during demo-client trial • Calculate kcal/min (e.g., chart or L/min × 5 kcal) • Recreational sport and active living (kcal chart) • Manipulate balance with duration (kcal/session) and frequency (kcal/week) to promote high kcal expenditure • Confirm consistency with goals and needs
5. Set aerobic volume (duration and frequency).	• Total work per session (intensity and duration) • 20-30 min, progressing to 45+ min • 250-500 kcal/session • Minimum 3 times/week; work toward 5-7 times/week • Total kcal deficit per week (intensity, duration, and frequency): 1000-2000 kcal/week • Supplement with active living recommendations • Kcal deficit from diet modifications
6. Select resistance training method.	• Standard (simple) sets • Circuit • Supersets • Compound set • Pyramids (ascending, descending) • Split routine • Negatives (forced repetition) • Plyometrics (with caution)

Decisions	Choices
7. Select exercises, equipment, and order.	• Choice suits goals, needs, preferences • Simple, complex, multijoint, single joint • Equipment (and brand) pros and cons • Constant, variable, accommodating resistance • Free weight, machine • Bands, tubes, balls, boards • Equipment features (e.g., ROM limited, pivot locations) • Exercise order
8. Set resistance intensity and volume.	• Based on goal (e.g., strength, hypertrophy) • Established from assessment or during demo (e.g., percent of 1RM [relative intensity] or trial and error [5- to 10RM]) • Interdependent with volume (sets × reps × load) • Match reps to load (based on goals) • Momentary failure for trained clients (greater neural activity) • Large muscle groups may require higher percent 1RM • Sets × reps × load = volume • See table 7.8, "Intensity and Load" • Rest between sets reflects objective, size of muscle group, and reps × load • Time under tension (e.g., slower movements) • Time under tension for workout affected by rest time • Minimum 2-3/week
9. Design progression and monitoring.	Aerobic: • Stage of progression (ACSM: initial, improvement, maintenance) • Methods of progression—FITT (e.g., increase time initially) • Rate of progression (build kcal deficit, e.g., 10%/week) • Monitoring to cue progression timing • Monitoring to suit client's objectives but avoid overtraining • Monitoring to motivate Resistance: • Volume first, intensity second • One volume factor modified at a time (Example 1: Increase reps: 2 × 12-15; then 3 × 10. Example 2 [strength]: 2 × 12 at 100 lb; then 3 × 8 at 110 lb; then 4 × 6 at 120 lb) • 5% increase in load is very tolerable (when upper limit of reps met) • Increase reps when tolerated in second set • Progress (e.g., machines to free weights) when good strength base • Monitoring, follow-up checks should cue progression timing • Related to client's objectives (motivation) • Primary safety precautions listed
10. Design warm-up and cool-down.	• CV warm-up and cool-down transitions (e.g., after aerobic segment) • Specific joint and muscle stretching • Suits nature of the prescription and client specifics (e.g., mode, time, intensity, monitoring)

Note: CV = cardiovascular; MET = metabolic equivalent; HR = heart rate; HRR = heart rate reserve; FITT = frequency, intensity, time, and type; ROM = range of motion.

global and then formulate several shorter-term goals that could be accomplished before there are major changes in assessment measures such as target weight loss, skinfolds, or body mass index. You play a vital role by helping your clients set realistic, measurable goals and recording them in clinical notes for the clients. As mentioned earlier, there should be a two-pronged approach to goal setting: "Eating behavior" goals may include food management habits and strategies for stress management, whereas "activity integration" goals may require flexibility in the program design, purchase of home equipment, or time management. Any test results from body composition or cardiovascular assessments (chapter 4) will be helpful in setting realistic goals and initial prescription levels.

Step 2: Select Aerobic Activities and Equipment

The client's own preferences and availability of equipment will often narrow the choices very quickly. We must be informed about equipment, including specific functions and brand differences, because a client's decision to use or to purchase should be based on comparisons of pros and cons. Even for equipment of the same type (i.e., treadmills, bicycles, or elliptical trainers), there are frequently different features on the information displays or in the braking mechanism that would be better suited to your client.

Aerobic exercise is the best type of program for losing body fat. It also provides significant other health and cardiovascular benefits. Aerobic exercise involves large muscle groups, so you can look beyond walking, jogging, stair climbing, and bicycling to activities that also incorporate shoulder and trunk muscles such as cross-country skiing, swimming, skipping, rowing, elliptical training, and aerobic dance. Weight-supported activities such as swimming and water aerobics are excellent choices, especially for deconditioned or restricted clients; however, complementary weight-bearing activities should be added when tolerated. A circuit involving a number of aerobic modes of exercise can add some variety and cross-training. Other activities such as tennis, squash, basketball, baseball, hockey, and occupational and home maintenance activities have an aerobic component to them, but skill levels and competitiveness can place these activities at excessively high intensity levels. The action should be continuous, maintaining the energy expenditure level. It appears that aerobic exercise modes are equally effective in altering body composition (Heyward 2010).

Even with all these choices, there remains a single mode of exercise that consistently maintains adherence, suits the overweight client, and has a proven track record for weight management. I refer to walking or its progressive extensions, walk–jog–run. Walking with hand weights can increase energy expenditure by 5% to 10%, nearly 1 kcal/min (Williams 1995). For hypertensive clients, carrying weights in the hands tends to increase blood pressure more than weights strapped to the wrist. Walking faster or on an incline may be an alternative.

Flexibility exercises targeted at the muscles used in the aerobic activity may be integrated within the session depending on the design (e.g., interval or circuit). Resistance exercises focused on large muscle groups are often part of a complete weight loss prescription for lower-risk clients.

Step 3: Select Aerobic Training Method

A variety of training methods allow us to match specific benefits to the appropriate client. Continuous training methods are well suited to low to moderate intensities and for clients initiating a weight loss program. Pacing and reduced injuries are advantages over interval training. However, the ACSM (2009) recommended interval training for higher-risk clients who can tolerate only low-intensity exercise for short periods of time (1-2 min). Shorter, more intense intervals with intermittent recoveries may be better suited to the temperaments of your former athletes—just monitor carefully. Peterson and colleagues (2004) demonstrated that caloric expenditure was similar with 30 min of intermittent exercise compared with 30 min of continuous exercise as long as both occur at a moderate intensity level (70% $\dot{V}O_2$max) and the intermittent sessions are at least 10 min in length.

An active lifestyle can effectively complement a more formal exercise prescription and make a significant difference in the speed of weight loss or the ease of weight maintenance. Active living may not produce profound cardiovascular benefits, but for energy expenditure, "every little bit counts." Every time your client is about to relapse from her exercise program, remind her that washing the car, mowing the lawn, vacuuming the carpet, garden-

The Zen of Walking

My 63-year-old neighbor was approaching retirement and knew he wanted to play golf every day. His weight and blood pressure had been creeping up, and he was concerned about his future quality of life. He bought a portable music device and set aside his "walking time" after work each day. Gradually adding loops to his walking route to progressively extend his time, my neighbor had lost almost a pound a week in the first 3 months. The walking time became a cherished time of sanctuary and rejuvenation. It would never replace golf, he told me, but it became more than just a means of losing weight. Surely there is a Zen of walking.

ing, or doing house repairs are bonus calorie burners that are every bit as valid as a trip to the gym.

Step 4: Set Aerobic Intensity and Workload

Every client has an optimal intensity, depending on her condition and the length of the exercise. At very low intensities, our bodies rely predominantly on fat metabolism. At higher intensities, carbohydrates are the predominant energy source. This has led some people to conclude that to lose fat weight, low-intensity exercise is preferable. The fact is that higher-intensity exercise burns more calories per minute. Even though the proportion of fat calories used is smaller during high-intensity exercise, the total number of fat calories used in high-intensity exercise greatly exceeds those used in low-intensity workouts of equal duration.

Other physiological factors also support higher-intensity activity. First, the RMR can stay elevated for hours after a bout of intense exercise. Second, the cardiovascular training effect created by higher-intensity training increases the activity of certain muscle enzymes involved in burning fat. These enzymes favor the burning of fat rather than glycogen (McArdle et al. 2010).

However, for an unfit client, higher intensities cannot be tolerated for a long enough duration to produce significant caloric expenditure. Nonetheless, there are many health benefits to regular lower-intensity exercise that may normalize metabolic disorders common in obese clients. We must always turn back to our clients in making prescriptive decisions—in many cases, lower-intensity (longer duration and frequent) exercise may be most suitable. Showing obese clients how to live more actively on a daily basis may prove more successful than regimented programs (see table 9.4). Many overweight clients have orthopedic limitations, and they will sustain fewer injuries with a lower intensity. If previously inactive clients can get into the habit of exercise, their fitness may gradually improve to the point that we can prescribe higher-intensity levels of activity (e.g., 70-75% HRR) without driving them away. Moderate-intensity activity is defined as 3.0 to 5.9 METs, and vigorous activity is greater than or equal to 6.0 METs (Donnelly et al. 2009). As our clients' cardiovascular fitness improves, so does their anaerobic threshold. This increases their ability to work at higher absolute intensities (e.g., speed on the treadmill) for longer and still burn fat and not just carbohydrate.

Step 5: Set Aerobic Volume

If losing weight is your client's priority, your prescription should stress duration or total energy expenditure (intensity × duration). One of your initial challenges is to bring your clients to a point of sufficient aerobic fitness that they can sustain moderate intensity for enough time to burn a lot of calories. If a client is jogging at an 8 min/mile pace and fatigues after 3 miles (4.8 km), she has burned approximately 336 kcal (24 min × 14 kcal/min). If she reduces her speed to a 9 min/mile pace, she can complete 4 miles (6.4 km) and burn 450 kcal (36 × 12.5 kcal/min). Duration and total distance are more important than speed (intensity) alone. The slower pace also avoids the inhibiting effect of lactic acid on fat mobilization.

Similarly, a jogger, because his activity is continuous, uses considerably more calories in an hour than a hockey player, who may be moving for only 40% of the game. Be aware of this principle if you base your prescription on a chart of caloric expenditures per minute for various activities. Skill levels, such as in racket sports, can significantly change the energy expenditure per hour.

The benefits of avoiding labor-saving devices—taking the stairs, walking to work, and generally living more actively—accumulate during the day and effectively extend the daily energy expenditure. This approach may be well suited to your client's lifestyle and level of commitment and may firmly place him in the action stage of change. It is possible to use frequent short bouts of moderate day-to-day activities to lose the equivalent of 2 lb (0.90 kg) of body fat per month (table 9.6).

It is quite evident that the more a person exercises, the greater his weekly caloric expenditure. Exercise frequency complements duration and intensity, and the combination of these three factors yields the *volume of activity,* often measured in kcal/week. Four sessions per week is satisfactory, provided duration and intensity are adequate. A frequency of three times per week usually requires such high intensities or very long sessions to reach sufficient weekly caloric expenditures that clients often get discouraged or injured. A daily program is most likely to establish a behavioral habit and promote adherence. The ACSM (Donnelly et al. 2009) recommends that adults participate in at least 150 min of moderate-intensity PA to prevent weight gain and reduce associated chronic disease risk factors. Weight loss and prevention of weight regain are likely with doses of PA that approximate 250 to 300 min per week of moderate-intensity PA.

Table 9.6 **Health-Related Fitness Prescription**

Day	Activity (150 lb [68 kg] person)	Kcal
Monday	30 min at fitness club—aerobic	250-300
Tuesday	Brisk walk to work—30 min Stairs—5 min	200-250
Wednesday	30 min at fitness club—aerobic	250-300
Thursday	Brisk walk to work—30 min Stairs—5 min	200-250
Friday	Brisk walk to work—30 min Stairs—5 min Wash and wax car—30 min	300-350
Saturday	Gardening—30 min House cleaning—30 min	300
Sunday	Mowing lawn—30 min Raking and yard work—30 min	400-450
	Total	**1900-2200**

Step 6: Select Resistance Training Method

Resistance training methods combine the selection of load, reps, sets, and rest (see chapter 7) with the sequence of exercises to produce specific muscular fitness outcomes. Depending on the type and availability of equipment, the time devoted to resistance training will limit the number of reps and sets and the number of exercises selected. For example, in a 50 min lunchtime workout, your client may only have 20 min for resistance work. Cullinen and Caldwell (1998) reported that moderate to intense resistance training 2 days a week for 12 weeks significantly increased fat-free mass and decreased percent body fat.

For the purposes of weight management and body composition, exercises are usually arranged to provide maximum work with sufficient recovery. Alternating push–pull exercises in a circuit or in standard sets allows good balance (agonist–antagonist) and recovery.

Step 7: Select Exercises, Equipment, and Order

The choice of resistance equipment or the type of exercise must suit the clients' goals, needs, preferences, and availability. Complex, multijoint exercises with large muscle groups allow a client to get a full-body workout with maximum caloric expenditure. Look also to maintain balance in your exercise selection: agonist–antagonist and bilateral symmetry. The order of the exercises may be somewhat predetermined by the training method.

In selecting equipment, consider the best method of resistance, the type of equipment, and the interface of that equipment with your client (ergonomics). Machines offer various types of resistance (e.g., gravity, variable resistance, hydraulics, pneumatics, isokinetics) that may or may not suit your client. Equipment features such as range of motion limits and adjustable seating are particularly important for large- and small-sized clients. When equipment is limited, a lot can be accomplished at home with bands, tubes, balls, boards, and gravity. For more detail see chapter 7.

Step 8: Set Resistance Intensity and Volume

Resistance can be expressed as either RMs (repetitions maximum: the maximum load that can be lifted the specified number of repetitions) or the absolute resistance (actual poundage). Throughout the training program, the absolute resistance is adjusted to match the changes in strength so a true RM target (e.g., 15RM) continues to be used. Training intensity is a critical prescription factor, providing the stimulus needed for improvement in specific muscular components. Low to moderate loads (60-70% 1RM) are a good preparation, emphasizing muscular endurance (10-20 repetitions). If your client is a beginner, 1 or 2 sets are sufficient to produce excellent benefits. Exercises with a larger muscle mass (to increase energy expenditure) and longer between-set rest intervals (to avoid early fatigue) allow greater training volume (Farinatti and Neto 2011). In a weight management workout, time is needed for a warm-up, aerobic activity, resistance work, and a cool-down. Depending on the type and availability of equipment, the time devoted to resistance training will limit the number of reps and sets and the number of exercises selected.

Step 9: Design Progression and Monitoring

For aerobic training, the perpetual challenge is to find a rate of progression that builds the caloric deficit without overtraining or reducing compliance. Duration is usually the first factor to increase. Volume is the goal, but often frequency is limited by other commitments and intensity should increase only when the cardiovascular or orthopedic condition permits. An increase of 10% in the weekly caloric expenditure (e.g., duration increased from 40 min to 44 min) is usually well tolerated. Peak exercise heart rates or perceived exertion scores that begin to decrease in successive workouts should signal a time to progress. Slower recoveries and increased signs of fatigue may indicate that the current level should be reduced or the progression was too rapid. Monitoring progress at follow-up sessions should begin by reviewing the steps taken toward goals. "You were going to try to get out for a walk on your lunchtime last week. Were you able to get away?" If the goals were specific and measurable, it is easy to focus on the projected outcomes, being careful to create a natural link between the client's behavior and his body composition and health goals.

For resistance training, it is advisable to increase volume first and then intensity. Modify only one volume factor at a time. For example: increase reps from 12 to 15 (2 × 12-15) and then increase sets to 3 but drop reps to 10 (3 × 10). Begin to increase the reps when they are tolerated in the second set. A 5% to 10% increase in load is very tolerable when the upper limit of reps has been met. Progressions with training methods or equipment (e.g., machines to free weights) should occur only when there is a good strength base. Regular monitoring or follow-up checks should cue the best time for progression. The rate and method of progression are related to the client's objectives and level of motivation. Techniques such as periodization are discussed in chapter 7.

Feedback should go beyond recognition and encouragement. Clients need to take ownership of their program by anticipating and strategizing for difficult situations, such as holidays, stressful work periods, or missed appointments. When clients feel discouraged, they need to focus on daily behaviors and short-term successes.

Step 10: Design Warm-Up and Cool-Down

The warm-up should include a gradual increase in the aerobic activity sufficient to raise the body temperature and approach the low end of the target heart rate. Selected stretching of active muscle groups is facilitated by the warmth and elasticity of the muscle and connective tissue. The length of the warm-up should be greater if the fitness level of the client is low, cardiovascular risk level is high, or there is a possibility of sporadic higher exertion (e.g., competitive sports).

The cool-down is important for overweight clients to avoid blood pooling, rapid changes in blood pressure, and postexercise muscle stiffness. If 10 min are devoted to the cool-down within a 45 to 50 min exercise session, this can include a 3 to 5 min gradual tapering after the aerobic portion of the workout with 5 to 7 min of specific muscle stretching afterward. Ensure that your client's heart rate is below 100 beats/min or within 20 beats/min of the original heart rate and that your client looks and feels recovered.

Case Study

A 42-year-old insurance broker, Fred, was a prime example of creeping obesity. He had coached basketball for 17 years but had done nothing for the last 5 years. He claimed that a busy insurance practice and a new cottage had left him little time for regular exercise. He had noticed the weight problem, but it was his last medical checkup (elevated cholesterol and borderline hypertension) that motivated him to seek help with an exercise program.

Case Study: Creeping Obesity

Our first task was to focus on his priorities—to determine what he wanted to achieve, not just what his doctor wanted. His objectives were to

- lose 12 lb (5.4 kg) in the first 6 months and a total of 24 lb (10.8 kg) in the first year, primarily through exercise;
- reduce his elevated cholesterol level to a normal range; and
- reduce the fat around his waist (if possible) and strengthen that area.

Assessment, Discussion, and Action

The assessment provided me with the data in table 9.7. After I explained the assessment results and the implications of his doctors' findings, Fred was committed to making some immediate changes. He decided to walk the 20 min to work each day and to set aside three 10 min sessions in his office each week to do muscle strengthening exercises. He planned to coach a basketball team and to be physically active in their 1 1/2 h practice once a week. We discussed the possibilities for cross-country skiing at his cottage during the winter. After Fred's wife attended the follow-up session, she agreed to eliminate her own high-cholesterol, high-fat snacks at night and reduce between-meal "junk" eating. This was important for Fred, because he feared that if these foods were available in the house, he wouldn't be able to resist them. The rest of their menu appeared reasonable except for the number of times they ate at fast food outlets.

Prescription

To see how I filled out Fred's prescription card, see figure 9.5. The prescription card will guide Fred or another personal trainer when I am not there. Specific workloads, times, and monitoring levels are listed for the warm-up and again for the aerobic workout. Upper and lower limits that include perceived exertions are useful with intermittent training methods such as basketball or the uneven terrain of cross-country skiing. After a brief aerobic cool-down, on the days that he has time, Fred can add his resistance exercises, checking his card periodically for descriptions, weight, reps, sets, and precautions. I would prefer to be there for decisions about progression.

Results

For the first month of the program, Fred followed the program and eating habits very closely and lost 4 lb (1.8 kg) (3500 kcal/week). He set up a corner of his office with a mat, tubing, some music, and a monitoring chart. His wife continued to be a good support, and besides a few meal celebrations, by the sixth month both had significantly modified their eating habits. Weather and work pressures permitted Fred to walk to work an average of 3 days per week for the remainder of the 6 months. By this time the weight loss was almost 15 lb (6.8 kg), his waist girth was down 2 in. (5 cm), his blood pressure was consistently 130/84, and the basketball was a lot of fun! Although the cardiovascular results showed no significant improvement (perhaps the intensity was too low), he felt less fatigued and generally more energized. Even if Fred's absolute aerobic capacity remained the same, his relative capacity improved with his loss of weight. He certainly "carried" himself better and avoided any injuries in the 6 months. His physician was pleased with the lowered weight and blood pressure and was confident that his blood cholesterol would soon follow. Fred's wife was the gatekeeper in the kitchen and she would often join Fred on a walk or ski. Not only was she instrumental in motivating Fred, she too lost about half the weight that Fred shed!

Table 9.7   Fred's Assessment Data

Risk factors	
Weight, cholesterol, borderline hypertension, and lifestyle (physician approval to continue was obtained—PARmed-X+)	
Body composition	
Weight	84.1 kg (185 lb)
Height	172.5 cm (5 ft 8 in.)
Body mass index	28 (overweight)
Body fat	24.5%
Abdominal girth	96.5 cm (38 in.)
Cardiovascular	
Resting heart rate	80 beats/min
Blood pressure	Resting, 135/88 (high normal); recovery, 135/84
Oxygen uptake	33 ml · kg^{-1} · min^{-1} = fair, with early leg fatigue and slow recovery
Musculoskeletal	
Strength	Weak abdominal muscles but average upper body strength on push-ups and grip strength
Posture	Lumbar lordosis and rounded shoulders

Client name: Fred		Trainer name: John	
Client goals		**Special considerations**	
• Lose 12 lb in the first 6 months and a total of 24 lb in the first year • Reduce elevated cholesterol level and BP to a normal range • Reduce fat around waist and strengthen that area		Basketball and cottage motivators Spouse support with meals	

Circulatory Warm-Up			
Equipment and mode	**Workload**	**Time**	**HR/PE objective**
Good walking and basket-ball shoes	Light to moderate	First 2-3 min of walk or ski	HR: 120-130 RPE: 11-12

Stretching Warm-Up	
Name and brief description	**Guidelines**
• Walking: stretch lower body (including hip flexors) • Skiing: chest stretches plus walking stretches or 15 easy lunges with arm action • Basketball: do along with team	• Walking: WU, gradually • Increase speed • Skiing: WU, start skiing slowly • Basketball: WU, ease into drills

Aerobic Workout
Intensity/training range

Lower limit: *50*% HRR *129* beats/min *12* RPE Upper limit: *65*% HRR *144* beats/min *14* RPE

	Equipment	Training methods	Frequency	Kcal/session
1	Walking shoes	• Continuous for walk-ing	10 trips/week	10 3 20 min 3 7 kcal/min = 1,400 kcal/week
2	Cross-country ski equip-ment Basketball shoes	• Continuous for cross-country • Intermittent for bas-ketball practices	1x/week	40 min 3 10 kcal/min = 400 kcal/week

Phase	Workload	Time	Phase	Workload	Time
Warm-up	See above		Warm-up	See above	
Peak	Walking: 7 kcal/min (7 energy points); 50-55% HRR (129-134 beats/min); RPE: 12-13	20 min each	Peak	skiing and bas-ketball: 10 kcal/min (10 energy points); 55-65% HRR (134-144 beats/min); RPE: 13-14	50 min
Cool-down	Keep moving at work		Cool-down	Gradually decrease inten-sity Allow HR recov-ery before resis-tance work	

Figure 9.5 Fred's prescription card. *(continued)*

- *Walking: increase the route length or vigor of the arm action (power walk) or speed*
- *Skiing and basketball: increase duration of active time*
- *Skiing and basketball: check heart rate (or RPE) at peak times and modify or active recovery*
- *Monitoring chart (modified calendar) recorded completed activities, weight, blood pressure, and waist girth on a weekly basis*

Resistance Workout	
Equipment type (e.g., free weights)	**Training method**
Tubing, mat, music, monitoring chart	*Standard sets for resistance work: three specific shoulder strengthening exercises and three core exercises*

Goals

- *Reduce fat around waist (if possible) and strengthen that area*
- *Work shoulders for skiing*

Guidelines

- *WU: do an easy set of 5-10 (50% 1RM)*
- *Two sets of 10-15 reps*

Exercise (brief description)	Muscles	Weight	Reps	Sets	Precautions
Shoulder strengthening 1 Lat pull-down (machine)	*Latissimus dorsi*	*65-75% 1RM*	*10-15*	*2*	
Shoulder strengthening 2 Bench press (machine)	*Pectoralis major*	*65-75% 1RM*	*10-15*	*2*	
Shoulder strengthening 3 Triceps pull-down (Theraband)	*Triceps brachii*	*65-75% 1RM*	*10-15*	*2*	
Specific core exercise 1 Twisting curl-up, knees bent	*Abdominal obliques*		*10-15*	*2*	*Stop if loss of form Maintain neutral spine*
Specific core exercise 2 Four-point alternate arm–leg extensions	*Erector spinae*		*10-15*	*2*	*Stop if loss of form Maintain neutral spine*
Specific core exercise 3 Reverse curl-up	*Rectus abdominis*		*10-15*	*2*	*Stop if loss of form Maintain neutral spine*

Progression and monitoring

Increase to 3 sets once 15 reps are reached consistently.
Use monitoring chart (modified calendar) to record completed activities, weights, reps, and sets weekly.

Cool-Down	
Name and brief description	**Guidelines**
Walking: stretch lower body (including hip flexors) Basketball: do along with team Skiing: do chest stretches plus walking stretches All exercises: gradually decrease speed Resistance: stretch back, chest, and hip flexors	*Feel recovered before ending cool-down Monitor BP periodically*

Note. BP = blood pressure; HR = heart rate; PE = perceived exertion; RPE = rating of perceived exertion; WU = warm-up; HRR = heart rate reserve.

Figure 9.5   *(continued)*

Justification of Weight Management Prescription

Each personal fitness trainer will have a slightly different approach to the case study prescription. However, as you make choices, be sure you have a strong rationale for each one.

1. **Review Client Needs and Confirm Goals**
   - Two pounds per month is safe and was projected from energy deficit.
   - Physician reported elevated cholesterol and borderline hypertension.
   - Waist girth and abdominal visceral fat are high risk and affecting posture.
   - Client's highest priority was creeping obesity.
   - Change was motivated by doctor and checkup results.
   - Client was concerned about appearance.

2. **Select Aerobic Activities and Equipment**
   - Walking is safe, well tolerated, and convenient.
   - Client can walk long enough to burn calories.
   - Walking is transportation and time efficient.
   - Skiing and basketball are enjoyable, so the client is motivated.

3. **Select Aerobic Training Method**
   - Continuous exercise provides for sufficient fitness and exercise tolerance.
   - Interval exercise includes active recoveries that are self-selected, allowing higher intensity.
   - Exercises provide high energy expenditure.
   - Client finds the exercises fun.

4. **Set Aerobic Intensity and Workload**
   - In walking, intensity and workload match, and monitoring is easy.
   - HR is easily maintained in appropriate range for objectives.
   - Skiing is self-regulated; rating of perceived exertion (RPE) is helpful.
   - Intensity and workload suit lifestyle.

5. **Set Aerobic Volume (Duration and Frequency)**
   - Total weekly caloric expenditure is good.
   - Recreation is a bonus and in time can be expanded.
   - Walking is an active lifestyle integration.

6. **Select Resistance Training Method**
   - Standard sets allow recovery of muscle groups.
   - Method is suited to recreational activities of interest.

7. **Select Exercises, Equipment, and Order**
   - Equipment works multijoint large muscles of chest, back, and trunk.
   - There is a minimum of equipment, which is easily substituted if no equipment.
   - Program is simple and short, which provides motivation.
   - Exercise 1: Monitoring chart (calendar) is motivational.
   - Exercise 2: Program is simple and short, which provides motivation.
   - Exercise 3: Provides third exercise isolation and assists basketball shooting and passing and ski poling.
   - Exercise 4: Provides core stability, back support, and strong flexion + rotation; improves lumbar lordosis.
   - Exercise 5: Balances abdominal muscles, stabilizes back, and assists lifting activities.
   - Exercise 6: Strengthens flexion and improves appearance; stabilizers fatigued last; improves lumbar lordosis.
   - Exercise 7: Balances abdominal muscles, stabilizes back, and assists lifting activities.
   - Exercise 8: Strengthens flexion and improves appearance; stabilizers fatigued last.
   - Two sets of 10 to 15 reps are sufficient for strength and body composition changes.

8. **Set Resistance Intensity and Volume**
   - 65% to 75% 1RM is a good preparation intensity emphasizing muscular endurance.
   - Two sets of 10 to 15 reps are sufficient for strength and body composition changes.
   - Time available for resistance training limits the volume.

9. **Design Progression and Monitoring**

   Aerobic: Progressive overload will improve CV system and ability to increase kcal/min at same RPE.
   - Exercise provides preparation for jogging (i.e., walk volume and basketball).
   - Power walking increases energy expenditure.
   - Increasing time and pace will increase weight loss and decrease CV risk factors.
   - Monitoring will guide time and extent of CV overload.
   - Monitoring chart (calendar) is motivational.

Resistance:

- Three sets are well tolerated and build volume.
- Monitoring will guide time and extent of resistance overload.
- Monitoring chart (calendar) is motivational.

10. **Design Warm-Up and Cool-Down**
    - Increases venous return
    - Provides gradual return to preexercise state
    - Carries less chance of dizziness, light-headedness
    - Increases myocardial perfusion
    - Clears metabolic wastes and lactic acid
    - Stretches target previously active muscles

Note: HR = heart rate; RPE = rating of perceived exertion; CV = cardiovascular.

Summary

We must help our clients accept a large range of healthy weights and variations in body size by taking a two-pronged approach to helping them lose weight: (a) modify eating behaviors and (b) integrate activity (not merely fitness prescription). This involves identifying the reasons for a client's weight problem, that is, what is eaten (e.g., overeating or eating the wrong foods) and why it is eaten (e.g., emotional eating). Some of the common issues or areas of confusion for clients are (1) counting calories, (2) the relationship of diet and exercise, (3) special nutritional concerns for active clients, and (4) the role of resistance training in weight management. Practical suggestions are integrated with the updated Dietary Guidelines and the position stand "Appropriate Physical Activity Intervention Strategies for Weight Loss and Prevention of Weight Regain for Adults."

Fat metabolism and energy expenditure are a combination of resting metabolism, metabolizing food (thermic effect of food), and physical activity (thermic effect of exercise). Trainers can encourage clients to become more active and to estimate the weight loss value of lifestyle changes by using the Energy Deficit Point System.

Whether your client's needs are weight loss, maintenance, health, or appearance, the 10-step model for weight management will guide your design decisions for a tailored program. The model is similar to that used in chapter 6 for cardiovascular prescription. Resistance exercise is incorporated into this weight loss prescription to minimize the reduction of lean body mass and to increase the RMR. The case study shows how the model for weight management guides the prescription with physiological justifications and client-centered (behavioral) justifications for each choice made.

FORM 9.1   Assess Your Energy Profile

Instructions: Make rough estimates, or measure, your food and beverage servings. It is a good idea to review what constitutes a serving size using the guidelines provided by your national health authority, such as the USDA Center for Nutrition Policy and Promotion (www.choosemyplate.gov) or Health Canada (www.hc-sc.gc.ca). The Health Canada guidelines here are given by age ranges and sex; the USDA guidelines listed are a general recommendation for a healthy adult with a 2000-calorie daily intake. For mixed foods, identify the key food ingredients, estimate the amount of each, and check the corresponding number of boxes. Make notes as to how you've tracked servings, and review your intake after three days. Are you eating enough to meet the recommendations? Did you choose nutrient-rich and healthy foods?

Recommended servings	Day 1	Day 2	Day 3

Fruits and vegetables
 Age 19-50   Women: 7-8
                    Men: 8-10
 Age 51+   Women: 7
                    Men: 7
 4 1/2 cups per day			

	Notes:		

Grains
 Age 19-50   Women: 6-7
                    Men: 8
 Age 51+   Women: 6
                    Men: 7
 6 oz. per day			

	Notes:		

Milk and alternatives
 Age 19-50   Women: 2
                    Men: 3
 Age 51+   Women: 3
                    Men: 3
 3 cups per day			

	Notes:		
Meat and alternatives Age 19+ Women: 2 Men: 3 5 1/2 oz. per day			
	Notes:		

From J.C. Griffin, 2015, *Client-centered exercise prescription,* 3rd ed. (Champaign, IL: Human Kinetics). Adapted from Dairy Farmers of Canada.

FORM 9.2 Weight Management Prescription Worksheet

Aerobic Segment

Component objective: _____

Decisions	Key points
1. Needs and goals	
2. Activities and equipment	
3. Training method	
4. Intensity and workload	
5. Volume (duration and frequency)	
6. Progression and monitoring	
7. Warm-up and cool-down	

Resistance Segment

Component objective: _____

Exercise (brief description)	Body area, muscles	Intensity and weight	Reps	Sets	Rest between sets	Precautions

Method of progression:

_____

From J.C. Griffin, 2015, *Client-centered exercise prescription*, 3rd ed. (Champaign, IL: Human Kinetics).

FORM 9.3 Weight Management Prescription Card

Client name   Trainer name

Client goal	Special considerations

Circulatory Warm-Up

Equipment and mode	Workload	Time	Objective

Stretching Warm-Up (Name and Brief Description)

Name and brief description	Guidelines

Aerobic Workout

Intensity and training range

Lower limit: _____%HRR _____beats/min _____RPE Upper limit: _____%HRR _____beats/min _____RPE

Equipment	Training method	Frequency	Kcal/session
1			
2			

Phase	Workload	Time	Phase	Workload	Time
Warm-up			Warm-up		
Peak			Peak		
Cool-down			Cool-down		

(continued)

(continued)

Progression and monitoring

_____

_____

_____

Resistance Workout

Equipment type (e.g., free weights)	Training method

Goals	Guidelines

Exercise (brief description)	Muscles	Weight	Reps	Sets	Precautions

Progression

_____

Cool-Down

Name and brief description	Guidelines

Note: HR = heart rate; RPE = rating of perceived exertion.

PART III

Exercise Prescription for Injuries and Older Adults

Our understanding of the effects of physical activity on human health has advanced in recent years, not only among fitness professionals but also in the general population. Consequently, fitness consumers increasingly want specific results, more choices, and more guidance about how to exercise, particularly when recovering from injury. Many of us—whether clinical kinesiologists, personal trainers, physical therapists, athletic trainers, chiropractors, physical educators, or fitness specialists in private or community settings—have noted the lack of resources for guiding these informed consumers. This section recognizes the expertise of individual professionals from different disciplines to deal with injury management, allowing for a comprehensive approach to prevention, assessment, and management of an injury. Defining the boundaries helps to identify the areas of expertise of personal fitness trainers and to ensure that overstepping these areas is avoided.

Part III examines the intrinsic and extrinsic biomechanical causes of soft tissue injuries. Each type of tissue has different biological properties that influence its mechanism of injury and adaptation to training. The most common types of fitness injuries are caused by repetitive microtrauma in which soft tissue becomes inflamed or degenerates with damage that can be cumulative, resulting in ligament strains, joint synovitis, muscle myositis, or tendinitis. All inflamed tissues follow the same basic pattern of healing involving inflammation, proliferation or repair, and remodeling. Specific objectives for range of motion, strength, and activity demands must be set to progress from one phase of healing to the next. To avoid new injuries, there is new evidence on the merits of reestablishing neuromuscular control, training that includes proprioceptive challenges, coordination, balance, and agility.

Part III also focuses on exercise prescription for clients recovering from or having a history of orthopedic injury. You will find a brief description and background information on functional anatomy for plantar fasciitis, Achilles tendinitis, shin splints (medial tibial stress syndrome), patellofemoral syndrome, hamstring strain, low back pain, rotator cuff tendinitis (impingement syndrome), and lateral epicondylitis (tennis elbow). You will also find probable causes and strategies for prevention as well as specific exercise designs for stretching and strengthening damaged tissues for each of these injuries. This section presents new approaches to injuries such as spinal stability and presents new preventive and rehabilitation merits of eccentric training.

Part III continues with the special needs of the older adult. Chapter 12 examines sarcopenia, osteoporosis, and osteoarthritis and then focuses on the role of specific exercise and activity, including precautions. Then it describes common soft tissue changes with aging and injury prevention. A new paradigm is required in training older clients that includes well-designed soft tissue strengthening, stretching, and mobilization exercises. The most effective client-centered approach is through gradual progression of volume and intensity, adequate recovery time, and the use of cross-training or interval training with functional progressions.

Chapter 13 is a comprehensive discussion of successful aging, physiological changes, and the effects of specific exercise or activity prescriptions for the wide range of clients in this demographic. The final chapter focuses on functional mobility and aging, identifying causes, providing screening tools, and applying functional exercise design principles.

Causes and Prevention of Overuse Injuries

Chapter Competencies

After completing this chapter, you will be able to demonstrate the following competencies:

1. Describe the causes of soft tissue injury to ligaments, tendons, cartilage, and muscles.
2. Describe the biomechanical characteristics of each kind of soft tissue that determine its vulnerabilities to injury.
3. Describe the phases of injury healing.
4. Prescribe exercise appropriately for each healing stage.
5. Describe how to minimize risk of injury or reinjury.

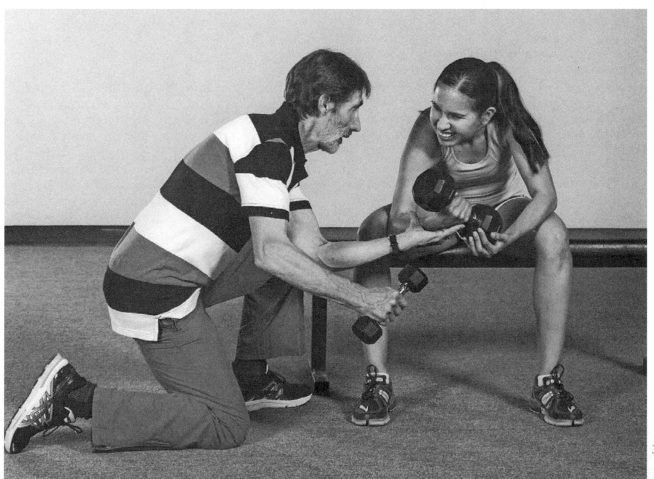

Injuries to ligaments, tendons, cartilage, and muscles are called soft tissue injuries. To help your clients deal with such injuries, you must be familiar with the causes of soft tissue injury, the biomechanical characteristics of each kind of soft tissue that determine its vulnerabilities to injury, the phases of injury healing, how to prescribe exercise appropriately for each healing stage, and how to minimize risk of injury or reinjury.

Team Approach to Injury Management

While participation in sport and physical activities is an important component of a healthy lifestyle, clients can expect to sustain an injury at some point in time. The team approach to injury management allows for comprehensive prevention, assessment, and management of an injury as it integrates the expertise of individual professionals from different disciplines and from different perspectives. Unfortunately, personnel and provisions are not always readily available to many participants in physical activity, exercise, recreation, and sport. Within the fitness industry, the areas of injury prevention and immediate management are often overlooked or relegated to personal trainers regardless of their background. Establishing the responsibilities of various members of the health care team and recognizing when to refer are essential to ensuring appropriate care. Responsibilities that generally fall outside the domain of the personal trainer may include clinical counseling and evaluation, diagnosis, immediate care or treatment of injury or disease, documentation and maintenance of health care records, prescription of diets or specific supplements, and the development of a comprehensive plan for treatment and rehabilitation.

The personal trainer or fitness specialist is responsible for teaching techniques and strategies related to goal-oriented exercise. These individuals are also responsible for administering and supervising activities or activity areas within a health club facility or personal training venue. They are responsible for injury prevention, on-site assessment, and management of injuries, including reducing the potential for further injury or harm. Although the role of the fitness specialist as a member of the injury management team varies depending on the setting and expertise of other staff, her responsibilities may include the following:

- Evaluation of the status of participants before activity (identification of risk factors)
- Supervision during activities
- Instruction in proper technique, skill development, and monitoring (document progress)
- Development and implementation of conditioning programs that are physiologically appropriate and suited to the individual client
- Provision of general information on healthy eating
- Coaching, providing behavior change information, and implementing motivational strategies
- Inspection of equipment, facilities, and activity areas to ensure safety

In the absence of an athletic trainer, physician, or physiotherapist, a personal trainer may

- determine the appropriate course of action in managing an injury,
- assess the nature and severity of the injury, or
- implement an appropriate course of action (e.g., administering basic first aid, initiating an emergency care plan, referring to another member of the injury management team) (Anderson and Parr 2011).

Once a personal fitness trainer recognizes risks related to injury history, the client should be referred to the appropriate medical or allied health practitioner. In addition, the personal trainer receives and follows exercise or health guidelines from a physician, physical therapist, registered dietician, and so on. IDEA (2001) has identified general conditions that may require a referral (table 10.1).

Causes of Soft Tissue Injury

The biomechanical causes of soft tissue injuries can be classified as intrinsic risk factors, extrinsic risk factors, or some combination of the two. The biological causes of overuse soft tissue injuries

Table 10.1 Fitness Referrals to Physician or Therapist

Condition or situation	Refer for preexercise screening	Obtain medical–therapy guidelines before exercise	Stop exercise and refer to physician
Past injuries, such as low back disorder or whiplash	x	x	
Recent injury or rehabilitation under medical care	x	x	
Taking prescribed medications	x	x	
Severe or chronic pain during exercise			x
Pain lasting more than a few hours postexercise			x
Difficulty maintaining coordination; dizziness			x
Chronic disease, such as arthritis, cerebral palsy, clinical depression, eating disorder		x	

can be explained as repeated microinsult to the tissues.

The following list of intrinsic and extrinsic risk factors identifies issues that can contribute to overuse injuries either alone or in combination. The cycle of overuse injury, healing, and reinjury is not broken until the contributing intrinsic or extrinsic factors have been addressed.

Intrinsic Risk Factors

- Malalignment
- Muscle imbalance
- Inflexibility
- Hypermobility
- Muscle weakness
- Instability
- Excess weight

Extrinsic Risk Factors

- Training errors (excessive or repeated forces)
- Equipment
- Environment
- Technique
- Sport-imposed deficiencies

Often but not always with overuse injuries, there is a final event in which the loading pattern exceeds the tissue strength and injury becomes apparent, but the circumstances leading up to

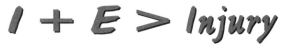

| Intrinsic risk (Predispose the client) | Extrinsic risk (Expose the client) | (Combination and interaction of I and E leave client vulnerable) |

Figure 10.1 Risk and cause of injury.

Reprinted by permission from Jozsa and Kannus 1997.

the injury may be just as important as the final mechanism (figure 10.1).

Intrinsic Factors

Intrinsic risk factors are biomechanical characteristics unique to an individual. Each client has a specific structure, alignment, movement mechanics, and injury history that constitute an "intrinsic" risk. Poor muscle strength or muscle imbalance, hypo- or hypermobility, excess weight, and malalignment all prevent the optimal distribution of loading. Subsequent exposure to extrinsic risk factors, such as type of training, equipment, or the environment, more readily affects those with a higher intrinsic risk.

For example, overpronation of the ankle produces a whipping action on the Achilles attributable to the excessive range of motion.

These torsion forces may be related to degenerative changes to the tendon (Achilles tendinitis). Saidoff and Apfel (2005) reported that almost 60% of injured runners overpronated. Excessive pronation has also been linked to higher incidence of shin splints attributable to the increased stretch of the tibialis anterior. In fact, torsion of the tibia that comes with pronation makes it difficult for the patella to track evenly during gait. Patellofemoral syndrome can result (see chapter 11). Careful observation of the Achilles and the subtalar joint while your client is standing and walking should reveal a pronation problem. A medial wearing pattern on the heel of your client's shoe is additional evidence.

Always screen clients as discussed in chapter 4, and carefully follow up after your prescription to monitor any potential risk. It also can be useful to do some sleuthing on your client's history of injuries—you may uncover an intrinsic predisposing factor that has not been corrected. Careful supervision and appropriate intervention can minimize the effects of a client's intrinsic risk factors.

Extrinsic Factors

Training errors are the primary extrinsic factor associated with overuse injuries. Saidoff and Apfel (2005) identified training errors in 75% of tendon injuries and overuse syndromes. Changes in duration, intensity, or frequency of activity are common mechanisms of extrinsic overload: too soon, too much, too often, or with too little rest. But risk increases with any kind of change in the loading pattern, for example, during transitions from preseason to competition, with a change of technique, or with something as simple as a new pair of shoes.

The risk factors most commonly introduced by these training errors are

- excessive force in the development of momentum,
- eccentric overload, and
- work volume overload.

Depending on the extent and frequency of the overload or excessive force, any of these three biomechanical risk factors can cause either

- repetitive submaximal tissue overload that leads to microtrauma with incomplete cellular repair and subsequent deterioration of connective tissue, or
- abusive tissue overload that causes acute injury attributable to macrotrauma and may initiate tendinitis or other injury that is resistant to healing and continues as an overuse injury.

Fitness activities often follow patterns of repetitive submaximal tissue overload. Initial studies of high-impact aerobic dance revealed a high incidence of lower extremity injuries (Griffin

Table 10.2 Common Sites of Overuse Tendon Injuries

Tendon	Common name
Adductor brevis, gracilis, pectineus, iliopsoas	Groin pull
Achilles	Achilles tendinitis
Patellar	Jumper's knee
Common wrist extensor tendon	Tennis elbow (lateral epicondylitis)
Common wrist flexor	Golfer's elbow (medial epicondylitis)
Supraspinatus	Swimmer's shoulder (impingement)
Other rotator cuff tendons (infraspinatus, teres minor, subscapularis)	Rotator cuff tendinitis
Tibialis posterior	Shin splints

1987): The inherent repetitive overload causes fatigue, loss of strength, and microtrauma to the tibialis posterior, soleus, and gastrocnemius. Without continuing rest and ice treatment, tissue repair is inadequate and subsequent performance is painful, weak, and restrictive. People in this situation suffer from shin splints or Achilles tendinitis. Overuse injuries to the muscle-tendon are so common in the fitness activities used for conditioning in specific sports that some of the injuries have taken on common names, such as tennis elbow, swimmer's shoulder, and jumper's knee. Table 10.2 lists the common sites of overuse tendon injuries (Hess et al. 1989).

Figure 10.2 shows how repetitive submaximal tissue overload injuries can percolate before any symptoms emerge. If training loads exceed the tissue's ability to repair itself between activity sessions, injuries will eventually result. Common situations in which this occurs are at the beginning of a program; at a point of progression; or at training camp when the duration, intensity, and frequency of training increase at the same time. Generally there are two kinds of fitness and sport activities that lead to repetitive submaximal tissue overload damage: endurance activities and those associated with repetitive actions.

Momentum

Excessive or uncontrolled momentum is a common technique error in sport, recreational activities, and occupational tasks. You should develop the ability to spot high-momentum movements that place clients at risk. Because momentum is the product of velocity × mass, momentum is high when a large part of the body moves rapidly. A joint experiences even greater forces as

- the mass of the moving part is farther away from the joint (longer lever) or
- the movement goes to the end of the range of motion.

At risk during actions such as these are the joint capsule, musculotendinous unit, and other soft tissue structures. The triceps kickback exercise design presented here illustrates progressive increases in exercise momentum.

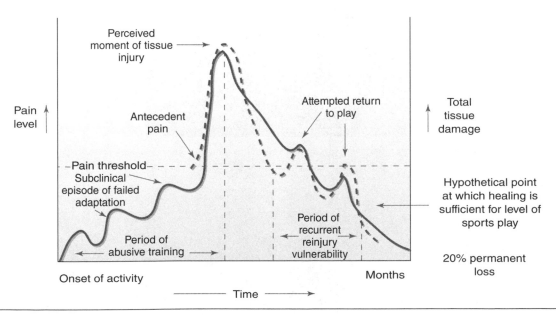

Figure 10.2 Chronic microtrauma.

Reprinted by permission from Leadbetter 1992.

Triceps Kickbacks

This example uses a kettlebell and shows three levels of progressive increases in momentum (figure 10.3).

Level A

This exercise uses a small body part and short lever. The momentum is low but depends on weight used.

- Upper arm stays by side of body.
- Elbow extends and returns.

Level B

This exercise uses additional arm weight and a longer lever. The momentum is greater and provides a greater range of motion.

- At the end of elbow extension, the entire arm extends at the shoulder; return.

Level C

This exercise is the same as level B with a rotation of the spine as the weight is lifted higher. Level C takes the range of motion of the shoulder and elbow beyond a safe point. The high-momentum actions described introduce a repeated tensile stretch to the muscle–tendon unit, including the low back.

- As the shoulder reaches end of its range of motion, momentum forces the trunk to rotate.
- The addition of any speed to force a heavy weight up would create dangerous torque strain on the back.

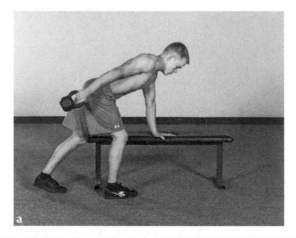

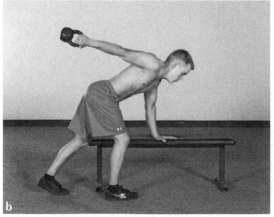
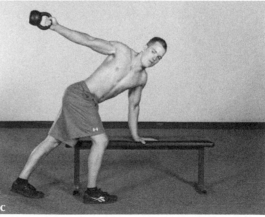

Figure 10.3   Triceps kickbacks: *(a)* level A, *(b)* level B, *(c)* level C.

Always stress quality of motion. Every individual has a unique **stop point** for each joint, linked to muscle tightness and muscle strength. This is the point in a joint's range of motion (ROM) that, for motion to continue, would require involvement of another joint. Identifying the stop point requires a learned "intuitive inhibition"; you can help your clients discover these stop points by carefully observing excessive movement as they exercise. Use form 10.1, Momentum Quiz, to practice recognizing the levels of momentum such as those found in the triceps kickbacks example and the risks that those increases may present.

Eccentric Contraction Patterns

You should also evaluate your clients' **eccentric contraction patterns**. Eccentric contractions generate the greatest muscular forces. Extreme strain is placed on connective tissue when it is elongated under tension, creating considerable potential for microtearing. Eccentric contractions can induce injury particularly in fast-glycolytic muscle fibers, and especially when the contractions are performed by muscles not previously conditioned with eccentric contractions. Furthermore, eccentric overload seems to be particularly associated with delayed-onset muscle soreness.

Eccentric contractions occur when

- muscles attempt to counter the force of momentum by slowing down the action—examples include ballistic arm action, especially with hand weights, and the follow-through action during racket sports;
- muscles attempt to counter the force of gravity—examples include any lowering of a limb or of the body, such as the lower body's strain during the support phase of running (figure 10.4).

Sports can overload musculoskeletal systems in predictable patterns. For example, sports involving throwing may leave the external rotators of the shoulder fatigued from continual eccentric deceleration of the arm. This chronic fatigue leads to a loss of flexibility, weakness, and eventual injury (figure 10.5). Eccentric overload is evident in the high incidence of lower leg injuries during many aerobic weight-bearing activities (Houglum 2001; Anderson and Parr 2011). Eccentric patterns also appear in dynamic front lunges, which require many eccentric contractions to counteract the force of gravity—gastrocnemius, soleus, and tibialis anterior to control the speed of ankle dorsiflexion; quadriceps to control knee flexion; gluteus maximus and hamstrings to control hip

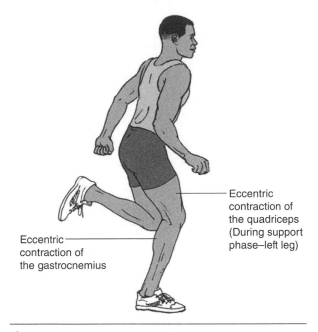

Eccentric contraction of the gastrocnemius

Eccentric contraction of the quadriceps (During support phase–left leg)

Figure 10.4   Eccentric contractions in running.

flexion; and probably the erector spinae, which controls the downward tendency of spinal flexion. It appears possible to prevent severe muscle damage by preconditioning muscles using a progression from slow- to fast-velocity eccentric exercise (Chapman et al. 2011).

Understanding Soft Tissue Injuries

Each type of tissue has different biological properties that influence its mechanism of injury and adaptation to training. The phases of recovery from injury involving inflammation are the same, however, no matter what tissue is involved. Understanding tissue type characteristics and the phases of healing will better equip you to prevent tissue degeneration and to promote proper healing.

Types of Soft Tissue

Soft tissue, such as ligaments, tendons, and cartilage, is susceptible to injury. Its structure is suited to its function, but the external forces often exceed its structural integrity.

Ligaments

Ligaments run from bone to bone, holding the bones together. Ligaments are like a flat mesh that reinforces the joint or joint capsule. The

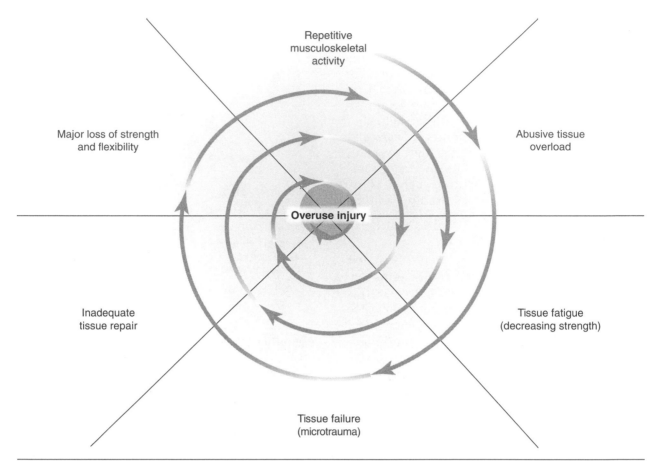

Figure 10.5   Spiral of overuse injuries.

organization of the tough collagenous fibers in the ligament can be parallel, oblique, or even spiral (as in the anterior cruciate ligament). The fibers are arranged to provide the best stabilization for the joint. Ligaments contain slightly more elastic fibers than do tendons.

Overuse injuries to ligaments are less common than the acute injury from a sudden overload or stretch in an extreme position. However, throwers (e.g., baseball players) may stretch their shoulder capsular ligaments and powerlifters their cruciate ligaments, reducing the joint's stability and leaving it susceptible to injury.

Providing more than passive stabilization, ligaments also contain proprioceptors that, when injured, reduce our ability to sense position or movements of the joint. Therefore, progressive kinesthetic activities are beneficial before return to full functional training.

Tendons

Tendons attach muscle to bone. They vary in length and can be round; if the muscle is broad and flat, the specialized tendon (aponeurosis) is also this shape. Structurally, tendons closely resemble ligaments. The main difference is the tendon's parallel collagen arrangement in successively larger bundles. Progressing from interior to exterior as well as smaller to larger, these layers are tropocollagen, collagen, subfibril, fibril, fascicle with an outer endotendineum, and finally the tendon with an outer epitendineum (figure 10.6).

Tendons consist primarily of collagenous fibers (70%) embedded in a gel. The endotendineum, which is the connective tissue sheath surrounding fibrils of collagen, carries blood vessels and nerves. The epitendineum (the outermost layer) is like an elastic sleeve allowing free movement of the tendon against surrounding structures.

Muscle and tendon function as one unit. Injury may occur at any point along this muscle–tendon unit: in the muscle belly, in the tendon, at the musculotendinous junction, or at the tendon–bone attachment. The connective tissue surrounding similar bundles of muscle fibers infolds and attaches to the tendon's collagenous projections within the myotendinous junction. At the other end, the tendon attaches to the periosteum and the bone's fibrocartilage, with a few fibers penetrating the bone itself.

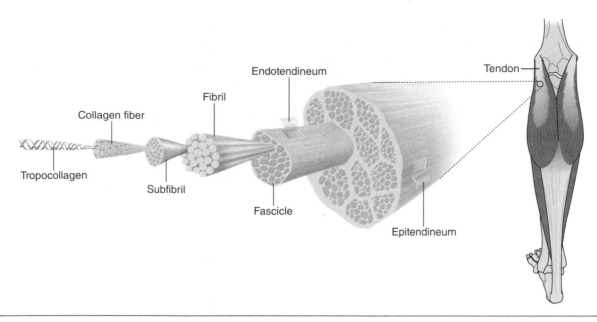

Figure 10.6   The structure of a tendon.

Tendons are the soft tissues most likely to incur overuse injury. Tendinopathies represent the most frequent type of musculoskeletal disorder, with the prevalence in the athletic population estimated to be 40% to 50% (Molina et al. 2011). Such injuries are typically recurrent, with symptoms of pain and functional disability. Advances in the understanding of tendon pathology indicate that Achilles, patellar, epicondylar, and rotator cuff tendinosis is often misdiagnosed as tendinitis. Because tendinosis is the sequel to unsuccessfully treated tendinitis and (unlike tendinitis) does not involve inflammation, treating tendinosis as if it were tendinitis will not help it (Kahn et al. 2000). Because these tendinosis conditions involve degenerative changes including loss of collagen, altered fiber organization, and vascular disruption, a treatment must be devised that will address these degenerative problems. Bracing and taping provides some mechanical relief of symptoms and may facilitate continued participation. There are no widely accepted recommendations for treatment of tendinosis (e.g., ultrasound, electrical stimulation); however, long-term benefits may come from active stabilization and progressive eccentric exercise (Hanson 2009).

Cartilage

Bones contact one another, forming a joint, but are separated by a layer of smooth, resilient hyaline cartilage. Some joints contain fibrocartilage structures that, together with the shape of the bone surfaces, influence movement.

Hyaline cartilage covers the articular surface of joints. Although 70% water, it has a meshwork of collagen fibers aligned horizontally on the surface, crisscrossed in the middle, and aligned vertically near the bone. Hyaline cartilage is not supplied with blood vessels or nerves, so the cartilage cells obtain oxygen and nutrients by diffusion. Regular loading maintains a cycle of nutrients in and around the cartilage. Injuries can be from acute joint trauma in which underlying bone is also injured (osteochondral). Degenerative changes can also occur because of cartilage failure or increased loading (osteoarthritis).

Fibrocartilage is found in the knee's meniscus, the wrist, labrum around the shoulder and hip, and the intervertebral disc. Fibrocartilage is strong yet resilient, helping to absorb shock and facilitate fit and stability. Although some fibrocartilage has blood supply, it has the same limited ability to heal itself as the nonvascularized hyaline cartilage.

Structural Strength of Tissues

"Terms of Structural Biomechanics" shows how tissues such as ligaments, tendons, and muscles react to stresses such as stretching (tensile stress). Initially, the wavy configuration of the collagenous fibers in the connective tissue straightens out. Relatively little force is needed to elongate the tissue, and the relationship between the load (force) and the deformation (stretch) is linear. In this "elastic range," the tissue can act like a spring, and once the load is removed, the tissue returns to near its original length (see figure 10.7). If the change in length exceeds a "yield point" (which is about 4% for a ligament), there is more permanent deformation (lengthening) with some slippage of collagen cross-links. The plastic range is the strain range between the yield point and rupture point where the material is deformed and may be damaged and injured if the strain goes beyond the tissue's ultimate strength. Eventually collagen fibers reach a rupture point and sever completely.

The relationship between stress and deformation of tendons is similar to that of ligaments. Some activities and sports, such as soccer, basketball, and rugby, require repetitive loading up to 8% change in length (Bahr and Maehlum 2004), potentially causing collagen fibers to rupture. Tendinitis is an inflammatory response within the tendon as a result of microstructural damage to the collagen fibers. The tendon is particularly vulnerable because the force of a contracting muscle is transmitted through the tendon.

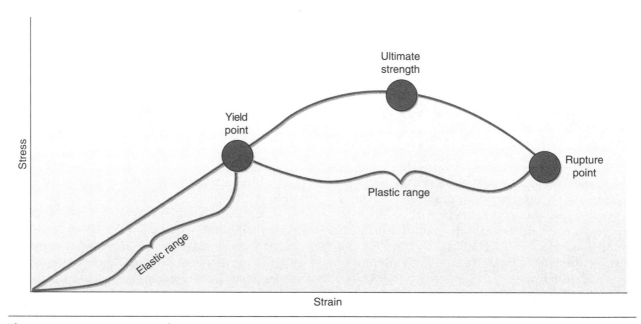

Figure 10.7 Stress–strain graph.

Terms of Structural Biomechanics

- **stress–strain curve (load deformation)**—The deformation (strain) increases proportionally to the stress resisting the load. The muscle–tendon complex has properties of elasticity up to a point (elastic range), after which permanent deformation (plastic range) and ultimately a rupture will occur.

- **stress**—Reaction forces to external loads set up within the tissues (e.g., stress created in bone, ligament, and tendon within the arch of the foot to support body weight).

- **strain**—Deformation; changes in tissue size, shape, length.

- **tensile**—Pulling apart (e.g., tendon, ligament, muscle).

- **shear**—Sliding apart (e.g., joint surfaces, L5-S1, epiphyseal plates).

- **compression**—Pressure (e.g., intervertebral disc, cartilage).

- **elasticity**—Ability to return to original dimension immediately.

- **plasticity**—Ability to retain changes in size or length when load is removed.

- **resilience**—Ability of tissue to vigorously return to its original size when unloaded.

- **damping**—Characteristic of tissue to return to its original size less vigorously than it was deformed (i.e., loss of energy).

- **absorbed strain**—Process that occurs if loading goes into the plastic range, when a considerable amount of energy may be lost (dissipated during permanent deformation).

To understand the relationship between loading and deformation of hyaline cartilage, remember that the collagen fibers are organized as a meshwork. Deformation increases linearly, straightening the fibers until tearing occurs rather abruptly.

Inflammatory Injury Healing and Reconditioning

The most common types of fitness injuries—and as many as 50% of all sport injuries—are caused by repetitive microtrauma in which soft tissue becomes inflamed or degenerates. The damage can be cumulative, resulting in ligament strains, joint synovitis, muscle myositis, or tendinitis. Injury occurs most often when a tissue like the tendon has been stressed repeatedly until it is unable to endure further tension. All inflamed tissues (ligament, tendon, muscle, cartilage, and bone) follow the same basic pattern of healing (table 10.3). Injuries need inflammation to heal, but inflammation does not always result in healing.

You must recognize the phase and the characteristics of the healing phases of injury involving inflammation. The process of returning to regular activity or competition involves this natural phased healing, preparation of the tissues for return to function, and the use of proper techniques to maximize reconditioning. Specific objectives for ROM, strength, and activity demands must be set to progress from one phase of healing to the next. The three phases of healing are inflammation, proliferation or repair, and remodeling. These stages are described next, and the appropriate exercise strategies for each phase are described in detail in the section "Exercise Prescription for Injured Clients". Because not much is known about either the process of or treatment for tendinosis, discussion is limited to healing involving inflammation (figure 10.8).

Phase 1: Inflammation

During inflammation, which generally lasts only a few days, the injury is stabilized and contained and debris is removed. The phase begins with bleeding and the release of blood products such as platelets into the injured area. Both vasodilation and increased capillary permeability are induced by histamine that is released by damaged cells (Germann and Stanfield 2002). These vascular changes cause the redness, warmth, swelling, and pain of inflammation. Platelets help stimulate the clotting mechanism, forming a meshwork of fibrin and collagen (Bahr and Maehlum 2004). Neutrophils move through the capillary walls to the injury, where they release enzymes that dissolve the damaged extracellular matrix. Later, macrophages remove debris and excess fluid partially caused by the rupture of cell walls. The damaged lymph vessels are unable to drain the excess fluid (edema) until the area becomes stable and the vessel is repaired (Houglum 2001). With a loss of blood flow and oxygen to other healthy cells, the area may experience hypoxia, cell damage, and further edema. The inflammatory substances and edema may cause function-inhibiting pain. Phase 1 inflammation needs to occur but should be minimized through application of ice, compression, elevation, and rest. Sometimes inflammation does not proceed to repair and remodeling, and the body remains in a chronic inflammatory state. Chronic inflammation may be caused by constant irritation by a mechanical stress; contamination by bacteria; antigen–antibody reactions; or invasion by microorganisms. Chronic inflammation can result in chronic pain (Denegar et al. 2010). Clients should be referred to their physician when inflammation is prolonged.

Table 10.3   Healing Phases of Inflammatory Injury

Phase	Characteristic	Duration
Inflammation	Localized redness, swelling (edema), increased temperature (warmth), pain (tenderness), loss of normal function	Up to 5 days
Proliferation or repair	Scar tissue red and larger than normal because of edema; increased collagen fiber production	3-21 days
Remodeling	Redness (vascularity) reduced, water content of scar reduced, and scar tissue density increased; collagen fiber alignment and increased tissue strength	7 days to >1 year

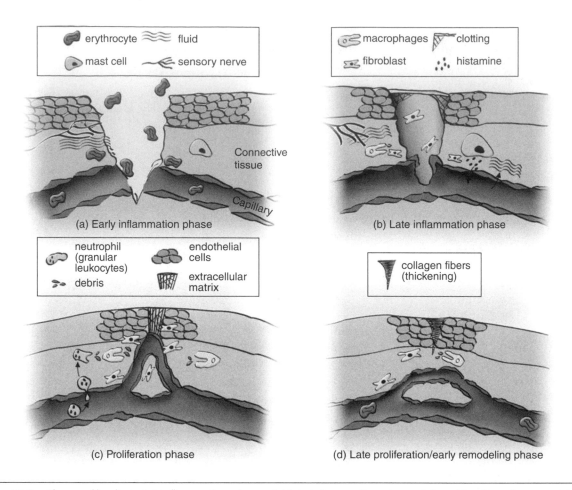

Figure 10.8   Phases of healing: *(a)* inflammation phase, *(b)* late inflammation phase, *(c)* proliferation phase, and *(d)* late proliferation and early remodeling phase.

Phase 2: Proliferation or Repair

Once the macrophages remove most of the debris from the area, the next step is the growth of new blood vessels (angiogenesis) and other tissue. Growth factors enter the area and are responsible for the local migration and proliferation of fibroblasts and endothelial cells. Fibroblasts are important for the development of new capillaries and the extracellular matrix (Houglum 2001), which has both a fibrous component (collagen and elastin) and a gel-like ground substance. The ground substance fills the spaces between the fibrous elements and reduces friction when stress is applied. At the same time, there is a continuous breakdown and removal of extracellular matrix and cellular debris (Bahr and Maehlum 2004). Also, the new matrix draws water into the area, increasing edema. As the injured tissue is repaired, its tensile strength increases.

Phase 3: Remodeling

With some overlap of phases, remodeling begins as some of the fibroblasts become myofibroblasts to shrink the wound (Houglum 2001). This scar tissue contraction and adhesion formation can cause a loss of motion at a joint. The number of macrophages reduces and mature blood supply is established by selective removal of capillaries with low blood flow. Swelling and wound sensitivity are reduced with the loss of extracellular matrix substances. Remodeling of the scar tissue involves the formation of thicker collagen fibers in the direction of tissue tension. As fluid is reduced in the area, the collagen fibers can produce more cross-links with each other. When the fibers are aligned in a parallel fashion, collagen can form the greatest number of cross-links to increase tensile strength, and the form and function of this scar tissue depend significantly on the degree to which the tissue is loaded by stretching and contractile exercises while the tissue is remodeling. Proprioceptors such as the muscle spindles and Golgi tendon organs, which monitor muscle length, tension, and rate of change, may be damaged and will start to repair in this stage.

Overuse Injuries

If your clients are to maintain long-term fitness, you must be able to recognize the signs and symptoms of overuse; prescribe appropriately for injured clients, taking the phases of recovery into account; and control risks of further injury. Although you need to understand the mechanisms of injury, the different types of injury, and the physiological healing process, in addition you must establish a communication network of health care practitioners to facilitate referral and dialogue.

Some clients do not take pain seriously and will mask it until it becomes acute. Ask clients about pain and be alert for signs of pain while they are exercising. Form 10.2, Pain Questionnaire, may be used during the assessment or monitoring stages of exercise prescription. Urge clients to seek help when they first experience pain. During movement, your client may show signs of feeling pain or warmth, or you may notice swelling or crepitus. Crepitus is a crackling sound similar to the sound heard when hair is rolled between the fingers near the ear. To ensure early intervention so that problems will not become serious, watch carefully for any of these symptoms of overuse.

The series of events that lead to overuse injury is remarkably predictable (O'Connor et al. 1992). When a movement is performed repeatedly and the tissue becomes irritated and inflamed, overuse injury occurs. Although inflammation from tissue damage is required for proper healing, an excessive or prolonged inflammatory response can become self-destructive. To prevent tissue degeneration and promote proper healing, you must interrupt the spiral of overuse discussed earlier (figure 10.5). The following situations often lead to tissue damage:

- A change in execution (e.g., joint alignment)
- A change in the client's interface with equipment (e.g., setup or starting position, change of shoes)
- Failure of execution with no spotting
- Increase in load or intensity
- Omission of warm-up or cool-down
- Resumption of training after a period of inactivity
- Addition or deletion of exercises from the original prescription
- Change in location of workouts (e.g., surface) or environment (e.g., temperature)
- Addition of supplemental activity such as a sport

Be aware of your client's comments or behaviors, as they may reveal an emerging overuse injury:

- Has she changed her gait or running pattern?
- Does she regularly take painkillers before exercise?
- Does her pain increase even after a good warm-up?
- Does her pain continue even after the intensity has been reduced?

Nirschl (1988) presented a pain phase scale for overuse injuries. This scale is useful for initial assessment and as a way to monitor a rate of progress in a program (see "Pain Scale for Overuse Injuries").

Pain Scale for Overuse Injuries

Phase 1: Stiffness or mild soreness after activity. Pain usually gone within 24 h.

Phase 2: Stiffness or mild soreness before activity that is relieved by warm-up. Symptoms not present during activity but return afterward, lasting up to 48 h.

Phase 3: Stiffness or mild soreness before activity. Pain partially relieved by warm-up. Pain minimally present during activity but does not alter activity.

Phase 4: Pain more intense than in phase 3. Performance of activity altered. Mild pain noticed with daily activities.

Phase 5: Significant (moderate or greater) pain before, during, and after activity, causing alteration of activity. Pain with daily activities but no major change.

Phase 6: Pain persists even with complete rest. Pain disrupts simple daily activities and prohibits doing household chores.

Phase 7: Phase 6 pain that also disrupts sleep consistently. Aching pain that intensifies with activity.

Exercise Prescription for Injured Clients

You must recognize the stages of healing and understand the characteristics of each. Only then will you be able to set appropriate objectives for ROM, strength, and activity demands to progress from one phase of healing to the next.

Tissue damage can come from a macrotrauma or sudden onset (acute injury) or from microtrama or repeated abnormal stress (overuse injury). In most cases, it is easy to classify an injury as either acute or overuse. However, some injuries have a sudden onset of symptoms but may have started much earlier with heavy training and little recovery. These should be treated as overuse injuries.

An important part of treating overuse injuries is preventing atrophy of the musculoskeletal system because of inactivity. Tendons, capsules, cartilage, and ligaments are just as affected by inactivity as muscles. It has been demonstrated that after 8 weeks of inactivity, 40% of strength and 30% of stiffness in the tendons are lost (Bahr and Maehlum 2004).

Overuse injuries can be very discouraging to clients. Recurrent injury often results from incomplete rehabilitation. To optimize clients' quick (and permanent) return to their programs, encourage the following three-stage progression: (1) acute response (inflammation control), (2) recovery (repair), and (3) functional progression (remodeling) (figure 10.9).

Stage 1: Acute Response

The goals for this stage are to control inflammation and manage pain. These guidelines also prepare for new tissue formation during healing and avoid worsening the injury. To achieve these goals, relative rest, anti-inflammatory treatment, and passive modalities including ice, compression, and elevation are the primary treatment options.

Inflammation can hamper reconditioning in many overuse injuries. Reduction and elimination of inflammation must be a priority of exercise prescriptions. To limit bleeding, relieve pain, decrease swelling, and improve healing, have the client begin effective PRICE (prevention, rest, ice, compression, elevation) treatment as soon as possible. Bleeding and plasma exudation continue for 48 h after an acute soft tissue injury, so to be effective, PRICE treatment must continue for 2 to 3 days.

- **Prevention and rest.** With overuse injuries, the affected muscles must be allowed to rest, sometimes for several weeks depending on the pain. Andrish and Work (1990) suggested stopping the offending activity until the pain subsides, usually in about 1 to 2 weeks. Correct any biomechanical abnormality or training error that may have caused inflammation—such as work-related overuse, continuation of a sport while injured, or aggravation caused by poorly designed exercises.

- **Ice.** The use of cold (cryotherapy) is not only effective immediately after an injury or flare-up; it should be continued as long as inflammation persists. Ice causes local vasoconstriction and slows metabolic activity; it relieves pain and muscle spasm. When your client has joint pain, stop all painful activities immediately and ice the joint. Kaul and Herring (1994) reported that ice chips in a plastic bag were the most effective local

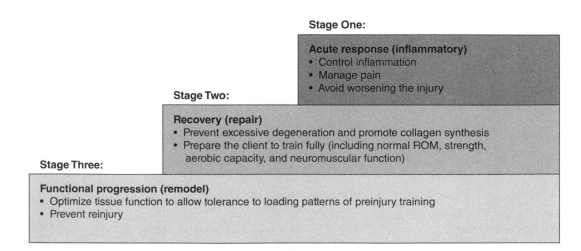

Figure 10.9   The three-stage progression to complete rehabilitation.

application method, followed by use of frozen gel packs and endothermic chemical reaction packs. Frozen gel packs are convenient and reusable and require a thin insulating towel coverage to avoid nerve damage and frostbite. Ice massage with water frozen in a foam cup can be used to produce analgesia. Excess pressure should be avoided and sessions should be short (5-10 min). With acute tendinitis, ice should be applied at the end of every activity session.

- **Compression.** Compression with an elastic bandage will limit the development of hematoma. Blood flow can be significantly reduced under the bandage and even more so when the fit is tighter. An ice bag under the compression bandage can increase local pressure over the injury site.

- **Elevation.** Elevation is recommended for the first 2 days whenever the client is lying down or sitting still. No reduction in blood flow occurs until the injured area is more than 30 cm (12 in.) above the level of the heart (Bahr and Maehlum 2004). Therefore, the injured limb should be propped up considerably, especially in bed at night. Cold application should be used in combination with compression and elevation for maximum benefit.

There is an argument that ice decreases the metabolic rate mainly by reducing circulation and that this will slow the natural inflammatory process. However, if ice application is brief (e.g., 5-7 min), when the ice is removed, there is an influx of circulation and lymphatic activity that comes to the area (similar to contrast bath treatments), which could reduce swelling and increase evacuation. My advice for many overuse-type injuries: brief, repeated applications of ice chips or a frozen Styrofoam cup with the injured tissue in an elevated position (gravity can assist evacuation), interspersed with moderate isometric contractions of the surrounding muscles (usually avoiding movement of the injured joint).

Pharmacological control of inflammation is often accomplished through NSAIDs (nonsteroidal anti-inflammatory drugs) such as aspirin (e.g., Bayer) and ibuprofen (e.g., Advil, Motrin). Nonsteroidal anti-inflammatory drugs prevent plasma proteins (e.g., prostaglandins) from acting by decreasing membrane permeability. However, prostaglandins provide a gastroprotective effect, and the use of NSAIDs may put the client at risk for gastrointestinal bleeding (Gillespie 2011). They may also help ease symptoms such as pain and spasm. Ibuprofen has been shown to decrease muscle soreness induced after eccentric exercise (Tokmakidis et al. 2003). Do not use NSAIDs to reduce pain in order to allow a more intense workout. Masking pain and potentially "pushing through" an injury may increase the risk of worsening an injury that would normally be limited by the sensation of pain. Ensure that your client has no medical contraindications. If inflammation persists or worsens, your client should see a physician. Keep a proper perspective regarding the role of NSAIDs, especially given their risk of side effects and their potential to blunt the normal healing process (Stovitz and Johnson 2003).

Stage 2: Recovery

The goals for this stage are to prevent excessive degeneration, promote collagen synthesis (repair), and prepare the client to train fully, including normal ROM, strength, aerobic capacity, and neuromuscular function.

Pain and swelling are the main considerations when prescribing how much and what to do. Cryotherapy may continue to be useful, particularly after an exercise session. The client will begin with low-load stresses to promote increased collagen synthesis and prevent loss of joint motion. Relative rest is obviously protective.

Soon after an injury, exercise enhances tissue oxygenation, minimizes atrophy, and aligns collagenous fibers to increase tissue strength. At first, have your client

- limit excessive stretching of damaged tissue;
- do isometrics (progressing from submaximal) at different joint angles; and
- start with midrange isotonics (daily), completing about 30 repetitions in 2 or 3 sets (may start with no weight).

Design activities your clients can do to enhance healing and maintain fitness. For example, if your client has a running injury, running in water with a flotation belt can be an effective alternative. Healing also involves increased vascularization through rehabilitative exercise and cardiovascular conditioning. During this stage, your clients should limit the ROM to that in which they remain pain free. Pain can activate neural mechanisms within the body that inhibit strength, flexibility, and function (Ralston 2003).

As your clients heal, have them progress to

- full effort on isometrics;
- isotonics in full ROM—gradually increasing weight by 10% to 20% and reducing

repetitions initially, and then gradually increasing them again; and

- a minimum frequency of three exercise sessions per week.

Stretching can be done two or three times per day; increased joint ROM can be retained for 4 to 6 h (Frontera 2003). As rehabilitation progresses, include strength exercises for muscle groups proximal and distal to the injured area. Use rubber tubing or elastic bands (if you deem them appropriate). Incorporate ROM exercises and moderate static stretching to regain muscle balance and to treat muscles that have tightened because of compensation. Prescribe light cardiovascular exercise that does not traumatize the injured tissue (e.g., aquafitness, hand ergometry, stationary bicycle).

At this point, your client may gradually resume training at about half the previous intensity and gradually increase the effort over 3 to 6 weeks. Returning too quickly is the most common reason injuries recur. Make sure that the warm-up and cool-down include complete stretching of the affected area.

Stage 3: Functional Progression

The goals for this stage are to optimize tissue function to allow tolerance to loading patterns of preinjury training. These guidelines also aim to prevent reinjury.

Functional progression is a planned, progressively difficult sequence of exercises that acclimatize the individual to training or competition demands or fitness needs (Ralston 2003). Thus, you must be able to evaluate exercises and categorize their levels of difficulty and appropriate applications.

With increased loading, the newly formed collagen fibers begin the process of hypertrophy and align themselves along lines of stress (Earle and Baechle 2004). Prescribe functional activities using closed-chain, dynamic, multijoint exercises that closely mimic the demands and movements of preinjury endeavors.

General Guidelines

General body conditioning—including cardiovascular, strength and endurance, muscle balance, and flexibility—enhances rehabilitation of any injury and will decrease the chance of its recurring. Introducing exercises specific to the injury, however, can provide neurophysiological stimulus and help redevelop proprioceptive skills.

During stage 3, follow whichever of these guidelines are appropriate for your client:

- Include full ROM strengthening, reaching momentary failure at the end of each set.
- Insist on a minimum exercise frequency of two or three times per week.
- Select other resistance equipment (e.g., isokinetic, hydraulic, variable resistance).
- Use heavier or thicker tubing or bands to isolate movements and muscles.
- Include partner-resisted exercise and proprioceptive neuromuscular facilitation with client-specific static stretches.
- Add activities specific to the client's sport or usual training activities (e.g., interval training; muscle isolations; drills for agility, speed, and skill).
- If the client is involved in a power-oriented eccentric activity, progressively build the eccentric strength and power of the involved muscle groups (e.g., eccentric Achilles exercises, plyometrics).

Neuromuscular Concerns

Clients will continue to improve function by adding more advanced, activity-specific exercises. In addition, the client must regain normal neuromuscular function. If not, changes in recruitment patterns of muscles around the injured joint may alter technique and produce unfavorable loading. To avoid new injuries, training must include proprioceptive challenges, coordination, balance, and agility once the client has regained at least 85% of his original strength (Bahr and Maehlum 2004). Neuromuscular retraining contributes to the body's ability to maintain postural stability. Houglum (2001) identified a four-part progression to reestablish neuromuscular control:

1. Proprioceptive and kinesthetic awareness (joint position sense)
2. Dynamic joint stability (balance, agility, coactivation)
3. Reactive neuromuscular control (e.g., plyometrics)
4. Functional motor patterns (specific, complex, sportlike activities)

The following is an example of a lower extremity neuromuscular progression:

1. Stork stand
2. Single-leg balance on a wobble board
3. Plyometric hops—alternating legs
4. Alternating single-leg lateral hops over a line (skier)

Delayed-Onset Muscle Soreness

Aside from the pain of a muscle or connective tissue injury, vigorous exercise can produce delayed-onset muscle soreness (DOMS). Delayed-onset muscle soreness can emerge 8 to 12 h after certain exercises, is generally at its worst within the first 2 days following the activity, and subsides over the next few days.

Delayed-onset muscle soreness is thought to be a result of microscopic tearing of the muscle fibers (Ross 1999). Others (Szymanski 2001) believe that the symptoms of DOMS are associated with damage to the connective tissue around the muscle, accumulation of calcium, release of intracellular proteins, and inflammation. In addition to microscopic tearing, swelling may take place in and around the muscle. This swelling increases pressure on nerves and other structures, resulting in pain and stiffness. The amount of damage depends on the intensity, duration, and type of exercise. As noted previously, activities in which muscles forcefully contract while they are lengthening tend to cause the most soreness. These eccentric contractions occur in activities involving a braking action such as running downhill, lowering weights, descending stairs, performing plyometrics, and performing the downward phases of push-ups and squats. Unaccustomed activities involving sudden major changes in the type or length of exercise may also cause delayed soreness.

Delayed-onset muscle soreness is not as serious as the injuries discussed previously, but it is a lot more common. To reduce soreness and speed recovery, encourage the use of ice, gentle stretching, and massage, although there is limited research evidence to guide management practices (Snyder et al. 2011). The use of a compressive sleeve can decrease perceived soreness, reduce swelling, and promote recovery of force production (Kraemer et al. 2001). Initially have the client avoid any vigorous activity. You may, however, work the unaffected areas of the body. If the client performs low-impact aerobic activity such as biking or walking, blood flow is increased to the affected muscles, which may reduce soreness. Also, NSAIDs such as aspirin or ibuprofen may temporarily help, although they won't speed healing. Of all the treatments, warm-up appears to be the most promising approach. Increasing muscle temperature reduces muscle and connective tissue viscosity, increases muscle elasticity, and increases resistance to tissue tearing (Szymanski 2001).

Start the client with a general warm-up designed to increase core body temperature (e.g., jogging, cycling, or aerobic activities for 5-10 min). Proceed to a specific warm-up including multijoint movements and skill application activity related to the activity (e.g., warm-up set on the weights; dynamic flexibility such as crossovers, lunges). Static stretching of the muscles used in the activity can be effective when it follows the low-impact aerobic activity. Encourage your client

Preventing Reinjury: Risk Control

Reexamine your client's history and assessment to uncover his unique combination of intrinsic and extrinsic risk factors for (re)injury. Controlling these forces is both an objective of stage 3 and an ongoing preventive strategy. You must know the client's limitations, as well as the inherent demands of his training, and keep both extrinsic and intrinsic risks in mind at all times.

- Minimizing extrinsic risks. Avoiding training errors can be the single most effective way to minimize extrinsic risks. In a typical exercise prescription, the client follows a format that may start with a warm-up, lead into cardiovascular activity (balanced by some muscular conditioning), and finish with a cool-down. Review the discussion of training errors ("Extrinsic Factors," earlier in this chapter) and copy and use form 10.3, Injury Risk Control Checklist, to ensure that each of these program segments is free of training errors.

- Minimizing intrinsic risks. As discussed previously, it is your job to assess the biomechanical or structural risks that each client brings to the initial exercise prescription. Always make it an objective of your prescription to correct malalignments, muscle imbalances, joint instability, and muscle tightness or weakness. A prescription must assess both initial and developing intrinsic risk to be truly client centered. In addition to this chapter, review chapters 4 (assessment) and 8 (muscle balance) to ensure that you are well prepared for this task. Careful supervision and appropriate intervention or referral to a clinical specialist can minimize the effects of a client's intrinsic risk factors.

to cool down thoroughly after activity. With activities such as plyometrics, start with low-volume training. Progress the intensity of the workout (e.g., gradually increase intensity and duration for at least 2 weeks and incorporate some eccentric multijoint exercises).

In a controlled trial comparing cold and heat therapy for the prevention and early-phase treatment of DOMS of the lower back, pain relief was 138% greater with the heat wrap at hour 24 postexercise (Mayer et al. 2006). Both cold and heat reduce the transmission of pain, and trainers can easily individualize these analgesic treatments for lower back DOMS.

Case Study

This case study examines the intrinsic and extrinsic factors of a common lower body injury and how to apply the guidelines for progression to avoid overuse injuries. Even after the initial recovery, it is important to look for other possible (intrinsic) factors that may trigger reinjury.

Case Study: Too Painful to Jog

A 35-year-old woman approached you about some pain she had recently felt in her Achilles and just below her patella. She had been jogging 20 to 25 min/session, 2 or 3 days/week for the last 5 weeks, and had been asymptomatic. Five days ago she participated in a 2 h volleyball tryout after a regular jog. The pain escalated over the next 3 days to the point where it was too painful to jog.

The repetitive eccentric motion of the volleyball activity was sufficient to irritate the muscle–tendon unit of the Achilles and patellar areas. A normal initial inflammatory process had taken place; icing and rest were advised until the symptoms disappeared. In the interim, an aquafit program, upper body resistance work with some tubing, and some therapeutic exercises for her lower legs would focus on some new and some parallel goals until she could resume jogging. Some counseling about overuse may be warranted.

This approach dealt with the extrinsic causes of the injury and could probably get the client back to jogging within a reasonable time. However, you have not yet addressed the potential for reinjury caused by a possible structural weakness (intrinsic). Once the discomfort has subsided, examine your client's muscle balance and alignment (chapters 4 and 8) to identify weak links and provide a basis for therapeutic exercise prescription.

You can combine these activity suggestions to correct intrinsic needs with guidelines emerging from the extrinsic causes of injury to design the core prescription for your client. From this point, progress with your client through the three stages of the overuse intervention progression: acute response, recovery, and functional progression.

Summary

Injuries to ligaments, tendons, cartilage, and muscles are called soft tissue injuries. Personal trainers must be vigilant for the causes of soft tissue injury and knowledgeable about the characteristics of soft tissue, the phases of injury healing, how to prescribe exercise appropriately for each healing stage, and how to minimize risk of injury or reinjury. Identifying the responsibilities of various health care professionals and recognizing when to refer are essential to the team approach to injury management.

Biomechanical causes of soft tissue injuries may be intrinsic (such as muscle imbalance or joint instability) or extrinsic (such as work volume or eccentric overload). Each type of tissue has different biological properties that influence its mechanism of injury and adaptation to training. The most common types of fitness injuries are caused by repetitive microtrauma in which soft tissue becomes inflamed or degenerates with damage that can be cumulative, resulting in ligament strains, joint synovitis, muscle myositis, or tendinitis. All inflamed tissues follow the same basic pattern of healing involving inflammation, proliferation or repair, and remodeling. You can guide your client's recovery by setting specific objectives for ROM and strength. Activity demands must also be set to progress from one phase of healing to the next.

Vigorous exercise, often eccentric in nature, can produce delayed-onset muscle soreness, which is thought to be a result of microscopic tearing of the muscle fibers or associated with damage to the connective tissue around the muscle.

Watch for symptoms of overuse, and anticipate and intervene as necessary in these situations, which often lead to tissue damage. Recognize your areas of expertise and identify who is qualified to address the client's needs. Develop a network of credible exercise and medical health professionals to use as referrals.

FORM 10.1 Momentum Quiz

The buildup of momentum is very common in fitness activities. Many of these high-momentum movements are contraindicated because of the eccentric overload or lack of control. To test your skill in recognizing momentum and the risk it may present, try the following quiz. The answers to the quiz may be found in the online resource for this book.

For each of the following exercises, identify

1. how the momentum is produced (mass × velocity) and
2. possible adverse effects.

Example

Full neck circles

1. The head is quite heavy; if circles are done quickly, momentum will affect the neck.
2. Facet joints of the cervical spine will be jammed during the hyperextension phase; may affect the neck arteries.

Quiz

1. Straight-leg speed sit-ups

   _____

   _____

2. Stepping down and up quickly from a high aerobic step (bench)

   _____

   _____

3. Full squat with barbell

   _____

   _____

4. Throwing a plyoball with one hand

   _____

   _____

5. Changing directions quickly in a squash game

   _____

   _____

6. Two-handed kettlebell swing

   _____

   _____

7. Forward-step deep lunge

   _____

   _____

From J.C. Griffin, 2015, *Client-centered exercise prescription*, 3rd ed. (Champaign, IL: Human Kinetics).

FORM 10.2 Pain Questionnaire

1. Do you have any current pain? _____

2. What are the symptoms? _____

3. How long have you had these symptoms? _____

4. Have you had any related conditions in the past, and what treatment was provided? _____

5. In what joint or area do you feel the pain? _____

6. In what positions do you feel the pain? _____

7. During what movement do you feel the pain? _____

8. Do you feel the pain more or less before activity? _____

9. Do you feel the pain more or less after activity? _____

10. How long does the pain last? _____

11. Do you get tired (muscularly) more easily than you used to? _____

12. Have you experienced a loss of strength? _____

13. Are you compensating in your movements to avoid pain or loss of strength? _____

14. Do you feel tight anywhere? _____

15. Have you changed your prescription? _____

16. Have you recently increased your exercise volume or intensity? _____

17. Have you changed your location of exercise, type of equipment, or other conditions? _____

18. Have you recently changed shoes or are your shoes worn? _____

19. Is the injury or pain getting worse? _____

20. What do you think is causing this problem? _____

21. How could it be alleviated? _____

From J.C. Griffin, 2015, *Client-centered exercise prescription*, 3rd ed. (Champaign, IL: Human Kinetics).

FORM 10.3   Injury Risk Control Checklist

Warm-Up

❏ Use smooth, dynamic ROM movements—reaching as far as the muscle comfortably allows.

❏ Avoid forced, prolonged, or rapid movements of the back.

❏ Avoid hyperextension of the neck or lowering the head below the heart.

❏ Avoid excessive reps with arms above shoulders; control arm speed.

❏ Introduce and progress low-impact movements to raise temperature and heart rate.

❏ After some warming, statically stretch the muscle groups to be used in the workout.

❏ Add supplemental stretches if muscles are tight or sore or if expecting higher intensity than usual.

❏ Progress to preaerobic level (lower end of target heart rate).

❏ If workout is to be high eccentric, build eccentric overloading gradually.

Cardiovascular

This checklist is particularly relevant if your client is unconditioned, just returning from a layoff, or moving up to the next level.

❏ Avoid excessive stress, especially to the lower body, by using intervals, pyramids up and down, split routines, or a circuit.

❏ Help the client find the "stopping point," where the feeling of burn replaces momentary fatigue (especially in eccentric work).

❏ Check for excessive pronation, forefoot weight bearing, turning with foot planted.

❏ Minimize impact shock by encouraging light feet and resilient knees, providing low-impact alternatives, and ensuring that footwear and floor surface are appropriate.

❏ Monitor intensity and duration, which are the training errors linked most closely to overuse injury. Look for signs of overtraining (e.g., decreased performance, lethargy, early fatigue, elevated heart rate).

❏ Provide a few minutes of cardiovascular cool-down for circulatory adjustments and to gain flexibility—have client hold static stretches for up to 30 s.

Muscular Conditioning

❏ In designing a program, consider previous injuries to structures providing joint stability (e.g., include avoidance or rehabilitation).

❏ Contend with the forces of momentum and gravity.

❏ Avoid excessive knee or back flexion, lifting arms with palms forward, and allowing hip extension to force the back into increased lumbar lordosis.

❏ Remember that progression may be rapid initially and then level off.

❏ Intervene with help or with an exercise alternative when technique or condition appears to be a problem.

❏ Suggest beginning with a light set and following with static stretch of the muscles used (especially if used eccentrically).

❏ Think muscle balance—remember, the cardiovascular activity has already worked selected muscles.

Cool-Down

❏ Relieve anticipated muscle tightness that may result from eccentric work—for example, in quadriceps, calves, and erector spinae.

❏ Stretch tight postural muscles—for example, anterior chest, hip flexors, hamstrings.

❏ Be sure client is relaxed and cool before heading back to daily routine.

From J.C. Griffin, 2015, *Client-centered exercise prescription,* 3rd ed. (Champaign, IL: Human Kinetics).

Exercise Prescription for Specific Injuries

Chapter Competencies

After completing this chapter, you will be able to demonstrate the following competencies:

1. Describe the functional anatomy and probable causes for each of the following conditions:
   - Plantar fasciitis
   - Achilles tendinitis and tendinosis
   - Shin splints (medial tibial stress syndrome)
   - Patellofemoral syndrome
   - Hamstring strain
   - Low back pain
   - Rotator cuff tendinitis (impingement syndrome)
   - Lateral epicondylitis (tennis elbow)
2. Describe preventive exercise strategies including precautions, beneficial activity indications, and exercise contraindications.
3. Assist with the postrehabilitation treatment plan for a client to minimize risk of reinjury or to speed recovery by designing specific exercises and activities for stretching and for strengthening injured tissues.

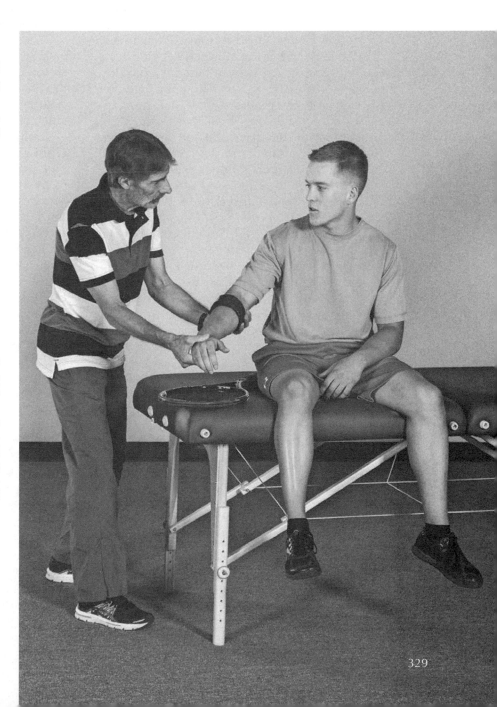

This chapter should help anyone who works with clients recovering from, or having a history of, orthopedic injury. It provides a brief description of and functional anatomy background for plantar fasciitis, Achilles tendinitis and tendinosis, shin splints (medial tibial stress syndrome), patellofemoral syndrome, hamstring strain, low back pain, and rotator cuff tendinitis (impingement syndrome). We also consider probable causes and strategies for prevention. Specific exercise designs for stretching and strengthening injured tissues are grouped together near the end of the discussion of each injury. This convenient format will permit easy reproduction for practitioners wishing to provide visual aids for their clients. Although the exercises were designed for specific injuries, they can also serve as a glossary of exercises that may be selected for any of the prescription models outlined in earlier chapters.

The specific conditions discussed comprise a sample of overuse injuries of tendons, muscles, and other connective tissue. These are common injuries seen in the fitness culture, but the chapter does not provide an exhaustive treatment of overuse injuries. Readers will find more extensive coverage of athletic injuries and therapeutic exercise in the Human Kinetics publications by Houglum (2010), *Therapeutic Exercise for Musculoskeletal Injuries, Third Edition;* Whiting and Zernicke (2008), *Biomechanics of Musculoskeletal Injury, Second Edition;* and Tiidus (2008), *Skeletal Muscle Damage and Repair.*

The chapter emphasizes overuse injuries resulting from repeated abnormal stresses. As we saw in chapter 10, this microtrauma may be caused by extrinsic factors such as faulty equipment (e.g., worn shoes) or training errors (e.g., too little recovery) or intrinsic factors such as malalignment or muscle imbalance. The following section examines the probable causes and strategies for prevention for overuse injuries of tendons (e.g., Achilles

tendinitis), muscles (e.g., hamstring strain), and other connective tissue (e.g., plantar fasciitis and shin splints). Table 11.1 defines common injuries to muscle and connective tissues.

Plantar Fasciitis

Plantar fasciitis is inflammation of the strong tissue that runs along the bottom of the foot and connects the heel to the base of the toes. Along with the muscles and bones, this connective tissue, the plantar fascia, forms the arch of the foot (figure 11.1). The plantar fascia is multilayered fibrous connective tissue. It arises from the calcaneus and forms five divisions that insert on the ball of the foot. By tensing like a bowstring on the plantar surface of the feet, the plantar fascia helps to support the arch.

What starts as a slight pain in a client's heel may gradually build. It is usually worse with the first step of the morning and can be quite intense when the area bears weight as in walking or running. A sufferer may limp or bear weight on the lateral side of the foot to ease the pain.

Plantar fasciitis is caused by excessive tightness within the fascia, producing microscopic tears and inflammation. Alignment problems such as overpronation or low arches may contribute. Pressure on the fascia may be caused by weak muscles—including the small intrinsic muscles in the foot and other muscles in the lower leg such as the flexor digitorum and tibialis posterior. Tight gastrocnemius and soleus muscles can also cause fasciitis by keeping the Achilles tendon tight, thereby making the ankle less flexible and forcing the plantar fascia to absorb more weight. Any activity in which the weight is taken on the ball of the foot—such as high-impact aerobics, basketball, sprinting, tennis, or bounding—can create excessive pull on the fascia. There is some evidence that chronic plantar pain may not be

Table 11.1 Common Injuries to Muscle and Connective Tissue

Injury	Description and definition
Ligament sprain	Trauma (often acute) to a ligament that compromises the stability of the joint. The injury can range from a first-degree sprain involving a partial tear and minor joint instability to a third-degree sprain involving a complete tear and full joint instability.
Tendinitis	Painful overuse tendon condition involving inflammation (Cook et al. 2000).
Tendinosis	Collagen degeneration rather than inflammation of a tendon (Hanson 2009). This tendinopathy often results from a lack of adequate repair of a tendinitis.
Muscle strain	Trauma to the muscle involving muscle fiber tearing. The injury can be a first-degree strain involving a partial tear, pain during muscle activity, but little loss in strength. A second-degree strain results in a loss of strength. A third-degree strain is a complete tear.

Certified Personal Trainers and Defining the Boundaries

Rehabilitation and reconditioning are a team-oriented process requiring all members of the sports medicine team to work together. You must recognize the responsibilities of different health care providers who may be needed throughout the healing and strengthening phases. Although you will need to understand the mechanism of injury, the different types of injury, and the physiological healing process, you must also establish a communication network of health care practitioners to facilitate referral and dialogue. Defining the boundaries helps to identify the areas of expertise of personal fitness trainers and to ensure that overstepping in these areas is avoided. In addition, most certification programs for personal trainers such as the American College of Sports Medicine, National Strength and Conditioning Association, and Canadian Society for Exercise Physiology have published competencies and a scope of practice in the area of injury prevention and treatment.

During the initial counseling session you should determine past injuries, current pain, and potential causes of injury. In many cases, your clients will approach you after they have started their program and experienced some discomfort. At this stage, effective questioning and probing are critical to determining your client's needs. Because of your unique knowledge and insight into exercise design, modification, demonstration, monitoring, and health promotion, you can serve a vital role during the final stages of an advanced rehabilitation and reconditioning program (Earle and Baechle 2004).

Understanding an injury and its potential cause can be the first step toward preventing it. The key to recovery is to recognize the problem and its causes in the early stages by monitoring symptoms carefully. Take time to listen to your client when you ask, "How are you feeling today?" You must understand preventive exercise strategies including precautions, beneficial activity indications, and exercise contraindications. However, it is also your responsibility to recognize when you need to advise your client to seek medical assistance.

You should advise your clients to consult their physician if their pain is significant, does not go away with rest, is accompanied by a noticeable hot and inflamed area, or is linked to an accident. Only a qualified medical professional can determine the precise cause of your client's pain and order the appropriate treatments.

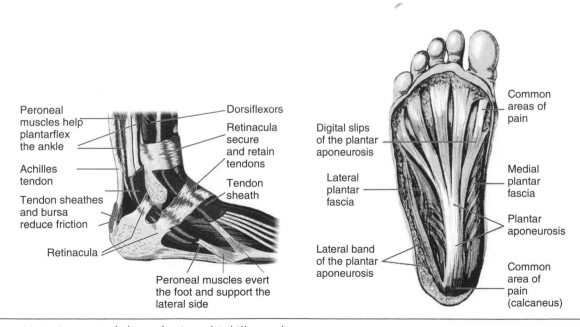

Figure 11.1 Anatomy of plantar fascia and Achilles tendon.

inflamed tissue; however, further research is needed on this issue (Sanders 2007).

Massaging with ice for 5 to 7 min several times a day can be effective. Apply cold packs for up to 20 min (Rizzo 1991). A good technique involves rolling the sole of the foot over a frozen water bottle to stretch, ice, and massage in one movement. Before advising clients to be fitted for an orthotic, help them look for good supportive footwear with distinct arch support, strong heel cup, and full sole cushioning. A heel lift may also be needed. Some clients may be helped with a heel cup, which forces more fat to remain below the heel. If a calcaneal spur (heel spur) is present, a foam or felt pad with a hole cut in it to release pressure may be helpful. Even lacing shoes tightly can assist with medial support and reduce pronation. The use of a night splint to relieve symptoms, by preventing the ten-dency for the plantar fascia to contract and shorten during sleeping, has become popular. Although people with plantar fasciitis should avoid some high-trauma activities, other activities such as recline cycling, swimming, pool running, rowing machines, or circuit weight training should not produce discomfort. Anything that produces pain should be avoided. Walkers should decrease their mileage, avoid hills, and look for softer surfaces.

Weak foot muscles may not be able to support the dynamic structure of the foot. Strong muscles are required to help maintain a sound arch and withstand the sometimes three- to fivefold load increase placed on the plantar fascia when, for example, the foot is landing during a moderate downhill run (Batt and Tanji 1995). Once the foot is pain free and flexibility is returning, your client should begin strengthening exercises.

Plantar Fasciitis
Stretching Guidelines and Prescription

Gentle, prolonged stretching should be pain free. Stretching exercises should focus on the Achilles tendon and the soleus and gastrocnemius muscles. Figure 11.2 shows a soleus stretch with the rear knee bent to further elongate the Achilles. Have client slightly bend the knee with the heel on the floor for the soleus.

A simple wedged heel-cord box (figure 11.3) can facilitate stretching. Your client can achieve more complete fiber elongation by using variations such as straight knees or toes inward or outward. Sanders (2007) reported

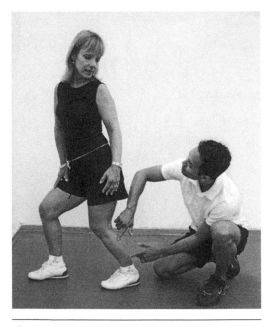

Figure 11.2 Achilles tendon stretch.

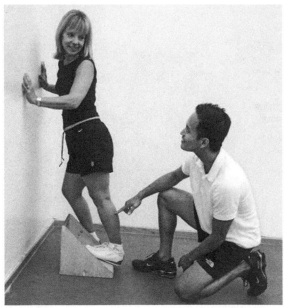

Figure 11.3 A straight-knee gastrocnemius stretch with a wedged box.

that patients performing plantar fascia stretching in the morning showed significant improvements in pain, activity limitations, and patient satisfaction. Ask your client to sit cross-legged and pull the toes back toward the shin until the arch feels the stretch (see figure 11.4). Have your injured client stretch at least twice a day.

Massage and foot manipulation can help relax tight, rigid connective tissue in the foot itself and in the intrinsic muscles. Using a foot massage bar or tennis ball, clients should apply pressure and slowly roll the bar or ball on the ground with their bare foot, feeling the pressure from the heel to the ball of the foot.

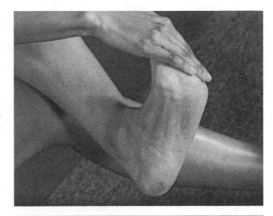

Figure 11.4   Plantar fascia stretch.

Plantar Fasciitis
Strengthening Guidelines and Prescription

By using her toes to pull a towel (figure 11.5) or to grasp a marble, your client can condition the intrinsic muscles of her foot and the toe flexors that help support the arch. Have your client work on a slippery surface and pull the towel in by curling the toes. Daily practice of this exercise may still take 6 weeks to improve the foot's configuration.

Balancing on one leg will help strengthen and reacquaint the lower leg muscles with the proper support alignment (figure 11.6). Direct clients to feel the muscles of the foot and lower leg working, then progress to holding their balance with their eyes closed. Many balance activities will train proprioceptive pathways that may have been damaged (Hanney 2000). The unilateral mini-trampoline balance with ball toss (figure 11.7) can be progressed with more difficult catches. While the client balances on one leg on a mini-tramp, toss an appropriately weighted ball back and forth to the client. Before you permit resumption of full-intensity activity, prescribe a progression using closed kinetic chain (weight-bearing) exercises including the ankle, knee, and hip (chapter 7).

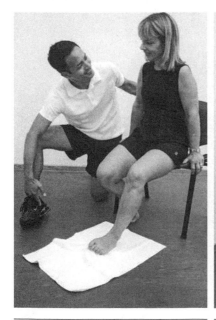 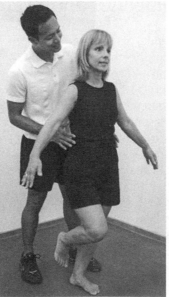 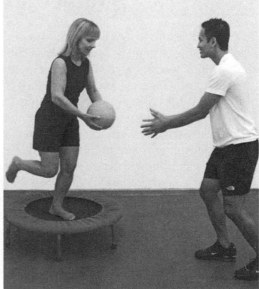

Figure 11.5   Toe curls with towel.   **Figure 11.6**   One-leg balance.   **Figure 11.7**   One-leg mini-trampoline ball toss.

Achilles Tendinitis and Tendinosis

Achilles tendinitis is inflammation of the tendon, its sheath, or the bursae (figure 11.1). Your client may describe pain located 2 to 5 cm (0.78-2 in.) above the calcaneus (Prentice 1994). In early, mild tendinitis, the foot loosens up at the beginning of activity but the pain gradually increases. If inadequately treated, the condition may result in adhesions between the tendon and the sheath or the scar tissue within the tendon (or both), which further decreases elasticity. More advanced, chronic **Achilles tendinosis** involves degenerative changes often attributable to uncorrected overpronation (Bahr and Maehlum 2004). This condition causes pain when your client climbs stairs or walks normally, escalates with activity and subsides with rest, and may be accompanied by weakness during plantar flexion. Morning stiffness, poor flexibility, and swelling or tightness of the calf muscles are common symptoms.

Racket sport players and longer-distance runners are particularly susceptible to Achilles tendinitis. The combination of repetitive microtrauma from these activities and excessive pronation is particularly risky. Insufficient stretching or rapid overstretching can lead to damage. Nonresilient flooring that is not springy and does not absorb the shock, or uneven ground, may contribute to the injury. The injury is often slow to heal because of poor vascularization in the lower part of the tendon, an issue with older clients (Myerson and Biddinger 1995). Have your clients avoid repetitive, weight-bearing dorsiflexion, particularly during high-impact eccentric contractions of the calf muscles such as the push-offs required by many sports. Once you have established the cause, prescribe specific changes to prevent further aggravation. With Achilles tendinitis, use cryotherapy immediately after the injury or flare-up, as well as into the reconditioning and management stages (anti-inflammatory agents are not as effective with tendinosis). Initial conservative management of mild to moderate Achilles tendinitis should involve a decrease in activity by at least 50%. Examine your client's running shoes for proper heel fit. If other biomechanical problems exist (chapters 4 and 10), consider adding a 1/4 to 1/2 in. (0.6 to 1.3 cm) heel lift or referring your client for orthotics. Low-impact activities such as cycling, rowing, swimming, low-impact aerobic dance, or most weight training—as long as they do not produce pain—can help your client maintain aerobic conditioning. Limit any toe push-offs.

Achilles Tendinitis and Tendinosis
Stretching Guidelines and Prescription

To avoid adhesions, your client should begin gentle, passive stretching as soon as pain allows. Have her stretch the Achilles tendon with a static dorsiflexion—knee straight (gastrocnemius) and bent (soleus) (figure 11.2). Turning the toes slightly inward during the stretches shown in figure 11.2 will enhance the Achilles stretch.

If these stretches create pain, have your client use partial or non–weight-bearing ankle dorsiflexion stretches. Figure 11.8 shows a seated ankle dorsiflexion using tubing or TheraBand. With the tubing or TheraBand securely wrapped around the ball of the foot with tension, have the client point her foot (plantar flex) and return slowly. This stretch may also be performed with a bent knee.

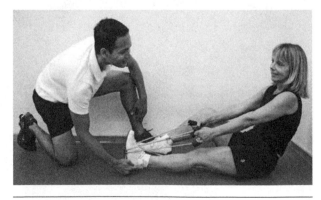

Figure 11.8   Seated tubing dorsiflexion.

Achilles Tendinitis and Tendinosis
Strengthening Guidelines and Prescription

Begin with light progressive resistance exercises for the calf muscles. One easy method is to work against tubing or an elastic band by placing the foot in the loop and pressing down (starting position as in figure 11.8). Dynamic plantar flexion with weights or a machine may start in a seated position (figure 11.9). With a resistance on the thighs, the client presses up to the toes and returns slowly to a flat foot. Note that single-leg balancing (figure 11.6) and standing toe raises are fully weight bearing with a closed kinetic chain.

The final progressive stage before return to activity should include progressive eccentric strengthening. This may be initiated with standing toe raises (figure 11.10). While the client is standing (with some support, if needed), have her raise up onto her toes and slowly return down. From the slow descent, she should move rapidly into plantar flexion. A progression of this exercise involves performing it on the edge of a stair and allowing the heel to lower.

Toor (2004) reported that clients in the final stage of recovery from Achilles tendinosis have responded well to regular progressive eccentric exercises such as the four-corner plyometric drill (figure 11.11). Set up four markers in a square, 3 m (10 ft) apart. From the center of the square, the client combines forward, backward, and lateral movements by touching various combinations of markers.

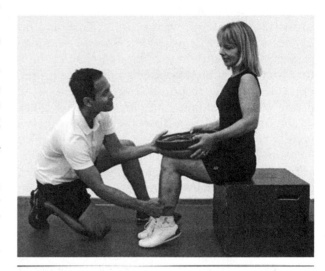

Figure 11.9   Seated heel lift.

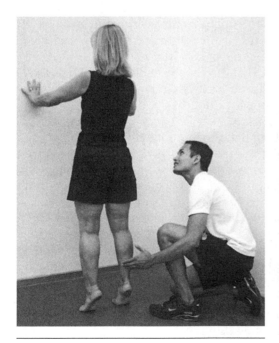

Figure 11.10   Standing toe raises.

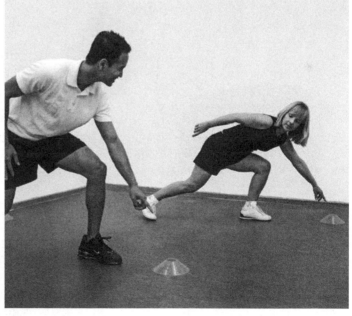

Figure 11.11   Four-corner plyometric drill.

Shin Splints

Shin splints, or more precisely **medial tibial stress syndrome** (MTSS), is an inflammation of the fascia, tendon, periosteum, bone, or a combination of these along the posterior medial border of the tibia (figure 11.12). Sometimes referred to as **posterior shin splints**, MTSS is probably associated with fatigue tear of fibers of the soleus or tibialis posterior muscle at its fascial insertion into the periosteum of the tibia (Korkola and Amendola 2001; Craig 2008). Recent evidence suggests that the pain may be due to microfractures in the medial tibia associated with a chronic bone remodeling response from fascial traction (Craig 2008). The pain can range from a slightly uncomfortable dull ache to an intensity that makes weight bearing difficult. Shin splints account for an estimated 10% to 20% of all injuries in runners and up to 60% of all overuse injuries of the leg (Couture and Karlson 2002). Shin splints are an overuse condition common to people who start a weight-bearing training program too vigorously, to jumpers (e.g., volleyball, basketball, high-impact aerobics), and to runners logging more than 30 miles (48 km) per week. Occurring in the upper anterior shin, **anterior shin splints** are aggravated by overuse of the tibialis anterior and in some clients may reveal a stress fracture (Fick et al. 1992).

Medial tibial stress syndrome pain is in the muscles that are active during the first 80% of the stance phase, such as the tibialis posterior and the flexors of the toes (Prentice 1994). The subtalar joint normally goes from a supinated position at heel strike to a pronated position during midstance and then returns to supination during push-off. Hyperpronation during midstance places these muscles under significant stress—they contract eccentrically (lengthening) to try to stabilize, but eventually the point of attachment (origin) will become inflamed. Even more significant may be the maximum velocity of the pronation (Craig 2008).

Other factors sometimes related to MTSS include a tight Achilles tendon, running on hard surfaces, progressing too rapidly in training, logging exceptionally long training hours, muscle imbalance between weak shin and strong calf muscles, and improper footwear. The 10% rule suggests that the workout volume or intensity should not increase by more than 10% per week. If a biomechanical abnormality or training error is the cause, it must first be corrected. Allow the affected muscles to rest, sometimes for several weeks, depending on the pain. Use this time to ice (8-10 min, two or three times a day) and apply light pressure from an elastic wrap and elevate. Perhaps investigate the need for orthotics or to ensure that the shoe is well cushioned in the heel and insole. Andrish and Work (1990) suggested stopping the offending activity until the pain subsides (usually about 1-2 weeks), resuming training at about half the previous intensity, and gradually working up to previous levels over 3 to 6 weeks. Returning too quickly is the most common reason shin splints recur. Be sure your client pays close attention to warm-ups and cool-downs, ensuring complete stretching of the lower leg. Consider prescribing cross-training, particularly with non–weight-bearing exercise such as swimming, stair climbing, cycling, rowing, or low-impact aerobic classes. Throughout the recovery, if your client is a diehard jogger, direct him to the grass or to flat bark-covered trails and increase mileage before increasing intensity.

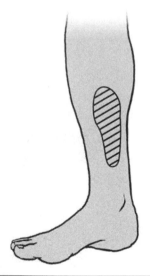

Figure 11.12 Pain location for shin splints (medial tibial stress syndrome).

MTSS
Stretching Guidelines and Prescription

Inflammation of the tibialis posterior and flexors of the toes causes tightness and decreased flexibility. After some rest and anti-inflammatory treatment, stretching exercises should target these muscles as well as the gastrocnemius, soleus, tibialis anterior, and peroneals. After some aerobic exercise to warm the muscles, your client should do static stretches several times, holding all the stretches at least 30 s and holding stretches for the Achilles tendon up to 60 s. The heel-cord box as shown in figure 11.3 is very effective. The bent-knee position aids in stretching the tibialis posterior as well as the soleus.

Figure 11.8 uses surgical tubing (or TheraBand) to stretch the calf muscles. The peroneal muscles on the lateral side of the calf are the ankle evertors and can be stretched by wrapping a TheraBand around the lateral side of the foot and pulling the ankle into inversion (figure 11.13). With the client in a seated position, have her invert her foot and wrap a TheraBand around the forefoot, placing tension on the band. She slowly everts her foot against this tension. Your client should relax at the end of the range of motion to feel the stretch. Using the TheraBand or a hand (figure 11.14), have the client pull the foot up behind, bringing the heel to the buttock. This shifts the stretch to the front of the shin to reach the tibialis anterior. Although this can stretch the quads, grasping the instep (not the ankle) and pulling up on the foot gives the shin an effective stretch.

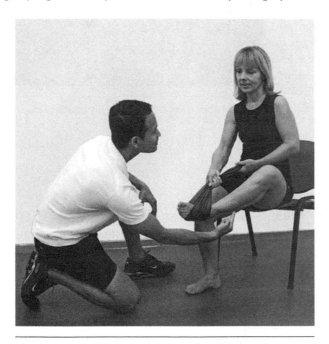

Figure 11.13   TheraBand peroneal stretch.

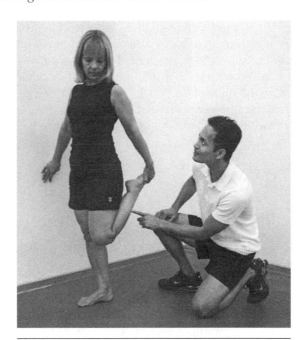

Figure 11.14   Heel-to-buttock stretch.

MTSS
Strengthening Guidelines and Prescription

Start a strengthening program when the pain is minimal. The affected muscles in shin splints usually show signs of weakness and early fatigue. Toe curls with a towel (figure 11.5) will strengthen the flexors of the toes and the tibialis posterior as well as strengthen the arch to minimize hyperpronation.

The anterior muscle groups are very often weak and out of balance with the posterior plantar flexors. Movements as simple as seated or standing toe lifts or drawing the alphabet with the feet usually present enough of an overload for the early stages of conditioning. The opposite foot, a partner's resistance, or surgical tubing can all be used to create added resistance to this dorsiflexion.

Clients with MTSS (posterior shin splints) should also strengthen their ankle evertors and invertors. A uniplane wobble board, which is simple to build (figure 11.15), can be used with the foot aligned with the half-cylinder keel under the board. In bare feet, the client rocks side to side on the wobble board in a controlled manner, touching the right edge and then the left edge. Although a well-cushioned shoe is mandatory for a return to training, most of the rehabilitation exercises provide greater benefit if done with bare feet. Have clients progress to keeping their balance on a multiplane wobble board.

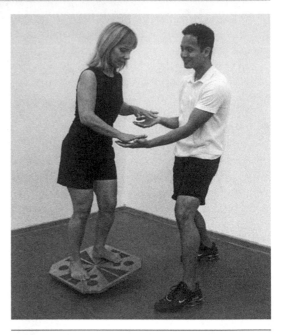

Figure 11.15   Wobble board inversion and eversion.

Patellofemoral Syndrome

The patella moves up and down within a groove at the front of the femur (figure 11.16, *a* and *c*). Deviation from this aligned tracking produces patellofemoral pain, resulting from irritation behind the patella and wearing of the articular cartilage. Sometimes called "runner's knee," this condition differs from "jumper's knee," which is a patellar tendon tendinitis with pain lower near the attachment of the tendon to the tibial tuberosity (figure 11.16*b*).

Clients may complain of pain in the front of the knee when they sit in a car or at the movies, kneel or squat, get up from a chair and start walking, or go up or down stairs. The pain may appear at the beginning or end of a workout and may result in swelling or fullness in the knee. Other symptoms may include giving way, popping, catching, or locking (Doucette and Goble 1992). Patellofemoral syndrome is one of the most common knee complaints, having been shown to account for 57.5% of the knee injuries in one group of runners (Taunton et al. 1987). It occurs most often in women, in the young, and in those who are active in running or in court sports such as basketball and tennis.

Improper alignment and tracking of the patella are major causes of patellofemoral pain (figure 11.16*c*). Your clients may notice such pain especially as they run up hills or straighten their knees with weights. Causes of poor tracking include the following:

- **Deficiency of supporting and stabilizing muscles.** Kneecap motion is guided by the quadriceps, particularly the vastus medialis. This muscle may be less resistant to fatigue than the vastus lateralis, creating an uneven pull on the patella (Earle and Baechle 2004).

- **Tightness of supporting structures.** If the vastus lateralis or the lateral retinaculum (figure 11.16*a*) is tight, lateral tilting or tracking of the patella may occur. Because the iliotibial band is connected to the lateral retinaculum, its tightness may affect tracking during flexion. Both the hamstrings and the gastrocnemius cross the knee joint, and tightness can increase patellar pressure. Tight hamstrings increase knee flexion and can change lower leg mechanics. A tight gastrocnemius muscle can limit dorsiflexion and produce excessive subtalar motion (Galea and Albers 1994).

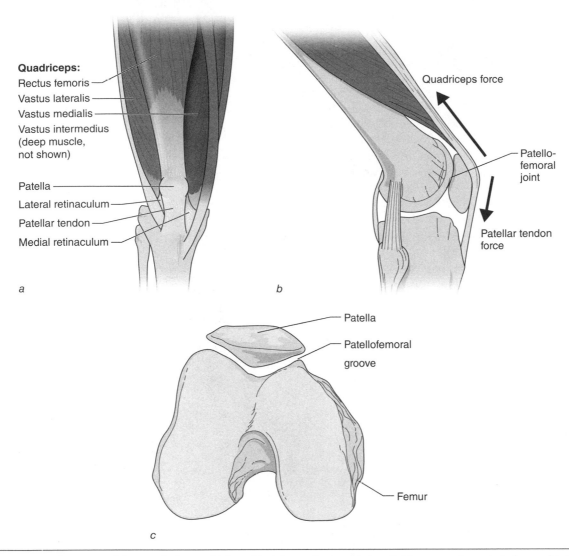

Quadriceps:
Rectus femoris
Vastus lateralis
Vastus medialis
Vastus intermedius
(deep muscle,
not shown)

Patella
Lateral retinaculum
Patellar tendon
Medial retinaculum

a

Quadriceps force
Patello-
femoral
joint
Patellar tendon
force

b

Patella
Patellofemoral
groove
Femur

c

Figure 11.16 Anatomy of the patellofemoral joint with *(a)* anterior knee joint, *(b)* forces on the patellofemoral joint, and *(c)* patellofemoral tracking.

• **Structural alignments.** Wide hips and knock-knees may contribute to lateral tracking of the patella (Bahr and Maehlum 2004). An awareness of this alignment problem can help you direct your client to alternative activities or reduce the prescription load. Excessive pronation of the foot usually causes a rotation of the tibia, which may result in increased lateral pull on the patella. Orthotics may be appropriate.

Besides poor tracking, patellofemoral syndrome may be caused by acute trauma, chronic repetitive stress such as running, sudden increases in workloads or mileage, uneven or hilly terrain, or poor running shoes. In addition, deep squats and other closed kinetic chain exercises requiring knee flexion greater than 90° increase compression and tissue stress between the patella and the femur.

To avoid this syndrome, have your client replace running shoes that are older than a year, have more than 500 miles (about 800 km) on them, or look worn out on the soles or broken down on the uppers. Ask at-risk clients if they have changed their intensity, distance, or terrain. Have them stay away from hills, switch to lower-impact aerobic activities, or decrease mileage. DePalma and Perkins (2004) reported that the substantial forces generated in landing can be reduced by 60% through absorbed forces in the ankle and foot. When the knee and hip go through a wider range of flexion, another 25% of the force is reduced when combined with forefoot landing.

However, when a client already has knee pain, stop all painful activities for at least 2 to 4 weeks. Aspirin or ibuprofen may help ease symptoms, as may icing. Clients should exercise caution in taking nonsteroidal anti-inflammatory drugs (NSAIDs) for more than 3 weeks to avoid side effects (Faltus 2009).

Patellofemoral Syndrome
Stretching Guidelines and Prescription

Tightness in a number of muscles may contribute to patellofemoral pain: vastus lateralis, iliotibial band, hamstrings, and gastrocnemius. Stretching the quadriceps (including vastus lateralis) can decrease patellofemoral compression during dynamic activities. However, stretching this muscle may be contraindicated if pain exists past the 70° position of knee flexion. Have your client stand with his right leg forward on a stair or chair and left leg back, keeping the torso upright and lower back flat. From this lunge position, direct him to lower and lean forward until he feels a moderate stretch in the front of the left thigh. He should allow the right knee to bend and rotate the pelvis under to increase the stretch, then hold (figure 11.17).

To stretch the iliotibial band, your client stands with legs crossed (with support if needed), crosses the affected leg behind the other leg, and pushes her hip in the opposite direction. The affected leg is close to an adjacent wall or table and behind the other leg. She then moves her pelvis toward the table, keeping the back leg straight (figure 11.18).

To stretch the hamstrings, your client places one leg onto a bench or table with knees straight. While holding her back straight, she bends forward from the hips to a point of tension. She moves her pelvis and trunk as a unit, slowly lowering her abdomen toward her thigh. After about 20 s, she lowers slightly, tilting the pelvis forward and holding for another 10 to 15 s (figure 11.19). The gastrocnemius can be stretched effectively with exercises shown in figures 11.3 and 11.8.

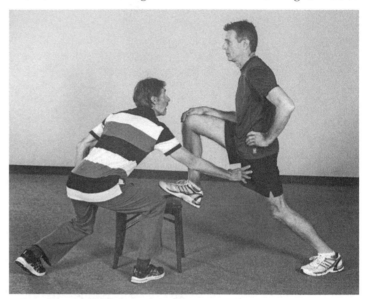

Figure 11.17   Vastus lateralis stretch.

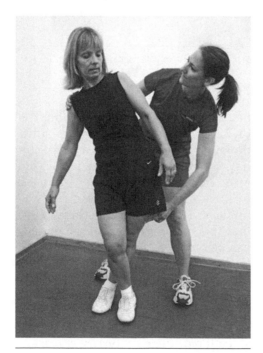

Figure 11.18   Iliotibial band stretch.

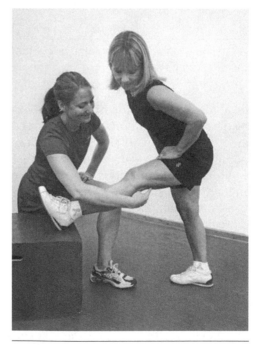

Figure 11.19   Hamstring stretch.

Patellofemoral Syndrome
Strengthening Guidelines and Prescription

To guarantee a safe return to normal activities, your client must fully regain strength in the injured leg. Have him do the following exercises every second day, stopping if there is any pain or if he is unable to do the exercise correctly. Most people do well by progressing from about 5 to 15 repetitions, then adding a second set and building from 10 to 15 reps. The client should allow a minute or two between sets, depending on his stage of recovery, eventually building to 4 or 5 sets. Exercises to strengthen the vastus medialis will promote a return to muscular balance and increase the medial stabilization of the patella.

Start with end range extensions, in which your client reclines with a firm pillow or rolled towel under her knee to create about 30° of flexion. With her hip slightly rotated laterally and the opposite knee flexed, she then straightens her knee and holds for 10 s. Small ankle weights can increase resistance.

Exercises with the foot in a fixed position on the ground (closed-chain exercises) are especially functional because they use common movement patterns and control the body's momentum (eccentric contractions), as well as teach kinesthetic awareness. Closed kinetic chain exercises are favored in therapeutic exercise prescription, particularly for the knee (Post 1998). Closed kinetic chain exercises include leg press, partial squats, stepping, stationary cycling, and plyometrics. With any closed kinetic chain exercise, ensure that the medial side of the knee is aligned with the inside of the foot and that the knee does not pass beyond the front of the foot. Watching your client's alignment is very important because the exercises are unforgiving if the biomechanics are faulty. Two specific examples of closed-chain exercises are forward lunges (figure 11.20) and step-downs (figure 11.21).

In a forward lunge, your client steps forward about 2 to 3 ft (0.60-0.91 m) from a standing position, keeping the knee over the foot and not allowing the front knee to flex more than 90°. At the same time, he lowers the back knee until it is 4 to 6 in. (10-15 cm) from the floor. Ensure that the knee does not go beyond the front foot. He returns to an upright position and alternates legs. As strength increases, he can hold small hand weights.

In a step-down, the client stands sideways on a bottom step or aerobic step box with the injured leg nearest the stair. Supporting the weight as the knee bends, he slowly bends the injured knee until the opposite foot lightly touches the ground and then slowly straightens it. As he progresses, he may add hand weights or use higher steps.

Working with a wobble board (figure 11.15) can strengthen supporting muscles of the lower leg. Open-chain exercises (the foot is free), such as those provided by isokinetic knee extension equipment, can isolate a muscle like the vastus medialis by using range of motion (ROM) stops for the last 30° of extension. These exercises can also introduce higher-speed contractions under stabilized conditions, which may be appropriate for athletes.

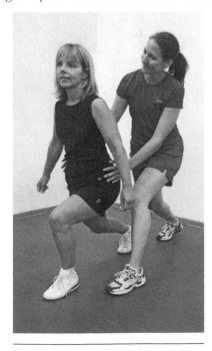

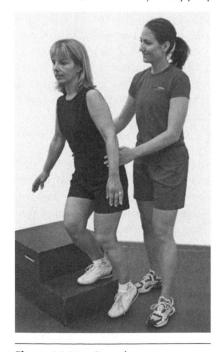

Figure 11.20   Forward lunges.   **Figure 11.21**   Step-downs.

Rubber tubing or TheraBands can also be used, especially when knee movement is still painful. From a supine position, with the tubing around both legs just above the knee, your client performs straight-leg raises to strengthen hip flexors (figure 11.22). Because most of the vastus medialis originates from the tendon of the adductor magnus (Doucette and Goble 1992), strengthening the muscles of the inner thigh may help pull the kneecap into alignment. For the inner thigh pillow squeeze (figure 11.23), from a recline position with knees bent and a pillow between them, have your client hold or pulse the squeeze for 15 to 20 s, repeating three to five times. Finally, progression of the program may involve multidirectional movement patterns with increased eccentric resistance.

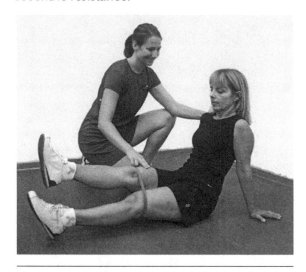

Figure 11.22   Straight-leg raises with tubing.

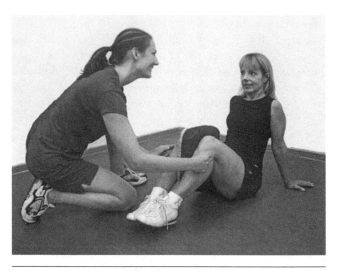

Figure 11.23   Inner thigh pillow squeeze.

Hamstring Strain

The hamstring muscle, located on the posterior thigh, comprises the semimembranosus, semitendinosus, and biceps femoris (figure 11.24). The hamstrings are biarticular (two-joint) muscles producing extension of the hip and flexion of the knee. As with other frequently injured biarticular muscles (e.g., rectus femoris or long head of the biceps brachii), the hamstrings are subject to stretching at more than one point. Injuries to this muscle complex usually affect the common origin on the ischial tuberosity and may affect the insertion behind the knee or the belly of the muscle. As with most muscle strains, symptoms include tenderness and, usually, a large area of swelling. An injured person feels discomfort when gentle resistance is applied against knee flexion and hip extension.

Hamstring strains are described in three grades. Grade I sufferers complain of tightness at the end range of hip flexion and some pain on palpation. People with grade II strains usually have adjusted their gaits, perhaps landing flat-footed with limited swing-through. Knee flexion and hip extension may cause moderate to severe pain with noticeable weakness. Recovery takes between 1 and 3 weeks. Grade III hamstring strains usually

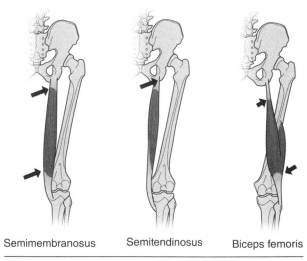

Semimembranosus   Semitendinosus   Biceps femoris

Figure 11.24   Anatomy of the hamstrings. Arrows indicate most common sites of injury.

require the use of crutches and require a 3- to 12-week rehabilitation period (De Palma 1994).

Hamstring strains are common with sprinters, gymnasts, and athletes in soccer, football, lacrosse, and basketball. These strains can result from a quick, explosive contraction while the hip is in flexion and the knee is extending. For those clients involved in running activities, the hamstrings may simultaneously work concentrically at the hip and eccentrically at the knee (e.g., striding before foot strike). The hamstring muscles decelerate the forward swing of the tibia, thus opposing the activity of the quadriceps. The imbalance of an overly strong quadriceps may cause the injury. Other causes may be hamstring fatigue or weakness, tight hamstrings, imbalance between the medial and lateral hamstrings, or improper running style.

The strong tendency for hamstring injuries to recur makes a solid case for a supplemental exercise prescription including stretching, strengthening, and cardiovascular maintenance. Best and Garrett (1996) reported that following a hamstring injury, flexibility and lower eccentric strength decrease. Some authors have suggested that hamstring injuries due to muscle imbalances can be reduced with eccentric training programs (Page et al. 2010). Initial treatment typically consists of rest, ice, compression (elastic wrap), elevation, and pain relief (e.g., acetaminophen for 7-10 days). After the acute stages, heat (hot packs, whirlpool, or heating pad) may be used before the stretching exercises (DeLisa 1998). All activities should be followed by ice treatments to decrease inflammation and discomfort. Although someone with a grade I hamstring strain may continue to be active, a supplementary prescription for extra stretching and strengthening should begin immediately to avoid further injury.

Hamstring Strain
Stretching Guidelines and Prescription

In addition to predisposing your client to a hamstring strain, tight hamstrings may cause low back pain. Because hamstrings attach to the back of the pelvis (see figure 11.24), tight hamstrings can prevent the pelvis from tilting forward when the spine flexes, forcing all movement to come from the low back. Avoid stretches such as standing or sitting toe touches, in which the lower body is static and the upper body is rounded and actively flexing.

The doorway hamstring stretch (figure 11.25) promotes a static upper body with lower body hip flexion. Your client lies on his back in a doorway with his buttocks close to the wall. One leg extends through the door while the other is raised up against the wall. He slowly moves his buttocks closer to the wall to increase the stretch. The heel slides up the wall, gradually straightening the leg; after the client feels a comfortable, pleasant stretch, he holds his position for 30 to 60 s. This may also be performed as a self-administered proprioceptive neuromuscular facilitation stretch (chapter 8).

The straddle hamstring stretch (figure 11.26) uses a table or chair for support. With feet pointing forward and one foot about 3 ft (0.91 m) in front of the other, your client bends forward at the hips (not the waist), feeling the stretch in the front leg hamstring. As the front leg stretches, he must avoid hyperextending the knee. He holds for 30 s, lowers slightly, and holds for another 15 to 30 s. Maintaining the lumbar lordotic curve in the low back isolates the hamstrings and safeguards the back.

You may need to delay these stretches until the second week for grade II hamstring strains. Active ROM movements in a prone or seated position can begin earlier or as soon as there is no pain (De Palma 1994). Work with a physician or physiotherapist for the timing on grade III strains; your client should be pain free.

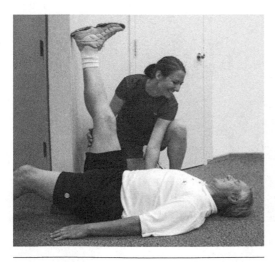

Figure 11.25 Doorway hamstring stretch.

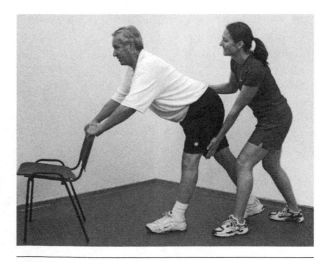

Figure 11.26 Straddle hamstring stretch.

Hamstring Strain
Strengthening Guidelines and Prescription

You can begin resistance strengthening exercises immediately for a grade I strain, after about 3 to 6 days for grade II, and after 10 to 14 days for a grade III strain (De Palma 1994).

Avoid resistance exercises using a machine (such as knee flexion in a prone position), because the hamstrings are less efficient in a shortened position. However, knee flexion from a seated position allows the hamstrings to start stretched at the buttocks, improving their mechanical advantage in working through a full ROM. An added advantage with some machines is the ability to change the lever arm and torque by adjusting the position of the lower leg pad. A straight-leg hip extension machine is also safe for strengthening hamstrings. If such a machine is not available, substitute elastic tubing or bands (figure 11.27). With a band or tubing around both ankles, the client extends one leg straight backward.

Eccentric exercises such as ball curls (figure 11.28) should be part of a preventive program. From a supine position, with both feet on the stability ball, the client raises hips until knees, hips, and shoulders are in a straight line. Using arms on the floor for balance, she pushes the ball forward and back.

To simulate the function of the hamstrings during running, Santana (2000) suggested a challenging stability ball exercise that combines a bridge, a leg curl, and some alternate leg action (figure 11.29). The client starts in a bridge position with one heel on the ball and the other leg on the ground flexed at the knee. He pushes downward with the heel on the ball, raising the hips and torso. The leg pushes against the ball, lifting the hips upward as the opposite leg curls forward; the client then returns to the ball and repeats with the other leg. He repeatedly raises and lowers the bent knee, building speed with recovery.

Isokinetic exercises, such as with an electronic Cybex knee flexion machine, are effective in conjunction with isotonic and isometric exercises. Progressions to faster speeds may be more sport specific for athletes.

In later phases of all three grades of hamstring strains, educate your clients to perform lightweight squats. Clients should do squats rather than leg curls because in a squat, the feet are fixed on the ground and the lower body joints form a closed kinetic chain.

If your client is pain free, have him swim or bike to maintain cardiovascular condition. Add jogging a few days later if appropriate. Simulate sport-specific activities for athletes, gradually introducing those skills that involve eccentric contraction of the hamstrings. It has been shown that a progressive agility training program with trunk stabilization exercises is more effective than an isolated hamstring stretching and strengthening rehabilitation program (Sherry and Best 2004).

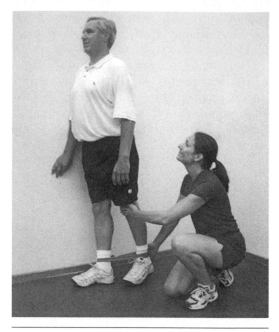

Figure 11.27 Straight-leg hip extension with tubing.

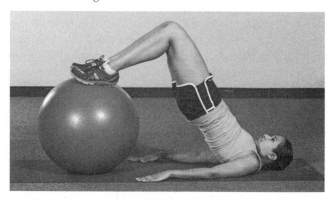

Figure 11.28 Ball curls.

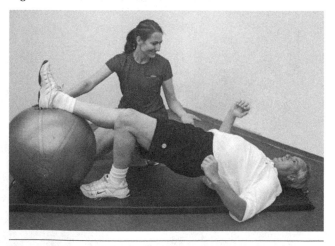

Figure 11.29 Stability ball simulated run.

Low Back Pain

Low back pain in active clients is common and often recurs. Estimates of lifetime prevalence range from 60% to 90%, and the annual incidence is 5% (Drezner and Herring 2001). Back pain usually arises in the soft tissues such as ligaments, fascia, and muscle and with most clients should last no longer than 3 weeks. Ninety percent of clients with back pain should lose their symptoms within 6 weeks with or without intervention (Waddell 1987). People whose pain persists beyond 6 weeks, or those who have exacerbated a previous injury, usually have not removed the stresses that created the original injury.

Back pain is usually attributed to strain of the lumbar muscles, inflammation of the facet joints, or degeneration of the intervertebral discs. Most back injuries are from movements causing microtraumas. Such movements may be performed for weeks or months until they cause failure of the tissue, resulting in a macrotrauma. Common movements that can cause microtraumas include repeated incorrect lifting, prolonged static postures (including sitting and flexion), and chronic physical stress on the spine or muscles.

Knowledge of the individual sport or training regimen can help us understand the injury mechanism. In skiing, throwing sports, weightlifting, and martial arts, the muscle–tendon insertions might become inflamed because of sudden or repeated loading. In football, the injury mechanism may be sudden loading (throwing), compression (falls or contact), or torsion (rapid turning). Dance and gymnastics involve increased lumbar lordosis and hyperextension, making these athletes susceptible to facet joint inflammation.

Tight hip flexor muscles initiate a common muscle imbalance pattern that affects lumbar motion. The result is an excessive anterior pelvic tilt and lumbar lordosis. These factors lengthen the hip extensors (e.g., hamstrings), placing them at a mechanical disadvantage and causing early recruitment of the spinal extensors (e.g., erector spinae).

Deep posterior muscles (e.g., multifidus muscles) work together with the deep abdominal muscles (e.g., transversus abdominis), the diaphragm, and the pelvic floor muscles as a functional stabilizing unit. But recent studies have indicated that pain has a reflex effect on muscle activity by inhibiting the deep stabilizing musculature while activating muscles like the iliopsoas and the erector spinae, which increases the anterior tilt forces (Bahr and Maehlum 2004).

Another common cause of back problems is simply aging. With increasing age, the nucleus pulposus decreases in volume and the vertebrae end up sitting closer to each other. The annulus fibrosus becomes more lax, and the increased play around the vertebral margins can cause osteophytes. These changes put more stress on the synovial facet joints and ligaments, leaving them inflamed and tender. Movements may become restricted and alignments altered (Liemohn 2001).

Long-term management consists of regaining muscle balance and joint ROM. Trunk muscles must be strengthened with exercises or swimming. You must also give each client personal counseling about suitable activities and advice on back care and lifting techniques. For example, Watkins (1999) showed a 33% reduction in the tension on the spinal extensor muscles during lifting from a squat rather than a stoop, and a 50% reduction of core stability was maintained.

Be aware of the stage of the injury. Gradually introduce appropriate exercises following the acute treatment stage (mainly modality treatment and pain relief). Be sure that your clients ask their therapists or physicians for any precautions or advice that will help you design a safe and effective exercise plan.

Base your exercise prescription goals for back rehabilitation on the specific diagnosis, history, and evaluation your client receives from his physician or therapist:

- Which structures and muscles need stretching?
- Which structures and muscles need strengthening?
- What deviations in posture, alignment, and stabilization need attention (see chapter 8)?
- What faults are present in movement mechanics in daily life, work environment, sport, or exercise routine (see chapters 5 and 10)?
- See the brief condition descriptions, with implications for exercise, in table 11.2. Remember, if your client has a back problem of any kind, she should consult a physician, physiotherapist, or chiropractor.

Table 11.2 Low Back Conditions and Exercise Implications

Condition	Description and cause	Exercise implications
Muscular strain	Clients report a history of sudden or chronic stress that initiates pain in a muscular area during the workout. Pain is provoked by contraction or stretching of the involved muscle. If an overuse injury, correct any improper posture or movement patterns.	Prescribe mild contraction followed by a stretch (figures 11.30-11.32). Progress with intensity. Include abdominal strengthening (figures 11.38, 11.41, 11.42) and active extension exercise (figures 11.36, 11.40, 11.43). At early stages of tissue healing, avoid direct contraction of the strained muscle (e.g., hyperextension) and passive lumbar flexion (e.g., knee-to-chest stretch) (Earle and Baechle 2004).
Piriformis or quadratus lumborum myofascial pain or strain	The piriformis muscle refers pain to the posterior sacroiliac region and buttocks. It is a deep ache that worsens during sitting with hips flexed or adducted or during weight-bearing hip rotation. Pain from the quadratus lumborum is an aching or sharp pain in the lateral back area and upper buttock. Pain is felt on moving from sitting to standing, during prolonged standing, or during sneezing.	Stretching is the main component in changing any myofascial pain. Exercises should include stretching exercises such as those in figures 11.31, 11.32, and 11.35. They should also include strengthening exercises such as those in figures 11.37, 11.39, 11.42, and 11.43.
Lumbar facet joint sprains	The client will report a specific event that caused the problem or a series of repetitive stresses that progressively got more painful. Pain gets sharper with certain movements. The pain feels deep and localized near the spinous process.	Stretching in all directions should be within a comfort range (figures 11.30, 11.31, 11.33). Exercises should involve joint mobility, trunk stabilization, and posture control. Pain-free abdominal and back strengthening is important (figures 11.36, 11.38, 11.40, 11.41).
Disc-related back problems	Pain is usually central but radiates across the back of one side. The client may describe a sudden or gradual onset after a workout that becomes more severe during resumption of activity. Forward bending and sitting increase pain, and a postural analysis may reveal a shifted hip and slightly flexed posture.	Unless working with a therapist, prescribe only gentle mobilization and postural exercises until the client is pain free (figures 11.30, 11.33, 11.34). At this point, abdominal and back extensor strengthening should be emphasized with an eye to preventing reinjury (figures 11.36, 11.38, 11.39, 11.40). Avoid exercises involving significant lumbar flexion such as bent-over rowing, full sit-ups, deadlift, standing toe touch, spinal twists, and flexion-based movements in aerobic dance.
Sacroiliac (SI) joint dysfunction	The client will describe a dull, achy back pain near the bone prominences of the SI joint. The pain may radiate to the buttocks or thigh, particularly during hip flexion, during side bending to the painful side, or during the stance phase of walking. Pain may also be felt during trunk rotations, landing heavily on one leg, kicking, and jumping.	If one side of the back is tight, stretching is important (figures 11.31, 11.32, 11.35). Exercises that help (re)gain alignment and stability of the pelvis are important. Appropriate exercises may include those in figures 11.37 through 11.40.

Low Back Pain
General Prescription

A comprehensive approach to low back pain should include lumbar stabilization exercises; correction of muscle inflexibilities; exercises to improve endurance of the lumbar spine, abdominal muscles, and kinetic chain; aerobic conditioning; and correction of faulty mechanics. Instability of a spine segment and poor endurance of trunk musculature contribute significantly to low back pain (Schilling 2008). Exercises should be done with a "neutral" spine (normal low back curvature) to limit the compressive loads on the intervertebral discs. The following exercises will increase both the strength and the flexibility of the back:

- **Kneeling back stretch.** Have the client tuck head and reach forward, rounding the back and moving the chest toward the floor (figure 11.30).

- **Single knee to chest.** The client lies supine with low back pushed down. The client pulls one knee to the chest—enough to feel a comfortable stretch in the low back (figure 11.31).

- **Lying knee rocking.** The client lies supine with knees bent 90°. The knees slowly rock from side to side through a pain-free ROM. The back will rotate slightly (figure 11.32).

- **Mad cat stretch.** The client arches the back while tucking the chin and tightening the stomach (figure 11.33).

- **Prone press-up.** From a prone position, the client extends elbows to raise upper body. Hips stay on the floor and the back is relaxed (figure 11.34).

- **Spinal twist.** The client sits with right leg straight and left leg bent and on the outside of the right knee. The right elbow is placed on the outside of the upper left thigh. The client slowly turns her head to look over her left shoulder (figure 11.35).

- **Back press.** Lying on back with knees bent, the client tightens the stomach by pressing elbows to floor (figure 11.36).

- **Diagonal curl-up.** Lying on back with knees bent at 90° and pelvis stabilized, the client raises the head and shoulders while rotating to one side, reaching with arms at sides (figure 11.37).

- **Hip lift bridge.** Lying on back with both knees bent 90°, the client lifts the buttocks from the floor and extends one knee, keeping stomach tight (figure 11.38).

- **Opposite arm and leg lifts.** From a prone position (or on all fours), the client raises the opposite arm and leg 4 to 6 in. (10-15 cm) from the floor. Firm pillows or rolled towels should be under the pelvis and forehead (figure 11.39).

- **Supported hip extension.** With the torso leaning flat over a table, the client raises legs alternately from the floor (figure 11.40).

- **Seated trunk rotation with tubing.** The client holds the band tight to chest (taut) and gently rotates away with pelvis and knees in place and back straight, exercising only within a pain-free ROM (figure 11.41).

- **Diagonal downward rotation with tubing.** Standing with feet shoulder-width apart, the client pulls tubing with both hands downward across the body (figure 11.42).

- **Diagonal upward rotation with tubing.** Standing with feet shoulder-width apart, the client pulls tubing with both hands, straightening the body and rotating away from the door or anchor (figure 11.43).

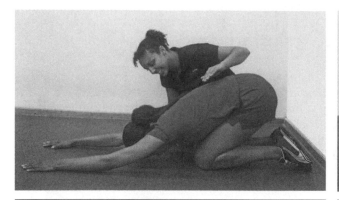

Figure 11.30 Kneeling back stretch.

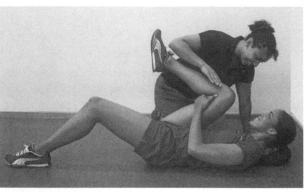

Figure 11.31 Single knee to chest.

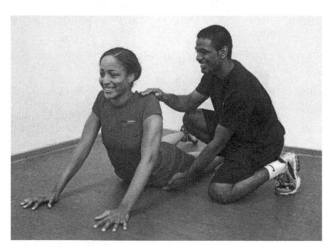

Figure 11.32 Lying knee rocking.

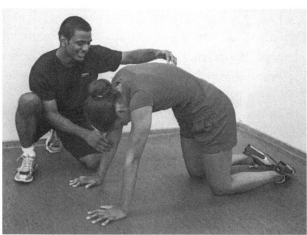

Figure 11.33 Mad cat stretch.

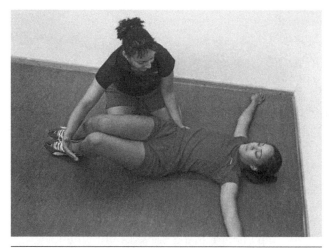

Figure 11.34 Prone press-up.

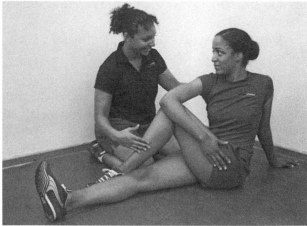

Figure 11.35 Spinal twist.

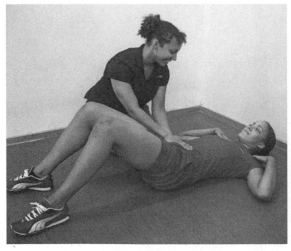

Figure 11.36 Back press.

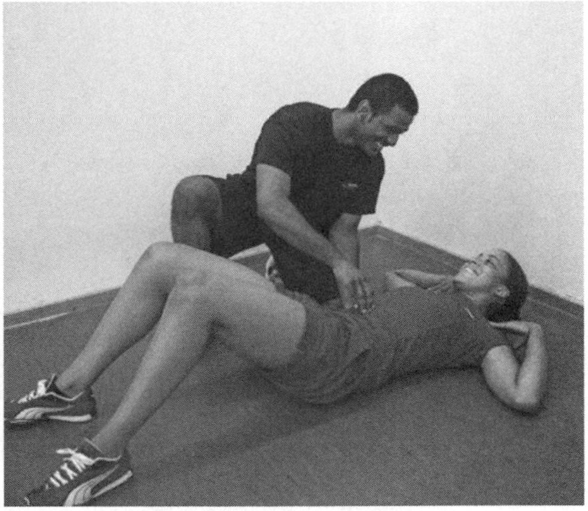

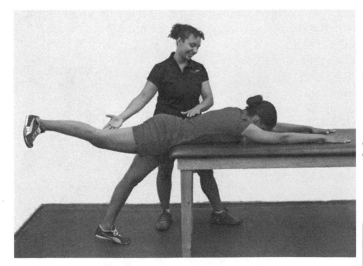

Figure 11.37 Diagonal curl-up.

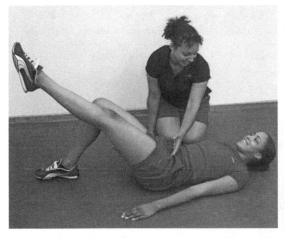

Figure 11.38 Hip lift bridge.

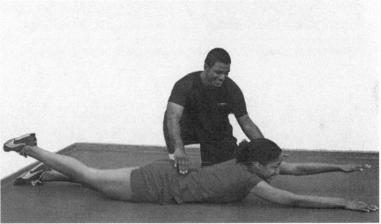

Figure 11.39 Opposite arm and leg lifts.

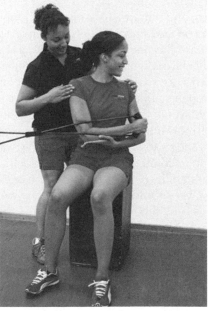

Figure 11.40 Supported hip extension.

Figure 11.41 Seated trunk rotation with tubing.

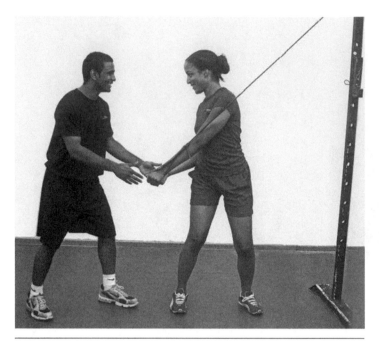

Figure 11.42   Diagonal downward rotation with tubing.

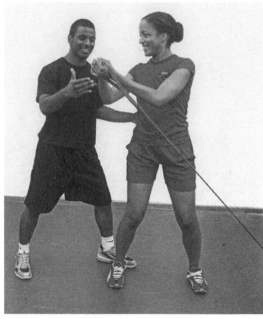

Figure 11.43   Diagonal upward rotation with tubing.

Low Back Pain
Spine Stability Prescription

Spine stability is provided by passive connective tissue restraints, active muscle contraction, and neural control mechanisms. Clinical instability is defined as a decrease in the capacity of the stabilizing system of the spine to maintain a motion segment within its physiological limits, which can lead to structural changes, neurological dysfunction, and incapacitating pain (Schilling 2008).

When teaching clients about how their backs work, I describe the structure as having three layers: deep, middle, and outer, each with its own function. The tiny muscles of the deep layer provide positional information to the brain. The middle layer provides the bulk of the routine stability and includes the quadratus lumborum, multifidus, and transversus abdominis (along with the diaphragm and pelvic floor muscles to create a "stiffen-

ing" effect on the lumbar spine). The use of a stability ball will increase the need to keep steady and will engage this middle layer of muscles to a larger degree. Research has shown a positive trend toward enhancing spinal stability through stability ball training (Carter et al. 2006). The outer layer of thick, long muscles provides for more powerful movements and includes the erector spinae, obliques, and rectus abdominis. It may be that the tension from the thoracolumbar fascia is also a contributing factor to lumbar stability (Schilling 2008). One or two exercises for each layer should be included in any well-balanced preventive program, as in the following example:

• **Deep layer (positional):** Ball sitting single-foot contact—the client sits tall with low back in natural curve and adds arm movements. The client sits in the center of the ball with hips and knees at 90° and tightens core. She gradually straightens one leg, leaving one point of ground contact. Once stable, she mixes various arm movements (e.g., side, forward, alternating). She can progress by closing eyes (figure 11.44).

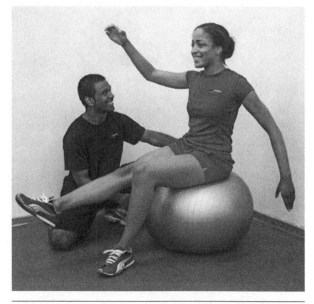

Figure 11.44   Deep layer (positional): ball sitting single-foot contact.

• **Middle layer (stabilization):** Belly blaster—the client lies on back with knees bent, pelvis tilted back, low back pressed into the mat, and abdominal core held tight. She lifts one leg with knee still bent. With shoulders on the mat, she extends the opposite arm and pushes the hand against the knee for 5 s. Repeat on the other side (figure 11.45).

• **Outer layer (power movements):** Dead bug run—the client lies on back with knees and hips at 90° and both arms directly up. She tilts pelvis back, presses low back into the mat, and holds abdominal core tight. She extends arms straight up and lifts both legs up with knees bent. She lifts one knee toward the chest and extends the other leg upward. When the one leg moves toward the chest, the arm on the same side is reaching over the head. Keeping back flat against mat, she extends one leg out and then the other in a cycling motion. She progresses by adding an alternating pumping motion of the arms. She continues until a smooth alternating pace is difficult (figure 11.46).

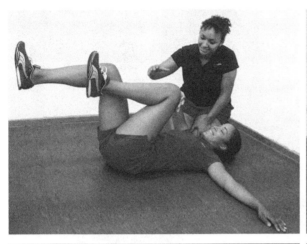

Figure 11.45 Middle layer (stabilization): belly blaster.

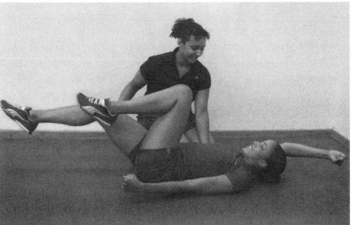

Figure 11.46 Outer layer (power movements): dead bug run.

Low Back Pain
Core Stability Prescription

Because lack of core stability can reinforce dysfunctional patterns of movement, you need to increase clients' postural awareness and conscious activation of the core stabilizers (figures 11.47-11.49). Proprioceptive (neuromuscular) training using closed kinetic chain exercises on a mobile surface is optimal for reactive stability (figures 11.50 and 11.51).

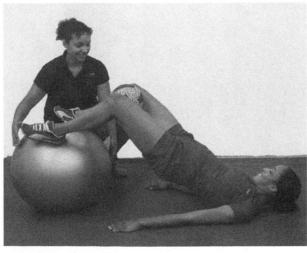

Figure 11.47 Buttocks curl.

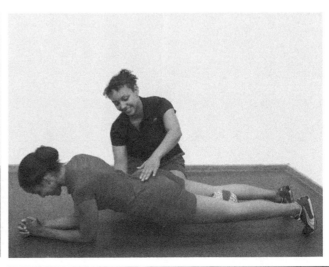

Figure 11.48 Plank.

Sit-ups, which are commonly prescribed to encourage healthy backs, have been shown to impose high compressive forces on the spine. McGill (2007) recommends exercises similar to the plank (figure 11.48) for the rectus abdominis, the side bridge (figure 11.50) for the lateral flexors such as the obliques and quadratus lumborum, and opposite arm and leg lifts (figure 11.39) for back extensors.

The following exercises will increase core back stability:

• **Buttocks curl.** The client lies on her back with hips and knees at 90° and a small ball between her knees. She then tightens her core. She curls the pelvis and lifts the buttocks off the floor. Have her avoid using the momentum of her legs. She holds for 5 s and slowly lowers (figure 11.47).

• **Plank.** The client kneels with forearms resting on the floor and the ball between the knees. She tightens her core. Have her lift knees and support the straightened body between her elbows and toes (figure 11.48).

• **Sitting hip rib lift.** The client sits in the center of the exercise ball with hips and knees at 90°. She places her hands on the top of the pelvis with her fingers on her abdominal muscles. Have her tighten her core (feel it!) and keep the rib cage elevated. She lifts one foot off the ground without allowing the level of the pelvis to drop. Have her progress by reaching arms above her head (figure 11.49).

• **Side bridge support on stability ball.** The client performs a side support position from the knees with the forearm across the ball. Have her maintain a straight line between the knees, hips, and shoulders. Progression may involve a side bridge from the feet and the addition of a top leg lift (figure 11.50).

• **Neuromuscular core.** Standing on rubber air pillows or wobble boards with a tight core, the client performs tosses to the trainer in a cross-body, diagonal direction. She uses the reverse movement when receiving the ball (figure 11.51).

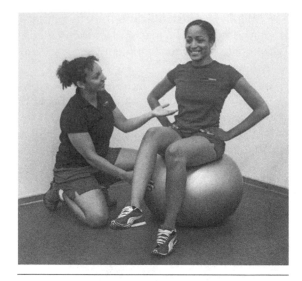

Figure 11.49 Sitting hip rib lift.

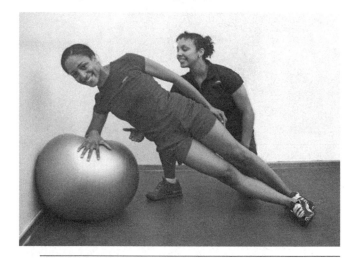

Figure 11.50 Side bridge support on stability ball.

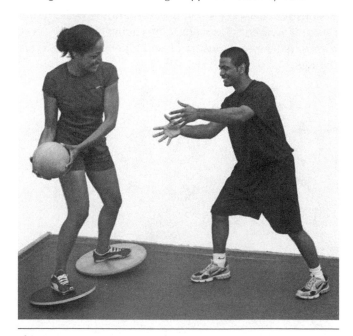

Figure 11.51 Neuromuscular core.

Rotator Cuff Tendinitis

Impingement in the shoulder is common because the space between the top of the humerus and the bottom of the acromion (the "roof" of the shoulder) is not particularly large (figure 11.52). Under certain circumstances, any of the structures running through the space—the supraspinatus tendon, the infraspinatus tendon, the tendon of the long head of the biceps, or the subacromial bursa—can be impinged on. Impingement usually occurs between the greater tubercle and either the acromion or the shoulder ligaments. Impingement impairs the ability of the supraspinatus to depress the humeral head, allowing the deltoid to pull the head up toward the acromion, worsening the impingement. Voluntary abduction ROM is reduced and painful, and scapulohumeral rhythm is altered (Bahr and Maehlum 2004). Faltus (2010) highlights the role of the infraspinatus muscle to depress the head of the humerus within the subacromial space in the range of 30° to 60° of arm abduction.

Impingement syndrome often originates with soft tissue trauma that sets up a cycle of pain, biomechanical changes, and weakness. Swelling of the tissues makes the space even smaller, further irritating the tendons. There also may be reduced blood supply and the start of tendon degeneration. Pain may occur when the shoulder is abducted while internally (medially) rotated as in the recovery phase of kayak paddling Any movement that calls for raising the arm overhead while internally rotated has the potential to impinge on the tendons and bursa and cause injury.

In clients without a history of trauma, repetitive overhead motion is usually the cause of impingement syndrome. As the muscles fatigue, tendon degeneration occurs. This is evident in activities with rapid eccentric contraction of the external (lateral) rotators such as throwing, swimming the butterfly, and serving in tennis. For example, someone doing an upright row exercise rotates his shoulder internally as he raises it. Raising the elbows high magnifies the danger of impingement. Another cause of impingement is muscle imbalance. The potential for muscle imbalance is high: Major muscles such as the pectoralis major and latissimus dorsi rotate internally, countered only by small muscles such as the infraspinatus and teres major (chapter 5). Tightness of the anterior shoulder musculature and weakness of the shoulder girdle stabilizers adversely affect glenohumeral rhythm during rapid and forceful movement patterns. Proper biomechanics requires a fine balance between joint mobility and stability. Overlooking such common causes may lead to progression of the impingement. As well, with scapular muscle weakness, compensatory activation and overuse of the upper trapezius during overhead motion are necessary to achieve the desired ROM and perhaps to avoid pain.

Modification of activities or of the workplace is critical for prevention and treatment. You can modify some activities to allow limited participation. It may be helpful to modify movements so that they are in the plane of the scapula, that is, with the humerus in abduction at about 30° of flexion anteriorly. Suggest swimming with fins and kicking only, or avoiding overhead serving when playing tennis or volleyball. Monitor your client's technique for faults such as upright rowing or lateral flys with the thumbs pointing down. To promote circulation in the shoulder area, prescribe upper body aerobics such as cross-country skiing, rowing, or arm ergometry.

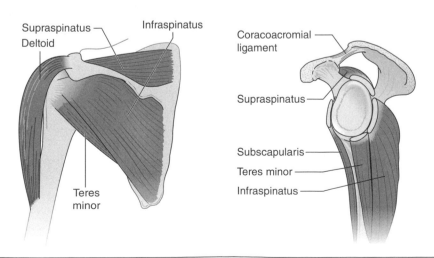

Figure 11.52   Anatomy of the shoulder rotator cuff.

Impingement Syndrome
Stretching Guidelines and Prescription

After testing for postural alignment and muscle tightness (chapter 4), address muscle imbalance with static stretches or proprioceptive neuromuscular facilitation stretches (chapter 8). Demonstrate proper execution of shoulder exercises, including ROM exercises as shown in figure 11.53. For this stretch, lying on table or floor, the client moves a wand toward the head and then down toward the waist through a pain-free ROM. Be sure that your client performs stretches with relaxed shoulder girdles and proper alignment and with elbows below shoulder height to avoid entrapment of the supraspinatus tendon.

Figures 11.54 and 11.55 illustrate specific stretches for internal and external rotators, designed to maintain muscle balance. For both of these stretches, with shoulder abducted 60° and externally rotated, the client turns his body gently away from the doorway and holds.

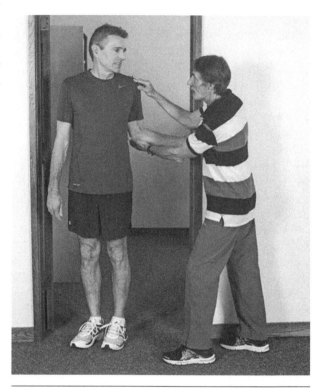

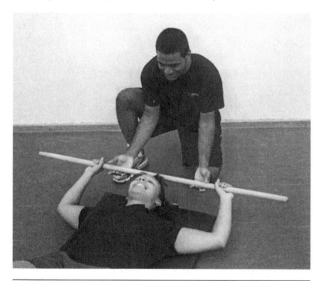

Figure 11.53 Lying wand shoulder rotations.

Figure 11.54 Doorway internal rotator stretch.

Overdevelopment or overtightness of the pectoralis major and anterior deltoid can force the shoulder into internal rotation. Figures 11.56 and 11.57 show exercises designed to stretch these muscles as well as the long head of the biceps. For the wall pectoralis stretch, with the arm horizontally abducted against a wall, the client turns his body away from the wall, then repeats with elbow bent (figure 11.56). For the anterior deltoid and biceps stretch, the client reaches behind with a straight arm and grasps the top of a chair. He moves his body forward and downward with arm directly back (figure 11.57).

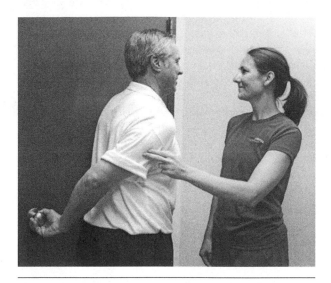

Figure 11.55 Doorway external rotator stretch.

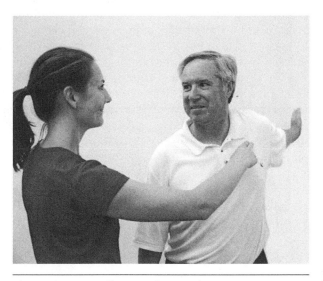

Figure 11.56 Wall pectoralis stretch.

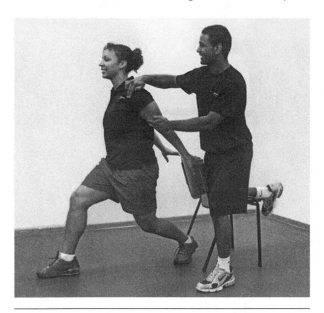

Figure 11.57 Anterior deltoid and biceps stretch.

Impingement Syndrome
Scapular Stabilization Guidelines and Prescription

Before progressing to specific shoulder joint resistive exercises, your clients should be able to lift their humerus (thumbs down) to 90° while maintaining the scapula stabilized in retraction (adduction). The exercise for this involves actively stabilizing the scapula in retraction while actively abducting the arms with elbows flexed. Figure 11.58 illustrates an exercise for this training as well as for strengthening the scapular retractors. From a supported prone or incline position, the client lifts dumbbells toward her chest with elbows bent and close to her side. Have her try to pinch the scapulae together. The wall-slide exercise (figure 11.59) stabilizes the scapula by recruiting the serratus anterior. With the scapulae depressed and protracted and the shoulder in 120° of flexion, the client slides a towel up and down a wall, providing pressure to the wall with the ulnar side of the wrist. Both these exercises may improve control of upward rotation while improving stabilization of the scapula against the chest wall, thereby avoiding impingement. Emphasize good coordination between movements of the humerus and the scapula (scapulohumeral rhythm). To achieve optimal results, postural correction including scapular stabilization exercises should be done before a rotator cuff or deltoid strengthening program (DePalma and Johnson 2003).

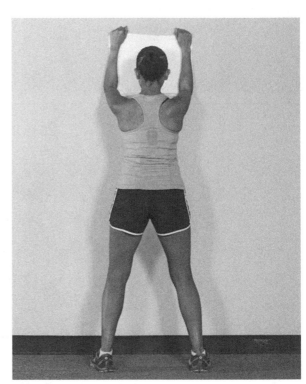

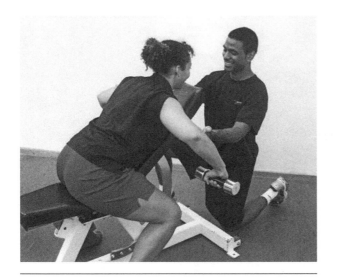

Figure 11.58   Scapular retraction with dumbbells.

Figure 11.59   Wall-slide exercise.

Impingement Syndrome
Shoulder Strengthening Guidelines and Prescription

A shoulder strengthening program for prevention or treatment of rotator cuff tendinitis centers around two activities: (1) strengthening the external rotators to maintain muscle balance and (2) strengthening the supraspinatus because of its role in impingement syndrome.

Figures 11.60 and 11.61 show resistance exercises for strengthening the external rotators. For shoulder external rotation with tubing, the client pulls tubing away from anchor point, keeping elbow bent at 90° (figure 11.60). For side-lying flys with dumbbells, from a side-lying position the client grasps a dumbbell or tubing with the top arm bent 90° at the elbow. He lifts the weight upward (keeping the elbow tight) and returns slowly (figure 11.61).

Releasing and catching a small ball in front of the body will eccentrically train the external rotators. For the eccentric ball catch the client's arm is abducted 90° and the elbow flexed, and a ball is held in the up position. The ball is released and the hand comes down quickly to catch it. The upper arm remains abducted (figure 11.62).

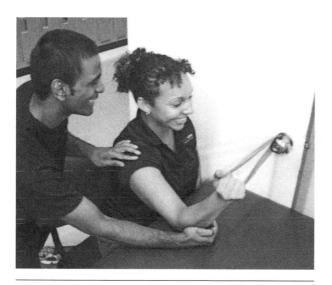

Figure 11.60 Shoulder external rotation with tubing.

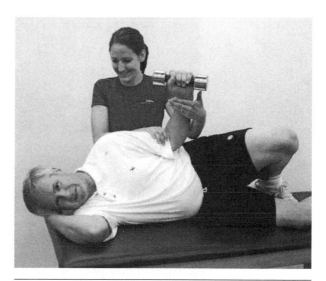

Figure 11.61 Side-lying flys with dumbbells.

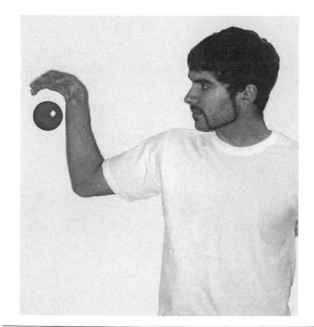

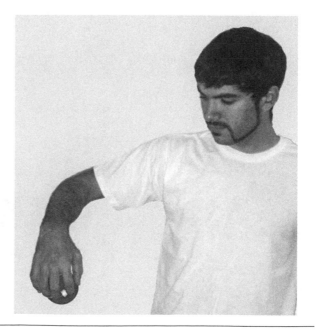

Figure 11.62 Eccentric ball catch.

The strengthening program should progressively increase repetitions, and then resistance, to build a strength and endurance base. Free weight exercises and a modified push-up on a wobble board train proprioception and stabilization. To perform a wobble board push-up, clients place their hands flat on the top of a wobble board and perform push-ups in a slow and controlled manner (figure 11.63).

Straight-arm lifts will strengthen the important supraspinatus muscle. Figure 11.64 shows standing straight arm lifts with the scapulae retracted, depressed, and stabilized. Clients hold light weights with their thumbs pointing upward and their arms raised in front of the body and lowered to the side. Next, clients lift their arms straight to the side and lower, then midway between front and side and lower. Take all lifts to the horizontal only.

Tubing, machines, and isokinetics help movement in various positions and speeds; such exercises can be customized to a chosen sport or employment task as a final phase of rehabilitation. Rapid transitions from concentric to eccentric (e.g., plyometrics) enhance muscle reactive capabilities that improve dynamic joint stability.

Always keep in mind the impingement zone and the stage of rehabilitation. Clients should continue on a maintenance program of core exercises several times per week and continue applying ice after workouts.

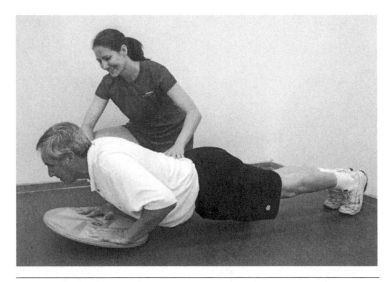

Figure 11.63   Wobble board push-up.

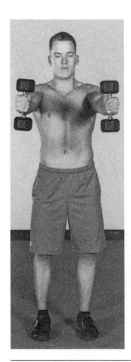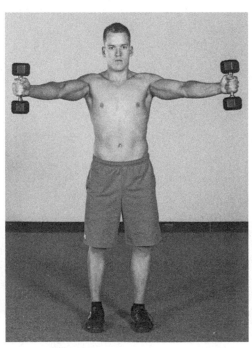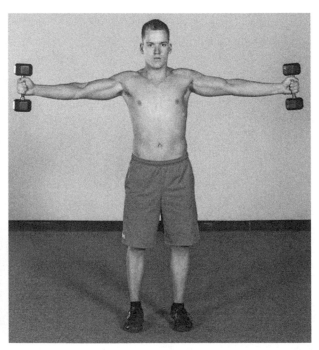

Figure 11.64   Straight-arm lift.

Lateral Epicondylitis

The elbow is the meeting place for strong arm action generated from above and enduring gripping strength from below. It is also the meeting place for three bones—humerus, radius, and ulna—forming a hinge joint allowing flexion and extension. Proximally the radioulnar joint allows the forearm to rotate with pronation and supination. Although the elbow is relatively stable, the lateral epicondyle of the humerus is a common point of origin for most of the wrist extensors and is vulnerable to strong, impact types of repetitive movements. Lateral epicondylitis, or tennis elbow, is the most common overuse injury of the elbow. A 50% prevalence is reported among tennis players older than 30 years, with a peak between the ages of 35 and 50 (Bahr and Maehlum 2004). It results from microtearing and degeneration of the wrist extensor tendon (mainly the extensor carpi radialis brevis) on the lateral epicondyle (figure 11.65). The client may complain of pain at the lateral elbow and grip weakness.

Lateral epicondylitis (tennis elbow) occurs with a number of activities that require repetitive extension of the wrist, including carpentry, painting, gardening, and word processing, as well as with golf, bowling, baseball, weight training, and racket sports. Injury from repetitive stress causes formation of scar tissue, and over time, strained tendons become thickened and weakened from the microtrauma. Management of tennis elbow begins with rest and avoidance of any activities that lead to pain. Inflammation should be controlled with ice, rest, and NSAIDs.

Apart from repetitive movements and repetitive shock, a common cause of tennis elbow involves overtraining or underconditioning: too much, too fast, and too soon without appropriate preseason conditioning or with improper warm-up and stretching. Improper stroke mechanics, especially if the elbow leads in a backhand shot, may place excessive stresses on the common wrist extensor origin. Equipment modification is also important. For example, in tennis, a larger racket head of lightweight material with medium string tension in a larger-diameter handle will reduce the occurrence of injury (Jackson 1997). Counterforce bracing offsets the angular acceleration of the muscle force, thereby reducing tension at the attachment of the extensor tendons. Strengthening, endurance, stability, and stretching at the shoulder are also necessary for prevention and will directly influence the elbow forearm and wrist.

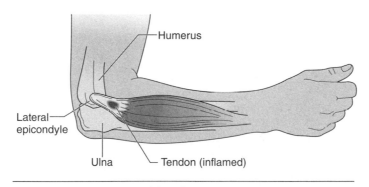

Figure 11.65   Anatomy of the elbow.

Tennis Elbow
Stretching Guidelines and Prescription

Stretching lengthens the muscle–tendon unit and decreases the strain during joint motion. Stretching the wrist extensors may best be achieved with the elbow fully extended and the wrist in flexion. Add some passive pressure with the opposite hand, then repeat with the wrist in extension. The stretch in figure 11.66 starts with the elbow extended and wrist fully flexed. With the arms straight in front and wrists flexed, slowly rotate the hands back and forth as far as possible. Repeat this movement with elbows slightly flexed, focusing more on the radioulnar muscles.

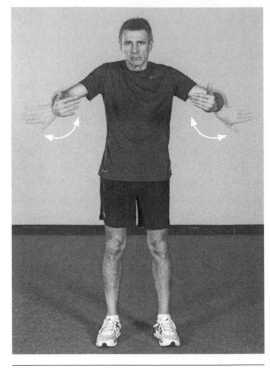

Figure 11.66   Flexed wrist rotation stretch.

Tennis Elbow
Strengthening Guidelines and Prescription

Strengthening causes muscle–tendon unit hypertrophy and increases the tensile strength of the tendon. Strength can be improved with tubing or light hand weights by wrist flexion, wrist extension, forearm pronation, and forearm supination. It is important to maintain this muscle balance. With the forearm supported, perform dumbbell wrist flexion with palms up, wrist extensions with palms down, pronations and supinations starting with a thumbs-up position. Perform the eccentric phase slower than the concentric phase (figure 11.67).

It has been suggested that eccentric strengthening induces musculotendinous hypertrophy, increases tensile strength, and provides stimulus for tendon cells to produce collagen (Martines-Silvestrini et al. 2005). Eccentric contractions should be performed at a slow velocity to avoid reinjury, as in the Flexbar twist. Reynolds (2009)

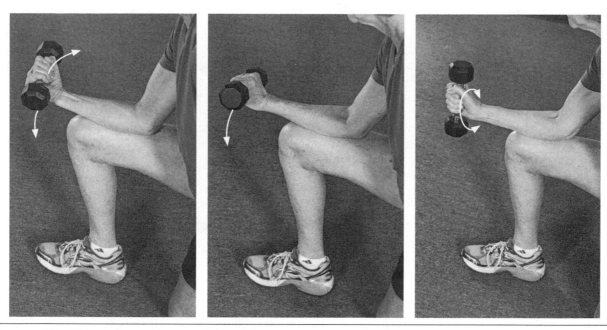

Figure 11.67 Wrist flexion, wrist extension, and forearm pronation and supination.

reported an 81% improvement in elbow pain and a 72% improvement in strength with 3 sets of 5 to 15 reps daily for 8 weeks using the Flexbar twist. Grasp the TheraBand Flexbar (available on Amazon.com) in the involved hand with maximum wrist flexion. Grasp the top of the bar with palm facing forward. Flex the top wrist (noninvolved) and bring the arms straight in front of body with the involved wrist still in full extension. Slowly untwist the bar to allow the involved wrist to move into flexion (eccentric contraction of wrist extensors) (figure 11.68).

Exercises for scapular–humeral stabilization (figure 11.58-11.64) are crucial to achieving stability in the elbow. Epicondylitis is known to be a lingering and sometimes chronic injury. It is important that clients progress in their exercise program without pain and under the supervision of a licensed health professional.

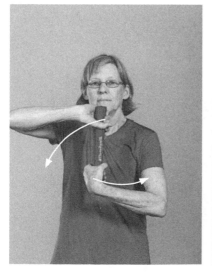
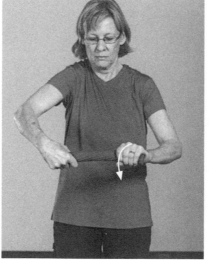
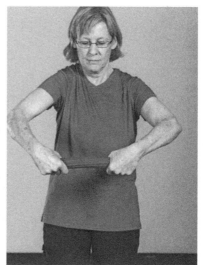

Figure 11.68 Flexbar twist.

Remember Your Scope of Practice

Recognizing their scope of practice and defining their boundaries help to identify the areas of expertise of personal fitness trainers and ensure that overstepping in these areas is avoided. The symptoms from most overuse injuries can be alleviated with relative rest, ice, mild stretching, NSAIDs, and appropriate modifications of contributing intrinsic and extrinsic factors. Overuse injuries are generally self-limiting. However, diagnosis of the cause of an injury or chronic pain requires specific attention from other members of the injury management team. For you to have a network for these referrals will be of great value to your client. Follow up on referrals and request specific guidelines to assist in the selection of the most appropriate exercise intervention to help your client quickly return to full function.

Summary

Personal trainers are often faced with clients recovering from, or having a history of, orthopedic injury. It is important to understand the functional anatomy background, causes, and prevention of common overuse injuries such as plantar fasciitis, Achilles tendinitis and tendinosis, shin splints (medial tibial stress syndrome), patellofemoral syndrome, hamstring strain, low back pain, rotator cuff tendinitis (impingement syndrome), and lateral epicondylitis (tennis elbow). Preventive exercise strategies including precautions, beneficial activity indications, and exercise contraindications should be tailored to the client.

Trainers and other exercise specialists will find specific exercise designs for stretching and for strengthening injured tissues immediately helpful for their clients.

For personal fitness trainers to recognize their scope of practice and define their boundaries helps to identify their areas of expertise and ensure that overstepping in these areas is avoided.

Exercise and Musculoskeletal Conditions in Older Adults

Chapter Competencies

After completing this chapter, you will be able to demonstrate the following competencies:

1. Explain sarcopenia, discuss the risk factors affecting the condition, and then describe the role of specific exercise and activity, including precautions.

2. Explain osteoporosis, discuss the risk factors affecting the condition, then describe the role of specific exercise and activity, including precautions.

3. Explain osteoarthritis, discuss the risk factors affecting the condition, then describe the role of specific exercise and activity, including precautions.

4. List the changes with aging in the following soft tissues: muscles, fascia, tendons, ligaments, joint capsules, articular cartilage, intervertebral discs, bone, and skin.

5. Develop strategies for soft tissue care and injury prevention in active older adults.

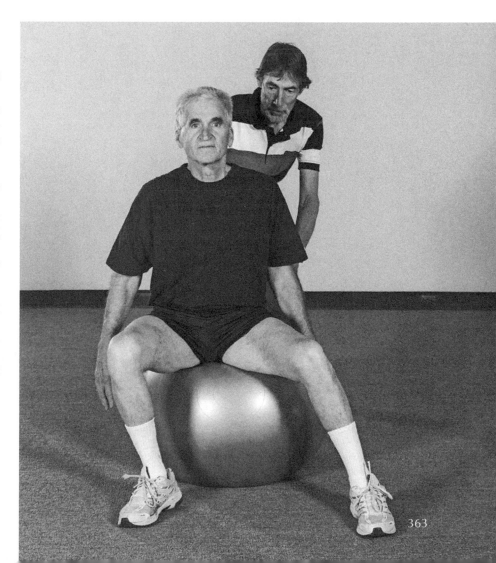

What do trainers need to avoid or include if their client has a musculoskeletal condition? This first part of this chapter describes each condition (sarcopenia, osteoporosis, osteoarthritis), discusses the risk factors affecting them, and then focuses on the role of specific exercise and activity, including precautions. Musculoskeletal conditions affect bones, muscles, and connective tissue around joints. Sarcopenia, osteoporosis, and osteoarthritis are three of the most common musculoskeletal conditions with aging adults.

The second part of the chapter examines common soft tissue changes with aging and follows up with a discussion of soft tissue care and injury prevention in an effort to elucidate why soft tissue injuries always seem to be an issue with older adults.

Sarcopenia

Some may hold that sarcopenia is not a musculoskeletal condition; however, the structural and functional declines linked to the loss of muscle tissue due to aging are a significant problem. In a Canadian study of over 4500 adults 60 years and older, sarcopenia was significantly and independently associated with functional impairment and disability, particularly in older women (Janssen et al. 2002). It has been estimated that from age 60 to 80 years, the prevalence of sarcopenia in the general population progresses from 15% to 32% for men and from 23% to 36% for women. After the age of 80, these values increased to about 51% for women and 55% for men (Signorile 2011). In this chapter we discuss the factors associated with declines in muscle performance, as well as the specific training strategies for losses in muscle mass and strength.

Sarcopenia is most prevalent in inactive clients; however, it also affects those who remain physically active, suggesting that physical inactivity is not the only contributing factor (see figure 12.1). Other contributing factors include the following:

- **Motor unit remodeling.** Motor neurons are responsible for sending signals from the brain to the muscles to initiate movement. A motor unit consists of the motor neuron and all of the muscle fibers that it innervates. Motor neurons die with age, resulting in a denervation of the muscle fibers within the motor unit. This denervation causes the muscle fibers to atrophy and eventually die, leading to a decrease in muscle mass. When a motor neuron dies, an adjacent motor neuron may reinnervate the muscle fibers, preventing atrophy. This process is called motor unit remodeling. Compared to fast-twitch (FT) motor units, remodeled slow-twitch (ST) motor units have less precise control of movements, less force production, and slower muscle mechanics (Roth et al. 2000). This may help explain the loss of balance and speed of movement with age.

- **Decreased hormone levels.** Several changes in hormone levels come with aging, including a decrease in the concentrations of growth hormone (GH), testosterone (T), and insulin-like growth factor (IGF-1). The development of sarcopenia may be linked to decreases in these hormones:

  - GH and IGF-1: dominant role in the regulation of protein metabolism

  - GH and T: required for protein maintenance

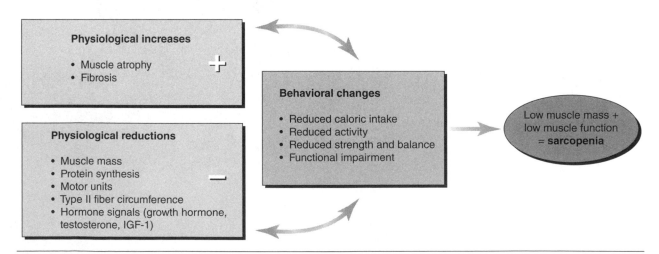

Figure 12.1   Contributing factors to sarcopenia.

- IGF-1: levels positively correlated with muscle protein synthesis rates

As well, changes in female estrogen levels may play a role in the development of sarcopenia during menopause.

- **Decreased protein synthesis.** The quality and quantity of protein in the body are maintained by a continuous repair process, which involves both protein breakdown and synthesis. With age, the changes in body protein turnover reflect a decreased synthesis rate rather than an increased catabolic rate. A decrease in muscle protein synthesis results in the loss of muscle mass. In addition, the muscles' ability to regenerate following injury or overload decreases with age (Roth et al. 2000).

Exercise Effects and Considerations

The development of sarcopenia is multifaceted, and many of the causative factors are uncontrollable; however, the easiest and possibly the most effective treatment within our control is progressive resistance training. Researchers have shown that resistance training positively influences the neuromuscular system, hormone concentrations, and protein synthesis rates. A properly designed resistance training program may increase motor neuron firing rates, improve muscle fiber recruitment, and create a more efficient motor unit leading to faster muscle contractions and greater force production.

The American College of Sports Medicine Guidelines for Musculoskeletal Fitness (ACSM 2010), presented in chapter 7, provide the key elements (FITT) for a resistance training prescription. However, the degree of change observed in sarcopenia is related directly to the type of resistance training employed. If we take a look at intensity or training load, most studies have employed resistance levels of 8RM to 12RM (repetitions maximum; 70% to 80% of maximum strength). High-intensity training, such as resistance and complex agility training, can actually increase the number of branches or the complexity of the neuromuscular junction and so decrease the effects of age-induced unraveling at the neuromuscular junction (Signorile 2011). In a study of men in their 60s, Candow and colleagues (2011) demonstrated that 12 weeks of heavy resistance training (3 sets of 10 repetitions to muscle failure, 3 days per week) was sufficient to eliminate deficits in muscle size and strength when compared with measures in healthy younger men. However, in the early stages of the training program, loads of 40% to 50% of maximum strength can produce improvements similar to those at higher intensities. It appears that progressive resistance training should include cycles of high-intensity, lower-volume training relative to the client's fitness level.

If we consider the number of repetitions to maximize strength-hypertrophy in older persons, 8 to 12 is usually recommended. However, lower repetitions with greater loads may prove more effective at increasing strength in well-trained older clients. Single sets may be effective during both the tissue adaptation and the early stages of strength training, but it may be necessary to use multiple sets to produce strength improvements in older clients who reach higher training levels (Signorile 2011).

Because we see sarcopenia in physically active clients (albeit to a lesser degree) and due to the selective decline in muscle fiber size (primarily in type II [fast-twitch] fibers), it is possible that the physical activity is not intense enough, long enough, or specific enough to recruit fast-twitch muscle fibers. Resistance training increases the cross-sectional areas of the muscle fibers of older persons, especially the areas of type II fibers, which are the fibers most dramatically affected by the aging process. From age 65 to 89, explosive lower limb extensor power declines 3.5% annually, while strength drops only 1% to 2% per year. Leg extensor power correlates significantly with a number of activities of daily living (ADLs), including rising from a chair, walking speed, and climbing stairs, as well as with recreational activities and fall prevention (Pizzigalli et al. 2011). It is also interesting that clients with higher power outputs show faster recovery rates after injuries and falls (Sayers 2007). While it may seem prudent to avoid eccentric contractions and potential muscle damage, there is evidence that eccentric contractions may be required for hypertrophy and improved neural activation strategies. Porter (2001) found that eccentric training alone led to increases in both concentric and eccentric ankle dorsiflexors, while 8 weeks of concentric training in the ankle plantar flexors of the same subjects did not change either concentric or eccentric strength.

Exercise Guidelines

General guidelines encourage targeting major muscle groups; however, muscle groups should also be targeted based on clients' inability to perform specific ADLs and their movement patterns. Because of the lower muscle mass, clients require more gluteus, quadriceps, and calf muscle activity to perform lower body functions such as climbing stairs. Ankle dorsiflexor strength is a major predictor of falling and should also be targeted for those with balance issues. As well, because of the high concentration of type II fibers in the back and thighs (quadriceps and hamstrings), these muscles are often the first to atrophy in older adults.

It is often a challenge to ensure safety when muscle power is an objective. Before beginning a high-speed training program, you should

- develop a strength base, including eccentric contractions necessary to decelerate a limb as the movement approaches the end range of motion;
- have clients perform these early strength movements through their full range to prepare connective tissues to deal with momentum and inertial forces;
- use devices that minimize momentum such as rubber tubing, bands, pneumatic devices, or a swimming pool; and
- screen clients carefully, making sure they have the strength and fitness to increase the speed of movement and are performing with proper technique.

Osteoporosis

Osteoporosis is a disease that drains bones of their mineral content and increases their susceptibility to fractures. It is characterized by low bone mass and microarchitectural deterioration of bone tissue. The National Osteoporosis Foundation (2008) reports that in the United States,

- 10 million people have osteoporosis;
- 34 million have low bone mass;
- 80% of these are women;
- osteoporosis is responsible for more than 1.5 million fractures annually; and
- of these, 700,000 are vertebral fractures, 300,000 are hip fractures, and 250,000 are wrist fractures.

The following risk factors for osteoporosis can help identify clients who are likely to develop the condition.

- **Menopause.** Before menopause, women lose approximately 0.3% of their bone mineral content each year. After menopause, the annual rate jumps to 2.5% to 3% (Kaplan 1995). Estrogen plays a vital role in bone mass and strength, and when it is no longer manufactured, calcium in the bones decreases at an accelerated rate. This leads first to osteopenia, which is decreased bone mass, and ultimately to osteoporosis. Estrogen deficiency also occurs in women who have had a hysterectomy or those with eating disorders.
- **Low peak bone mass.** One of the main causes of osteoporosis is a low rate of bone mineral accumulation during maturity. Think of bone mineral as like money in the bank: The more money you accumulate in your peak years, the lower your risk of depleting your financial resources (or bone density) when you grow older.
- **Low calcium intake.** Adequate calcium intake may be as crucial for maintaining peak bone mass as it is for attaining it.
- **Genetics.** Family history plays a role in osteoporosis.
- **Smoking.** Cigarette smoke interferes with the body's ability to produce estrogen and can also affect men.
- **Sedentary lifestyle.** Reduced weight bearing, as seen with bed rest, in astronauts, or with simple inactivity, leads to progressive thinning and eventual loss of bone.

Typical interventions for preventing osteoporosis include diet (adequate calcium and vitamin D intake), exercise, and medication. Our focus is on exercise. Since many older adults have not been tested for the condition, it is important to interview the client and determine if screening by a physician is needed. Clients who answer "yes" to any of the following questions should see their physician:

- Do you have a family history of osteoporosis?
- Do you smoke?
- Have you had a previous fracture?
- Are you taking any medication that can increase bone loss?

For female clients, determine:
- Did she go through early menopause?
- Has she had a hysterectomy?
- Are there visible signs of osteoporosis such as stooped posture?

Exercise Effects and Considerations

Exercise has a dramatic effect on bone mass in the growing skeleton and can improve bone mass, which will reduce the risk of osteoporosis.

Even in both pre- and postmenopausal women, exercise training programs were found to prevent or reverse almost 1% of bone loss per year in the lumbar spine and femoral neck. As well, exercise training appears to significantly reduce the risk and number of falls. Among 3,262 healthy men (mean age 44 years) followed for 21 years, intense physical activity was associated with a reduced incidence of hip fracture. The benefits of the higher-intensity exercise clearly outweigh the potential risks, particularly in older clients (Warburton et al. 2006).

The loads or stresses placed on the bones during exercise needs to be great enough to stimulate them. For example, if your client can perform an exercise with 15 repetitions, she is not stressing the muscle enough to encourage bone building (Martin 2010). Elastic bands and light hand weights are preferred in the early stages of a program, as many weight machines start at too high a resistance and are difficult to get in and out of. The effect of exercise on bone is specific to the location of the stresses caused by the exercise. For example, if stronger leg bones are desired, then brisk walking, squats, and lunges will help. For clients who exhibit no pain, target the shoulder retraction muscles with a rowing action, ensuring no slouching that might increase upper back curvature.

Exercise Guidelines

A typical exercise prescription for older clients with osteoporosis should include resistance training, flexibility, balance, and cardiovascular training.

The National Osteoporosis Foundation (www.nof.org) recommends regular weight-bearing activities for 45 to 60 min, four times per week. Tips for **resistance training** include the following:

- Strengthen back extensor muscles and abdominal muscles while avoiding spinal flexion exercises, which may increase the risk of compression fractures.

- Avoid exercises that may increase the risk of falling.

- Aquatic exercises are helpful for muscle conditioning and range of motion but will not help maintain bone mineral density.

- Strengthen large leg muscles to help prevent falls and subsequent fractures (Brennan 2002).

Many older adults become round-shouldered, and flexibility exercises can help improve posture. **Flexibility training** does not load the bone, but it can relieve tightness, maintain mobility, and improve posture. Target the chest for clients with rounded shoulders and stretch the hip flexors, since these muscles become tight in older adults from sitting or walking with a stooped posture.

Balance and agility training improves motor coordination and can prevent falls. Balance is best improved through exercises that involve multiple systems, for example, motor, sensory, and cognitive. In an excellent resource, *FallProof!*, Debra Rose describes in detail four approaches to balance and mobility training (Rose 2010):

1. Center of gravity control: Assisting clients to stand steadily in space, lean through their limits of stability, or perform a variety of weight transfers (figure 12.2*a*)

2. Multisensory training: Improving clients' ability to select appropriate sources of sensory information to control balance and generate an appropriate motor response (figure 12.2*b*)

3. Postural strategy training: Improving clients' ability to select the appropriate movement strategy when the task or the environment demands (figure 12.2*c*)

4. Gait pattern variations: Assisting clients to develop a gait pattern that is more efficient, flexible, and adaptable (figure 12.2*d*)

Figure 12.2 illustrates exercises that represent each of Rose's four approaches to balance and mobility training. These exercises have an important role in promoting balance confidence as well as performance.

Older adults with osteoporosis often become deconditioned from lack of activity. For this reason, **cardiovascular training** is recommended 3 to 5 days per week. Find a mode of training that the client will do regularly (e.g., walking or recumbent stepper). Clients with osteoporosis should avoid jumping activities. For those unfamiliar with regular cardiovascular activity, an interval training design alternates bouts of the activity with rest intervals (e.g., 60 s activity, 30 s rest) and can delay fatigue and help sustain a longer period of activity. For those who have trouble with long periods of repetitive movements, circuit training may also be a useful alternative. As well, bones respond best to different stresses and new challenges provided by a progressive circuit (see highlight box "Osteoporosis Circuit Training Program").

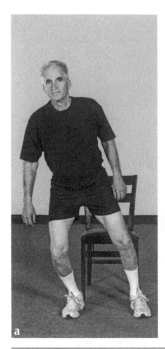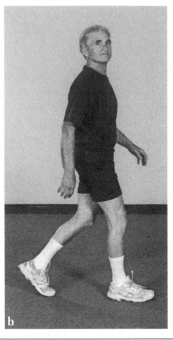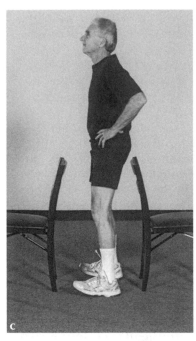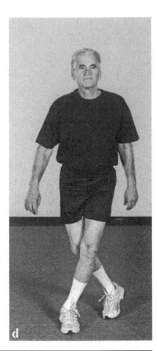

Figure 12.2 Balance and mobility training through *(a)* lateral weight shifts; *(b)* walking with head turns to right, center, and left; *(c)* ankle strategy; and *(d)* side stepping, braiding, and tandem walking.

Osteoporosis Circuit Training Program

The total exercise time for this program is 12 min. Have your client rest 30 s between each station, or longer if needed.

Station 1
Step on and off a step or platform 6 in. high (15 cm) for 2 min.

Station 2
Perform wall push-ups for 1 min.

Station 3
Perform step touch movements with lightly swinging arms for 2 min.

Station 4
Perform rhythmical partial squats with repeated touches to a chair seat for 1 min (music helps).

Station 5
Take a broom and hold it a horizontal against your thighs; in a smooth movement, bring it above your head and back down to your thighs. Continue for 1 min.

Station 6
Take a light weight (e.g., a can) from a bureau or counter to a stool or chair; take it from the stool or chair to the floor and stand straight; pick it up and place it on the chair; move it from the chair back to the counter. Continue for 2 min.

Osteoarthritis

Osteoarthritis (OA) is a functional disorder of the joints that increases in prevalence with age. It affects approximately one of every two adults over the age 65 and 85% of those 75 years and older (American Geriatrics Society Panel on Exercise and Osteoarthritis 2001). Among all causes of disability in Canada, arthritis ranks first among women and second among men (www.arthritis.

ca). Osteoarthritis accounts for more mobility problems, such as walking and climbing stairs, than any other disease and is the most common reason for total hip and knee replacements. It tends to affect hands as well as weight-bearing joints such as hips, knees, feet, and back and can range from mild to very severe. The causes of OA are not completely understood, but it seems clear that hereditary, environmental, and lifestyle factors are involved. Risk factors such as age, sex, and family history cannot be modified; however, others, such as muscular weakness, obesity, repeated heavy physical activity, and inactivity, can be changed. Participation in occupations requiring strenuous physical activity or intense competitive sports throughout life may contribute to the development of OA. Other risk factors for developing OA include muscular weakness and reduced joint proprioception (Spirduso et al. 2005).

As a degenerative joint disease localized to the affected joint, OA appears first as deficits in articular cartilage (see figure 12.3). As the damaged hyaline cartilage begins to break down, it changes from a smooth gliding surface to a rough network of frayed collagen fibers, causing increased friction and further damage. Eventually, the articular surface may disappear, exposing the two bones to direct contact. A thickening of the bone endings and growth of bony spurs (osteophytes) at the edges of the joints occur. An X-ray can reveal this altered joint anatomy and the narrow joint spaces due to the loss of cartilage. Other changes may include fissures in the cartilage, inflammation of the synovial membrane, thickening of the joint capsule, and increases in synovial fluid (Taylor and Johnson 2008). The client may experience the following signs and symptoms:

- Pain that worsens following exercise or immobility
- Pain and stiffness on weight-bearing joints such as the hip, knee, spine, and feet
- Some inflammation, usually mild
- Crepitus or a grating sound when roughened cartilage rubs together

Because the cartilage is damaged, the nerve endings on the bone sense pain from the weight-bearing forces of bones rubbing against one another. To protect the joint from movement, the tendons, ligaments, and muscles contract in spasm, resulting in pain. The synovial membrane lining the joint capsule can also become irritated and inflamed because of floating cartilage in the synovial fluid.

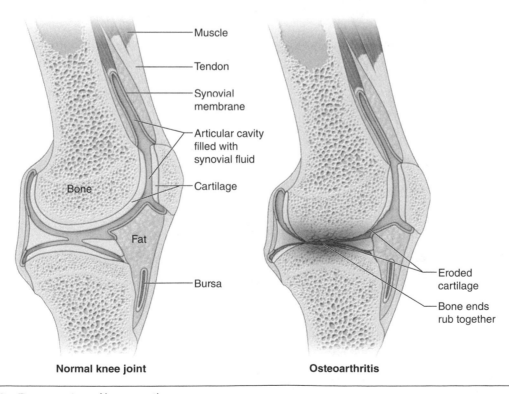

Figure 12.3   Degeneration of knee cartilage.

Exercise Effects and Considerations

Exercise does not exacerbate pain or disease progression and can decrease pain and improve function (American Geriatrics Society Panel on Exercise and Osteoarthritis 2001). The management of OA includes exercise, ice or heat, medication, and patient education (including diet and weight control). The primary aims for an exercise program are to mitigate pain during activity, reduce joint stress, maintain active joint motion and alignment, normalize gait, and improve shock attenuation through increased strength. Appropriate and regular physical activity can improve sleep, which is often difficult for people in pain.

As a runner, I am also pleased to report that running does not accelerate the development of OA among healthy older individuals (Chakravarty et al. 2008).

Exercise Guidelines

The following guidelines for exercise design should prove helpful:

- Start slowly, including warm-up and cooldown sessions to reduce joint stiffness.
- Use cross-training to avoid overuse of certain joints.
- Resistance training should use smooth motions or may begin with isometric contractions such as straight-leg raises for a painful knee.
- Avoid overuse of the damaged joints (e.g., use techniques such as isometrics).

- Consider using braces or straps, then ice after exercise.
- Select shoes and insoles for maximum shock attenuation during the weight-bearing activities.
- Emphasize low-impact, non–weight-bearing activities (e.g., bicycling or warm water exercise, 28-31 °C) if joint pain is already prevalent.
- Walking may be aided by poles or a cane to partially unweight joints.
- Discontinue or modify any exercise that causes pain during or shortly after exercise.
- Progress by time rather than intensity in most cases.
- Use pain tolerance to help set intensity levels.
- Keep the exercise intensity in the "optimal intensity zone" (see figure 12.4). For most, this is low to moderate intensity; however, tolerated activity for regularly active clients can be at higher intensities.

The exercise program should include aerobic conditioning as well as flexibility, strength, postural stability, and neuromuscular exercises (including balance) designed to prevent disability and permit the client to perform ADLs. Muscular weakness is a common finding with OA, and attempts at increasing strength play an important role in reducing activity-related symptoms. For example, strengthening the quadriceps and hamstrings will provide support to arthritic knees.

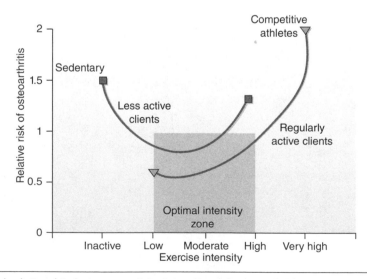

Figure 12.4   Theoretical relationship between activity intensity and osteoarthritis.

Exercises may focus on maintaining common activities such as transferring from sit to stand or step-ups to maintain independence in daily living. The increased strength and flexibility will help stabilize joints and reduce stiffness and pain. The aerobic exercise can encourage weight loss, which will reduce the forces produced at the joints and thereby reduce pain.

Some joint stiffness at the onset of exercise and soreness or aching in joints and muscles during or after exercise are normal. If joint swelling or a feeling of "hotness" increases or gets worse at night, send your client to her health care provider.

Musculoskeletal Injury

Despite the benefits of increased activity, injury has been identified as the second most common barrier to sport participation in older age groups. Clients over the age of 60 take twice as long to heal as younger adults, while those over the age of 75 years take three times as long (Jones and Rose 2005). Obviously, injury prevention is a worthy goal.

Researchers at the University of British Columbia documented the clinical pattern of overuse injuries in 685 physically active individuals (mean age = 56.9 ± 6.1 years) over a 5-year period and compared these findings to those for a younger group averaging 30 years old. Running, fitness classes, and field sports were commonly associated with injury in the younger group, while racket sports, walking, and low-intensity sports were more commonly associated with injury in the older group. The frequency of tendinitis was similar in the two age groups, while metatarsalgia, plantar fasciitis, and meniscal injury were more common in the older population. Anatomically, injury sites in the foot were more frequent in the older group, and injury sites in the knee were more frequent in the younger group. In the older population, the prevalence of OA as a source of activity-related pain was 2.5 times higher. In the older group, 85% of the diagnoses were overuse injuries known to respond to conservative treatment, and only 4.1% required surgery (Matheson et al. 1989). Scott and Couzens (1996) reported that the most common injuries in those aged 50 to 80 years were overuse injuries compounded by OA of the knee, hip, thumb, wrist, and spine. Bursitis of the hip and shoulder were also common, as were tendon problems such as lateral epicondylitis of the elbow, Achilles tendinitis, and rotator cuff tendinitis.

If the client participates in a particular sport or recreational activity, the injury may be specific to these joint actions. Swimmers commonly injure their shoulders; cyclists suffer upper body and neck injuries; and runners injure their lower extremities. Older athletes are more susceptible to injury as a result of the age-related changes in connective tissue, bone, and muscle.

To try to clarify why soft tissue injuries always seem to be an issue with older adults, this section first examines common soft tissue changes with aging and follows up with a discussion of soft tissue care and injury prevention.

Soft Tissue Changes With Aging

Soft tissue includes muscles, joint capsules, ligaments, tendons, fascia, articular cartilage, intervertebral discs, and bone (see figure 12.5). It can function to support, stabilize, and reinforce and can restrict mobility. Let's examine the effects of aging and the implications for musculoskeletal injury.

The bony structures that make up a joint undergo gradual decrease in blood supply with aging. This can lead to arthritic changes (e.g., osteophyte formation) with an effect on joint function and motion. Osteoporosis and OA (discussed earlier) are major pathological processes that occur in bone as a result of aging. Radiographic

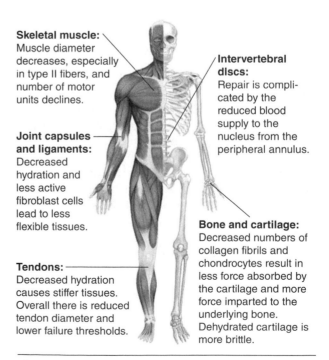

Skeletal muscle: Muscle diameter decreases, especially in type II fibers, and number of motor units declines.

Joint capsules and ligaments: Decreased hydration and less active fibroblast cells lead to less flexible tissues.

Tendons: Decreased hydration causes stiffer tissues. Overall there is reduced tendon diameter and lower failure thresholds.

Intervertebral discs: Repair is complicated by the reduced blood supply to the nucleus from the peripheral annulus.

Bone and cartilage: Decreased numbers of collagen fibrils and chondrocytes result in less force absorbed by the cartilage and more force imparted to the underlying bone. Dehydrated cartilage is more brittle.

Figure 12.5   Soft tissue.

evidence of OA does not necessarily indicate that degenerative joint disease is the cause of activity-related pain in the older athlete. Careful attention must be given to ruling out other soft tissue injuries that occur coincidently with OA (Matheson et al. 1989). Bone fractures heal much more slowly because of the decreased activity of the bone-forming osteoblasts.

Skeletal Muscle

Skeletal muscle decreases slowly between 25 and 50 years of age; after this, the rate of muscle atrophy increases. The muscle diameter decreases especially in the type II fibers. The number of motor units is diminished, with loss of fast motor units first. There is a reorganization of the other motor units, which may explain the reduction of reaction time and functional mobility in aging clients. The reduction of blood supply to the bone at the point of insertion leaves the bone with decreased quantity and quality of cells, rendering it more susceptible to avulsion of the muscle from the bone (Speers 2005). All these aging factors make it even more important for joints not to be immobilized for too long in older persons. Even decreased average activity associated with aging is detrimental to muscle strength and the ability to absorb energy before failure. Disuse and immobilization accelerate the loss of strength and endurance, early fatigue, and increased stiffness. This may be one reason it is more common to see an increase in muscle tears such as rotator cuff strains. Muscles in older persons also have a decreased ability to heal after any kind of trauma.

Age increases susceptibility to eccentric contraction–induced skeletal muscle injury and also impairs the ability to recover from injury. The capacity of a muscle to respond efficiently to a mechanical stimulus such as eccentric loading determines either successful adaptation or maladaptation in the remodeling-regeneration of myofibers. Recent evidence has indicated that muscles from older clients can be conditioned to be protected from eccentric contraction–induced injury, although slower speeds and rest between exposures are important factors in muscle adaptation (Baker and Cutlip 2010). Contraction-induced injury causes damage to small groups of sarcomeres as a result of eccentric contractions. The injury or delayed-onset muscle soreness generates an inflammatory response. Older clients are more susceptible to muscle injury and delayed recovery. This may lead to degeneration and atrophy (Taylor and Johnson 2008).

Capsule and Ligaments

Capsule and ligaments are specialized, dense fibrous connective tissues. Their main role is to provide stability to the joints. The capsule forms a complex structure that covers the joints and contains synovial fluid. It is reinforced with thickenings or capsular ligaments attaching bone to bone. The ligaments act to stabilize the joints during motion, particularly at the end of the range of motion. As ligaments age, structural and material properties change in response to loading conditions. In older clients, midtissue tears are more common, whereas in younger individuals injury is more common at insertion sites. With age, there is a decrease in water, and the fibroblast cells become less active. The ligaments become more stiff and less flexible, with a lower threshold to failure. During repair, collagen fiber alignment remains less organized in older people, usually resulting in a functional loss.

Tendons

All soft tissue suffers from a lack of hydration with age, which generally limits mobility. As with ligaments, tendons and fascia demonstrate excessive collagen cross-bridging, which holds the tendon's collagen fibers together and results in increased stiffness. With age, the overall diameter of the tendon decreases. These changes contribute to making tendons drier and stiffer in older clients, reducing their overall tissue plasticity, and lowering the failure threshold (Seto and Brewster 1991).

Cartilage

Articular (hyaline) cartilage provides a smooth gliding surface for the joints by reducing friction. This cartilage also acts as a major site of shock absorption and dissipation of joint forces. With age come decreases in the number of collagen fibrils and chondrocytes (cartilage cells); therefore less force is dissipated and absorbed by the cartilage and more forces are imparted to the underlying bone. Cartilage shows an age-related loss of water, and as it becomes more brittle, it cracks and abrades more easily. Further deterioration of the vascular supply results from decreases in joint synovial fluid and compromises healing (Speers 2005). An area of injured cartilage may result in increased loads on the surrounding normal cartilage. The accumulated effects of small cartilage injuries over the decades can cause serious problems in the older active client.

Another type of cartilage, fibrocartilage, is found in the knee (meniscus) and surrounding the periphery of the shoulder's glenoid fossa (labrum). The main role of the menisci is to distribute joint forces within the meniscus itself and to act as a shock absorber. The meniscus increases the surface area of contact and helps equalize the distribution of forces to the underlying articular cartilage. With aging, collagen as well as the noncollagenous contents of the meniscus increase with a decrease in cellularity and water content. The declining vascular supply and nutrition give rise to complex tears involving both the circumferential and horizontal collagen fibers (Speers 2005). The shoulder's labrum provides load transmission, shock absorption, stabilization, and probably proprioception. In addition, it acts as a rim to limit humeral head gliding and serves as an attachment site for the glenohumeral ligaments. With age, the depth of the labrum decreases due to its degeneration, forcing the cartilage to bear increasing forces across the joint.

Intervertebral Discs

Intervertebral discs are cartilaginous structures that contribute greatly to normal spine function with load absorption and the provision of stability. With age, the nucleus pulposus undergoes the most change. There is a loss of gelatinous material as well as a decline of water content in the nucleus, which is reduced further by pressure borne by the disc. By the sixth or seventh decade the nucleus becomes fibrocartilage, and it becomes difficult to separate the inner disc from the transition zone or the outer annular disc. Repair of the disc is further complicated by the reduced blood supply to the nucleus from the peripheral annulus (Speers 2005).

Soft Tissue Care

Active older clients must be aware of the physiological changes in soft tissue with aging and be proactive in maintaining healthy soft tissue strength and mobility. These changes ultimately affect not only strength and joint mobility but also locomotion, posture, balance, and coordination. We have seen that soft tissue in the joint area is weaker and less extensible with aging. Muscle attachments must accommodate to this lack of range of motion; and if they are inflexible, the potential for injury is greater. Soft tissue that has been impaired through disuse, injury, or a disease process such as OA may have irregular collagen fiber orientation in the repaired tissue, resulting in further limitation to movement and forces (Seto

and Brewster 1991). A new paradigm is required for training older clients that includes well-designed soft tissue strengthening, stretching, and mobilization exercises. The benefits of resistance training for seniors has been well documented (see earlier in the chapter). Its injury prevention benefits extend to the correction of muscle imbalances, posture improvement, and the development of joint stability statically and dynamically.

A regular flexibility program will maintain good muscle elasticity and help prevent injuries to muscles, tendons, and ligaments. Based on the age-related soft tissue changes discussed earlier, low-intensity and long-duration stretching of warm tissue is extremely important in creating somewhat permanent plastic changes in tissue length. For example, before a stretch, soft tissue should be warmed with low-level physical activity. Low intensity means low force or mild stretch with no pain. To overcome collagen deposition and muscle stiffness, Feland and colleagues (2001) found that holding a hamstring stretch for 60 s was most effective in clients aged 65 years and older. Each stretch should be repeated several times, and daily stretching of frequently used muscles is most effective.

The key to keeping older clients active is to enable them to work out as painlessly as possible. Even those with OA can benefit from regular movement that speeds the rate of cartilage replacement, thereby making it stronger. Although adolescents heal faster, when it comes to adults the tissue repair mechanism works similarly whether they are 40 or 70 years old. There are relatively few distinctive rehabilitation differences between older and younger patients, especially with longtime exercisers who tend to have a good understanding of the rehabilitation process. Many active older clients want to continue their sport or a favorite activity while they are injured. Each case is different, but there may be an opportunity for safe compensation through modification of the activity. For example, advise tennis players who have supraspinatus tendinitis to hit ground strokes, serve underhand, and switch from singles to doubles. In this way, they don't lose too much strength and coordination, which allows them to pick up where they left off once they resume their activity at full strength. You may also consider the REST approach: Resume Exercise below the Soreness Threshold. To accomplish this, you may need to advise some clients to consider a new activity or exercise routine. This may mean taking their running workouts into a swimming pool or switching to bike riding to reduce stress on painful knees or hips. The key is to find the activity or exercises that your client wants to do on a regular basis but that are within their physical abilities. Cross-training activities during rehabilitation maintain aerobic conditioning and muscle strength while the client heals: walking, bicycling, swimming, water and traditional aerobics, cross-country skiing, and strength training.

Finally, in terms of soft tissue care, nonsteroidal anti-inflammatory drugs (NSAIDs) are widely used to reduce inflammation and fever and to relieve pain. Ibuprofen (including Advil and Motrin) and other drugs such as aspirin or Celebrex are generally considered effective for mild to moderate pain and inflammation. However, NSAIDs are associated with numerous adverse effects. The most significant complications include gastrointestinal toxicity (peptic ulcer disease, gastrointestinal bleeding) and modest worsening of underlying hypertension (Taylor and Johnson 2008). If NSAIDs are used to mask pain during activity, there is risk of further injury.

Glucosamine sulfate and chondroitin sulfate are also commonly used by active older adults and those with arthritis. These are naturally occurring substances found in the connective tissues of the body, including the hyaline cartilage that covers the ends of the bones in the joints. Both substances have been shown to provide elasticity and resiliency to cartilage. They may also slow cartilage damage and provide relief of pain in people with OA while having few side effects (Taylor and Johnson 2008).

Injury Prevention Strategies

Soft tissue injury may result from exercising too often, at too high an intensity, or for too long, as well as from using improper form or progressing too quickly. The most effective means of preventing injury is through gradual progression of volume and intensity, adequate recovery time, and the use of cross-training or interval training (see discussion of functional exercise design and functional progressions in chapter 13). Proper equipment, technique, and nutrition also play an important role in reducing the chances of injury.

For most older clients, moderation in everything is wise, so encourage them to listen to their body signals as they exercise. They should feel refreshed and not lethargic after the session, with no undue fatigue or soreness the day after. These would be signs that they need to cut back or take a day of rest. A major part of injury prevention is recognizing pain. You need to teach your client how to differentiate between "OK" pain and "bad" pain. OK pain typically develops shortly after starting a new exercise program or after increasing the intensity or duration of current exercise. It is not severe, should not involve a joint, is usually delayed muscle soreness, and should not last more than a few days. Bad pain is usually felt in a joint or tendon and typically stems from an overload on the tissue. It might produce joint stiffness or reduced mobility such that ADLs are affected. It is important not to continue to exercise in the same fashion with this type of pain. Find an activity during the injury recovery that will not further the pain. Stretching is most often prescribed to avoid injury and during recovery from injury. These are some important stretching precautions worth noting:

- Avoid forcing a joint past its normal range of motion.
- Avoid intense stretching if joint or muscle soreness persists beyond 48 h.
- Avoid stretching an area of a recent bone fracture.
- Avoid stretching tissue that is swollen or painful.
- Avoid excessive stretching of soft tissue that has been immobilized (e.g., in a cast or splint).
- Avoid excessive forward flexion of the spine or neck.
- Avoid rapid or ballistic bouncing to stretch tissue.

In the next chapter in the context of client-centered functional exercise prescription, we raise two questions: *How do functional progressions make the prescription more client centered? How should clients feel and when should they progress?* Review these sections because the best strategies for injury prevention come when you are in tune with your client's needs.

Injury should be no more of a deterrent to exercising in the elderly than it is at any age. And age should not be a deterrent in the prescription of a rehabilitative program for overuse injuries. While it was once thought that the body would "wear out" with activity and that lower physical capacity was a natural accompaniment of aging, it is now recognized that activity will add years to life and life to years.

Summary

Sarcopenia, osteoporosis, and OA are three of the most common musculoskeletal conditions with aging adults. Sarcopenia is most prevalent in inactive clients, with other contributing factors including (1) motor unit remodeling, (2) decreased hormone levels, and (3) decreased protein synthesis. The easiest and possibly the most effective treatment is progressive resistance training.

Osteoporosis is a disease that drains bones of their mineral content and increases their susceptibility to fractures. Exercise has a dramatic effect on bone mass in the growing skeleton and can improve bone mass, which will reduce the risk of osteoporosis. A typical exercise prescription for older clients with osteoporosis should include resistance training, flexibility, balance, and cardiovascular training.

As a degenerative joint disease localized to the affected joint, OA appears first as deficits in articular cartilage. Osteoarthritis accounts for more mobility problems, as in walking and climbing stairs, than any other disease. The primary aims for an exercise program are to mitigate pain during activity, reduce joint stress, maintain active joint motion and alignment, normalize gait, and improve shock attenuation through increased strength.

Despite the benefits of increased activity, injury has been identified as the second most common barrier to sport participation in older age groups. Soft tissue includes muscles, fascia, tendons, ligaments, joint capsules, articular cartilage, intervertebral discs, and bone. With aging come changes in specific soft tissues. These changes in soft tissue with aging ultimately affect not only strength and joint mobility but also locomotion, posture, balance, and coordination. A new paradigm is required for training older clients that includes well-designed soft tissue strengthening, stretching, and mobilization exercises. The most effective means of preventing injury is through gradual progression of volume and intensity, adequate recovery time, and the use of cross-training or interval training (see discussion of functional exercise design and functional progressions in chapter 13).

Exercise Prescription for Older Adults

Chapter Competencies

After completing this chapter, you will be able to demonstrate the following competencies:

1. Discuss the concepts of aging, biological age, quality of life, successful aging, and physical activity.

2. Develop strategies for appropriate lifestyle integration and behavioral change for increased activity in older adults.

3. Describe the physiological changes with aging and the effects or benefits of exercise specifically for the cardiovascular–respiratory system, the musculoskeletal system, and locomotion.

4. Outline a process for client screening and assess physical impairments (including declines in cardiovascular or musculoskeletal systems) and functional limitations (restrictions in physical tasks or behaviors of everyday life).

5. Describe general training principles suitable for the older adult for cardiovascular and musculoskeletal fitness, balance, flexibility, and functional mobility.

6. Select exercises that simulate movement patterns used in active daily living and recreation (functional training).

7. Apply personal and appropriate exercise modifications, successful demonstration, careful monitoring, and progressions.

8. Design elements around client activity that provide safety through effective preparation and through ongoing awareness.

9. Determine your clients' level of physical function and modify any exercise or activity to suit their needs and capabilities and to reinforce proper technique.

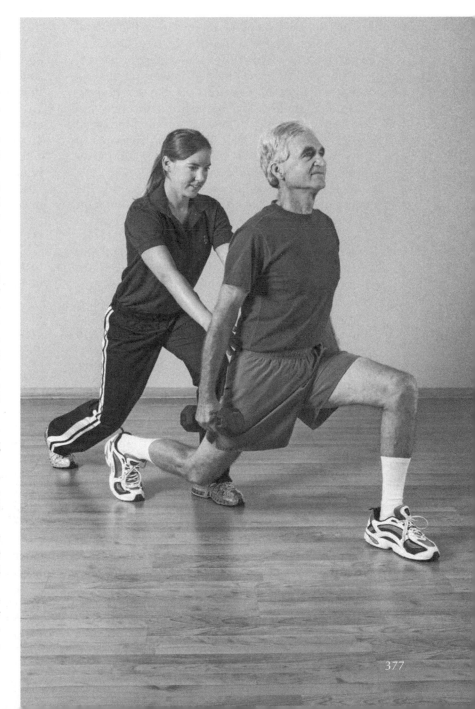

The chapter begins with an overview of successful aging, quality of life, and physical activity. There is now strong evidence that regular and systematic exercise throughout life, when accompanied by reasonable health habits, increases the quantity and quality of life.

There are both structural and functional changes in the body systems with age, and it is difficult to pinpoint if the changes are due to disease, physical inactivity, or normal aging. The chapter outlines physiological changes with aging and the effects or benefits of exercise specifically for the cardiovascular–respiratory system, musculoskeletal system, and locomotion.

Following the screening process and before people become active, assessment of physical impairments (including declines in cardiovascular or musculoskeletal systems) and functional limitations (restrictions in physical tasks or behaviors of everyday life) should be performed.

A large part of the chapter focuses on general training principles for cardiovascular and musculoskeletal fitness, body composition, balance, and flexibility, although depending on the functional status or disease of the client, modifications to the program should be made. Chapter 14 focuses more on functional mobility.

The prescription process continues with the selection of exercises that simulate movement patterns used in active daily living and recreation (functional training). The final layer of exercise or activity design should come with personal and appropriate exercise modifications, successful demonstration, careful monitoring, and progressions providing a client-centered approach. Trainers working with older adults must determine their clients' level of physical function and modify any exercise or activity to suit their needs and capabilities and to reinforce proper technique.

Aging

Is age defined simply as the length of time you've lived? How do we age, and can aging be slowed? Some people live longer and have a higher quality of life than others. So it appears as if we can define life in terms of quantity and quality. Aging refers to a number of processes within us that over time cause a loss of adaptability, impairment of functionality, and eventually death (Spirduso et al. 2005). This process of aging refers to the clinical symptoms and the loss of reserve capacity to adapt effectively and includes the effects of disease and the environment. For example, an older person who has poor functional mobility, reduced peripheral vision, and slower reaction time may not be able to prevent a sudden fall that may cause injury and loss of independence. Disease, accident, and lifestyle choices can all change the rate of deterioration and thus the rate of aging.

Although there are many theories of aging, in all likelihood, aging is not caused by any single factor but is due to a combination of causes. Physiological functions of the human body decline with age after their peak at relatively standard rates. For example, lean body mass declines at a rate of 10% per decade, nerve conduction velocity by 15%, and vital capacity by as much as 50% per decade (Taylor and Johnson 2008).

The "graying" of the population is not limited to North America, as the phenomenon of extended life expectancy occurs in most developing countries. The largest cohort in the United States and Canada is the baby boomers, born between 1946 and 1960; in fact, one in three people in Western society is a baby boomer. By 2026, about 20% of this population will be over the age of 65.

Age categories vary considerably in the literature. Some view the "middle-aged adult" as 40 to 55, others 45 to 64 years. A relatively new category called "young-old" has been used and typically refers to those in their late 60s to early 70s, a reflection of the increasing number who have maintained performance levels.

Biological Age

In addition to chronological age, larger differences in function may better be described by biological age or functional age. Biological aging refers to the progressive functional changes that take place at the cellular, tissue, and organ levels and eventually affect performance levels of all body systems. Strictly speaking, biological age would require measurement of time-related decline in physical systems irrespective of chronological age. However, practically, it can be defined by how clients function in their daily lives, in their jobs, and in community interactions. Functional age is affected by how well clients function physiologically and has been used to explain the individual differences seen in physiological variables within chronological age groups. Biological age has been defined statistically as the distance of an individual from the average score for his age group. For example, clients whose scores on a variable were higher than the average of their age group would be described as younger for their age. This is a measure of the client's aging status relative to his cohort age group and may not represent a measure of the rate of aging of the person. However, people certainly have different patterns of aging, and comparisons of the function and performance of clients serves many important purposes in professions such as physiotherapy, nursing, and health promotion specialties. Average values provide an idea of the capacities of a large number of people at a given age.

One of the most important factors influencing the quality of life in very old people is the maintenance of sufficient aerobic power to allow independent living. Aging is typically associated with a decrease in maximal oxygen uptake of about 5 ml · kg^{-1} · min^{-1} per decade. Eventually maximal oxygen uptake becomes low enough that ordinary activities of independent living become extremely fatiguing. When maximum oxygen uptake decreases below a threshold of about 15 to 18 ml · kg^{-1} · min^{-1}, there is a probable loss of independence. Following a regular endurance exercise routine through middle age can delay biological aging by up to 12 years (Barclay and Lie 2008).

Quality of Life

Of what value is quantity of life if the quality of life is not maintained? The World Health Organization has identified a number of components of a person's perception of her quality of life, including health, physical function, social relations, occupation, standard of living, and sexual functioning. The term health-related quality of life (HRQL) reflects more the functional effects of an illness on patients and the therapeutic effects of improving health status. Health status and HRQL are measured by both physical and mental scales. Physical health includes physical function, bodily pain, and general health. Mental health includes emotional health, vitality, and social function (ALCOA 2006). The World Health Organization Quality of Life Instrument–Older Adults Module was used with a large number of Brazilian adults over 60 years, with the results indicating that increases in the levels of physical activity can contribute to improvements in quality of life of older adults (Dartagan et al. 2012).

It has been said that the quality of life is the difference between active living and just being alive. Quantity of life is of value only if the quality of life is maintained. Living longer without changes in health habits will only extend the period of morbidity. Morbidity is a condition of absence of health in which the individual is so physically or mentally disabled by a chronic disease that she becomes immobile and dependent on the care of others (Vita et al. 1998). Living with a single or with multiple chronic diseases predisposes an individual to a very poor quality of life. The major chronic diseases that eventually lead people into a condition of morbidity are atherosclerosis, cancer, osteoarthritis, diabetes, emphysema, and cirrhosis of the liver. These diseases generally start early in life and progress through the life span, going through subclinical, problematic, severe, and eventually terminal stages. More than 25% of those 65 years and over are limited in their activities due to a long-term health problem. Figure 13.1 illustrates the percent

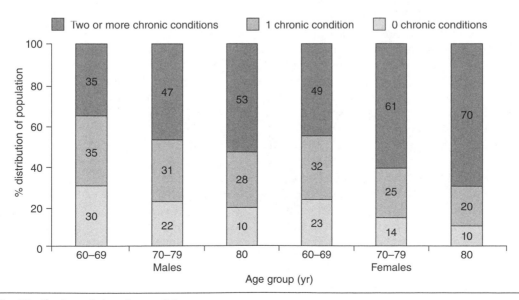

Figure 13.1 Distribution of chronic conditions.

Reprinted by permission from Taylor and Johnson 2008.

distribution of the population 60 years and older by the number of chronic conditions, according to age group and sex. Older males experience more heart disease, cerebrovascular disease, and emphysema. Although women live longer, they have more nonfatal chronic conditions such as arthritis, colitis, and soft tissue disorders. As a result, older women have higher incidences of disability and are more dependent.

Emphasis has shifted from lengthening life to increasing years of health. Maintaining health and postponing the onset of a debilitating disease as long as possible is called "compression of morbidity." A healthy lifestyle may prevent or delay symptoms of diseases such as osteoarthritis and cardiovascular disease. Vita and colleagues (1998) demonstrated that a group of older nonsmoking adults who had low body fat and good exercise habits not only extended their longevity from 1 to 4 years but also decreased their morbidity in the last year of life by 50%. Persons with better health habits may survive longer, but more importantly, disability is postponed and compressed into fewer years at the end of their life.

The primary contribution of regular physical activity to quality of life varies with age in middle-aged adults (45 to 64) and the young-old (65 to 74); good health habits and exercise can maintain near-peak performance and postpone premature aging. In the old (75 to 84), mobility is the primary role of physical activity and can substantially enhance the quality of life, enabling the elderly to continue to participate in many of the most challenging experiences of life. Physical ability and functional mobility are the basis for performing activities of daily living and job-related tasks, as well as participation in sport and recreation. There is a strong contribution of health, energy and vitality, and physical function to the quality of life. Integration of these three factors has a significant influence on a client's active life expectancy.

Several measures of old-age disability and limitations have shown improvements in the last decade; however, it is unclear whether medical expenditures have fueled the health improvements. Census Bureau reports and systematic reviews are barometers of the well-being of our population. Disability and underlying physical limitations are not inevitable consequences of aging. Yet almost 20% of older U.S. adults have chronic disabilities, and roughly one-third have mobility limitations. In addition, the cost of medical care for disabled older persons averages three times that for a nondisabled senior (Freedman et al. 2009). A Canadian survey of over 2325 men aged 55 to 97 found that health issues of greatest concern included those compromising independence and quality of life, with the greatest percentage of respondents specifying mobility impairments. It was alarming that risk factors and screening for mobility impairment were discussed with only 13% of them. As older clients' health priorities become better understood, a shift in the way health care is delivered should also be a priority. "It is time for our health care system to invest in strategies for older adults to preserve their autonomy, well-being, and quality of life" (Tannenbaum 2012).

In a review of the literature that has examined the relationship between physical activity and quality of life (QOL) in old age, the evidence indicated that physical activity was positively associated with many but not all domains of QOL (Rejeski and Mihalko 2001). The authors pointed out that performance-based assessments of function were more likely to be related to QOL, as such improvements were much more relevant to older adults. It appeared that when physical activity was associated with increases in self-efficacy, there were clear improvements in HRQL. The demographics of our aging society dictate that QOL will continue to be a very important health promotion objective. The relationship between QOL and physical activity appears to be positive and relatively consistent in older adults despite the problems with its measurement.

Successful Aging

The notion of successful aging is an attractive one and directly addresses QOL during aging. What does successful aging mean to your client? With the increasing number of individuals over the age of 65 worldwide, it is critical for society to recognize the importance of helping seniors maintain their health and physical and cognitive functioning as well as their engagement with life. These three dimensions provide the foundation for successful aging (SA) (Liffiton et al. 2012). The concept of successful aging was introduced by Rowe and Kahn (1987) in the context of separating the effects of disease from the aging process itself. Successful agers were people who were more satisfied with life and had better than average physiological and psychological characteristics in late life as well as healthy genes. Rowe and Kahn proposed that those aging "successfully" would show little or no age-related decrements in physiological function, while those aging "usually" would show disease-associated decrements, often interpreted as the effects of age. Sabia and colleagues (2012) defined successful aging as good cognitive, physical, and cardiovascular functioning, in addition to the absence of disability, mental health problems, and chronic disease. These authors found that participants engaging in four healthy behaviors had 3.3 times greater odds of successful aging. They defined healthy behaviors as never smoking, moderate alcohol consumption, physical activity (≥2.5 h/week moderate activity or ≥1 h/week vigorous activity), and eating fruits and vegetables daily. With all four individual healthy behaviors combined, the impact on successful aging was substantial when measured over a 16.3-year follow-up.

In an attempt to develop a positive aging phenotype for women over 65, Woods and colleagues (2012) used an 8-year follow-up to determine that "physical-social functioning" was the strongest predictor of outcomes related to positive aging, including years of healthy living, years of independent living, and time to mortality. Strawbridge and coauthors (2002) studied 65- to 95-year-olds over a 6-year period. They defined successful aging as needing no assistance and not having difficulty on any of 13 activity–mobility measures plus little or no difficulty on five physical performance measures. These authors found that persons more likely to age successfully had close personal contacts, had no depression, and walked regularly for exercise. In their discussion, they painted a picture of the 75-year-old man or woman who had aged successfully. This individual would do more volunteer work, exercise more, and attend more community activities than counterparts who had not aged successfully. She would see physicians less, spend less time sick in bed, and be less apt to feel too tired to do things she enjoyed doing. She would more often feel excited or pleased and find more meaning in her everyday activities.

Another dramatic measure of successful aging is the compression-of-morbidity phenomenon in which persons with lower health risks (often defined in terms of smoking, body mass index, and exercise) have disability later in life, have less disability at any given age, and have less cumulative disability than persons with greater health risks. The onset of disability was postponed by more than 5 years in a low-risk group as compared with a high-risk group (Vita et al. 1998). These results are encouraging because they suggest that with improvements in modifiable health risks, elderly persons will have greater vitality.

The American Association of Retired Persons has identified a series of relationships of physical activities to life priorities (Sloan 2001). With pre-retirement adults aged 60 to 69 years, the investigators found that PA (physical activity) would prolong active life and protect QOL by keeping people healthy. The retired group embraced activity to keep their function and independence and to compensate for a more sedentary life. Successful aging depends on the interaction of genetics, personal and social environment, lifestyle factors, attitudes, adaptability, social supports, and certain personality characteristics. The key to successful aging is to integrate positive physical, social, mental, emotional, and spiritual activities into our daily lives.

How many "healthy life years" will you have left at age 65? A recent report presented statistics from 27 European Union countries on "healthy life years," defined as the number of years that a person can expect to live in a healthy condition. A healthy condition was defined by the absence of limitations in functioning/disability, measured by a self-perceived question asking for the extent of any limitations caused by a health problem in activities that people usually do. Healthy life years was defined as the number of years a person of a specific age is expected to live without any severe or moderate health problems, which means that the respondent can maintain usual activities. People who were 65 in 27 European Union countries in 2010 were expected to live an estimated 21.0 years if they were women and 17.4 years if they were men. Within that time frame, women would have 8.8 healthy life years and men 8.7 healthy life years. The highest number of healthy life years at age 65 for women was recorded in Sweden at 15.5 years. The longest life expectancy at age 65 was in France (23.4 years), and healthy life years at 65 was 9.8 years for women (Eurostat Press Office 2012).

Regular physical activity can favorably influence a broad range of physiological systems and may be a lifestyle factor that discriminates between those individuals who have and have not experienced successful aging.

Benefits of Physical Activity in Older Adults

As an unprecedented number of baby boomers enter their 60s, the role of exercise as a "health promoter" has become very evident. Increased physical activity can reduce the effects of aging that lead to functional declines and poor health. However, Canada's Physical Activity Guide to Healthy Active Living for Older Adults suggests that about 60% of older adults are inactive and thus unable to enjoy health benefits of regular exercise (Health Canada 2001). Statistics in the United States indicate that few older adults engage in physical activity on a regular basis, estimating that only 31% of people age 65 to 74 participate in 20 min of moderate physical activity three or more times a week. As well, the United States ranks 50th among 225 countries in life expectancy (Fern 2009). Clearly, deleterious behavioral patterns, including physical inactivity, represent a major contributor to premature death and a reduced QOL.

Moore and colleagues (2012) pooled the results of six studies involving people 40 years and older to determine if leisure-time physical activity predicted longer life. Compared to people with no leisure-time physical activity, those who reported that they got the recommended level of physical activity (2.5 h of moderate intensity or 1.25 h of vigorous intensity) lived 3.4 years longer. People who were obese and inactive had a life expectancy that was between 5 and 7 years shorter than that of people who were normal weight and moderately active.

For a personal trainer, it is important to ask if it is aging or lack of activity that causes loss of functional capacity. Aging and the loss of functional capacity are affected by disease and disuse (reduced physical activity). It is difficult to distinguish physiological changes attributable to aging per se from those attributable to declining physical activity, the occurrence of disease, or other factors. However, in many cases in those 50 to 75 years of age, symptoms that may be attributable to aging are actually the result of sedentary living. That is, physical activity will exert its primary influence on disease and disuse as opposed to age-related loss of functional capacity. There is now strong evidence that regular and systematic exercise throughout life, when accompanied by reasonable health habits, increases the quantity and quality of life. By exercising modestly and regularly, elderly patients can substantially lower their risk of death from coronary artery disease, colon cancer, and complications of diabetes but also make performance of the many tasks of daily life, as well as participation in a variety of recreational activities, considerably easier.

Even for people who start between the ages of 60 and 75, regular exercise can reduce overall mortality rates. One of the most definitive studies of exercise and mortality examined over 30,000 men and women and the effects of fitness and physical activity on longevity (Blair et al. 1989). The authors found that men in the lowest fitness category died at 3.5 times the rate of the most fit, and women at 4.5 times the rate. Another outcome was that exercise seemed to have the beneficial effect of countering some diseases. Both men and women in the least fit category had higher incidences of cancer as well as cardiovascular disease. As well, hypertensive men who exercised had half the mortality rate of hypertensive men who did not exercise. The most important predictor of longevity was avoidance of the lowest fitness category (i.e., lowest 20% as measured by oxygen uptake).

The benefits derived from a regular exercise program in later years can mean the difference between institutionalization and independent living. These benefits are best seen with a combination of aerobic training and resistance training. Exercise professionals should also have a proactive focus on components of fitness influencing balance because of the strong connection with fall prevention. According to the National Safety Council (2009), the leading cause of disability and injury deaths for individuals 65 years and older is falls. The cost of the medical treatment related to falls for persons older than 65 years in 2020 is projected to be $43.8 billion in the United States. Ironically, changing to a cautious lifestyle to protect ourselves from falls can increase our likelihood of falling by drastically cutting back on one of the most effective preventive therapies: physical activity.

The body's cardiovascular capacity decreases 5% to 15% per decade after the age of 25. Muscle mass decreases by nearly 50% between the ages of 20 and 90. On the psychological front, cognitive function and perception of control or self-efficacy are susceptible to declines with aging, and depression is one of the most frequently reported mental health disorders in older adults. The good news is that regular physical activity can reduce and even prevent a number of these functional declines associated with aging. In older adults, aerobic training leads to the same 10% to 30% increases in cardiovascular function as seen in young adults. Strength training helps to offset the loss of muscle mass and strength. Regular exercise also improves bone health, postural stability, and flexibility. It provides a number of psychological benefits such as the preservation of cognitive function, alleviation of depression symptoms, and improved sense of personal control.

Canada's Physical Activity Guide to Healthy Active Living for Older Adults (Health Canada 2001) describes an exercise and aging cycle that demonstrates the relationship between physical activity and physical deterioration with aging. So strong is the relationship between the amount of regular physical activity and the amount of health benefits that in the mid to late 1990s the Surgeons General in both Canada and United States issued statements identifying inactivity as an independent risk factor for cardiovascular disease.

Transtheoretical Model Applied to Older Adults

To help integrate positive health behavioral changes, we can revisit the Transtheoretical Model (see chapters 1and 2) with some increased sensitivities to our clients who are 50+. Prochaska's well-documented Transtheoretical Model suggests that a client's readiness to engage in behaviors such as exercise can be described on a continuum of stages known as the stages of change (Prochaska and DiClemente 1982). Only about 20% of people with a less than ideal behavior are prepared to change at any one time. In senior living facilities, the average rate of participation in physical activity classes is around 20% to 25% (Van Norman 2010). Barke and Nicholas (1990) found adults between ages 59 and 80 more likely to be in the contemplation, action, or maintenance stages than in precontemplation. This suggests that even the least active older adults were thinking about engaging in physical activity or were already preparing to be active. Older adults are more likely to be motivated to be physically active when the activity is at a moderate intensity, is inexpensive, and is convenient and, especially for older women, when it includes a social aspect. Motivation should also be geared to your client's stage of change.

A client's stage of change will determine what messages are relevant and what programs will best meet his needs toward increasing regular physical activity. The model is especially helpful to fitness professionals because it acknowledges the client-centered approach regarding individual differences in readiness to exercise. What strategies or recommendations would you make to your client based on his stage of change?

Precontemplation Stage Strategies

Clients who have not yet begun to think about starting a program of physical activity can benefit from discussions about the pros and cons of physical activity. Perhaps the client has a chronic health condition such as osteoarthritis but does not realize that physical activity could have a positive effect. To help clients get started with physical activity, it is necessary to be realistic about their negative expectations regarding exer-

cise. For the older adult, these "cons" or costs vary from person to person, but could include the time they would have to find in order to exercise; the difficulty of getting to the exercise location; the expense of a membership or special equipment; feeling self-conscious in front of others; and fatigue, muscle soreness, or a general feeling of discomfort. In the early stages of change, for the older adult it may be therapeutic to discuss relevant topics and ask questions related to personal health issues and concerns. The "pros" or benefits of physical activity are client specific. Although you may be able to expound on numerous benefits, only those benefits that are personally valued will be effective motivators. It may be effective to explain that some of these benefits are immediate, such as feeling more alert or energized on exercise days. Others may be cumulative, such as the reduction of blood fats with as little as 500 kcal per week of activity. People in the precontemplation stage will not seek you out, so information should be provided to them over the general course of their day. Many of the strategies and benefits could be used in an advertising campaign at the local community center to encourage potential clients to set up an initial appointment. Then their concerns can be more directly addressed, helping to minimize their perceived costs. Once they believe that potential benefits of physical activity outweigh the potential costs, they will be more likely to move to a contemplation or even preparation stage. For example, if feeling tired after exercise is an issue, perhaps your client could schedule her activity in the evening, when feeling relaxed would encourage better sleep.

Contemplation Stage Strategies

Continued discussion of the pros and cons of physical activity may be warranted for those who intend to begin a program but have not yet started. Many older adults are faced with the challenge of coping with multiple losses that often restrict the amount and nature of social contact. As well, clients who are recently retired may have relied on the work setting as a primary source of social contact and now miss this time and support. Physical activity programs can serve a dual function by meeting both exercise and social needs. Many community agencies and programs offered by churches or social groups can provide the physical benefits of an exercise program with the psychological value of social interaction. Another social support strategy involves adding a social element before or after the activity; that is, people can arrive early to chat with others or meet at a local coffee shop after a class or tennis match. One of the strongest potential supports for regular activity is the person's spouse. Recruiting social support from friends or family members is almost always an effective strategy for physical activity motivation, particularly during the contemplation and preparation stages when clients are attempting to establish regular patterns of physical activity.

Preparation Stage Strategies

When clients have decided that they want to begin a physical activity program and may have begun to engage in some activity, it is a good time to set specific goals. In the preparation stage, communications should include questions regarding their short- and long-term goals. These may involve improving balance and muscle strength related to activities of daily living, or, from a practical perspective, more easily carrying a basket of laundry or bag of groceries up a flight of stairs. Exercise specialists can play a pivotal role in teaching clients how to set and evaluate their goals; however, it is important that clients' goals be their own. Exercise prescription may seem to imply that an exercise plan is imposed by an expert. However, if the client does not feel that she has played a primary role in choosing her own goals and providing input to her program, adherence is unlikely. The challenge is to identify one or two goals that match the current needs, abilities, and lifestyle of your client. Ask your clients how they feel about the proposed goals and how long they think they could continue to meet these goals. Lifestyles, motivations, and stage of readiness for physical activity differ with older adults. Take time to understand your older client's concerns, motivation, and comfort level with proposed goals. Be sensitive to the fact that for some older adults, goal setting may need to revolve exclusively around increasing lifestyle activity. These goals should be designed to produce success, increasing clients' confidence in their physical abilities and their ability to incorporate the exercise routine into their lifestyle. Goal setting may be part of an introductory session and continues to be an important strategy for clients after preparation, during the action or maintenance stages. The specific steps of goal setting are described in chapter 2.

Action Stage Strategies

Even after clients have been engaged in regular physical activity, it is helpful to review their initial goals and adjust them as necessary. Help your clients feel good about what they have accomplished, evaluating successes and problems, and then have them commit to a new set of short-term goals. Provide encouragement and reinforcement with ongoing positive messages. Also, encourage exercise to become more intrinsic at this stage. An effective strategy is the use of positive self-talk related to the client's exercise goals as an exercise motivator. Statements such as "I can do it" or "I'll feel much better once I've stretched" can help clients to begin or continue exercising. Thoughts that help them feel good about exercising can be recalled at times they feel discouraged. Negative self-talk such as "This is a lot of hard work" is likely to occur. Remember, the action stage has the greatest risk for relapse. Be realistic and encourage clients to try to make their self-talk positive and personalized. Motivating self-talk often emphasizes the beneficial effects of exercise: "I will have more energy later in my day" or "This will help me improve my balance."

Maintenance Stage Strategies

Clients exercising regularly for at least 6 months have started to make exercise part of a more active lifestyle. For the older client, relapse prevention strategies, such as planning for potential barriers and recognizing minor lapses, can help prevent lapses (brief periods of inactivity) from turning into relapses (extended periods of inactivity) (Bryant and Green 2005). Tracking progress and improvements and introducing a variety of activity opportunities have been proven effective (Van Norman 2010). In the action or maintenance stage, the client's computer or other device has been shown to be an effective motivator. A systematic review of 12 studies found that e-mail feedback was one intervention among multiple others that aided lifestyle changes with people aged 50 and older (Aalbersa et al. 2011). If clients use e-mail, try sending reminders and tips periodically. Older clients at this stage can also benefit from strategies that keep physical activity both convenient and interesting. Activity that is too inconvenient will be stopped as soon as the effort outweighs the rewards. But there is always a balancing act. Downhill skiers, for example, buy expensive equipment, drive hours to the ski hills, wait in line for tickets and tows, brave harsh weather, and ski to fatigue by the end of the day. This inconvenience is happily tolerated because they are having fun. Clients are willing to deal with hardships if an activity is extremely enjoyable or rewarding. Ways to integrate exercise into lifestyle include a regular routine called "daily dose" and special times called "social adventures," discussed later in the chapter. These should be part of the strategy for older adults in the maintenance stage. There are two important lessons:

1. Engage in exercise plans that are convenient. Routines such as the daily dose can be done even on days when clients have little time or energy for elaborate plans. Hopefully these will be somewhat enjoyable, but they don't have to be blissfully fun if they are relatively convenient and easy to do.

2. Engage in enjoyable exercise activities such as "social adventures" even if they are somewhat inconvenient. For example, one client may be willing to drive for an hour to a favorite hiking spot while another may dress up for ballroom dancing.

Aging Effects and Exercise Training Benefits

Even in the absence of disease, changes associated with aging affect all the major organ systems. Aging is associated with visible and sometimes dramatic changes in the body. There are both structural and functional changes in the body systems, and it is difficult to pinpoint if the changes are due to disease, physical inactivity, or normal aging. As personal trainers, we must be prepared to work with the bodily changes in our older clients.

Aging Effects in the Cardiovascular and Respiratory Systems

Our ability to perform physical work is dependent to a large extent on the proper functioning of the cardiovascular and respiratory systems. The heart's ability as a reservoir and pump, the vascular system of arteries and delivery vessels, and the respiratory function of oxidizing tissues and eliminating carbon dioxide all work together to allow physical work.

With age, the heart's ability to circulate blood diminishes as both heart size and volume capacity drop. A decrease in sympathetic nerve activity to the heart results in a lower maximal heart rate, weaker contractions, and a decreased ejection fraction. Generally with aging, a longer time is needed for heart rate, blood pressure, ventilation, and oxygen consumption to reach equilibrium at any given work rate. Structural changes in the cardiovascular system with age include increased

thickening of the walls of the blood vessels and left ventricular wall and increased stiffness in the arteries. As a result, systolic and diastolic blood pressures increase with age, attributable primarily to a thickening and hardening of the aorta and arterial tree but also to an increase in total peripheral resistance. This may also cause postural hypotension, which predisposes seniors to dizziness, confusion, weakness, or fainting. Maximum heart rates decrease with age at a rate of approximately 5 to 10 beats per decade after the age of 20. As well, heart rates tend to recover more slowly after strenuous exercise. Cardiac output during maximum exercise decreases by about 30% between the ages of 20 and 80, primarily due to a reduction in stroke volume (Taylor and Johnson 2008).

These normal changes impair the elderly client's ability to tolerate an aerobic exercise challenge. This strain is especially evident at the start of an exercise session if the period of warm-up activity before beginning higher-intensity exercises is inadequate. One measure of work capacity or aerobic power is maximum oxygen uptake, a measure of the maximal rate at which the body can use oxygen. It declines about 5% to 25% per decade after the age of 25. In cross-sectional studies of peak oxygen uptake in older adults, a decline of 16% per decade has been observed, with a minimal value of 18 ml $\cdot$ kg^{-1} $\cdot$ min^{-1} in men and 15 ml $\cdot$ kg^{-1} $\cdot$ min^{-1} in women observed for living independently. As well, a 14% increase in the risk for dependency is seen with each 1 ml $\cdot$ kg^{-1} $\cdot$ min^{-1} decrease in maximal aerobic power (Barclay and Lie 2008). This decline has been attributed to a decreased cardiac output, a decreased arterial–venous (a-$\bar{v}$ O$_2$) difference, and a loss of muscle mass. Older adults may start to fatigue within a few minutes if the exercise intensity is at 70% to 75% of maximum oxygen uptake (perceived exertion of 14 or 15).

Factors other than age, however, account for 84% of the decline (Williamson 2011). The primary contributor is loss of lean muscle mass, so if people maintain lean muscle mass, the rate of decline slows dramatically. Age-related reductions in $\dot{V}O_2$max and strength also suggest that at any submaximal exercise load, older adults are often required to exert a higher percentage of their maximal capacity (and effort) when compared with younger persons.

Aging is an independent risk factor associated with several disorders of the cardiovascular system including coronary artery disease, hypertension, and hypercholesterolemia. There are basic aspects of the cardiovascular structure and function that change with age and contribute to the development of these diseases.

Pulmonary efficiency also declines with age. This is seen in a reduction in elastic recoil of the lungs; a gradual decline in the number of alveolar sacs; a decrease in some volumes and capacities, particularly FEV_1 (forced expiratory volume in the first second of a maximal expiration); increased chest wall stiffness; decreased strength of the respiratory muscles; small-airway closure; and decreased sensitivity to the respiratory centers in the nervous system. As well, a change in the surface area of the alveoli reduces gas exchange, and in combination with a decrease in alveolar capillary density, leads to a reduction in diffusion capacity. The vital capacity of the lungs (the maximum volume of air that a person can exhale after maximal inspiration) decreases progressively up to 40% or 50% by the age of 70 (Jones and Rose 2005). Pulmonary gas exchange does not usually limit exercise performance in older people; however, shortness of breath can occur when the volume of individual breath reaches about 50% of the vital capacity. This often causes older adults to voluntarily end their exercise sessions, particularly if they are not familiar with higher levels of activity.

Cardiovascular Training Benefits

The decline in maximum oxygen uptake is much less in regular exercisers. It is not unusual to find actively training seniors over 60 with a higher oxygen uptake and physical work capacity than in sedentary 20-year-olds. The benefits of regular aerobic exercise with adequate intensity, duration, and frequency include the following:

- Decreased resting and working heart rate
- Increased stroke volume, which maintains cardiac output
- Reduced vascular resistance and increased tone of peripheral veins
- Decreased systolic and diastolic blood pressure
- Reduced levels of blood lipids and increased glucose tolerance and insulin sensitivity

Improvement in maximum oxygen uptake with seniors following training is explained by an increase in cardiac output because of the gains in stroke volume. With moderate-intensity exercise, elderly people can expect gains of 20% to 30% in maximum oxygen uptake (Taylor and Johnson 2008). At any given age, physical activity can maintain a higher level of aerobic power (figure 13.2).

A suitable progressive program of endurance training of sufficient intensity ($\geq$60% $\dot{V}O_2$max) and frequency ($\geq$3 days/week) could increase the maximum aerobic power of middle-aged and older adults by 5 to 10 ml · kg^{-1} · min^{-1}. This effect could offset an age-related loss of 5 ml · kg^{-1} · min^{-1} per decade and reduce the effective biological age by 10 years or more, thereby allowing a correspond-

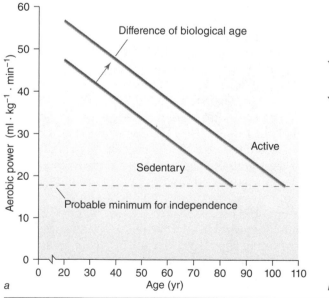

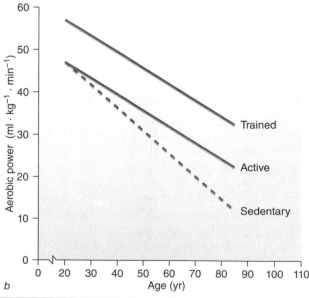

Figure 13.2   Aerobic power and age.

Reprinted by permission from Taylor and Johnson 2008.

ing prolongation of independence. Programs of aerobic training show a trend toward greater gain in aerobic power with longer duration: 12.9% with an 8- to 10-week program, 14.1% with a 12- to 18-week program, and 16.9% with a 24- to 52-week program (Barclay and Lie 2008). Larger improvements in $\dot{V}O_2$max were typically observed with longer training periods (20-30 weeks) but not necessarily higher training intensities (i.e., >70% of $\dot{V}O_2$max) unless an interval-type training regimen was used (Chodzko-Zajko et al. 2009). As well, participation in a group exercise program can counter the social isolation of elderly persons, in addition to maintaining maximal oxygen uptake contributing to the retention of functional independence.

Murias and colleagues (2008) compared younger adults (average age 24 years) with older adults (average age 68 years) training on a bicycle ergometer for 3 days a week for 45 min at 70% of $\dot{V}O_2$max. The amplitude and rate of increase in maximum oxygen uptake and lactate threshold were similar in the two groups after 12 weeks. It appears that the time course and amplitude of adaptations to cardiovascular fitness are similar in older and younger clients.

Aerobic training has significant beneficial effects on maximal exercise, such as increased oxygen uptake, cardiac output, ventilation, and gas exchange. In older men and women, endurance training elicits peripheral adaptations (delivery and extraction of oxygen to increase work capacity) and to a lesser extent, compared to younger clients, central adaptations (e.g., stroke volume) (Cerny and Burton 2001). At submaximal exercise levels, benefits include decreased heart rate, stroke volume, ventilation, and blood pressure. As well, the positive impacts of an active lifestyle can significantly affect activities of daily living.

Changes to structure and function of the cardiovascular system can lead to the development of disease; however, these effects can be influenced by regular physical activity. Regular physical activity increases average life expectancy through its reduction of secondary aging effects resulting from chronic disease and lifestyle behaviors (Chodzko-Zajko et al. 2009). In addition, regular physical activity reduces the risk of heart disease, hypertension, and diabetes and increases longevity and decreases disability. For example, regular physical activity of moderate intensity can negate the age-related decline in endothelial function and improve vascular compliance (Taylor and Johnson 2008). An active lifestyle both prevents and remediates disease and in this sense postpones many symptoms of aging in the cardiovascular and respiratory systems.

Even under heavy exercise conditions, pulmonary function is not usually a limiting factor in maximal physical work capacity. Moderate- to high-intensity physical training may prevent age-related decline in resting lung function until about 60 years of age (Jones and Rose 2005). With training, the older client will be able to use a larger fraction of the available vital capacity before stopping exercise because of shortness of breath. The shortness of breath is reduced because of increased respiratory muscle strength and changes in perception of exertion.

Nieman (2009) has shown that a brisk walking program, 5 days a week for 12 weeks, lowered sick days with the common cold by more than one-half in elderly subjects. During each walking bout, important immune cells were increased temporarily in the body, providing enhanced protection from viruses; this implies that near-daily activity is optimal for acute immune benefit. Nieman also found much lower rates of illness from upper respiratory tract infections (8% for the fit subjects and 50% for sedentary controls). There is growing consensus that moderate exercise training can counter chronic low-grade inflammation and offset at least part of the decline in the immune function with advancing age.

Long periods of disuse and sedentary living dramatically accelerate aging of the cardiovascular and respiratory systems. On the other hand, regular exercise postpones many symptoms of aging in those systems. Regular aerobic training improves coordination between the cardiovascular and respiratory systems. When physically challenged, these systems become more efficient at transporting gases to and from tissues, so demands placed on them become easier. It is also encouraging that the cardiovascular system responds to training regardless of previous physical activity patterns.

Aging Effects in the Musculoskeletal System

The most noticeable changes observed with aging are those involving the musculoskeletal system, and your clients will frequently want to set goals in this area. Lean body mass decreases, interstitial fat content increases, joint motion diminishes, muscle blood flow declines, and muscle strength and endurance decrease. Muscle power, or the rapid generation of force, declines earlier and more precipitously with age than strength does.

Aging effects are also prominent in the areas of joint flexibility, bone mass and mineral content, and body composition.

Muscle Strength

Muscle strength is maintained well up until the fifth decade of life, but in each of the next two decades, it is normal to see up to a 15% drop in muscle strength. After 70 years of age, strength loss may be as much as 3% per year. Severe loss of muscle mass and strength can result in loss of functional independence. For example, those with low ankle strength have a higher risk of falling (Van Norman 2010). Much of the strength loss with age is attributed to a loss of muscle mass. Muscle atrophy or decreased cross-sectional area of the muscle is caused by a loss of fibers, a decrease in fiber area, or a combination of these factors operating at the same time. Sarcopenia is the loss of skeletal muscle mass, strength, and contractile properties (e.g., time to peak tension) associated with aging. Causative factors may include selective muscle fiber atrophy (including a reduced capacity for hypertrophy), reductions in protein synthesis rates, slowed contractile shortening, and injury or neuromuscular diseases as seen in figure 13.3 (Spirduso et al. 2005). As well, older clients have a decline in anabolic hormone levels (e.g., testosterone, insulin), which influences hypertrophic capacity and strength. Loss of muscle strength may also be attributed to an unequal decline in number of type I and type II fibers (Taylor and Johnson 2008). There is a selective decline in muscle fiber size, primarily in type II (fast-twitch) fibers. Because of the high concentration of type II fibers in the back and thighs (quadriceps and hamstrings), these muscles are the first to atrophy in older adults.

Muscle Power

Peak power requires timing and coordination in the application of maximum velocity. For example, leg power more than strength is needed in older adults for activities such as climbing stairs, rising from a chair, fast walking, or fall recovery. Because of the preferential atrophy of type II (fast-twitch) muscle fibers that occurs with advancing age, the remaining muscle mass is not only smaller and weaker, but slower as well. Strength and power declines may also be explained by changes in the nervous system with age, including a loss of motor units and a larger innervation ratio in the motor units that remain. Recall that a motor unit is the motor nerve and all the muscle fibers it innervates. As we age, our motor nerves and their associated muscle fibers die off at an increasing rate. The motor units that we lose are mainly the fast-twitch variety, so aging muscles show a predominance of slow-twitch fibers; therefore, the slower and less powerful we become. The neural reorganization affecting muscle activation is also associated with a reported unsteadiness during dynamic eccentric contractions, which may be associated with a higher incidence of falling during stair decent compared with ascent (Cerny and Burton 2001). Age- and sex-related differences in muscle power may partially explain the impairments in muscle function that occur with

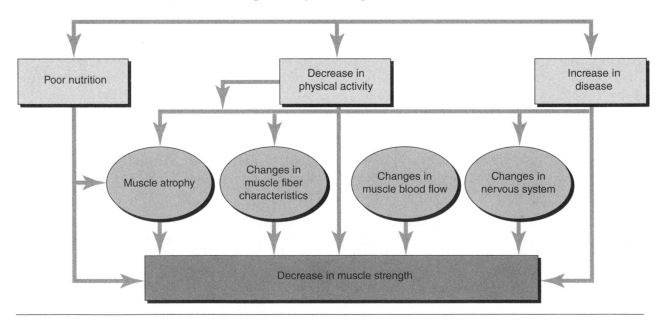

Figure 13.3   Factors that may cause loss of muscle strength with aging.

Reprinted by permission from Spirduso, Francis, and MacRae 2005.

aging and the greater muscle impairment observed in older women than in older men.

Joint Flexibility

Joint flexibility decline is influenced by decreases in muscle fiber flexibility and the elasticity of connective tissue. Flexibility and joint stability are also related to changes in the components of the connective tissue within the joint's cartilage, capsule, ligaments, tendons, and fascia. These become stiffer and lose elasticity and strength because of structural changes in the connective tissue as we age. For example, collagen is a structural protein providing strength within connective tissue. Collagen becomes irregular in shape due to cross-linking with increasing age. There is also a tighter meshing and decreased linear pull in the collagen tissue, which leads to a decrease in flexibility in older clients. Collagen changes in the annulus fibrosis of the intervertebral disc result in reduced spinal flexibility (Williamson 2011). Elastin is a far more elastic protein in connective tissue but degenerates at a much faster rate, making it harder to move, decreasing flexibility, and providing a general feeling of stiffness. These changes in connective tissue can produce reduced range of motion, decreased stored elastic energy, reduced mobility, increased joint contracture, and increased risk of injury. By the age of 70, the average adult may have lost 25% to 30% of his flexibility. Spirduso and colleagues (2005) cited research indicating a loss of flexibility (measured by the sit-and-reach test) of 15% per decade. A loss of flexibility can lead to performance issues with daily tasks such as getting in and out of a car, climbing stairs, or dressing. For example, combing one's hair requires flexion of the elbow, abduction and external rotation of the shoulder, pronation of the forearm, and flexion of the wrist and fingers. If the range of motion deteriorates in any of these joints, combing hair becomes difficult or impossible. Reduced range of motion can affect both balance and stability and presents a risk for injury to the joint structure or muscles. Another factor that reduces flexibility is the development of osteoarthritis, a degenerative disease of the joints involving loss and damage of cartilage, thickening of bone endings, growth of spurs or osteophytes, thickened joint capsule, and inflamed synovial membrane, causing substantial pain and impaired mobility.

Bone

The loss of structural integrity of the musculoskeletal system comes primarily from the decline in bone mass and bone mineral content. The losses in bone mass, bone density, and bone geometry are largely attributable to hormonal changes, dietary deficiencies, and physical inactivity. Women maintain bone density until age 35, while men do so until about age 55. By age 70, most people have lost 10% to 15% of their peak bone density. Fractures to the spine, hip, and wrist from minor stresses are the primary issues of osteoporosis. For example, those suffering hip fractures often experience a loss of independence because of incomplete recovery. The higher rate of bone loss in women contributes to the higher rate of osteoporosis and bone fractures among older women, with 50% of women and 13% of men in the United States experiencing an osteoporosis-related fracture sometime in their life (Spirduso et al. 2005).

Body Composition

Age-related changes in body composition also have implications for physical function and health. The redistribution of an increase in fat and the loss of muscle mass result in decreases in basal metabolic rate and substantial decreases in aerobic capacity. Moreover, increased body fat, particularly abdominal fat (expressed by a higher body mass index), is associated with increased risk for cardiovascular disease, diabetes, and earlier mortality.

Musculoskeletal Training Benefits

Exercise plays a critical role in maintaining a strong, efficient musculoskeletal system, which promotes lifelong functional independence and QOL. How can your older clients reverse their decline in strength? Adults of any age, even the very old, can experience significant gains in strength following a resistance training program. With increased muscle strength and joint stability come added beneficial outcomes such as improved walking speed, ability to rise from a chair, ease of stair climbing, and decreased frequency of falls.

Muscle Strength

One of the first high-intensity strength training studies in older adults (Frontera et al. 1988) trained 60- to 72-year-old males at 80% of one-repetition maximum (1RM) with 3 sets of 8 repetitions, 3 days per week, which was very similar to many protocols used today in clinical, community, and home-based settings. After 12 weeks the authors observed significant increases in strength (150%) and muscle mass (10%). Signorile (2011) offers a schematic representation of what generally happens to the neuromuscular aging curve with an intervention of appropriate exercise (figure 13.4).

Figure 13.4 shows the normal neuromuscular aging curve as a solid line. With 30% improvement in a client at 60 years of age, a 50% improvement in the client at 75 years of age, and an 80% improvement at 90 years, the dashed curve bends upward, demonstrating improvement in comparison to the solid line. If a client has been training his entire life (dotted line), there will still be an exponential drop in neuromuscular performance with age; however, the curve begins much higher, the decline begins later, and the drop is not as abrupt. There is still a decline with aging, but now the client is at a level equivalent to that of an untrained person years younger.

Muscle mass is increased with individual muscle fibers increasing in size and protein content. Muscle regeneration following the mechanical stress of resistance exercise creates an increase in strength through neural and hypertrophic mechanisms (i.e., increased fiber diameter). In a study of men in their 60s, Candow and coauthors (2011) demonstrated that 12 weeks of heavy resistance training (3 sets of 10 repetitions to muscle failure, 3 days per week) was sufficient to eliminate deficits in muscle size and strength when compared to measures in healthy younger men. With an additional 10 weeks of training, the remaining deficits in lean tissue mass were eliminated. With similarly aged clients and a 12-week program, Kalapotharakos and colleagues (2005) compared the effects of heavy (80% of 1RM) and moderate (60% of 1RM) resistance training (three times a week) on strength and functional performance. Significant differences in improvement were found between heavy and moderate resistance training with 1RM strength measures on the lower limbs. However, the two training systems showed similar improvements in functional performance as measured by walking velocity, chair rising time, stair climbing time, and sit-and-reach flexibility.

Fall Prevention

The neuromuscular benefits of exercise also play a significant role in potential falls prevention. Older adults who have the ability to protect or catch themselves during the act of falling have a reduced risk of injury. Strength training programs that specifically emphasized eccentric training in muscle groups such as the quadriceps, hip extensors, and foot plantar flexors have been shown to decrease the magnitude of unsteadiness during contractions. Balance training activities such as lower body strengthening and walking over difficult terrain have been shown to significantly improve balance and are thus recommended as part of an exercise intervention to prevent falls. Older adults identified as at the highest risk for falls seem to benefit from an individually tailored exercise program that is embedded within a larger, multifactorial falls prevention intervention program of balance, strength, flexibility, and walking (Chodzko-Zajko et al. 2009).

Functional mobility training incorporating strength and balance exercises has also demonstrated success in reducing the risk of falls (Pizzigalli et al. 2011). In an effort to examine how strength training could affect muscle weakness

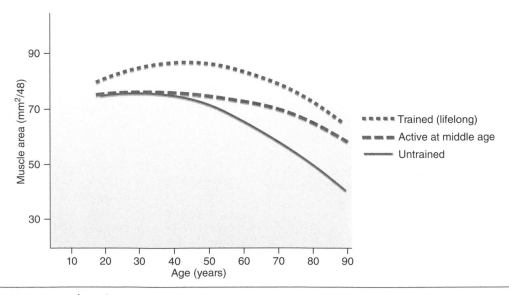

Figure 13.4 Neuromuscular aging curve.
Reprinted by permission from Signorile 2007.

and impaired mobility in relation to functional limitations and risk of falls, Zhu and Chodzko-Zajko (2006) reported on the effects of an 8-week strength training program. In addition to strength gains of 174% on average and a 9% increase in midthigh muscle area, the researchers observed a 48% improvement in tandem gait speed. It is clear that strength training can reduce or delay functional limitations as well as reduce physical impairment and falls.

Power

Resistance training designed to improve power has demonstrated good results with regard to maintaining physical function and mobility, for example in stair climbing, walking, and recreational activities. High-intensity physical activity promoting hypertrophy and maximizing the recruitment of motor units needed to activate type II muscle fibers has been effective in the trunk and lower body (Jones and Rose 2005). Strength training recommendations often neglect velocity, opting for slow, controlled movements. This is unfortunate, since the successful completion of many functional tasks requires the ability to generate force quickly, for example crossing a street before the light changes, driving a golf ball, even getting out of a chair. Certainly there are some important considerations around momentum and excessive eccentric work; however, it is not surprising that several studies show power to be more highly correlated with functional abilities than strength alone. Foldvari and colleagues (2000) reported that leg power was a stronger predictor of functional status in elderly women than any other physiological measure they assessed, including lower body strength. Gonzalez-Rave and colleagues (2011) examined changes among 60- to 70-year-old athletes and nonathletes after 16 weeks of contrast training that used a combination of heavy resistance and explosive exercises. There was an improvement in vertical jump performance and muscle mass in both groups regardless of the training history and current physical activity of each. This contrast training method for men in their 60s elicited an adaptive response without acute fatigue or overtraining. It appears to be safe and demonstrates the benefits of increased hypertrophy and power for functional activities and QOL in older clients.

Joint Flexibility

People can maintain musculoskeletal flexibility in later years by using joints through the full range of motion. Static and dynamic stretching, as well as aerobic exercise and resistance training in older adults, has been shown to increase joint range of motion (Fatouras et al. 2002). Older adults who maintain an active lifestyle are more flexible than inactive seniors, particularly in weight-bearing joints. Similar improvements in flexibility have been recorded between young and older participants in the same training programs (Spirduso et al. 2005). Regular activity has been shown to reduce pain and improve mobility in those with degenerative joint disease (Brennan 2002). The ability to live with osteoarthritic changes depends on how the stresses around the joint are shared by the muscle and the remaining articular cartilage. Stronger muscles and increased joint stability generally reduce the stress placed on the joint surface. In 2010, Baker and Cutlip published data on 4-month home-based strength training in individuals 55 and over with knee osteoarthritis. Patients in the exercise group experienced significant reductions in pain and improvements in flexibility, muscular strength, functional performance, physical abilities, QOL, and self-efficacy.

Bone

Physical activity is essential for maintaining bone mass and functional mobility. Weight-bearing aerobic endurance exercise and resistance training have been proven to help prevent bone loss and increase bone mineral content, contributing to the prevention of osteoporosis (Van Norman 2010). Although certain spinal flexion and rotation exercises should be avoided by patients with osteoporosis, there is little validity to reducing physical activity to prevent fractures. A progressive resistance training program that strengthens the back extensor muscles can reduce pain and improve functional mobility in patients with vertebral osteoporosis (Marcus 2001). Activity such as walking, jogging, and stair climbing, in which the skeleton incurs ground reaction forces, appears to be most effective for building bone in the femoral neck, a common fracture site (Jones and Rose 2005). Evidence appears to indicate that higher intensities are needed for bone modeling to result. Greater loads versus low to moderate intensity have shown better changes in bone density especially in the hip, spine, and wrist (Vincent and Braith 2002). Similarly, brisk walking showed better bone building than walking at a more leisurely pace. Most of the impact of the step is absorbed through the foot, ankle, knee, and hip. As a result, walking is good for building and preserving bone in the lower body and provides less stimulus to the spine or upper body (Martyn-St. James and Carroll 2008). However, the use of Nordic poles can incorporate more spinal muscle and upper body activation into walking while providing additional support that may help make brisk walking more secure. Recent studies also found that Nordic walking led to significant improvements in cardiovascular capacity, muscle strength, flexibility, and dynamic balance after a 9-week program (Parkatti et al. 2012).

Weight training for older adults should target specific muscle groups such as the knee extensors and hip extensors because these muscles are used in day-to-day activities and tend to deteriorate more quickly than upper body muscles. Muscles of the calf such as the dorsiflexors are important for walking and fall prevention. Forearm strengthening will assist with gripping, carrying groceries, and other manipulation tasks. Resistance exercise improves physical function by decreasing the relative intensity of tasks performed in daily life. It can also decrease the stress placed on the heart during tasks such as lifting moderately heavy boxes, activities that have been implicated as causes of heart attacks.

Changes in Locomotion

Why do older clients have trouble crossing the street before the light changes? There are clear differences in gait patterns when older adults are compared with younger adults, but it is difficult to ascertain how much of the change is attributable to aging alone or the effect of a disease process. These changes affect an older adult's ability to maintain her independence and can also increase her risk for falls. She may find it more difficult to cross the street before the light changes, get on and off moving walkways, or deal with other situations requiring rapid modifications of her gait cycle.

Various motor pattern compensations take place probably due to caution during the weight-bearing stage of gait. We tend to see a flatter foot-to-floor contact, less forward progression of the limb during single-limb support, and reduced knee flexion during the preswing and swing phases. These compensations are coping mechanisms used by older adults when they begin to experience more variability in their walking patterns or discomfort (Rose 2010). The most obvious change is gait speed. Measures are often recorded as preferred speed or maximum speed. Gait speed declines on average by 12% to 16% per decade in adults 70 years and older. The preferred speed is approximately 20% slower than in younger adults. During walking at a fast speed, the difference in gait speed is 17% (Spirduso et al. 2005). This loss of speed is primarily due to decreases in stride length as opposed to stride rate. This change alone appears to reduce arm swing; reduce rotation at the hips, knees, and ankles; increase

double-support time; and reduce ankle range of motion during the stance phase (Elble 1997). These changes may also be due to muscle weakness, joint instability, or loss of balance. Aging alters the speed–cost relationship; as preferred walking speeds decrease, energy costs increase. Jones, Waters, and Legge (2009) compared the energy cost of walking at a self-selected speed for 30 min in older and younger women. Energy costs at a self-selected pace were significantly higher in the older women. These authors found maximal $\dot{V}O_2$ to be the primary determinant of walking speed when all age groups were combined, and recommended the assessment of aerobic fitness before the initiation of an exercise plan for older women. The increase in the energy cost of locomotion, one reason gait becomes slower, may also be due to changes in posture such as increased thoracic kyphosis, forward head position, rounded shoulders, and increased hip and knee flexion. A deterioration of the sensory systems and poor anticipation of changes in the environment also adversely affect gait speed and a smooth walking pattern. Reduction in gait speed and shorter steps are common when older adults approach obstacles, especially if they are nervous about tripping. Rose (2010) reported that older adults with a history of falls demonstrated decreased stride length, ankle plantar flexion, hip extension, and lateral body sway as well as increased stride frequency when compared to older adults with no history of falls. Those with a falls history also show greater variability in their pattern of walking from strike to strike.

Locomotion Training Benefits

Although some of the age-related changes in locomotion are inevitable, much can be done to prevent or slow declines through careful selection of gait pattern improvement in various exercises. In combination with balance activities, older adults can achieve a gait pattern that is efficient, flexible, and adaptable to changing task and environmental demands.

Working on gait improvement should include activities designed to vary the gait pattern and progressively challenge the client by manipulating the environment. For example, begin with directional changes with abrupt starts and stops, changes in the length and width of the stride, or walking on toes and heels. Progress to variations such as sidestepping, crossovers, tandem walking, and turning on demand. This varies the temporal and spatial characteristics of the gait pattern, allowing clients a greater repertoire of movement options and increased confidence. Having clients practice avoiding obstacles or barriers within the environment will improve visual control of locomotion. Clients become more skilled at anticipating the changes and challenges in the physical environment. Such activities may include stepping over obstacles, on and off different surface types, or up and down inclines. As confidence and balance improve, activities can be used that demand division of attention between two tasks; for example, reaching for or catching objects, turning the head while walking, or navigating obstacle courses. Rose (2010) has effectively adapted gait pattern enhancement training to emphasize both balance and mobility with a focus on preventing falls.

Locomotion itself in the form of walking or running may be the single most important activity to maintain health as people age. Researchers at the Stanford University School of Medicine have been tracking 500 older runners over age 50 for more than 20 years. Their data show that regular running slows the effect of aging; older runners have fewer disabilities, have a longer span of active life, and are half as likely as nonrunners to die prematurely. Initial disability in runners was 16 years later than in nonrunners (Fries et al. 2008).

Preexercise Screening and Assessment

When taking on a new older client, how do you know when it is safe to begin an exercise program? General screening procedures are discussed in chapter 4; however, the level of risk is often higher with an older client, and this should be reflected in our approach.

Screening is done before any assessment or exercise program to identify chronic disease, acute illness or injury, pains, impairments, medications, cardiovascular risk factors, overall health status, and physical activity and exercise patterns. However, if the first thing you do is probe with reams of paperwork or prod and induce fatigue, clients who are not totally committed may leave with less resolve to change than when they entered. Take sufficient time to establish your clients' commitment, question them carefully, and focus on their areas of concern.

Counseling Interview

The interview process is a comfortable way to begin gathering information and establishing a relationship. What should you ask in the screening interview? By having your clients describe their past, present, and future activities and goals, whether they be recreational, occupational, or training, you can gain an overall appreciation of their health status. If you know what they have been doing, you can better determine what they're able to do. Information you gather from this initial conversation will not only help you determine where potential weaknesses may exist but what assessments should be done to help you decide where the training program should begin.

As we discussed in chapter 2, individual questions should be asked regarding the client's wants, needs, and lifestyle. Begin by addressing your client's present level of daily activity. Find out if he is still working, is retired, or what his occupation is or was. Whenever he mentions any activity, be it recreational, household chore, fitness training, or active social, always ask for the FIT (how frequently, how intensely, and for how long [time]). Most often you will be surprised when you begin with a simple request like "Tell me about a typical week in your life."

If the client is working, ask, "Is any part of your work physical?" and "How do you spend your time away from work?" If he is not employed or works part-time, you will need to ask questions about his lifestyle at home, such as "What specific things do you do for the upkeep of your home inside and out?" Housecleaning usually follows a consistent pattern, so ask about specific household tasks. A client who can clean the tub, wash the windows, or shovel snow is likely to have better muscle conditioning in the legs, trunk, or arms and therefore more likely to be able to start the program at a slightly higher level. Recreational activities and active social activities enjoyed by the client are positive areas on which to gather more information for both potential assessment items and the eventual exercise prescription.

Most active seniors have a history of injuries. Before any testing or exercise prescription, ask, "Have you had any recent injuries? Did you undergo any rehabilitation?" A good health and lifestyle questionnaire can gather considerable information in this area. Walking is the most common of all activities. Be sure to probe for detail: "How often do you walk?" "When was the last time you went for a walk?" "For how long do you walk?" "Is it a brisk walk or a stroll?" "Do you walk your dog?—describe the nature of those walks." Regardless of what types of activities are reported by your client, be sure to ask. "Do you experience any pain during the activity?" "How long does it take for the pain to subside?" "Is your doctor aware of this pain, and has your doctor ever restricted your activity because of the pain?"

Information about a client's overall health status, physical activity patterns, and readiness to exercise, as well as procedures and consent, may all be part of the screening process. Pertinent information can be obtained from an interview, forms, and questionnaires administered before the assessment or activity. Traditionally known as preexercise screening or health risk appraisal, this process is one way we can more positively present a health and lifestyle information session that may help clients on their first step to behavioral change. These screening tools may include the following:

- Form 1.1 FANTASTIC Lifestyle Checklist
- Form 1.4 Activity Preferences Questionnaire
- Form 1.9 Activity Counseling Model Checklist
- Form 4.1 RISK-I
- Form 4.2 Physical Activity Index
- Form 13.1 Functional Mobility Informed Consent

Other useful lifestyle appraisal screening tools can be found in chapter 4 or in Rose (2010), Jones and Rose (2005), Speers (2005), and Rikli and Jones (2001).

Almost anyone, at any age, can do some type of exercise and physical activity. According to the American College of Sports Medicine (ACSM 2010), the term "older adult" refers to people who are ≥65 years old or those who are 50 to 64 years old and have similar clinically significant conditions or physical limitations that affect their ability to participate in activity. Men ≥45 and women ≥55 or those with two or more cardiovascular disease risk factors are considered at moderate risk but can participate in moderate-intensity exercise that elevates their heart rate between 60% and 80% maximal heart rate (HRmax) (ACSM 2010). The National Institute on Aging (2009) says you can still be active even if you have a long-term condition like heart disease or diabetes but that you should talk with your doctor if you aren't used to energetic activity. This publication lists a number of reasons to check with your doctor before changing your activity:

- Any new symptoms you haven't yet discussed
- Dizziness or shortness of breath
- Chest pain or pressure

- Feeling that your heart is skipping, racing, or fluttering
- Blood clots
- An infection or fever with muscle aches
- Unplanned weight loss
- Foot or ankle sores that won't heal
- Joint swelling (especially ankles)
- A bleeding or detached retina, eye surgery, or laser treatment
- A hernia
- Recent hip or back surgery

The American Heart Association (AHA) and the ACSM have established similar screening criteria for the aging population (ACSM 2010). In addition to those just mentioned, they list the following risk factors associated with cardiovascular or metabolic disease:

- Unusual fatigue with usual activities
- Known heart murmur
- Intermittent claudication (cramping or unusual fatigue of the legs and buttocks during exertion)

The preamble to the Canadian Physical Activity Guidelines for Older Adults (65 and older) (Canadian Society for Exercise Physiology [CSEP] 2011) points out that potential benefits far exceed the potential risks associated with physical activity. The guidelines are appropriate for older adults with frailty, a disability, or a medical condition; however, people are warned to consult a health professional to understand the types and amounts of physical activity appropriate for them based on their exercise capacity and specific health risks or limitations. Screening information that provides your client's current physical activity level (frequency, duration, and intensity) and the types of activities your client enjoys helps you to choose appropriate functional testing and to develop an individualized exercise prescription suited to your client's abilities and interests.

Canada's Physical Activity Guidelines for Older Adults (CSEP 2011) include the following:

- To improve functional abilities, adults aged 65 years and older should accumulate at least 150 min of moderate- to vigorous-intensity aerobic physical activity per week, in bouts of 10 min or more.
- It is also beneficial to add muscle and bone strengthening activities using major muscle groups, at least 2 days per week.

- Those with poor mobility should perform physical activities to enhance balance and prevent falls.

Medical problems may range from mild to severe and can reduce the sharpness of the senses, slow motor actions, impair the brain's ability to translate sensory stimuli into the appropriate movement responses, and impair the ability to adapt quickly to sudden changes in the environment. Maintaining safe balance and mobility may be affected by medications that impair balance and motor functions, history of inner ear disorders or head injury, and conditions known to affect the senses (such as diabetes) and the brain (such as cardiovascular insufficiency). Previous or current injuries that place the client at greater risk of an accident or reinjury during exercise can also be identified during screening. Screening helps you determine contraindicated exercises that place the client at risk of reinjury. In addition to having deficits in strength, endurance, and flexibility, many new exercisers fatigue quickly because they are forced to consciously monitor actions that would otherwise be effortless and automatic (Nashner 2002).

In general, most elderly clients who are found to have low to moderate risk do not need a current medical examination or a stress test before beginning a low- to moderate-intensity exercise program (Morrison 2001). However, 4 out of 10 adults over 65 have a chronic disorder that may result in a functional limitation. These problems must be identified through the preexercise screening process. Any medical conditions that would cause the client to be at risk during exercise or physical assessment should require specific consent from the client's physician. Providing information about how to know when it is safe to begin an exercise program further empowers individuals to be responsible for their health. Some clients are already active and are just looking for some refinement. Others may never have exercised consistently and have no idea where to start. Not knowing if it is all right to exercise may stop people from continuing with their plans. Is important that the underlying cardiovascular health be known before any program begins. The algorithm in figure 13.5 (Brennan 2002) can help in assessment of a client's ability to start an exercise program.

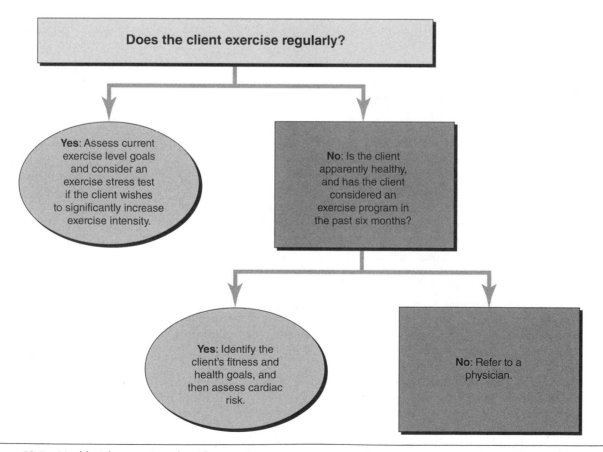

Figure 13.5   Health risk screening algorithm.

If high risk:
Refer to a physician.

If moderate risk:
Conduct a stress test before vigorous activity if the client has two or more cardiac risk factors.

If low risk:
Trial a low- to moderate-intensity exercise program.

Physical Screening Procedures

Check that pretest instructions to clients have been followed (see chapter 4) and that Functional Mobility Informed Consent (form 13.1) and PAR-Q+ were administered before the assessment begins (see chapter 4). Lusardi, Pellecchia, and Schulman (2003) suggest the following criteria to exclude individuals who have not obtained physician approval:

- Acute illness or injury
- Advised by their physicians not to exercise
- Have had congestive heart failure
- Currently experience during-exercise chest pain, dizziness, significant joint pain, or frequent use of inhaler
- Have uncontrolled high blood pressure (greater than 160/100)
- Within the previous 6 months, have had cardiac surgery, abdominal surgery, stroke, spinal or hip fracture, total joint replacement, chemotherapy, or radiation therapy

Screening helps you to identify clients who may need additional attention or accommodation in your program. Screening and assessment facilitate the early identification of functional fitness impairments in the older adult and can help you develop more tailored exercise prescription. Furthermore, documenting the information gathered during screening reduces your risk of liability and improves the safety and effectiveness of the program.

Test Selection Criteria

Following the screening process and before people become active, it is recommended that physical impairments (including declines in cardiovascular or musculoskeletal systems) and functional limitations (restrictions in physical tasks or behaviors of everyday life) be assessed. Functional mobility and health in later years are supported by a number of physiological components: strength and muscular endurance, aerobic capacity, flexibility, agility and dynamic balance, and body composition (Signorile 2011; Fern 2009). These components should be represented in the battery of tests.

According to the ACSM, the healthy senior can perform standard fitness testing procedures with suitable slight modifications (ACSM 2010). For any cardiovascular assessments, ASCM suggests initial workloads of 2 to 3 metabolic equivalents (METs) with increases not exceeding 0.5 to 1.0 METs for anyone with a low work capacity. Treadmill speed should be based on walking ability, and a cycle ergometer should be used if balance, muscle weakness, or other problems are present; however, often a walking test is more appropriate since more people walk during their normal activities. The ACSM warns that elderly individuals typically take one or more medications, many of which influence heart rate and blood pressure response to exercise. Others argue that field tests and the use of the client's perception, such as ratings of perceived exertion (RPE), during submaximal aerobic tests provide information that is most beneficial for establishing an exercise program and provides a positive experience more likely to facilitate a change in lifestyle (Bryant and Green 2005). The exercise specialist needs to know what exercise tests are most appropriate for testing a particular client and how the equations used for a given test were developed. For example, a multiple regression equation developed using healthy well-trained college-age males should not be used to predict $\dot{V}O_2$max for sedentary elderly men or women.

Rikli and Jones (2001) described a physical performance framework called the Functional Fitness Framework that demonstrates the progressive relationship between physiological components, functional performance, and functional activity goals. For example, a functional activity goal such as gardening cannot be achieved without functional performance of bending or lifting, which in turn requires physiological components such as strength and flexibility. These authors' Senior Fitness Test followed a list of selection criteria:

- It represents a cross section of functional fitness components associated with functional mobility.
- It has acceptable validity and reliability.
- It has the sensitivity to detect physical changes due to training.
- It is easy to administer and score.
- It requires minimum equipment and space (e.g., can be administered in clinical, community, and home settings).

- It is safe.
- It is reasonably quick to administer (e.g., no more than 30 to 40 min per client).

Many seniors and first-time clients will not be ready to move beyond an initial counseling and lifestyle appraisal: Pushing on to a full battery of exhaustive tests can destroy what little motivation they have. It is okay to use certain tests, such as standard screening tools, for first-time clients. When your client has expressed a specific interest or need, be sure to include test items for that component. If your client is intimidated by the idea of exercise, you can gather information from simple field-based tests that may be less threatening than more complex assessment tools. Field tests can still enable you to design an initial prescription that suits your client's immediate needs. The very process of administering a fitness assessment draws attention to the "client-centered" nature of the relationship. The testing process and the test results help to educate and motivate clients and stimulate their interest in exercise and other health-related issues. However, the primary function of measurement is to determine status.

How do you judge an effective test? Numerous physiological or functional fitness tests examine functional mobility tasks. In evaluating performance testing, it is important to be sure that the test is specific and relevant to the functional task or training program. When training and testing use a similar exercise (movement) and mode, test results will more accurately reflect improvements. For example, if the 30 s chair stand test is used to evaluate strength, endurance, and functional mobility of the lower body, and partial squats are a key part of the exercise prescription, the test should be sensitive in picking up performance improvements. As discussed in chapter 4, any fitness assessment protocol should also meet the criteria of being valid, reliable, objective, and probably economical (Hoffman 2006).

Fitness or Functional Assessments

Although physical functioning is of vital concern to the clients themselves and has implications for national health care costs, the assessment of physical function is not yet a routine clinical procedure. Functional assessments usually are conducted when there is evidence that basic activities may be compromised. However, the importance of regular physical health and function merits the establishment of a baseline of physical capacity at least by the age of 65. This benchmark of performance can accurately assess the degree and rate of change of physical function of our aging population. Periodic functional assessment provides a way to determine the extent of functional decline.

Determine first what you want to test: fitness or functional performance. **Functional fitness** refers to the fitness components (strength, power, flexibility, balance, and cardiovascular endurance) necessary to perform normal everyday activities safely and independently without undue fatigue. **Functional performance** is the observable ability to perform tasks of daily living or field tests that emulate tasks of daily living (climbing stairs, carrying objects) (Spirduso et al. 2005). Sometimes trainers sample a large cross section of fitness components or perform a functional mobility performance test battery. At other times, they may assess only high-priority components or selected items within a performance battery.

The test should suit the client's ability. Not surprisingly, there is a large hierarchy of physical function between the young-old and the old-old. The challenge is to find an appropriate test for the ability level of the client. Five broad categories have been identified:

1. Physically elite, capable of sport competition
2. Physically fit, capable of moderate physical work
3. Physically independent, capable of light physical work
4. Physically frail, capable of light housekeeping and basic activities of daily living
5. Physically dependent, cannot perform some or all basic activities of daily living (Spirduso et al. 2005)

Physically elite persons are very active and can be assessed safely by tests that are routinely used for young adults (see chapter 4; Speers 2005; or ACSM 2010). **Physically fit** persons maintain good health and activity habits, may be participating in activities with people much younger than themselves, and generally enjoy a biologically younger age. Most of the physically fit elderly could complete an assessment protocol similar to that used for the physically elite. The ACSM recommends that the modified Balke treadmill protocol be used with the elderly because it involves slow but constant walking speeds and a very gradual increase in grade increments (ACSM 2010). The physically fit elderly provide 50% to 75% of the upper scores on laboratory strength muscular endurance tests on the general public of that age. For clients in the physically fit category, several field tests are available to measure functional fitness (Rikli and Jones 2001) and functional mobility (Griffin 2011). Rikli and Jones' Senior Fitness Test (SFT) is presented in table 13.1. Norm-referenced and criterion-referenced performance standards were developed for the STF, and older adults can perform these test items safely without the need for a medical release in most cases. The items assess a wide range of physical components underlying functional mobility by using functional tasks of daily living. For example, instead of measuring lower body strength with a 1RM leg press, the 30 s chair stand is used. The SFT uses continuous-scale scoring (i.e., times or repetitions) so that significant differences can be detected. Other similar tests (Griffin 2011) use an ordinal scale and attempt to identify specific mobility issues within the performance of such functional tasks.

Physically independent elderly persons are those who do not exercise and do not focus much on beneficial health habits but have few functional limitations. They remain independent, but many of them would have difficulty completing more vigorous test items. They may have orthopedic complications that affect physical performance testing, with early termination leaving assessors unsure if the cause is a fitness limitation or joint pain. Of the groups at the five levels, the physically independent group is the largest, with 66.8% of men but only 49.7% of women over the age of 70 having no difficulty with basic physical functions (Spirduso et al. 2005). These clients have enough physical function to participate in some advanced activities of daily living (AADL), such as gardening, woodworking, travel, golf, and some recreational exercise, but they are vulnerable to unexpected physical stress. Activities of daily living (ADL) and instrumental activities of daily living (IADL) questionnaires regarding their physical difficulties and abilities are used at this level. It is important to find a valid way to assess physical reserve in the physically independent in order to know how far from frailty they may be. Functional fitness components such as lower limb strength are important to measure since these are necessary for shopping, housekeeping, and getting in and out of a car. The Senior Fitness Test would be appropriate for the higher-functioning members of this group. The American Alliance for Health, Physical Education, Recreation and Dance Functional Fitness Test is appropriate for sedentary independent-living elderly people over 60 who are not physically fit but are not yet physically frail (Osness 1996). The test includes measures of muscular strength and endurance, coordination, trunk and leg flexibility, and aerobic endurance. The physically independent group is at a higher risk of falling than the physically fit group. As mentioned earlier, parts of functional

mobility test batteries may be appropriate (Rikli and Jones 2001; Griffin 2011). For balance, in addition to the Fullerton Advanced Balance Scale, the Berg Balance Scale (BBS) has been shown to be highly reliable and valid when used across a broad spectrum of functional levels and is recommended for older adults with lower levels of function (Berg et al. 1995). The BBS assesses the client's ability to perform a series of functional tasks of simulated activities encountered in daily life (e.g., transfers, object retrieval, turning).

The **physically frail**, the second-lowest level, includes those with a condition that results from a multisystem reduction in reserve capacity to the extent that a number of physiological systems are close to, or past, a threshold of symptomatic clinical failure. As a consequence, the frail person is at an increased risk of disability from minor external stresses (Friedman et al. 2009). Although frailty and disability frequently coexist, they are different concepts. Frailty indicates instability and risk of loss. Disability indicates loss of function. With this group it is important to determine their risk of disability. Several different assessment batteries have been developed to determine the extent of their physical function, including surveys, life inventories, and diaries. As with the physically dependent group, assessment typically uses ADL–IADL tests with questions that relate more to complex physical abilities such as light housecleaning and shopping. Performance tests for the frail elderly measure primarily gross or large muscle groups and are often administered by physical or occupational therapists in hospitals or nursing homes. One such physical performance test for this level is Tenetti's Test of Mobility (1986), which assesses the client's ability to get around in the environment (e.g., bending over from a standing position and picking up a small item, placing a light object on a high shelf, sitting and rising from a chair). **Physically dependent**, the lowest level, is primarily assessed with ADL–IADL inventories.

With the risk of falling of such importance, assessment of mobility and balance may be your focus. In terms of mobility, the 8 ft (2.4 m) up-and-go test from the Senior Fitness Test battery has been used frequently. A second test used to identify functional limitations in mobility is the 30 ft (9 m) walk test (Hernandez et al. 2008). It measures walking stability and can demonstrate whether older adults are able to adapt their gait speed to changing task demands. In terms of balance, the Fullerton Advanced Balance (FAB) Scale measures multiple dimensions of balance in different sensory environments (Rose 2010).

Table 13.1 Senior Fitness Test Items

Exercise	Purpose	Description	Risk zone
30 s chair stand test	To assess lower body strength needed for numerous tasks such as climbing stairs; walking; and getting out of a chair, tub, or car (increased ability in performing this exercise may reduce the chance of falling)	Number of full stands from a seated position that can be completed in 30 s with arms folded across chest	Fewer than 8 unassisted stands for both men and women
30 s arm curl test	To assess upper body strength needed for performing household and other activities involving lifting and carrying (e.g., groceries, suitcases, grandchildren)	Number of biceps curls that can be completed in 30 s holding a hand weight—5 lb (2.3 kg) for women, 8 lb (3.6 kg) for men	Fewer than 11 curls using correct form for both men and women
6 min walk test	To assess aerobic endurance, which is important for walking distances, climbing stairs, shopping, sightseeing while on vacation, and so on	Number of yards (or meters) that can be walked in 6 min around a 50 yd (45.7 m) course (see chapter 4 for a diagram of the course layout)	Fewer than 350 yd for both men and women
2 min step test	Alternative aerobic endurance test for use when time restraints, space limitations, or weather prohibits giving the 6 min walk test	Number of full steps completed in 2 min, raising each knee to a point midway between the patella (kneecap) and iliac crest (top hip bone); the score is the number of times the right knee reaches the required height	Fewer than 65 steps for both men and women
Chair sit-and-reach test	To assess lower body flexibility, which is important for good posture, normal gait patterns, and various mobility tasks such as getting in and out of a bathtub or car	From a sitting position at the front of a chair, with leg extended and hands reaching toward toes, the number of inches (centimeters) (plus or minus) between the extended fingers and the tip of the toe	Men: minus 4 in. or more Women: minus 2 in. or more
Back scratch test	To assess upper body (shoulder) flexibility, which is important in tasks such as combing one's hair, putting on overhead garments, and reaching for a seat belt	With one hand reaching over the shoulder and one up the middle of the back, the number of inches (centimeters) between the extended middle fingers (plus or minus)	Men: minus 8 in. or more Women: minus 4 in. or more
8 ft up-and-go test	To assess the agility and dynamic balance important in tasks that require quick maneuvering such as getting off a bus in time, getting up to attend to something in the kitchen, going to the bathroom, or answering the phone	Number of seconds required to get up from a seated position, walk 8 ft (2.4 m), turn, and return to the seated position	More than 9 s
Height and weight	To assess body weight relative to body height because of the importance of weight management for functional mobility	Involves measuring height and weight, then using a conversion table to determine body mass index	Body mass index higher or lower than the healthy range values of 19 to 25

Adapted by permission from Jones and Rose 2004.

The test was developed for higher-functioning older adults and is made up of 10 items including standing on foam with eyes closed, walking with head turns, stepping up and over obstacles, and jumping for distance.

Interpretation of Results

How results are interpreted relates to the goals of the testing program. If health assessment and disease risk are the primary goals of the fitness assessment, interpretation should be made in that light. Results can be compared to those of previous tests to evaluate the progress in the conditioning program. It is helpful to the client if these are presented as a percentage change. Results can be compared to findings for others in the given age and sex sector if normative tables or performance norms are available for the test. An important feature of the Senior Fitness Test is the fact that the performance standards are also criterion referenced—that is, the standards represent a criterion behavior or goal, such as having the fitness level needed to perform a specific everyday activity. For example, a score below 8 on the chair stand test (SFT) is associated with loss of functional mobility (Jones and Rose 2005). Regardless of the score, time, number completed, or percentile, it should be clear to the client what exactly was being measured by the test. Be sure to include the specific component, such as lower body strength, upper body flexibility, or dynamic balance. Rikli and Jones (2001) include a personal profile form (figure 13.6) that records scores, percentile ratings, and comments—infor-

PERSONAL PROFILE FORM

Name _____ Test Date _____

Age _____ M ____ F ____

Test item	Score	Percentile category			Fitness standard met? Yes/No	Comments
		Below average 25th %	Normal range 75th %	Above average		
Chair stand (# of stands)	17	_____	_____	__X__	_Yes_	Keep up the good work!
Arm curl (# of repetitions)	20	_____	_____	__X__	_Yes_	Also good!
2-minute step (# of steps) or 6-minute walk (# of yds)	740 yd	_____	_____	__X__	_Yes_	Excellent! Keep up your walking program.
Chair sit-and-reach (# of inches +/–)	–4.0	__X__	_____		_N/A_	Flexibility needs work. Add stretches for calf and hamstring muscles.
Back scratch (# of inches +/–)	–8.5	__X__	_____		_N/A_	Should add exercises for shoulder flexibility.
8-foot up-and-go (# of s)	4.2	_____	_____	__X__	_Yes_	Very good mobility.
Body mass index (see BMI chart)	Ht. _67 in._ Wt. _154 lb_	BMI _24_	≤18 Underweight; may signify loss of muscle or bone 19-25 Healthy range ≥26 Overweight; may cause increased risk of disability or disease			

Figure 13.6 Sample personal profile form.

Adapted by permission from Rikli and Jones 2013.

mation that can help interpret personal strengths and weaknesses and track progress.

Test results are means to an end. Results can also be used to prescribe exercise, develop training goals, and motivate clients. They should not distract you from the purpose of serving your clients. It is better to undertest than to overtest so that you can devote more time to counseling and demonstrating the program.

Safety

It is always good practice to manage the risks by applying your knowledge and experience of exercise science and your training in safety procedures. How does the trainer ensure safety within a program of challenge and variety? Safety is partly preparation and partly ongoing awareness.

In terms of preparation, the best preventive strategy is to be aware of the potential safety issues and have a safety plan in place. Review your employer's emergency procedures or make formal action plans for preventing, responding to, and following up on emergency situations. Maintain your cardiopulmonary resuscitation (CPR) certification and your instructor or personal training certification, which usually carries with it some level of liability insurance. As indicated earlier in this chapter, for the protection of your participants and your own personal liability protection, ensure that basic health information has been collected, informed consent has been administered, criteria to exclude individuals without physician approval have been applied, and personal interviews or functional assessments have been completed. Ensure that the information about clients with high risk of medical conditions is easily accessible during sessions. Keep written records of any health incident or accident occurring in the session, including the date, time, possible cause and description of the injury or illness, and what actions were taken.

Ongoing awareness begins with the environment of your workout facility. Exercise surfaces that are slick, sticky, or uneven may cause a client to fall or trip, which can be very serious for adults with conditions such as osteoporosis. It takes much longer to warm up in a cold room, and clients who have been sedentary often have reduced flexibility. This has implications for longer, more aerobic warm-ups and presents difficulties for proper cool-down. For outdoor activities, clothing needs to be layered to adjust to cold and wind. Water intake needs to be encouraged, as older adults have a lower proportion of total body water. Those with cardiovascular risk may be unsafe in an overheated room when doing aerobic activity.

When creating exercises or movement patterns, weigh the risk against the benefits across the range of functional abilities. This implies that you have identified the client's current level of ability. Recall that despite the chronological age of the client, her level of function may range from elite to fit, independent, frail, or dependent (Spirduso et al. 2005). People at each level of function have specific needs and activities that are most appropriate for them. Well-selected activities or exercises can be more enjoyable and improve self-esteem and self-efficacy. Clients with previous joint injuries are at higher risk of sustaining an injury from a strength training program (Requa and Garrick 1996).

Contraindicated exercises, or those that may predispose a client to injury, need to be eliminated or modified. Activities that require quick footwork with rapid changes in direction demand high levels of coordination and dynamic stability and could lead to falls, trips, or lower leg injuries for many seniors. Inappropriate exercises typically involve issues of alignment, speed or momentum, joint loading, or shifting of weight. The Canadian Centre for Activity and Aging has published a series of potentially inappropriate exercises for elderly participants as seen in table 13.2.

Monitoring

Particular challenges with both aging and disease require our attention as exercise designers, leaders, and trainers. Do you monitor for safety or improvement? We need to be vigilant and monitor what we are asking our clients to do and how they react when they attempt the activity. The following monitoring recommendations follow naturally from the safety guidelines mentioned earlier:

• Know the medical history of your clients and the symptoms most often seen with their disease or relative age.

• Modify the exercise environment with good space for movement, adjustments of equipment, and personal positioning for effective sight lines or spotting.

• Provide special consideration related to sensory defects (e.g., acceptable noise or music levels, easy-to-read signs or charts, clear audible speech and instructions).

• Monitor positions and movements that might create greater joint stress (e.g., use caution when clients are performing exercises that involve shoulder joint stability or loaded knee movements involving shear or rotational stress).

Table 13.2   Potentially Inappropriate Exercises for Elderly Participants

Exercise example	Physiological factor	Safe alternative
Hyperextension of the neck	Alignment issue	Forward and lateral flexion
Full neck rotations	Compression of vertebrae and blood vessels supplying the brain	Rotation in the front only
Straight-leg sit-ups	Alignment issue	Isometric abdominal exercises
Lying on back and lifting straight legs up	Strain on lower back	Curl-up
Full sit-ups	Alignment issue	Isometric abdominal exercises
Sit-ups with feet or legs held, so that the hip flexors do most of the work	Strain on lower back; person may pull on head or neck to complete the sit-up and injure cervical vertebrae	Curl-up
Toe touches	Alignment issue	Modified hurdler's stretch
Feet shoulder-width apart and alternating toe touches (twisting)	Strain on lower back muscles and hamstrings	Modified hurdler's stretch
Sitting with legs stretched in front and reaching for toes	Strain on lower back muscles and hamstrings	Modified hurdler's stretch
Deep knee bends	Shearing force on knee joint	Sit-to-stand exercise
Duck walk	Shearing force on knee joint	Squat to 90° maximum
High-impact activities	Joint loading (compression)	Low impact (walking, dancing, and so on)
Bouncing while stretching	Issue with joint movement; may injure muscles, tendons, ligaments, and joints	Static stretching
Hurdler's stretch	Issue with joint movement at the knee; shearing force	Modified hurdler's stretch
Rapid torso twists	Issue with joint movement	Twist and hold to stretch obliques
Lateral flexion beyond 20°	Alignment issue	To stretch obliques and lats, reach up with one arm and bend slightly to the side
Side bends with weights	Compression of vertebrae	To stretch obliques and lats, reach up with one arm and bend slightly to the side

Reprinted by permission from the Canadian Society for Exercise Physiology 2003.

• Monitor your clients' reaction to intensity levels (e.g., RPEs are valuable for aerobic exercise but may also prove helpful during activities emphasizing muscular effort).

• Observe your clients and teach them to recognize (Taylor and Johnson 2008)

- chest pain,
- joint or muscle pain,
- sharp leg pain,
- nausea,
- light-headedness or dizziness,
- shortness of breath,
- pallor, or
- confusion.

Once your client has begun implementing your initial prescription, careful monitoring under standardized conditions can allow you to gain information about his status. This may also decrease the need for regular, formal reassessment in several component areas. For example, tracking of load and reps with a standardized exercise will clearly and reliably indicate increments of improvement. Similarly, monitoring heart rate and perceived exertion during a bicycle ergometer warm-up at a standardized load and speed will give information about how your client is doing that day and how he has progressed over the last few weeks. Monitoring throughout your client's exercise program shows this improvement and indicates when progressions should be made. Most exercise prescription for seniors should take a functional approach to progressions. This involves a series of basic movement patterns used in active daily living and recreation, graduated according to the difficulty of the exercise and the tolerance of the individual. The functional progressions proceed from simple, safe exercises to more complex skills that mimic functional activities and place the same demands on your clients that they will encounter with the task. Specific exercises and their progressions should vary depending on your client's needs, abilities, injuries, and goals. Functional progressions may involve gradual changes in intensity, duration or number completed, overloads, mechanics or leverage changes, movement variations or additional joints involved, or alternate exercise designs. The discussion of functional progressions later in this section addresses how much and when to progress. As a stepping stone to meet the Canadian Physical Activity Guidelines for Older Adults (65 and older) (2011), the suggestion is to start with smaller amounts of physical activity and gradually increase duration, frequency, and intensity.

Our clients who are experiencing difficulty in completing exercises or other functional tasks may develop these physical limitations because of pain. Therefore monitoring the types of activities or intensities that create pain is very important. A physician's evaluation for functional limitations may need to be part of the routine evaluation of all patients with significant pain. Treatment strategies may need to focus on both pain management and functional rehabilitation. Covinsky and colleagues (2009) studied the epidemiology of pain and functional limitations across middle and late life and found a strong association between pain and functional limitations. In terms of their degree of limitation, subjects with pain were similar to subjects without pain who were two to three decades older. However, in a study of longitudinal patterns of musculoskeletal pain over a 6-year period, it was found that despite high prevalence, the musculoskeletal pain in older adults was often intermittent (Thielke et al. 2012). These findings seem to refute the notion that pain is inevitable or unremitting or is a progressive consequence of aging. This is all the more reason we need to monitor our clients carefully and adjust our prescriptions on a day-to-day basis.

The health care practitioner or a clinician such as a physiotherapist must monitor pain and the condition of any injured tissue. If pain occurs with any exercise, that particular activity should be avoided. Pain, muscle spasms, muscle tension, and muscle weakness are all valuable protective systems. Pain is often counterproductive to exercise because it changes how we contract our muscles and sometimes how we perform a movement. It is a bad idea to ignore pain; more pain will likely ensue in the long run. However, it may be an equally bad idea to intentionally avoid activities because of a fear of pain (Jam 2010). Muscles, spinal discs, and joints become unhealthy and weak when they are underused. They thrive on tolerated movement and reasonable compression. Pain does not always indicate damage or harm to the body. All tissue has a pain threshold that is lower than its damage threshold (figure 13.7).

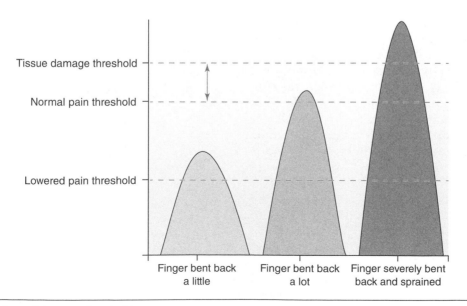

Figure 13.7   Pain and damage thresholds.
Adapted by permission from Jam 2010.

Precautions and Referral

Being more active is safe for most people. Functional mobility tests can help to screen for general mobility issues. However, some individuals may require further evaluation by a health care practitioner. If your client has significant pain or increasing pain with exercise, she should discontinue and seek advice. If she was following an exercise prescription, encourage her to show it to her health care provider and request direction on avoidance, modifications, or other treatments. Clients should be aware of the signs of ischemia, undue stress with breathing, sudden weakness, dizziness, vision or speech issues, or headache and seek medical attention immediately.

Exercise Component Guidelines

Training guidelines for older adults are not always the same as for younger adults. Exercise prescription for older adults should include the following primary goals:

- To improve basic fitness components with particular emphasis on aerobic activity and muscular strengthening activity
- To provide a functional approach to exercise involving meaningful daily activities with particular emphasis on flexibility, balance, and coordination
- To prevent or retard the progression of chronic diseases
- To prevent or retard disabilities caused by progressive functional limitations
- To ensure symptom-free exercise—no sharp pain, no increasing discomfort, and no tingling or numbness

Exercise prescription for the older adult should incorporate primary systems of the body: cardiovascular-respiratory (aerobic activity), musculoskeletal (resistance training), and neurological (flexibility, balance, and functional mobility exercises). To maintain independence, older adults need activity using multiple body systems. For example, a client who has a lower body musculoskeletal injury will limit his volume of aerobic activity, and the injury may limit his mobility (e.g., flexibility, agility). Improvement of the body systems need not be at a formal fitness center with machine-driven exercise. Depending on your client's current condition, exercise could include daily tasks, recreational activities, active hobbies and social interactions, active transportation, and active living.

Exercise prescription for older adults involves an awareness of the physiological aspects of aging at rest and at various intensities of exercise, as discussed earlier in the chapter. To provide a framework for the exercise prescription, the FITT approach can be employed (frequency, intensity, time or duration, and type or mode of exercise). Each of these elements can be adjusted in a prescription for the older adult to enhance selected fitness components. As seen in chapter 3, basic principles of adaptation, overload, progression, regression, and specificity apply in similar ways for young and old.

The broad strokes of exercise prescription are seen in the *component guidelines* for older adults (figure 13.8). The next layer is *functional exercise design,* which involves the selection of exercises that simulate the movements of everyday activities encountered by your client and are designed to make tasks and activities of daily living easier, safer, and more efficient. The final layer of exercise or activity design should come with exercise modification, successful demonstration, and careful monitoring providing a *client-centered approach.*

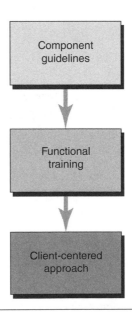

Figure 13.8 Layers of prescription design.

Cardiovascular Training

The American College of Sports Medicine in *ACSM's Guidelines for Exercise Testing and Prescription* (2010) recommends the component guidelines presented in table 13.3.

The Canadian Physical Activity Guidelines for Older Adults (CSEP 2011) are similar, emphasizing 150 min of moderate- to vigorous-intensity aerobic physical activity per week in bouts of 10 min or more to achieve health benefits and improve functional abilities, adding that more physical activity provides greater health benefits. These guidelines define moderate-intensity physical activities as those producing a little sweat and harder breathing, such as brisk walking or bicycling. Vigorous-intensity physical activities, such as cross-country skiing and swimming, will cause older adults to sweat and be out of breath.

Within the FITT principle for aerobic training, intensity is the critical factor. Although health benefits may be realized at lower intensities, aerobic fitness requires a greater stimulus. Because of the increased range in actual maximal heart rate with age, it may be better to use a percentage of heart rate reserve (%HRR) with maximal heart rate predicted using the following equation (Tanaka et al. 2001):

$$\text{HRmax} = 208 - 0.7 \times \text{Age}$$

An inactive or low-fitness client might start at 40% to 50% HRR, which is classified as "light," and an RPE of 10 or 11 (see table 13.4). Average fitness level corresponds to about 50% to 60% HRR, which is classified as "moderate" or "somewhat hard" with an RPE of 12 to 14. A high fitness level corresponds to 70% to 80% HRR, which is classified as "hard" with an RPE of 15 or 16.

Table 13.3 Cardiovascular–Respiratory Fitness Component Guidelines

Component	Guidelines
F: Frequency	At least 5 days per week if moderate intensity or 3 days a week if vigorous intensity or an equivalent combination of the two.
I: Intensity	If inactive, start at a tolerated level near 40% heart rate reserve and progress according to tolerance. Age-predicted peak heart rate may be variable after 65 years and medication can affect heart rates, so the use of ratings of perceived exertion (RPEs) can be valuable.
T: Time (duration)	If moderate intensity, 30-60 min per session or 150-300 min per week; if vigorous intensity, 20-30 min per session with a total of 75-100 min per week. These totals may be accumulated with shorter 10 min bouts of exercise throughout the day. When progressing, increase duration before intensity.
T: Type (mode)	Walking is excellent; however, stationary cycling, recumbent stepper, and aquatic exercise, for example, may reduce weight-bearing stress. Group settings provide social reinforcement. The modality of choice should be convenient and enjoyable.

Adapted from ACSM 2010.

Table 13.4 Sample Aerobic Prescription to Reach ACSM Guidelines Within 3 Months

Stage	Week	Frequency (sessions/week)	Duration (min)	Intensity (%HRR)	Intensity (RPE)
Initial	1	3	3 × (5 + 5)*	40-50	10-11
	2	3-4	4 × (5 + 5)	40-50	10-11
	3	3-4	2 × (10 + 5)	50-60	11-12
	4	3-4	2 × (10 + 5)	50-60	11-12
Improvement	5-7	3-4	20-25	50-60	11-12
	8-10	3-4	25-30	55-65	12-13
	11-13	3-5	30-35	55-65	12-13

The client is healthy, deconditioned, and young-old. The type of activities includes brisk walking, cycling, hiking, cardio machine, and an aerobic dance video. Warm-ups, cool-downs, and other training components are also incorporated into the program.

*Interval-type aerobic training, work-to-rest ratios 1:1 (i.e., 5 min work followed by 5 min light activity, easy walking, or stretching).

Musculoskeletal Training

The Canadian Physical Activity Guidelines for Older Adults (CSEP 2011) are similar to those of ACSM (2010), encouraging muscle and bone strengthening activities using major muscle groups at least 2 days per week (see table 13.5).

If a client is deconditioned, initial stages of training should keep intensity and duration low. As improvements are made, increase the number of repetitions before increasing the resistance. Machines or resistance bands are preferable to free weights if balance is an issue. If resistance training is new to the client, it may be easier to organize the exercises in a circuit, emphasizing proper technique at each station. Include multijoint exercises and move joints through a full pain-free range of motion, controlling both the concentric and eccentric movements. Excessive physical fatigue and muscle soreness can occur in the early stages, especially when the client has done too much too soon. When clients complain of these symptoms, lower the intensity during the sessions and increase the duration between sets and sessions. Avoid resistance training during flare-ups of arthritis, hot humid weather, or times of acute injury.

An intensity of 50% to 60% 1RM has been shown to be effective in improving muscle strength and endurance in community-dwelling older adults and residents of long-term care centers (Taylor and Johnson 2008). Once a period of initiation has taken place (4-12 weeks), a moderate to high load may be applied, represented by 70% or 80% 1RM or a resistance that can be repeated 8 to 12 times just before fatigue affects good form. Once a single set of 10 to 15 repetitions for that exercise has been successfully completed over several sessions, add a second set at the same weight but reduce the number of repetitions initially. Major muscle groups that should be targeted for older adults are those needed for lower body functioning (hip extensors, hip abductors and adductors, knee extensors, and ankle plantar flexors and dorsiflexors), for upper body functioning (biceps, triceps, shoulder stabilizers and movers), and for trunk stability (abdominal muscles and back extensors).

Balance, Flexibility, and Functional Mobility Training

The Canadian Physical Activity Guidelines for Older Adults (CSEP 2011) encourages those with poor mobility to perform physical activities to enhance balance and prevent falls. *ACSM's Resources for the Personal Trainer* (2010) recommends balance training 3 days per week for 10 to 15 min each session, potentially integrated into various phases of the exercise session. Activity examples to enhance dynamic balance include walking on an uneven surface, hiking, tandem walking, sidestepping, walking on toes or heels, or tai chi. The number of repetitions per exercise and rest intervals will depend on client conditioning and functional status. Four approaches to balance and mobility training that involve the motor, sensory, and cognitive systems are highlighted in the section on osteoporosis in chapter 12 (see figure 12.2). Balance training should be progressed from simple to complex. Examples are (a) surface progressions such as chair to balance disc to foam pad to physioball and (b) tasking progressions such as single tasking to multitasking (e.g., balance exercise while passing and catching a ball). Some balance training components can also be added progressively as part of a lower body strengthening routine. More capable clients may participate in aerobics classes or recreational sports such as tennis that involve higher levels of balance, coordination, and agility. Care should still be taken with some clients to avoid activities that carry a high risk of falling, such as those requiring rapid changes in direction.

Table 13.5 Musculoskeletal Fitness Component Guidelines

Component	Musculoskeletal fitness prescription
F: Frequency	Two or more nonconsecutive days per week.
I: Intensity	Load should be moderate, progressing to high.
T: Time (duration)	One set of each exercise (adequate rest between exercises). Perform 10 to 15 repetitions per exercise.
T: Type (mode)	May include machines, free weights, weight-bearing calisthenics, resistance bands, and so on. Target major muscle groups within 8 to 10 exercises.

Reprinted by permission from Spirduso, Francis, and MacRae 2005.

Balance and mobility are enhanced by flexibility training. Flexibility is also important for maintaining good posture and reducing the risk of injuries and back problems. Williamson (2011) encourages static stretching of all major joints (hip, knee, ankle, upper and lower back, neck, shoulder, and elbow) held for 15 to 30 s with 2 to 4 repetitions per stretch. Stretches are held to a point of tightness but not pain. Stretching can be incorporated at the end of the warm-up, after strength training, or during the cool-down when the muscles and core temperature are warm. Flexibility exercises should be included as part of daily exercise routines and could be done in conjunction with most activity sessions during the week.

Functional Exercise Design

Having followed the component guidelines, the prescription process should continue with the selection of exercises that simulate the movements of everyday activities encountered by your client. This *functional training* involves physical activities that are designed to make tasks and activities of daily living easier, safer, and more efficient.

Older clients themselves have repeatedly stated that their goals are to maintain functional fitness and independence in their chosen daily activities. Functional training makes older adults more aware of the connection between their exercise prescription and activities or tasks they perform in their daily lives. People can make many daily tasks and recreational activities easier by performing well-designed functional exercise. Griffin (2012) identified three primary domains of function:

1. Up and down activities: lower body focus
2. Locomotor activities
3. Carry–push–reach activities: upper body and trunk focus

Table 13.6 identifies specific functional tasks that are related to these domains.

Functional mobility involves movement patterns used in active daily living and recreation. Chapter 14 discusses this in more detail. Functional exercises, tasks, or activities allow the client to progress to a level of effective and efficient movement patterns. These should be paired with functional assessment to identify accurately the level of the client's ability to perform daily activities or more advanced recreational activities. For example, in the Senior Fitness Test, upper body flexibility is measured by the back scratch test and may reflect the ability to put on tight

Table 13.6   Functional Tasks, Training, and Functional Domains

Functional domain	Type of training	Functional tasks
Lower body	Resistance	Climbing and descending stairs; squatting down; using legs to lift an object; getting in and out of a chair or car; stepping onto a curb; recreational activities such as curling or golf
Lower body	Flexibility	Putting on socks and shoes; cutting toenails; picking up an object; recreational activities such as gardening
Locomotor	Mobility	Quick maneuvering; walking and looking elsewhere; dynamic balance while moving; getting to the door or phone quickly; responding to unexpected losses in balance; recreational activities such as tennis or playing tag with the grandchildren
Locomotor	Aerobic	Walking briskly for exercise, errands, events; bicycling; swimming and water aerobics; social dancing; activities requiring stamina, for example yard work, hiking, stair climbing; recreational activities such as bicycling or social dancing
Upper body, trunk	Resistance	Lifting or moving objects, for example furniture (or grandchildren); opening heavy doors; carrying groceries and luggage; washing windows or the car; recreational activities such as volleyball or cross-country skiing
Upper body, trunk	Flexibility	Putting on garments overhead; reaching for seat belt; viewing behind while driving; reaching overhead to a cupboard; combing hair; recreational activities such as baseball or yoga

overhead clothes. The exercise program should include range of motion exercises for shoulder joint abduction and rotation. In another example, several researchers (Griffin 2012; Rikli and Jones 2001) have used the timed up-and-go (TUG) test to measure agility and balance, components needed for avoiding obstacles while walking quickly or hiking. Those having difficulty should include motor coordination activities involving control and speed (suited to their level).

The term *functional* refers to basic required activities of daily living, as well as those that allow us to engage in recreational and meaningful activities related to work or leisure and to move effectively and efficiently in our environment (Taylor and Johnson 2008). As with traditional structured exercise, functional exercise also fulfills the development of essential fitness components of strength, dynamic stability, flexibility, motor mechanics, and so on. So how do you make your exercise design more functional? Several authors refer to this outcome as "functional fitness" (Rikli and Jones 2001). Functional exercise is also designed to restore clients' confidence and ability to achieve normal speed, power, control, and balance without the risk of injury. Ultimately, we want to give the client basic and advanced exercises and activities that will encourage increased participation in lifelong active living.

Essential in the design of functional exercise is the inclusion of certain elements:

- Dynamic stabilization (some muscles working to stabilize while other muscles work to accelerate or decelerate)
- Reactive movements to help maintain postural stability (relate to one of the primary causes of falls)
- Functional range of motion (without which, stress on structures and movement compensations can occur)
- A progression of challenge mimicking the speed, power, and agility required for continued participation in many activities

It is optimal if activity and exercise become not only a part of your client's lifestyle but also an element that enhances his QOL. Most days are completed with a series of routine tasks; some of these we may enjoy (like reading a newspaper), and others are a part of maintenance, such as sweeping a floor. Our lives are also made up of events that are usually longer in duration and take a little more planning. They often involve other people and may involve transporting ourselves to a different location.

Exercise, particularly starting an exercise program, is a challenge, and approximately half of all exercise plans end in failure within 6 months. Integrating activity within patterns of living can lead to more success. The first part of the lifestyle activity plan we call the daily dose is linked to activities of daily living. The second part of the plan is social adventure.

Daily Dose

Most of us have standard routines in our daily lives, things that we need to do or want to do almost every day. This may include activities such as preparing meals, shopping, light housecleaning, computer time, and reading. Researchers call these activities of daily living (ADLs). For one reason or another, most days these activities are completed at a certain time that is convenient or habitual. These activities may not be at the top of our list in terms of QOL, but their completion often gives us a sense of satisfaction. Integration of "daily dose" exercise within our routine must be just as convenient and most often at the same time every day. Daily dose exercise is our exercise habit or routine and may be once a day or several short bouts within the day. It is the cornerstone of an active lifestyle and prepares us for the challenges that may come with our "social adventures." Take a serious look at integrating one of the following three approaches as your daily dose exercise:

1. **Daily program.** It could be a walk, a yoga video, a series of stretches and calisthenics, a routine from your physiotherapist as a follow-up from an injury treatment, resistance training with light weights or TheraBands, or some time on a home exercise device such as a treadmill, bicycle, or stepper.

2. **Active living.** You may recall from chapter 6 that active living is an enhancement of the simple activities in a daily routine, like walking to the store instead of taking the car, or climbing stairs instead of riding the elevator, active playing with the grandkids, or selecting a more vigorous chore for the day. Active living may replace a daily program on certain days or further complement exercise. However, active living is about making choices and should extend beyond an exercise routine with the potential of becoming a way of

life. Table 13.7 provides a few more practical ways to integrate active living into your daily activities.

3. **Daily dose routine linkages.** Daily dose routine linkages are dynamic movement mini-routines that can be done at the same time as one of our activities of daily living, for example, when you are standing in the washroom about to brush your teeth. These are activities that happen every day, perhaps several times a day; and each time they do, they cue the client to do a specific daily dose routine.

Three different sample daily routine linkages are presented in the drills that follow. The first is for the lower body daily dose, the second is for the core and trunk area, and the third is for the upper body. These mini-routines are designed to improve flexibility, muscular endurance, strength, joint stability, and balance.

Table 13.7   Activities of Daily Living Boost Suggestions

ADLs and IADLs*	Active living "boost"
Housework	Rethink the stairs as something you want to use regularly during your "chores" time.
Shopping for groceries	Use abdominal core when reaching or lifting below waist and when loading car or unloading at home; use shoulder stability when reaching or lifting above waist.
Laundry	Carrying, bending, stairs, reaching, lifting: Laundry involves many functional activities; do it often and ensure a safe work area.
Lawn maintenance (gardening)	Continue to do what you can without overdoing it. "Labor-saving" devices are available; use them to be able to stay engaged, but don't use them if you can safely manage without.
Home maintenance	"Get your sweep on": Pick an area inside or outside the house that needs sweeping every day.
Oral care	Different hand positions and angles will work the rotator cuff muscles; manipulate the brush to activate the smaller hand muscles.
Transferring (such as moving into or from bed)	Use proper technique; be conscious of how you move, ensuring strong core and stabilized shoulders.
Walking	Look for opportunities for even short walks; for example, take garbage out, pick up mail.
Bathing	The warm water of a shower or bath will raise your tissue temperature enough to make a mini-stretch routine very effective; always remember, safety is first!
Putting on clothes	Extend the stretches when you put your arms or legs in or out of your clothes; have a chair or bed close, but work your balance when possible.
Grooming	Start with elbows low, then move them higher with each brush stroke; different hand positions and angles will work the rotator cuff muscles.
Meal preparation	Do a half squat each time you put a dish into the dishwasher.
Care of pets	Regular walks; bend at knees (squat, don't stoop when you scoop!); squat when you change water or food.
Care of others	Whether it is grandkids or a pet, find some time for "active" play (get down with them if possible).
Driving	Turn fully to look behind you both ways before you start the car; be conscious of how you get in and out of the car, ensuring strong core and stabilized shoulders.
Using technology (computer)	No longer than 30 min sitting at a screen; get up and move around (not to the refrigerator).
Use of a telephone	Walk around house while on the phone.

*ADLs and IADLs represent the skills that people usually need to be able to manage in order to live as independent adults.

Lower Body Daily Dose

This routine is linked to standing in the washroom before teeth brushing. Instruct your client to do 3 sets per day.

1. Partial squat (10 times), figure 13.9
2. Alternating hamstring curl (10 times), figure 13.10
3. Alternating side leg lift (10 times), figure 13.11
4. Knee-up hip roll (10 times), figure 13.12
5. Alternating toe (foot) lift (10 times), figure 13.13

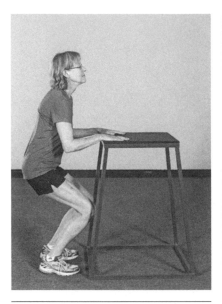

Figure 13.9 Partial squat.

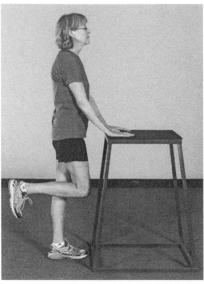

Figure 13.10 Alternating hamstring curls.

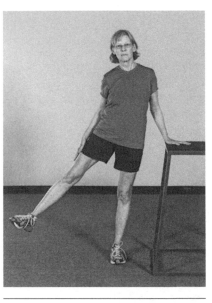

Figure 13.11 Alternating side leg lift.

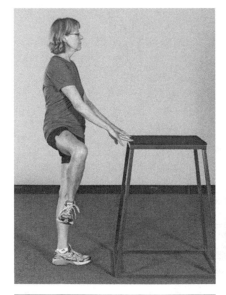

Figure 13.12 Knee-up hip roll.

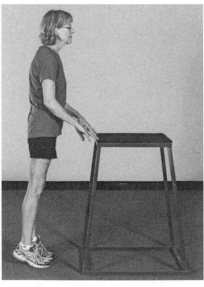

Figure 13.13 Alternating toe (foot) lifts.

Core and Trunk Daily Dose

The second daily dose routine is linked to either a bed or a sofa. While on the bed or while lying on the sofa, maybe watching TV, your client can do the following routine for the core and trunk area. Instruct your client to do 3 sets per day.

1. Core activation (2 × 15 s), figure 13.14
2. Knee-to-chest stretch (2 × 15 s each side), figure 13.15
3. Hip bridge lift (5 times, slow), figure 13.16
4. Bent knee lower (5 times each side), figure 13.17
5. Bent elbow push-up (5 times, slow, hold at top), figure 13.18

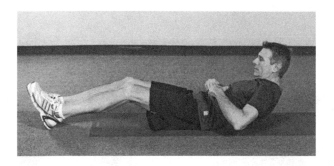

Figure 13.14   Core activation.

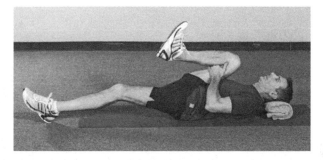

Figure 13.15   Knee-to-chest stretch.

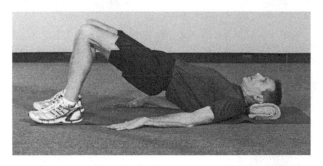

Figure 13.16   Hip bridge lift.

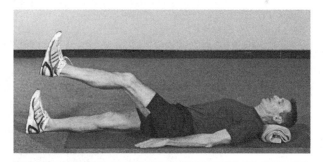

Figure 13.17   Bent knee lower.

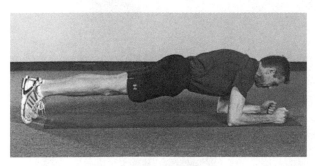

Figure 13.18   Bent elbow push-up.

Upper Body Daily Dose

The third daily dose routine is linked to the bedroom and getting dressed or undressed. Your client will be standing near the bed, and this activity will cue him to do the following routine. This routine may also be done during showering (stretches only) or immediately after. The warm water of a shower or bath will raise tissue temperature enough to make the routine very effective. Remind your clients to know their balance limits; always remember, safety first. Instruct your client to do 3 sets per day.

1. Single-arm wall stretch (2 × 15 s each side), figure 13.19
2. Back scratch stretch (2 × 15 s each side), figure 13.20
3. Tight-grip shoulder circle (10 each direction), figure 13.21
4. "Stick-em-up" pull-back (10 times), figure 13.22
5. Wall push-up (10 times), figure 13.23

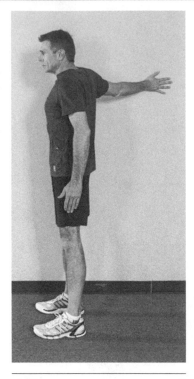

Figure 13.19 Single-arm wall stretch.

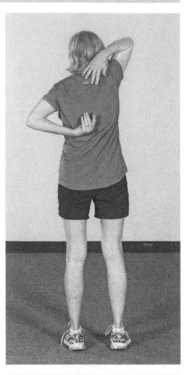

Figure 13.20 Back scratch stretch.

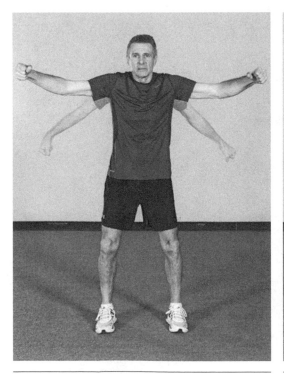

Figure 13.21 Tight-grip shoulder circles.

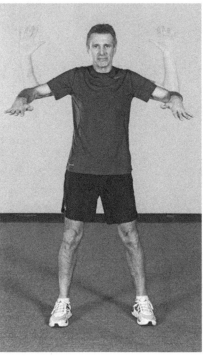

Figure 13.22 "Stick-em-up" pull-back.

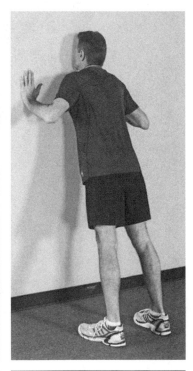

Figure 13.23 Wall push-up.

Social Adventure

Daily exercise is the core and the heart of a lifestyle activity plan. However, the real joy that people feel with activity may come from a different source. Apart from the plethora of research on the benefits of physical activity from a psychological or sociological perspective, it is a wonderful feeling when we share an active event with a friend or group of people—a "social adventure." For some it may be more social; for others it is the thrill of the mini-adventure. In any case, when you ski, golf, hike, curl, or bowl with someone else, you continue to create new stories of shared experiences. This is important at any stage of life; however, to feel renewed as an older adult is extremely refreshing. For some the experience may involve a change of geography, climate, and perhaps an adventurous exposure to the elements. For others it may be a game of doubles tennis with lots of laughter and time for coffee when all is done. If we can plan four or five of these events every month (a weekly social adventure), we add to the physiological benefits of the lifestyle activity plan. In some ways, the daily dose can keep us fit and mobile enough to be able to feel confident with the social adventures. For many of us, our QOL is defined in no small part by the nature and frequency of our social adventures.

Client-Centered Functional Exercise Prescription

The final layer of exercise or activity design should come with personal and appropriate exercise modifications, successful demonstration, careful monitoring, and progressions providing a client-centered approach. A client-centered approach includes the clients' goals, expectations, needs, and lifestyle as the focus of a personalized exercise prescription. The approach brings about a sense of what is important to the individual, his attitude, stage of commitment, and personal obstacles, which in themselves suggest unique strategies for motivation. There is always a human element to intervention, and we should never lose sight of the fact that what we do as health care professionals or personal trainers can have a huge influence on the quality of the intervention and ultimately its effectiveness. In a meta-analysis of intervention outcomes designed to increase physical activity, it was found that the most effective interventions were behavioral instead of cognitive interventions and face-to-face delivery versus mediated interventions (e.g., via telephone) and that they targeted individuals instead of communities (Conn et al. 2011).

Accommodating Levels of Fitness and Function

Clients of similar age can vary significantly in their fitness levels, which has implications for how they will respond to an exercise prescription. Nelson and colleagues (2007) defined older adults as 65 years and older, as well as adults 50 to 64 years with clinically significant chronic conditions or functional limitations that would affect their physical activity or functional mobility. The rate and magnitude of variance in performance depended on exercise history, disease, current injury, and genetics. The more information you have about clients' physical status through effective counseling and assessment, the more effective you can be in providing the most appropriate exercise prescription. Structured or targeted exercises are especially important for clients who had lower scores on specific fitness components. For example, a poor score on a chair stand test would indicate lower body weakness, leading to targeted exercises in the prescription to strengthen those muscles. This may also be a prerequisite for many activities leading to improvement in aerobic fitness.

Trainers working with older adults must determine their client's level of physical function and modify any exercise or activity to suit her needs and capabilities. Recall that there are five levels in the hierarchy of physical function in older adults (Spirduso et al. 2005). The definitions in table 13.8 provide descriptions and relevant needs within each level and assist in making the program relevant to the client. Personal relevance is the backbone to motivation.

My personal experience acting as a client for my undergraduate fitness students was to witness their difficulty in estimating a training stimulus that would avoid injury and overtraining but keep me motivated and produce a training effect. Chronological age is not as relevant as physiological age. Adjustments to the FITT approach, training format, and progression of the program should not be based on age. Once the FITT for each component of the program has been established, it is critical to monitor the unique individual responses of the client, both physiological and in terms of personal enjoyment. For example, the rate of progression in an aerobic training prescription is appropriate if your client feels refreshed and

Table 13.8 Categories of Physical Function

Category	Description
Physically elite	Individuals who train on an almost daily basis to compete in senior sport tournaments or work in a physically demanding job or recreational activity.
Physically fit	Individuals who exercise at least two times a week for their health, enjoyment, and well-being or work regularly at a physically demanding job or hobby. Their health and fitness reserves put them at low risk for falling into the physically frail category.
Physically independent	Individuals who live independently, usually without debilitating symptoms of major chronic diseases. However, many have low health and fitness reserves placing them at risk for becoming physically frail after illness or injury.
Physically frail	Individuals who can perform the ADLs but cannot perform some or all of the activities necessary to live independently, generally due to a debilitating disease or condition that physically challenges them on a daily basis.
Physically dependent	Individuals who cannot execute some or all of the ADLs, including self-dressing, bathing, transferring, toileting, feeding, and walking. These seniors depend on others for food and basic functions of living.

not exhausted after the session. And regardless of component guidelines that may seem appropriate, there should be no undue fatigue or soreness the day after and no onset of injury.

One of the reasons for the limitations to the component approach to exercise prescription for the older adult is that health status and physical functioning of many older clients fluctuates from day to day. Pain from arthritis or other musculoskeletal disorders also fluctuates from session to session. A client may feel comfortable on a hike one day but experience painful knees and difficulty walking on the flat sidewalk on another day. So we must establish a balance between designing a challenging overload in our prescription and appreciating the individual capabilities of our client for the current workout. On any day the client may have strong capabilities in some areas, such as strength, but feel challenged with flexibility because of temporary stiffness in certain joints. Besides having an ongoing dialogue, which is absolutely necessary with an older client, we must plan for variations in the level of challenge. We can adjust difficulty by changing individual or multiple aspects of the FITT, or by changing the demands of the task or activity (e.g., reducing a multijoint exercise to a single joint), or by modifying the objectives or rules of a recreational game. The environmental demands may also be changed to accommodate the client through such things as the type of surface, the lighting, or the ergonomics of a household task. For example, a simple walking activity is more challenging on a grass surface and more challenging when distract-

ing conversation is added. The following section on functional progressions (see discussion in chapter 14 also) provides more concrete ideas on establishing appropriate levels and progressions for your client.

A **functional progression** is a series of basic movement patterns used in active daily living and recreation graduated according to the difficulty of the exercise and the tolerance of the individual. Physiotherapists and other health care professionals have long known that muscle, joints, and other body tissue must be stressed gradually according to the manner in which they function. You need to teach your client to take responsibility to determine the degree of difficulty and change the parameters of a functional exercise program. The functional progressions proceed from simple, safe exercises to more complex skills that mimic functional activities and place the same demands on the client that she will encounter with the task. Specific exercises and their progressions should vary depending on needs, abilities, injuries, and goals. Functional progressions may involve gradual changes in intensity, duration, or number completed; overloads; mechanics or leverage changes; movement variations or additional joints involved; or alternate exercise designs. Functional progressions make the prescription far more client centered.

As a personal trainer, you must look for indicators of when to progress, which includes close monitoring of how your client feels. The exercise should feel "moderately difficult." If it is too easy, try a modification that makes it more difficult;

if it is a bit too difficult, try an option to make it easier. Clients should not move up a level until

1. they can complete the full number of reps and sets with good form,
2. they feel that the exercise is of low to moderate difficulty,
3. and there is no pain or undue discomfort.

When doing aerobic training, clients can continue at the current training stimulus if

1. they are able to breathe comfortably and rhythmically and are able to talk although probably unable to sing,
2. they feel refreshed and not exhausted after the session, and
3. there is no undue fatigue, soreness, or onset of injury the day after the session.

Risk takers need to progress more slowly, and other clients often need to challenge themselves a little more. Participants should be encouraged to "perform exercises to the best of their abilities, but to never push themselves to a point of overexertion, pain, or beyond the level they consider to be safe" (Jones and Rose 2005). We need to help clients become more skilled at listening to their bodies and understanding the signs and symptoms of overexertion. This is of greater importance in a group exercise setting but still presents a challenge to the personal trainer.

Exercise Demonstration

Demonstrating an exercise requires a balance between your technical knowledge and your people skills. The technical issues associated with the science of exercise demonstration are reviewed in chapter 5. Skills in designing multiple variations in technique to suit the abilities of your client and to reinforce proper technique are critical technical skills that are needed regardless of the age of the client. Skills involved in demonstration are also based on psychosocial aspects as outlined in table 5.11. From the time we meet our clients for the program demonstration until later in the program follow-up, we use our counseling skills to observe body language, question the client effectively, provide clarifications, and encourage two-way feedback.

Many older adults come to believe that they cannot perform the exercises that younger clients can. Unfortunately, this may discourage them from integrating fitness into their lifestyles. Fitness professionals have a real challenge in guiding older adults who are exposed to a barrage of new gimmicks, gadgets, apparel, gym settings, and the latest industry offerings. They may be anxious based on their past exercise history, your judgment of their abilities, or the inability to perform to their own standards. From experience, clients have developed images of what they believe they can achieve. This belief in one's abilities is called self-efficacy. When older adult clients know they have to perform, this belief in their ability is critical to feeling positive about attempting to complete the task. When we demonstrate an exercise, we have an amazing opportunity not only to teach a new skill but also to improve our client's confidence to overcome barriers.

Numerous studies have identified self-efficacy as both a key element in predicting physical activity behavior and a positive outcome of physical activity participation (Van Norman 2010). The belief in one's ability begins when we demonstrate or teach the exercises and have our client attempt them. The following four factors affect self-efficacy; and if we are aware of them and can control them, our clients will develop confidence in their abilities.

1. **Where are we starting?** If your client's past exercise history is limited or unsuccessful, he may be starting with a lack of confidence. The exercise may seem complex, the equipment may be unfamiliar, or your client may have an old injury about which he is concerned. Draw on information from the initial counseling or testing that may relate to the exercise you are about to demonstrate. Discovering exactly what your client may be concerned about will help establish a framework of goals wherein any anxieties are confronted and hopefully overcome.

2. **How can clients be successful?** The key to improving self-efficacy beliefs lies in identifying tasks that can be performed to facilitate success. Unrealistic expectations or setting the bar too low will result in failure or lack of progress, respectively. Identify actions that your client can control. Start by avoiding information overload, select your language carefully, and reduce the steps involved in doing the task—make it seem simple. If you can identify for your client similar tasks that he has done successfully, he will feel as though he can do the exercise that you are

teaching. Your first-session goal may be to achieve a pain-free range of motion at a controlled speed with no resistance applied.

3. **Practice makes perfect.** Repeat the "client trial" phase of the demonstration a number of times, providing clear and concise feedback specific to the physical action. Concentrate on teaching mastery of the task rather than simply building up the client's ego.

4. **Positive imagery.** Encourage imagery through the use of positive action words such as "feel," "squeeze," or "activate." For example, "During this rowing action, *feel* your shoulder blades *squeezing* together. When you do that, you know that you are *activating* the right muscles." This will allow you to emphasize specific movement patterns critical for safety or successful performance. Older clients are more likely to succeed if they can use positive imagery for their position, movement, and task completion.

Case Study

This client has an active background and fitness level and is interested in a resistance training program. The goals are that mesocycle 1 will build a training base and establish good exercise techniques; mesocycle 2 will build muscle mass to stimulate better function (see table 13.9).

Resistance Training Program for a Young-Old Client

Warm-ups, cool-downs, and flexibility training should be incorporated into the program.

Mesocycle 1 includes the following exercises for microcycles 1 through 6:

- Squat, leg press
- Bench press
- Leg curl (double)
- Seated row

Microcycles 7 and 13 are active rest. Mesocycle 1 includes the following exercises for microcycles 8 through 12:

- Squat, leg press
- Bench press
- Leg curl (single)
- Seated press
- Arm curl
- Seated row

Day 1 and 3 of mesocycle 2 includes the following exercises for microcycles 1 through 10:

- Squat, leg press
- Bench press
- Leg curl (single)
- Seated press
- Seated row
- Heel raise

Day 2 of mesocycle 2 includes the following exercises for microcycles 1 through 10:

- Dumbbell internal rotation (arms)
- Dumbbell external rotation (arms)
- Heel raise
- Arm curl
- Modified sit-up (10-15)

Table 13.9   Sample Resistance Training Prescription

Stage	Week (microcycle = 1 week)	Frequency (days/week)	Load	Reps	Sets	Rest (minutes between exercises)
Mesocycle 1	Microcycles 1-6	2	40% 1RM#	8	1	2-3
	Microcycle 7	2	Active rest			
	Microcycles 8-12	Day 1	60% 1RM*	8	1	2-3
		Day 2	60% 1RM	8	2	2-3
	13	2	Active rest			
Mesocycle 2	Microcycles 1-10	Day 1	80% 1RM^	8	2	2-3
		Day 2	40-50% 1RM	10-15	2	1-2
		Day 3	80% 1RM	8	2	2-3
	11	3	Active rest			

A weight that can be lifted for 20 reps or more; * a weight that can be lifted for 15 to 20 reps; ^ a weight they can be lifted for 10 to 12 reps (Kraemer and Harman 1998).

Summary

Aging refers to a number of processes within us that over time cause a loss of adaptability, impairment in functionally, and eventually death. In addition to chronological age, larger differences in function may better be described by biological age or functional age. Quantity of life is of value only if the quality of life is maintained. Maintaining health and postponing the onset of a debilitating disease as long as possible is called "compression of morbidity." Successful agers are people who are more satisfied with life and have better than average physiological and psychological characteristics in late life. There is now strong evidence that regular and systematic exercise throughout life, when accompanied by reasonable health habits, increases the quantity and quality of life. Older adults are more likely to be motivated to be physically active when the activity is at a moderate intensity, is inexpensive, is convenient, and, especially for older women, includes a social aspect.

There are both structural and functional changes in the body systems, and it is difficult to pinpoint if the changes are due to disease, physical inactivity, or normal aging. Although physiological changes with aging are inevitable, the effects and benefits of exercise are remarkable, specifically for the cardiovascular–respiratory system, musculoskeletal system, and locomotion.

Screening is done before any assessment or exercise program to identify chronic disease, acute illness or injury, pains, impairments, medications, cardiovascular risk factors, overall health status, and physical activity and exercise patterns. Following the screening process and before the individual becomes active, assessing physical impairments (including declines in cardiovascular or musculoskeletal systems) and functional limitations (restrictions in physical tasks or behaviors of everyday life) is recommended. Periodic functional assessment provides a way to determine the extent of functional decline and can be used to prescribe appropriate exercise. We need to be vigilant and monitor what we are asking our clients to do and how they react when they attempt the activity.

Depending on the functional status or disease of the client, general training principles should be modified for cardiovascular and musculoskeletal fitness, balance, flexibility, and functional mobility. The American College of Sports Medicine (2010) and the Canadian Physical Activity Guidelines for Older Adults (CSEP 2011) recommend similar guidelines, emphasizing 150 min of moderate- to vigorous-intensity aerobic physical activity per week in bouts of 10 min or more; encouraging muscle and bone strengthening activities using major muscle groups at least 2 days per week; and, for those with poor mobility, performing physical activities to enhance balance and prevent falls. Balance and mobility are enhanced by flexibility training. Flexibility is also important for maintaining good posture and reducing the risk of injuries and back problems.

The prescription process should continue with the selection of exercises that simulate movement patterns used in active daily living and recreation (functional training). The final layer of exercise or activity design should come with personal and appropriate exercise modifications, successful demonstration, careful monitoring, and progressions providing a client-centered approach. Trainers working with older adults must determine their client's level of physical function and modify any exercise or activity to suit the client's needs and capabilities and to reinforce proper technique.

FORM 13.1   Functional Mobility Informed Consent

I, (please print) _____ have read and understood the information on the Functional Mobility Exercise Program and all questions have been answered to my satisfaction.

I agree to voluntarily participate in this preassessment for the program and give my consent freely. I understand that the assessment will be conducted in accordance with the information letter, a copy of which I have retained for my records.

I understand I can withdraw from the assessment or program at any time, without penalty, and do not have to give any reason for withdrawal.

I consent to:

- Complete all parts of the Functional Mobility Screening. These tests include three activity focus areas ("domains"): up and down activities (lower body focus); locomotor activities; and carry–push–reach activities (upper body and trunk focus).
    - Functional Mobility Self-Rating Questionnaire (5 minutes)
    - Functional Mobility Performance Tests (30 minutes)
- Performing a combination of everyday activities such as bending down, reaching, balanced walking, turning, standing from a chair, walking around obstacles, carrying shopping bags, and so on.
- Performing the activities at my own pace.
- Work with the trained assistant who will be there to teach me and then will count or time or observe my trials.
- Immediately inform the staff of any symptoms during or after the testing.
- Stop or delay activity causing undue distress at any time.

Print name: _____

Signature: _____

Date: _____

From J.C. Griffin, 2015, *Client-centered exercise prescription,* 3rd ed. (Champaign, IL: Human Kinetics).

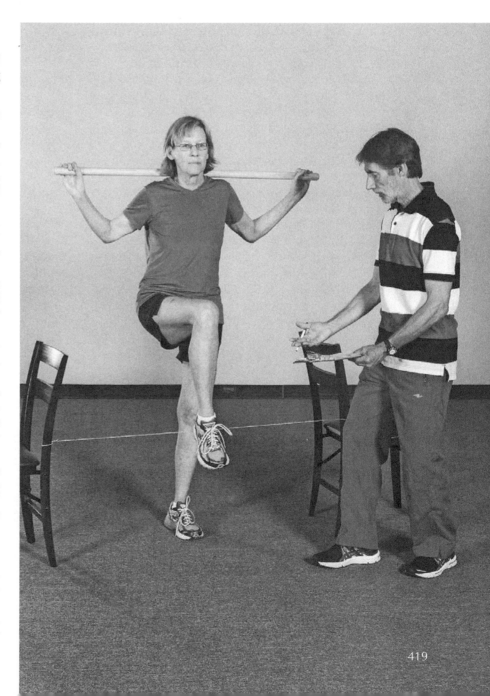

Functional Mobility and Aging

14

Chapter Competencies

After completing this chapter, you will be able to demonstrate the following competencies:

1. Identify the relationship between health and mobility.
2. Describe the implications of early functional mobility limitations, identify the predictors of disability, and explain the role of a functional mobility reserve.
3. Define and differentiate mobility, functional movement, functional fitness, functional mobility, impairment, and disability.
4. Explain the difference between bad and good compensation and provide a situational example for each.
5. Describe types of functional mobility assessment tools and the data on mobility function they provide.
6. Once the client's functional mobility issue has been identified, design an intervention that addresses the limiting components and how they may affect each client individually.
7. Design exercises and tasks that are functional, that is, basic activities of daily living that are required and those that allow us to engage in recreational and meaningful activities related to work or leisure.
8. Critique and apply the Functional Mobility Screening Tool for Adults 50-70 Years of Age and the subsequent interpretation of clients' results in the development of a personalized preventive exercise prescription.

To be successful and safe in performing the skills of daily activities, everyone needs the essential abilities in one or more aspects of physical function. Alterations in functioning in terms of performance or capacity may be seen as impairments (e.g., altered mobility, altered muscle strength-power, altered gait pattern, pain). Functional mobility is the ability to carry out activities one needs and wants to do (daily activities and recreation) efficiently for quality of life without undue fatigue or pain in order to stay healthy, safe, and active.

Most people value the importance of being able to get around. This is the basis for our independence and our freedom to choose what we want to do. Functional mobility is an aspect of everyday life, whether for the athlete, senior, student, or average adult. Early deficits in functional mobility have become a highly prevalent public health concern. Up to 50% of persons aged 65 years and older have disability in mobility-related tasks such as walking or climbing stairs (Chaves et al. 2000). Disability usually occurs first in mobility, and mobility difficulty predicts the onset of disability in tasks essential to living independently in the community.

A wealth of new information indicates that declines in mobility are not inevitable consequences of aging. If this is so, why do so many older adults lose their mobility, and what can we as personal trainers do to help prevent this loss? Mobility is restricted by an inactive lifestyle resulting in physical deconditioning. Combined with minor declines in our senses, losses in strength, balance, stability, flexibility, agility, and coordination are leading lifestyle-related causes of mobility decline. Mobility limitation has been shown to be an early predictor of physical disability, falls, loss of independence, and institutionalization (Hall and McAuley 2011).

Mobility is closely linked to both physical and psychological health. Difficulty with functional mobility is a major risk factor for dependency in other domains of physical functioning, causing decreased quality of life and substantial social and health care needs. Within a broad health promotion framework, it is the determinants of health that make and keep people healthy (PEI Health and Community Services Agency 1996). Conversely, these determinants of health can also have a dramatic impact on mobility. The following are some examples of specific needs for older clients within each of the determinants of health:

- Social support and networks—loss of activity partner
- Socioeconomic—inability to afford programs or equipment
- Physiological—injury or pain
- Behavioral—lifestyle choices and priorities
- Health services—disease prevention and therapy
- Psychological—inactivity due to depression
- Education—awareness of the health implications of mobility loss

As professionals we may find our role moving fluidly between those of the physical and the lifestyle coach for optimal effectiveness.

Preclinical diminished functional mobility is an intermediate stage of early functional loss and may be identified by an alternative manner of task performance (compensation). Compensation has the potential to lead to further mobility and stability imbalances; however, it is not necessarily a bad thing if it results in efficient movements that avoid normal pain patterns.

With the assistance of an effective screening tool, we can achieve early identification of changes in physical ability before overt limitations in functional behavior present themselves. Evaluation must consider clients' efficiency in performing certain movements. Any functional movement (activity) difficulties in turn may reflect a deficit in one or more of the essential components of functional mobility, such as balance and proprioception, muscular strength (stability), muscular endurance, muscular power, flexibility, speed, coordination (mechanics), agility, and aerobic and anaerobic capacity.

The interventions that are planned need to recognize the limiting components and how they may affect each client individually. Exercises and tasks should be functional; that is, they should simulate basic activities of daily living that are required and those that allow us to engage in recreational and meaningful activities related to work or leisure and to move effectively and efficiently in our environment.

This chapter chronicles the design and validation of the Functional Mobility Screening Tool for Adults 50-70 Years of Age and the subsequent interpretation of clients' results in the development of a personalized preventive exercise prescription (Griffin 2011a, 2011b, 2012).

Early Functional Mobility Limitations

Functional loss may be identified by difficulties in task (activity) performance. A high proportion of independent adults 50 to 70 years of age do not have a particular limitation but are at risk for functional mobility loss. Typical of the natural history of disability are changes before its onset that define a critical point when preventive measures would be most effective. That is, there is a preclinical state, usually asymptomatic, characterized by the development of early functional mobility impairment before it either is clinically apparent or interferes significantly with effective functioning (figure 14.1). The existence of a preclinical stage of disability that may be nonsymptomatic constitutes a major risk factor for the progression of mobility difficulty. People generally seek medical evaluation of functional problems only when they have passed a threshold beyond which they can no longer tolerate a functional decrement (Griffin 2011a). However, it is before this point that we, as personal trainers and health promotion advocates, need to intervene with good client-centered strategies.

Diminished functional mobility is an early stage of identifiable functional loss and may be seen in changes in task performance (impairment) such that the individual performs the task in a modified manner. With such adaptations, the person may not recognize difficulty in task performance and completes the task with an altered mobility pattern. It is incumbent on us to watch the movement techniques of our older clients carefully.

Because physical disability has such a negative impact on quality of life, substantial attention has focused on identifying predictors of disability so that interventions can be designed to prevent or postpone dysfunction. Physical function has proven to be a powerful predictor of independent living. When measures of physical performance are combined with self-reported physical activity level, the odds ratio for predicting loss of independence is dramatic.

Client screening should identify functional mobility difficulties by examining a hierarchy of difficulties of activities. Eventually, clinical disability progresses in predictable ways. It appears that difficulty with physical functioning may progress along a spectrum of activities requiring physical abilities from the most to least demanding (Siu et al. 1990). There may be a hierarchy of functional loss within the spectrum. What is currently preclinical may well become a clinical issue. For example, a preclinical observation may be the alteration of a movement pattern (compensation) such as excessive movement of the spine

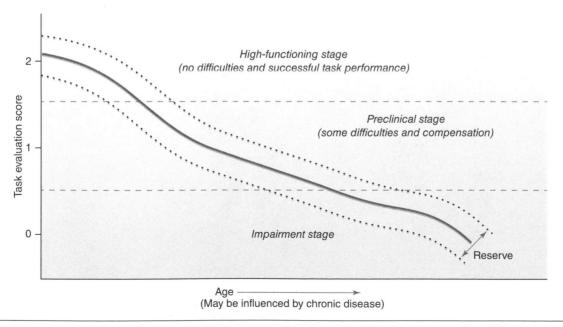

Figure 14.1   Decline of physical function with age.

rather than the hips to pick something up. This may progress to a loss of balance or a clinical issue of back pain with the same activity.

Mobility disability begins in a patterned way and should be reflected by ordered differences in demand among mobility tests. Siu and colleagues (1990) evaluated four hierarchical measures of physical function and produced two new self-evaluation scales. They noted that measures incorporating more complex and difficult physical tasks can be reliably collected and are valid.

Clients as young as 50 years find that many everyday activities require near-maximum effort. This may be referred to as a low **functional mobility reserve** (Nashner 2002). As functional mobility reserves decline over time, your client becomes less able to deal with changes in his physical environments. Functional mobility reserve may be seen as the difference between a client's maximal capacity to perform a task successfully and the minimal capacity required to perform that task or to maintain a specific level of activity (see figure 14.2). When designing programs for your older clients, remember that different tasks impose varying demands on the underlying components (e.g., cardiovascular, strength). Therefore your client's reserve is only as large as his weakest component for that task. For example, climbing stairs

demands leg strength and aerobic capacity—ask yourself which would be the limiting factor for your client.

Even though many older clients are physically independent, they are hovering very near the threshold of physical abilities below which they would be impaired. Others may not recognize that they have impairments but may be very close to functional limitations that would be more obvious such as those involved in climbing stairs or moving quickly. A very small setback in health—a minor disease, a small accident, or simply the passage of a little time—could change them from physically independent to partially dependent. In other words, they have little if any functional reserve. Screening for functional mobility should determine the physical reserve of older clients within functional domains such as locomotion or upper or lower body. We should take the time in our training sessions to examine the minimal capacity in components such as strength, flexibility, balance, or motor coordination to perform functional tasks.

Changes in the body's physical environment are regulated by an interactive network of feedback mechanisms that hold each system within specific physiological limits. When the functional reserve within any of these systems declines to a point

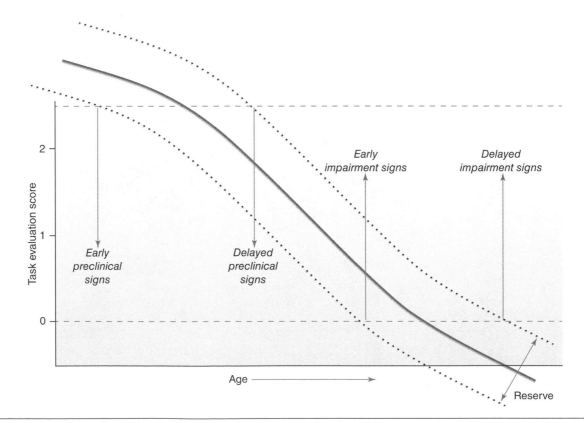

Figure 14.2 Functional mobility reserve.

Predictors of Disability

Ebrahim and coauthors (2000) found that obesity and physical inactivity in men aged 40 to 59 were strong predictors of locomotor disability in later life independent of the presence of diagnosed disease. Locomotor disability was defined as having difficulty walking 400 m, performing outdoor activities, climbing stairs, maintaining balance, and bending down and straightening up. Improved mobility and healthy lifestyle were associated with independence and less disability later in life. Others have argued that measures of lower body function alone are effective predictors of dependency (Guralnik et al. 1995). Low physical activity level and muscular weakness are predictors of disability later in life (Spirduso et al. 2005). Levelle and Iezzoni (2004) examined persons aged over 45 years from the early 1990s to 2000. They found that arthritis was associated with a 300% to 400% increased risk in mobility difficulties. The study warns of a surge in the prevalence of arthritis and mobility problems in the coming decades. Mobility may be impaired by problems such as arthritis or overweight that result in restricted activities.

that the system can no longer compensate for changes, we fall outside of our reserve, increasing the potential for injury or loss of independence. Health care practitioners working with older clients have a unique opportunity to prevent and even reverse their declines and improve their lives rather than waiting for those events to happen and then trying to deal with them through extended health care or nursing home care because the client has declined outside of her reserve.

Small changes in our ability to move are important in middle age. By the age of 50 years, most individuals are aware that they are losing muscle strength (mass) and endurance, limiting mobility. Increased life expectancy has led to public health concern about the increase in prevalence of disability in old age. Personal trainers have the challenge of reducing the prevalence, which requires identifying preventable or modifiable risk factors earlier in life.

The message is that the benefits of functional exercise and healthy lifestyle choices are a key foundation for our health. Traditionally those in the medical community, in general, have been poor promoters of functional exercise and improved functional mobility. All too often they have looked to pills, surgery, or retirement from physical activity as a solution to pain and increased deconditioning. For those who have an interest in exposing the myths of aging, a great deal of evidence now exists on specific benefits that older adults gain from functional mobility-based exercise:

- Increased bone density
- Improved balance, reducing the risk of falls
- Increased strength related to successful task execution and independence
- Improved agility, which encourages lifelong recreational activity

- Improved coordination and motor mechanics
- Improved appetite and gastrointestinal function
- Increased caloric expenditure and improved weight management
- Increased energy and decreased sleep loss
- Better pain management (Coalman 2002)

Functional Mobility Classifications

The World Health Organization has published the International Classification of Functioning (ICF). Functioning refers to all body functions, activities, and participation. Alterations in functioning in terms of performance or capacity may be seen as **impairments** (e.g., altered mobility, altered muscle strength-power, altered gait pattern, pain). Impairment in function would affect the execution of an activity. An **activity** is defined as the performance of a task or action (e.g., body position, carrying, walking, household tasks). Activity limitations would be manifested by a change in the performance of a given activity. If an individual's involvement in her life situations is affected (e.g., work, recreation, community life), the limitation is referred to as a **participation** limitation (Fried et al. 1991).

For example, a client may be asked to perform an activity such as climbing stairs. If the client has difficulty with the activity, it would be due to an impairment or an alteration in function such as reduced leg strength.

Loss of mobility and disability have catastrophic consequences on the quality of life of older individuals. According to Nashner (2002), chronic loss of balance and mobility is a geriatric syndrome in which multiple medical problems—none severe enough to earn a diagnosis—combine to give rise to a disability. Mobility involves the cooperative interactions of many biomechanical, muscular, and sensory coordinating mechanisms. In healthy individuals, these processes work together with little, if any, conscious effort. From the biomechanical standpoint, the muscles and joints are flexible and strong. From the sensory motor perspective, a sensitive precision translates a constant barrage of incoming stimuli that in turn are translated into appropriate movement responses of the muscles.

DiPietro (1996) at Yale University School of Medicine performed studies to determine the modifiable factors related to the plasticity of higher physical function, as opposed to merely the presence or absence of disability. The author examined the relationship between physical activity and maintenance of day-to-day functioning. The basic components of strength, balance, coordination, flexibility, and endurance were the building blocks needed to allow performance of more integrated functional tasks. Other sensory, cognitive, and motor abilities were employed in more advanced physical functioning. Physical activity was associated with better functioning even among older people at accelerated risk of functional loss—that is, those with already existing chronic disease.

Okada and colleagues (2011) looked at the relationship between core stability, functional movement, and performance. Functional movement was defined as the ability to produce and maintain a balance between mobility and stability along the kinetic chain while performing fine motor patterns with accuracy and efficiency. Muscular strength, flexibility, endurance, coordination, balance, and movement efficiency were components necessary to achieve functional movement, which is integral to performance and sport-related skills. The functional movement screen used in this study was applied to younger adults and included the hurdle step, in-line lunge, shoulder mobility, trunk rotation, and others as designed by Cook in his Functional Movement Screen (Cook 2006a, 2006b).

The Canadian Centre for Activity and Aging (CCAA) has defined functional mobility as the ability to interact with one's environment effectively. At its highest levels, it is measured as physical fitness. Full function requires flexible joints, adequate bone and muscle strength, and sufficient energy reserves. For the individual living independently in the community, adequate functional mobility is essential for activity such as changing a light bulb, climbing stairs to enter a building, or taking out the garbage. The loss of independence due to decreased functional mobility may pose a greater perceived threat to normal aging than the fear of death itself. Many elderly individuals recognize that a simple fall may bring an end to their precarious independence and therefore to their present lifestyle. According to the CCAA, people who are sedentary lose 30% of functional fitness ability at ages 45 to 55 and up to 60% at ages 55 to 65. Approximately half of this can be regained with fitness.

According to Rikli and Jones (2001), leaders in the area, functional fitness involves specific elements of fitness (strength, flexibility, endurance) that underlie their functional mobility screening. Tests involving quick turns during walking are helpful screening tools for functional mobility. However, tests like this that provide percentiles for functional fitness should also be broken down into their component functions, and performance should be evaluated on each component.

Coalman (2002) defined a functional fitness program as a physical activity and lifestyle modification program promoting self-determined goals that enhance the lifestyle of the participant. For example, it could involve having enough flexibility and balance to put on socks while standing. A focus on physical activity versus fitness is important to success. The most important feature of a successful functional fitness program is an individual exercise prescription, tailored to preferences, desired outcomes, and current needs and unique to each participant. The difference between traditional group senior-focused activity programs and functional fitness programs is the focus on a participant's individual assessment, exercise prescription, and goals.

The word "functional" has been loosely used in exercise training programs to refer to exercises relevant to specific functional activities that we perform on a daily basis and to higher levels of functional activity required for work or recreational pursuits. We can think of functional movement in terms of a pyramid (Rogers and Page 2004).

At the top of the pyramid is skilled activity such as lunging to hit a tennis forehand. This is built upon domains or compound movements that are not task specific; rather, they are multiple joint areas involved in planes of motion and generic movement patterns. They include

1. lower body with movements such as lunge, squat, step;

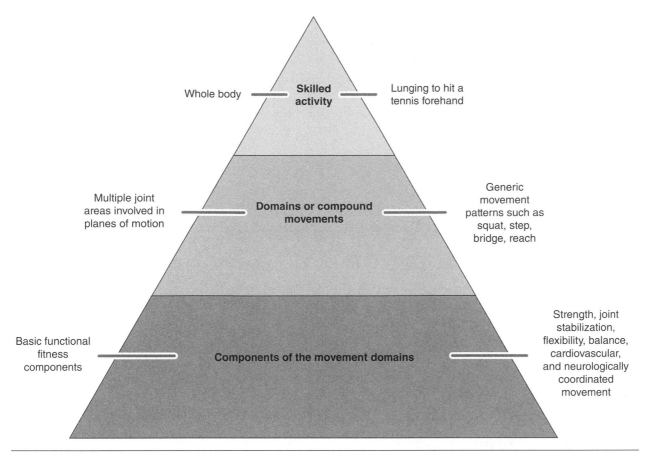

Whole body — **Skilled activity** — Lunging to hit a tennis forehand

Multiple joint areas involved in planes of motion — **Domains or compound movements** — Generic movement patterns such as squat, step, bridge, reach

Basic functional fitness components — **Components of the movement domains** — Strength, joint stabilization, flexibility, balance, cardiovascular, and neurologically coordinated movement

Figure 14.3   Functional movement pyramid.

2. spine or trunk with movements such as bridge, twist, bend, stabilize; and

3. upper body with movements such as push, pull, reach, press.

At the base of the functional pyramid are the components of the movement domains such as strength, flexibility, balance, cardiovascular, and neurologically coordinated movement and joint stabilization. Any skilled activity can be broken down into the domains and components using this functional pyramid (figure 14.3). This approach helps in identifying weak links in the chain of movement that can contribute to dysfunction. Deficits can then be addressed with therapeutic exercise. For example, the functional activity of standing from a sitting position in a chair is similar to a squat movement. The domain movement of a squat requires trunk stabilization, adequate hip and knee extension range of motion and power, and postural stability.

In summary, we can define functional mobility as the ability to carry out activities one needs and wants to do (daily activities and recreation) efficiently for quality of life without undue fatigue or pain in order to stay healthy, safe, and active. Physical abilities in later middle-age and older-age groups may range from a high level of physical fitness to a loss of independence in activities of daily living. With the assistance of an effective screening tool, we can achieve early identification of changes in physical ability before overt limitations in functional behavior appear. Further, the tool will assist the health practitioner in (1) targeting specific areas (activity domains) that present difficulty and (2) identifying physical components that may underlie mobility problems leading to loss of function. Ultimately, these findings can be employed by personal trainers and other health care practitioners in the design of individual programs to improve functional mobility.

Maintaining their physical capabilities gives clients the opportunity to have choices to determine how independent they want to be. The ability to identify impairment or alteration in function, whether in early or later stages, enables one to design interventions for health promotion (prevention), health maintenance (reducing or stabilizing impairment), or chronic disease management (arresting further impairment).

Exercise and Impairment Reduction

Simonsick and colleagues (1993) found that continued physical activity offered benefits to physically capable older adults primarily in reducing the risk of physical impairment and mortality. Moderate to high activity appeared to reduce the likelihood of developing limitations in physical functioning over 3 years, particularly in the areas of walking and doing heavy housework.

Groessi and colleagues (2009) compared physical activity and an educational intervention. After 12 months, the physical activity group was less likely to reach disability as defined as not being able to complete a 400 m walk. In addition, participants in the physical activity group had significantly higher scores in the performance of balance and chair stands and had a faster mean walking time in the 400 m walk.

In terms of delivery of the activity intervention, Fisher and coauthors (2007) found that class- and home-based exercise interventions were equally effective in producing improvements in level of physical activity and measures of physical function in older adults (50+) with chronic conditions. Whitehurst and colleagues (2005) found that a circuit format including functional exercises proved beneficial for functional mobility and was both time- and cost-effective.

A systematic review of 66 studies was conducted recently by Paterson and Warburton (2010) relating physical activity function limitations in older adults to Canada's Physical Activity Guidelines. The authors found that moderate and high levels of physical activity appeared effective in conferring a reduced risk of functional limitations or disability. Exercise training interventions of older adults showed improvement in physiological and functional measures and suggested a longer-term reduction in incidents of mobility disability.

Domains of Functional Mobility

In their model of a functional movement pyramid, Rogers and Page (2004) referred to synergies as regionalized, multijoint movements involving basic movement patterns. The three regions they identified were the lower body, the trunk and spinal area, and the upper body.

Defining the domains as groupings of related tasks and activities with similar components allows some awareness of similar activities that may present difficulties in the future, as well as identifying risks involved with that impairment. If the domains can be carefully described, it is possible to screen for people with early decrements within specific domains of physical functioning to identify those at high risk for further decline. The assessments within a domain should be sensitive enough to detect differences in performance and measure meaningful change after an intervention.

Critical to the design of a functional mobility screening tool are the identification and grouping of common functional movement patterns. A panel of experts used an ordinal scale to judge the test items and domain specifications in the validation of the development of a recent functional mobility screening tool (Griffin 2011b). These were the three domains:

1. Up and down activities
2. Locomotor activities
3. Carry–push–reach activities

Domain 1

Up and down activities with a lower body focus, such as these:

- Putting on socks
- Climbing and descending stairs
- Squatting down
- Using legs to lift an object
- Getting in and out of a car or chair
- Getting off a bus
- Doing yard work, gardening
- Strength- or muscular endurance-demanding tasks using the lower body (e.g., resistance training)
- Recreational activities involving getting in and out of a crouch position

Domain 2

Locomotor activities, such as these:

- Brisk walking, jogging
- Accelerating
- Quick maneuvering

- Walking and looking elsewhere
- Moving at different levels
- Stepping over an obstacle
- Dynamic balance (balance while moving)
- Reactive movements around the house (e.g., getting to the door or phone quickly)
- Hiking or exercise classes
- Recreational activities involving locomotion and agility

Domain 3

Carry and push–reach activities with an upper body and trunk focus, such as these:

- Lifting garments overhead
- Reaching high
- Reaching for seat belt
- Viewing behind while driving
- Lifting objects
- Moving furniture
- Raking leaves
- Carrying groceries
- Holding children and pets
- Heavy activities, chores around the house
- Feeling secure while standing on public transit
- Strength- or muscular endurance–demanding tasks using the arms or trunk

One limitation of any attempt to define broad domains is the probability of overlapping variables, which may confound the uniqueness of each domain. The essential physical components for functional mobility may overlap from one domain to another. For example, a domain including the ability to bend down and return upright may not be totally exclusive from another domain including lifting and carrying, since most lifts start with a bending action. In any case, the identification of domains as groupings of related tasks or activities assists significantly in the design of remedial interventions.

Components of Functional Mobility

There are common fundamental aspects of human movement that occur throughout many activities and applications. Evaluation must consider the client's efficiency in performing certain movements, therefore identifying fundamental movement deficits within the body's kinetic linking system (Cook 2006). Many normally functioning clients will be unable to perform a well-designed functional mobility test with full success because they use compensatory movement patterns, sacrificing the most efficient or mature performance execution. These functional movement difficulties in turn may reflect a deficit in one or more of the essential components of functional mobility, such as

- balance and proprioception,
- muscular strength (stability),
- muscular endurance,
- muscular power,
- flexibility,
- speed,
- coordination (mechanics),
- agility, and
- aerobic and anaerobic capacity.

Each functional movement test should have inherent in its design a combination of these essential components. When a client achieves less than a perfect score, the limiting factors (i.e., the essential components for that test) should be identified.

Okada and colleagues (2011) defined functional movement as the ability to produce and maintain a balance between mobility and stability along the kinetic chain while performing fundamental patterns with accuracy and efficiency. They identified a number of components required to achieve functional movement in this sense: muscular strength, flexibility, endurance, coordination, balance, and movement efficiency.

The Canadian Centre for Activity and Aging (2004) has shifted back toward the traditional exercise–fitness model to address performance measures of functional mobility. The CCAA sees the following as the components underlying functional mobility: cardiorespiratory endurance, anaerobic capacity, muscular strength, muscular endurance, flexibility, balance, coordination, and body composition.

Rikli and Jones (2001) suggested that certain physiological parameters were important in supporting functional mobility in later years: muscular strength, aerobic endurance, flexibility, agility/dynamic balance, and body composition. After identifying these physiological components, they selected specific test protocols that could measure these parameters. The items in their Senior Fitness Test (SFT), as well as the physical components tested by the items, are presented in chapter 13 (table 13.1).

Component-Specific Interventions

There is a significant, positive relationship between physical activity and physical function in older adults, with older adults who are more physically active less likely to experience functional limitation than their more sedentary counterparts. Physical activity intervention can vary widely in methodology, type of activity or goal, intensity, and method of measuring success. Most programs running two or three times per week over a 12- to 16-week period have demonstrated improvements in the specific functional fitness components targeted, regardless of age. The type and level of engagement in physical activity constitute an important predictor of physical function in older clients. Trainers should focus on reducing limitations to physical functioning.

Functional mobility difficulties, the inability to manage daily activities, are risk factors for becoming dependent on others and subsequent institutionalization. Despite widespread awareness of this among health care practitioners, very few studies have investigated the efficacy of interventions specifically aimed at improving mobility function and the integration of its key components. We have defined functional mobility in terms of its parameters or components, including strength, dynamic stability or balance, flexibility, and motor mechanics or ability. For example, to rise or lower from a chair, an 80-year-old person may require more than 100% of the strength of her quadriceps muscles and a full range of motion in ankle dorsiflexion. A strong person can get up in 0.6 s, but a weak person may require 6 s. Limited ankle flexibility may cause an uncontrolled drop into the chair. Many older people can no longer perform this functional task because of limits in specific components.

Strength, Power, and Motor Fitness

On average, strength decreases 10% per decade after 50 years of age. Strength and power are key predictors of functional performance and disability (Signorile 2011). Hanson and colleagues (2009) demonstrated that strength training can improve physical function when measured using standardized activities of daily living (ADLs), climbing stairs, walking, and chair stand performance. The gradual loss of muscle strength results in functional impairment and an increased risk of falling. The ability to rapidly develop high force

contributes to successful performance in everyday activities such as climbing stairs, regaining balance after a trip or slip, rising from a chair, and speed walking. These findings may be explained by a selective atrophy of type IIb fibers with age such that strength reduction occurs earlier in lower extremities than in upper extremities (Pizzigalli et al. 2011). The eccentric component of muscular strength is critical in many physical tasks; moreover, it provides the deceleration forces necessary for maintaining balance in static and dynamic conditions. The scientific evidence for the role of resistance training in maintaining physical functioning is well established; however, evidence is emerging regarding the positive role of neuromuscular training. Motor components of functional fitness can be enhanced with neuromuscular training (e.g., dancing, ball games, weight training, tai chi, skiing, keep-fit exercise, and other active lifestyle activities). A large group of adults aged 30 to 69 years who engaged in neuromuscular exercise had better motor and muscular skeletal fitness in terms of balance and functional leg extensor power, the two major fitness factors related to mobility functioning in aging adults (Lindstrom et al. 2009). In addition to muscle strength, rapid force production of the leg extensors has been shown to contribute to many tasks of daily life such as walking and stair climbing and even the prevention of falls. Foldvari and coauthors (2000) reported that leg power was a stronger predictor of functional status in elderly women than any of the other physiological measures they assessed, including lower leg strength. Leg power has also been highly correlated with stair climb time, rise time, maximal walking speed, and timed up-and-go. Holviala and colleagues (2006) demonstrated that high-volume and high-intensity strength training (including low-load exercises for explosive actions) twice a week for 21 weeks was associated not only with increased maximal strength, but also with improvements in explosive force production, dynamic balance, and functional mobility such as walking speed in middle-aged and older women. Power has been more highly correlated with functional abilities and strength.

Strength and Balance

Although sometimes difficult to define and measure, balance is basically the ability to maintain the body's position over its base of support, whether the base is stationary (static balance) or moving (dynamic balance). Dynamic balance includes maintaining balance while walking and stepping over or around objects. In older adults, static balance is maintained until significant functional declines occur, but losses in dynamic balance are evident much earlier. Based on the importance of strength and dynamic balance, particularly to reduce the risk of falls in older adults, training of postural muscles along with dynamic balance training is important. Researchers at Simon Fraser University found that 41% of falls occurred when older participants incorrectly shifted their weight outside of the base of support and did not have sufficient dynamic stability (strength) to correct their balance (Robinovitch et al. 2012). A systematic review noted that various methods of training appeared to improve static balance on stable and unstable surfaces as well as dynamic (moving) balance ability if performed at least 10 min per day, 3 days per week, for 4 weeks (DiStefano et al. 2009).

Several types of exercise programs (including exercise focusing on gait, balance, coordination, and functional tasks; strengthening exercise; tai chi, yoga, or dance), when conducted three times a week for 3 months, have been moderately effective in improving clinical balance outcomes such as timed up-and-go, one-legged stand, walking speed, or the Berg Balance Scale. In a recent study, Fujiwara and colleagues (2011) used simple heel raising to strengthen the plantar flexors and increase postural control during arm flexion. The earlier and stronger activation of the soleus restored equilibrium function and improved dynamic balance; deficits in both of these are considered to be primary causes of falls among the elderly.

Even though strength and balance are related, resistance training alone has only a modest effect on improving balance (Rogers 2003). In part, this is because the ability to maintain balance involves a set of processes that require the successful integration of multiple sensory systems. Besides the visual system and the vestibular system, the somatosensory system monitors the body's position in contact with other objects (floor) using muscle receptors that detect body movement and position. With advancing age, muscle strength and sensory function decrease, contributing to losses in balance. Rogers describes a program developed by researchers at the Center for Physical Activity and Aging at Wichita State University, Kansas, that combines strength training with balance-specific exercises to target the muscular system as well as the sensory control systems. After 3 months of performing these progressive balance exercises three times a week, participants improved both their strength and balance by approximately 20%.

My personal experience with balance training for adults in their fifth and sixth decades suggests placing special emphasis on

- maintaining functional muscular strength particularly in the lower body,
- retaining proprioception by controlling factors that influence balance such as base (in) stability, and
- maintaining neuromuscular pathways with coordination tasks.

Strength and Flexibility

The loss of muscular strength and flexibility with age is associated with a decline in functional abilities and health status. It is often assumed that strength training will improve flexibility as long as exercises are performed through a full range of motion and both agonist and antagonist muscle groups are being trained. Results in this area appear to be conflicting. One study found that independent of flexibility exercises, strength training increased flexibility in multiple-joint motions in inactive older males. The authors theorized that resistance exercise improves not only the tensile strength of tendons and ligaments but also the contractility of muscles to increase joint range of motion (Fatouros et al. 2002). However, in another study involving only shoulder abduction, flexibility training by itself was more effective than the same exercises incorporated with strength training, suggesting that strength training alone will not increase range of motion even when the action is through the full range of motion. These authors concluded that extensive stretching should be included in heavy resistance strength training programs among older individuals (Girouard and Hurley 1995). Developing flexibility with resistance techniques usually involves eccentric work (lowering phase) in which the muscle is elongated while it is contracting. Near the end of the eccentric range of motion, the number of contracting muscle fibers decreases, increasing the tension in each active muscle fiber. This may produce a greater stretch, resulting in enhanced flexibility; however, eccentric training is associated with delayed-onset muscle soreness.

Strength and Cardiovascular Endurance

Several studies have shown that declines with age in strength and cardiovascular endurance capabilities can be slowed down by proper training. Holviala and colleagues (2010) examined the effects of twice-weekly, 21-week total-body strength training combined with endurance cycling in men in their fifth and sixth decades. In addition to strength and cardiovascular assessments, the authors employed a unique load-carrying walking protocol on the treadmill to characterize functional performance. The improvements produced by the combined training may also be beneficial for aging workers in physically demanding occupations.

Step aerobics has been a popular exercise mode since the 1980s. In addition to cardiovascular and lower body muscular work, most group-led classes also involve dynamic arm movements, balance and agility, and various stretching exercises. Hallage and colleagues (2010) included functional fitness outcome measures such as the chair stand test, timed up-and-go, chair sit-and-reach, and arm curl test. Twelve weeks of step aerobic training increased functional fitness components of strength, balance, agility, and flexibility.

Looking for consistencies in 42 previous studies, Lopopolo and coauthors (2006) reviewed the effects of therapeutic exercise on gait speed. Therapeutic exercise was defined as strength training or as aerobic training combined with other exercise. Exercise had a significant effect on the habitual or self-selected gait speed. Gait speed was significantly affected by high-intensity and high-dosage exercise, but was not affected by low- or moderate-intensity or low-dosage exercise. Maximal gait speed was not significantly affected by therapeutic exercise.

What is functional training for an older client? Exercise that is functional often involves daily activities—walking rather than taking the car, or taking stairs and not the elevator. Within this context, the exercise has been described as "active living." Canada's Physical Activity Guide to Healthy Active Living for Older Adults (www.csep.ca/CMFiles/Guidelines/CSEP_PAGuidelines_older-adults_en.pdf) suggests activities such as vacuuming, gardening, walking, washing the floors, or climbing stairs and encourages their incorporation into the daily routine.

As noted previously, the term *functional* refers to basic ADLs that are required and those that allow us to engage in recreational and meaningful activities related to work or leisure and an ability to move effectively and efficiently in our environment (Taylor and Johnson 2008).

The term *functional exercise* implies the use of the whole body and primary systems of the body, that is, the musculoskeletal, cardiovascular, and neurological systems. Loss of mobility due to an injury or joint pain (musculoskeletal system) may limit the amount or speed of walking or other cardiovascular activity and in turn present fewer of the challenges necessary to keep balance performance well tuned (neurological system).

Functional exercise has three main goals. The first goal is to reach full functional ability in the basic components of strength, dynamic stability, flexibility, and motor mechanics. The second goal is to restore the client's confidence in and ability to achieve normal speed, power, control, and balance without the risk of injury. The final goal is to have the client perform basic and advanced exercises and activities that will encourage increased participation in lifelong active living. Optional functionally integrated exercises follow the guidelines for prescription described in chapter 8.

LIFE Approach

Functional exercises, tasks, or activities allow the client to progress to a level of effective and efficient movement patterns. They should be paired with functional assessment to identify accurately the level of the client's ability to perform daily activities or more advanced recreational activities.

An Australian study examined the LIFE approach, which involves movements specifically prescribed to improve balance or increase strength embedded into everyday activities (Clemson et al. 2012). For example, the strategy to improve balance included "reduce base of support" or "turning and changing direction." Prescribed activity incorporating a reduced base of support might involve a tandem stand or one-leg stand while working at the kitchen counter. Strategies to increase strength included "bend your knees," which might involve squatting instead of bending at the waist to pick things up from the floor. Compared to a structured program involving seven exercises for balance and six exercises for lower limb strength performed 3 days a week, LIFE produced similar improvements in dynamic balance. Compared to results in controls, LIFE demonstrated significant improvements in participants' static balance, ankle strength, function, and number of falls.

Disablement Process Model

The disablement process model described by Nagi (1991) outlines how pathology (chronic health conditions, injury) can lead to impairments in body systems (cardiovascular, musculoskeletal, cognitive, sensory, and motor). Lifestyle, inactivity, and aging can also lead to these types of impairments even without pathology. Eventually, the accumulated impairments can lead to limitations in physical functioning (e.g., walking, stair climbing) and ultimately to disability. Disability is usually defined as difficulty in performing or inability to perform daily activities such as work, recreation, household tasks, socializing, and self-care (Jones and Rose 2005).

The traditional models explaining the disabling process (Nagi 1991) describe five main stages in the progression to disability:

1. Disease/pathology

2. Lifestyle/inactivity

3. Physiological impairment, that is, a decline in body systems (e.g., muscular)

4. Functional limitations such as in climbing stairs or rising from a chair

5. Disability or the inability to perform normal daily activities (figure 14.4)

This model has allowed health researchers to examine the extent to which physical activity is associated with subsequent performance on functional tests, and in turn how changes in functional performance influence limitations. Physical inactivity can be a primary cause of impairment and functional limitation leading to disability. Increased physical activity results in improvement of fitness components (strength, flexibility, and so on) as well as functional abilities such as lifting, walking, and recreational activities. Figure 14.4 also identifies that not all limitations result in a disability or impairment. One possible reason is that physical limitations causing task difficulty may be somewhat avoided or modified to allow continued execution of functional tasks.

Hall and McCauley (2011) found that self-efficacy, or an individual's belief in her ability to successfully complete a task, also had a significant effect on self-reported limitations and subsequent disability. They found that individuals who were more physically active had higher self-efficacy and demonstrated better functional capacity, both of which were associated with fewer functional limitations. It appears that self-efficacy plays a pivotal role in formulating perceptions of disability, suggesting a complex series of interactions between confidence and task performance. These results are important when we consider

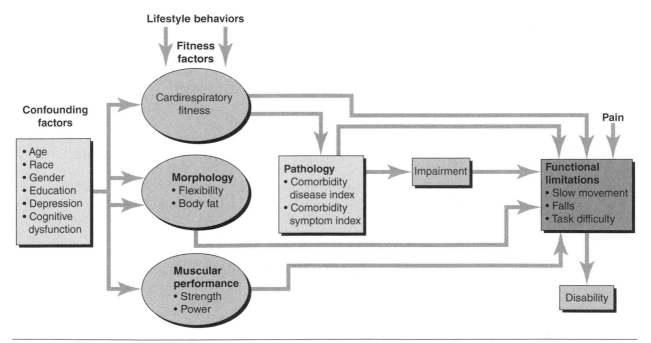

Figure 14.4   Pathway to disability.

Circus Self-Efficacy

In a recent discussion with an aerial instructor from a circus company, I was curious to find out if self-efficacy had much of an effect on outcome performances in the oldest clients, who were in their 40s. Classes were designed to involve cumulative task mastery over a period of time. The instructor said that there were two types of successful clients. The first type comprised those who could see the progressive, staged nature of the tasks and were comfortable working within those parameters. The second type consisted of those who were confident enough to try the task even if they modified it to suit their abilities or their strengths (compensation). Clients who were unsuccessful often showed a lack of confidence and would generate doubts in their own abilities because they could not picture themselves executing the task. These clients were also more likely to drop out of the class. I asked the instructor if she made efforts to modify the task difficulty or provided extra encouragement. She told me that she always did so and that these efforts could help renew a client's sense of ambition but that older clients' own confidence in their ability also had a significant effect on their success.

the influence that a personal trainer or a well-designed exercise prescription may have on participation and success in functional movements.

Compensation Strategies

The functional status of an individual can change even when there is no change in the severity of an underlying impairment. This commonly occurs through the use of compensatory strategies, which are often altered mobility patterns (Fried et al. 1991). The compensation serves to minimize the functional impact of an impairment and to maintain independent functioning without perception of difficulty—for example, when people use a different method to get in and out of a car. Compensatory strategies appear to be used in both conscious and unconscious ways by individuals with preclinical mobility problems. The following are types of compensation strategies:

- Physical modification—a change in the method of performing a task.
- Physiological modification—an increase in the reliance on other physiological systems to support the performance (e.g., strength compensating for balance).
- Behavioral modification—alteration of expectations about the performance of a difficult task. Individuals often report "doing less" than they used to. This restriction of activity may result in further decreased exercise tolerance and functional mobility (Fried et al. 1991).

Strategies of compensation may be efficient and safe or inefficient and potentially harmful. Once

people have some difficulty with an activity, it is a critical time for intervention. Early functional mobility problems may take a number of natural courses:

- **Compensation** or the alteration of a movement pattern that may be inefficient. This could lead to an increased risk of injury (Cook 2006).
- **Retraining or repairing** in order to regain performance or proprioception of the given aspect of the kinetic linking system. This could lead to regaining full functional mobility or use of a task modification that would be a safe compensation.
- **Cessation** of a group of activities dependent on the given aspect of functional mobility. This could lead to a more sedentary lifestyle or an increased functional loss in that area.

Individuals using compensatory movement patterns during activities may be sacrificing efficient movements for inefficient ones in order to perform at higher levels. If compensation is continued, then poor movement patterns are reinforced, leading to poor biomechanics and ultimately the potential of micro- or macrotraumatic injury (Cook 2006). The individual creates a poor movement pattern that he will use whenever he performs the task. Programmed altered movement patterns have the potential to lead to further mobility and stability imbalances. For example, avid hikers as they age may experience transient pain in their knees particularly during steep descents. A common compensation is to use Nordic walking poles. However, without proper instruction, this may place excess strain on the shoulder for stabilization during flexion.

This compensation may create anterior shoulder strength imbalances and excessive shearing forces, increasing the risks for injury.

Compensation is not necessarily a bad thing if it results in efficient movements that avoid normal pain patterns. Harris-Hayes and colleagues (2008) demonstrated that patient education to modify symptom-provoking functional activities through restriction of abnormal motions and alignments was very successful. In addition, they prescribed exercises to address impairments in muscle length, muscle strength, and motor control that they felt contributed to the pain.

In a study of adaptive changes in gait, older adults took more steps in a given distance, allowing them to compensate with more time in double-limb support and a more stable gait pattern. This demonstrates that older adults exhibit adaptive balance strategies to maintain a sufficient level of dynamic balance (Rogers et al. 2008).

Clients modify their movements for a number of reasons, sometimes in order to decrease pain in another area. Van Dillen and coauthors (2001) found that patients reporting increased back pain modified their limb movements while performing functional tasks in order to reduce pain. Similarly, in a case study, pain limited the ability to perform reaching movements and the ability to cycle; issues with alignment, muscle length and strength, and shoulder pain were shown. Screening is not diagnostic, but deviations in movement (e.g., of the shoulder) may leave patients at risk or may be the cause of pain. To be pain free, patients may modify their shoulder movements during demanding tasks (Caldwell et al. 2007).

Some functional movements have been studied carefully, helping us to determine the functional mobility of the client (Janssen et al. 2002). The ability to go from a sitting position to a standing position is an important skill especially in elderly people. Measurements have been obtained using techniques such as force plates, video analysis, and goniometry. Janssen and coauthors describe four distinct phases of the sit-to-stand movement. Phase 1 (flexion-momentum phase) starts with the initiation of the movement and ends just before the buttocks are lifted from the seat of the chair. Phase 2 (momentum-transfer phase) begins as the buttocks are lifted and at the start of the extension phase (phase 3). Phase 4 is the stabilization phase. Any deficit in these phases is reflected by adaptations, leading to compensations and dysfunctional movement patterns. Dysfunctional movement patterns in individual phases may involve components such as ankle flexibility,

leg strength, coordinated motor mechanics, and hip stabilization. De Brito and colleagues (2013) found that the ability to sit and rise from the floor was a significant predictor of mortality in 51- to 80-year-olds. Unfortunately, getting down to the floor and then up off it to do things like play with a child, clean out a kitchen cabinet, or participate in floor exercise may fall off the daily repertoire of possible movements. Lack of confidence and fear of embarrassment, in addition to physical decline in the form of decreased upper body and lower body strength, decreased range of motion, and balance issues, could limit success in this important mobility task. Moxley (2012) has described a technique that takes advantage of mechanical deficiencies that make getting up off the floor much easier (figure 14.5). This technique is appropriate for individuals who do not have a total knee replacement, hip replacement, or other significant issue.

We know that the rate of loss of strength may accelerate beyond the age of 50. Trudelle-Jackson and colleagues (2006) compared muscle strength of different lower extremity muscle groups and postural stability in women age 50 and older. The largest strength declines occurred in the plantar flexors, followed by the hip abductors and flexors. During stand-to-sit movements, the trunk inclined an average of 10° less; that is, older adults leaned forward less when sitting. This may have been due to a compensation that addressed reduced postural control and decreased the muscle forces needed at the hip while increasing the forces of the knee extensors. The quadriceps remained strong while the other hip stabilizers (e.g., abductors) lost their strength due to the habitual movement modification.

Mobility function has been shown to be the first area in which most older adults become disabled (see figure 14.1). Fried and colleagues (2000) were among the first groups to show definitively that preclinical disability could predict the onset of disability and provide insight into the critical points of transition to higher risk. They identified self-reported modification of the method of doing a task as a strong predictor of risk of incident mobility disability. The individuals reporting modification of their method of performing mobility tasks were compensating for the impact of underlying health changes. These modifications may well successfully minimize the effects of impairments on function and thus slow decline or maintain function in the short run so that little or no difficulty with the task performance is perceived. Rehabilitation focuses

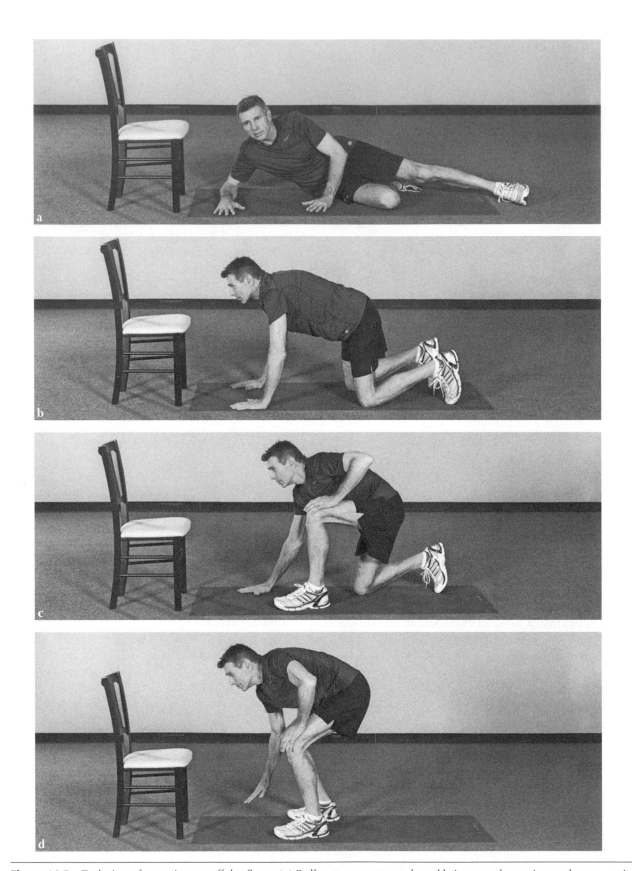

Figure 14.5 Technique for getting up off the floor: *(a)* Roll onto your stomach and bring your knees in one by one, using your upper body, to a position of all fours; *(b)* bring one leg up and forward under your chest, foot on the floor; *(c)* bring your hands in closer to your feet and then bring one arm or hand to your thigh; *(d)* pressing your hand(s) on your thigh, roll up all the way. It is advisable to have a sturdy chair nearby for support or dizziness.

Aerobic Tennis: Extending the Life of a Tennis Player

Thirty-six years ago I started playing tennis with my wife. We were both very competitive and soon found that without instant replay, the quality of our games suffered and the frequency of our debates increased. Thirty-five years ago we started to play "aerobic tennis"—we love it and are still married! There is no serving and no scoring. Each player starts with three or four balls, so ball retrieval time is kept to a minimum. The first four or five hits are usually directly to the opponent, allowing time to feel the movement pattern at a reasonable pace. Rallies often extend beyond 20 hits, with both sides feeling successful. Now that we are in our 60s, we continue to play aerobic tennis in order to accommodate friends we bring to the court who vary in fitness and ability. In a typical doubles scenario, we adjust the speed and difficulty of the shot to accommodate the player we are hitting it toward. Aerobic tennis is a cooperative game accommodating many levels of play, and it reduces the barriers that might be a part of a competitive tennis match. Most of the play is near to the baseline, with less aggressive volleys at the net. The self-efficacy of newer players rises quickly, as does their quality of play, with so many more shots per hour. They stay with the activity when they achieve this success. Their fitness also improves due to the continuous nature of aerobic tennis. If the game is between just my wife and me, she plays the singles court and, since I like to run, I play the doubles court. I try to get the ball closer to her, but hard, and she moves me around relentlessly. It is easy to keep heart rates elevated, dynamic balance challenged, and reaction and response time quick, with power and agility integrated into every rally. And to top it off, neither of us has lost a game in 35 years!

heavily on maximizing compensation and preventing further decline.

Perhaps the exercise health practitioner should not only attempt to correct poor compensations but also seek to implement effective compensations with people who may benefit from them. How should instructors plan for such safe compensation? Higher-functioning seniors or older middle-aged clients can develop effective compensations for mobility difficulties. Those at higher risk or those with a reduced reserve capability are less likely to be able to effectively compensate or to prevent the progression of the disability. We need to recognize that in some cases the transition to disability occurs when additional declines in health overwhelm the compensations being employed. Effective compensation may prove useful in disability prevention.

Designing successful age-appropriate programs opens the trainer to dealing with the challenges relating to their clients' aging body. Inspired creative programming through modifications and compensation must occur with personal trainers, health club owners, and any health care workers (Milner 2001). Special needs do not arise just because of changes in the physiological systems of balance, coordination, and muscular deficits but also relate to the environment of the exercise, safety issues, and personal relevance. To meet these needs, our planning should include assessments appropriate for clients' functional ability; safe and appropriate types of exercise at

the right intensity; exercise design in relation to function; and proper form, which may include some modification of compensation.

Functional Mobility Screening and Assessment

Screening of older clients for risk of mobility difficulty is an important step toward prevention of costly impairments limiting activity and eventual participation in an active lifestyle. Jette and Cleary (1987) refer to screening and assessment as a detailed review of data on function to guide decisions about the nature of the problem and specific treatment plans. They add that the clinical significance of different scores should be specified in the screening instrument. Difficulty with mobility is a marker of a high-risk group. A major obstacle to screening for early functional mobility problems is the lack of a method that identifies those who are at high risk.

Personal trainers can benefit from an overview of research findings that identify assessment tools and data on mobility function to guide decisions about the potential design of conditioning plans:

• **ADLs.** Commonly used terms are ADLs (activities of daily living) and IADLs (instrumental activities of daily living). The ADLs are the basic tasks of everyday life such as eating, bathing, dressing, toileting, and transferring.

IADLs extend these basic functions to include things like shopping, transportation, stairs, and housework. Difficulties in ADLs and IADLs can predict future functional decline, disability, and institutionalization (Aronow et al. 2008; Creel et al. 2001; Fries 2005).

• **Questionnaires.** Questionnaires addressing ADLs relevant to older adults provide an opportunity to capture a broad assessment of older participants' current physical activity habits (Saliba et al. 2000; DiPietro 1996). Having a good list of IADL and ADL items can facilitate consideration of high-risk individuals in population-based rapid health screens. Many studies have combined self-reported questionnaires and performance-related assessments (Chaves et al. 2000; Gill et al. 1995; Gill and Gahbauer 2008; Murtagh and Hubert 2004; Ostchega et al. 2000; Strawbridge et al. 2002).

• **Self-reported measures.** Fried and colleagues (2000) set out to determine whether potential self-report and performance measures of preclinical disability could predict incident mobility disability in high-functioning older women. In their study, physical disability was ascertained by self-report of difficulty in performing any of 27 tests of daily life, including mobility, upper extremity, household management, and basic self-care tasks. Participants were asked whether they had modified the method or had changed the frequency with which they performed the task as a result of underlying problems. Persons reporting such modification but no difficulty in a task were characterized as potentially in a stage of preclinical decline in function in that task or preclinical disability. Other objective measurements used included (1) dynamic balance, assessed by the functional reach test, and (2) maximal isometric strength of the knee extensors. The main outcome measure was walking 0.5 miles (0.8 km), climbing up 10 steps, lifting and carrying 10 lb (4.5 kg), and heavy housework. Stair climb speed was a sensitive predictor of difficulty. Overall, these findings suggest two types of indicators for preclinical disability, self-report and performance measures.

• **Performance measures.** A Canadian study identified greater flexibility and activity levels (especially outdoors) and faster normal walking speed as those variables most strongly associated with an independent lifestyle (Cunningham et al. 1993). Some researchers have found intermediate end points in the mobility disability pathway, such as lower extremity strength, peak walking velocity, and postural stability (Chaves et al. 2000; Weiss et al. 2007). Guralnik and colleagues (1995) looked at the ability of certain objective measures of lower extremity function to predict disability 4 years later. The participants reported no disability in ADLs and were able to walk 0.5 miles (0.8 km) and climb stairs without assistance. The tests included standing balance, a timed up-and-go walk, and a timed test of 5 repetitions of rising from a chair and sitting down. Those with the lowest scores on the performance tests were 4.2 to 4.9 times as likely to have disability at 4 years as those with the highest scores. The authors concluded that objective measures of lower-extremity function were highly predictive of subsequent disability.

• **Senior Fitness Test.** One of the best-validated tests is the Senior Fitness Test (SFT) (Rikli and Jones 2001). The SFT was developed to measure the basic physical abilities required to perform functional ADLs, as well as functional mobility. It is currently the only functional fitness test battery that has national norms. Each of the six test items is a functional measure of a combination of physical parameters, including muscular strength/endurance, aerobic fitness, flexibility, balance, coordination, speed/agility, and power (see table 13.1). In developing the SFT manual, Rikli and Jones (2001) referred to the Functional Ability Framework (chapter 13), in which they illustrate the progressive relationship among physical parameters such as muscular strength, functional abilities such as stair climbing, and activity goals such as gardening or housework. The SFT items were administered in 21 states to 7183 men and women between the ages of 60 and 94, with reliabilities ranging from 0.80 to 0.98.

• **Functional Mobility Screening Tool.** Recently, Griffin (2011a) designed the composite Functional Mobility Screening Tool, which includes a 24-item questionnaire, four basic mobility tests (flexibility and balance), and six performance mobility tests (functional movement patterns reflecting three domains). The three domains assessed are up and down activities, lower body focus; locomotor activities; and carry–push–reach activities, upper body and trunk focus. The content validity, or the degree to which the test battery reflected the defined domains, was rated either 3 or 4, rendering the validity significant (Waltz and Bausell 1981). The reliability of the screening tool was tested in a sample of 45 men and women. Intra-rater reliabilities were substantial or excellent, with correlations of $r = 0.72$ to 1.00, and were slightly higher than the interrater reliabilities (Griffin 2011b).

- **Functional Movement Screen (FMS).** The use of fundamental movements as an assessment of function with athletes is an attempt to pinpoint deficient areas of mobility and stability that may be overlooked in an asymptomatic active population. The FMS is designed to identify individuals who have developed compensatory movement patterns in the kinetic chain. Cook and colleagues (2006) have used fundamental movements and deficits during preparticipation screening as an assessment of function that may limit performance and predispose the athlete to microtraumatic injury (see "Functional Movement Screen," chapter 4).

Functional Mobility Screening Tool

The full Functional Mobility Screening Tool includes

- one questionnaire,
- four basic mobility tests,
- and six performance mobility tests (two tests per domain).

Clients begin with the Functional Mobility Self-Rating Questionnaire (form 14.1), which includes a few simple questions that help them identify mobility difficulties. A series of eight questions for each domain (area of difficulty) was based on a review of the ADL and IADL questionnaires in the literature, extensive client interviews, and reflections from a focus group of experts. Clients answer "No trouble," "Some trouble," or "Lots of trouble" to each question. If the client answers "Some" or "Lots" of trouble, she is asked to select one or two reasons (from a list of four) as to why the item is difficult for her. The four choices listed as reasons are the four components identified as critical for functional mobility.

After filling out the questionnaire, the client is encouraged to attempt a series of four self-rating basic mobility tests, listed in table 14.1, that center mostly on flexibility and are included in the domain scoring. Within the performance mobility testing, clients can begin with a test or activity (performance level 1) that may involve different components of the activity domain, including strength, agility, balance, or another parameter addressed in that test. Performance level 2 tests involve more complex, multiple tasks, integrating and expanding on the components of the first level.

Most tests in the Functional Mobility Screening Tool may be administered with minimal or no assistance and have a simple standard interpretation. This permits clients to begin by attempting a relatively simple basic mobility test that incorporates a functional range of motion before performing a higher-level, more complex performance mobility test. The principle of hierarchy is reflected in progressively more complex related activities (e.g., domain 1: lower body, sit-and-reach [B1]; chair stand [C1]; lunge and hurdle step [C2]).

Table 14.1   Functional Mobility Screening Tool Organization

Section	Part A: questionnaire	Part B: basic mobility	Part C: performance mobility
General content	A few brief questions to discover any difficulties with activities and reasons	Simple mobility tests emphasizing flexibility	More complex tasks involving various physical components; outcome measure involves movement evaluation
Domain 1: lower body	8 questions	B1: chair sit-and-reach (flexibility) (Rikli and Jones 2001)	C1: chair stand (Rikli and Jones 2001) C2: lunge and hurdle step (Cook et al. 2006)
Domain 2: locomotor	8 questions	B2: tandem pivot and walk (balance)	C3: timed up-and-go (Rikli and Jones 2001) C4: agility course
Domain 3: upper body and trunk	8 questions	B3: back scratch (flexibility) (Rikli and Jones 2001) B4: seated trunk and neck rotation (flexibility)	C5: side bridge (McGill et al. 1999) C6: lift–carry–reach course

Data Analysis

The Functional Mobility Screening Tool (Griffin 2011b) was subjected to the following statistical criteria.

Content Validity

The CVI (content validity instrument) and domain specifications were presented to a panel of experts for their judgment of the items using a 4-point ordinal rating scale (Waltz and Bausell 1981). All items received either a 3 or 4 rating, rendering the validity significant. Two items from the SFT that were used had criterion validity measures of 0.83 for chair sit-and-reach and 0.77 for the chair stand based on a one-repetition maximum leg press (Rikli and Jones 1999a).

Intra- and Interrater Reliability

The reliability of the screening tool was tested in a sample of 45 men and women. Test–retest reliability with the same tester (intrarater reliability) provided the degree to which scores on each test item were similar when repeated 1 week later. Twenty-two clients were retested by the same tester, and 23 clients were retested under the same conditions but by a different tester (interrater reliability). Other researchers looking at similar screening or test batteries have reported only intrarater reliability (Rikli and Jones 1999a). Another group (Minick et al. 2010) has reported interrater reliabilities based on four raters all viewing the same videotaped execution.

- Part A, questionnaire: Clients were consistent in answering the questionnaire from one week to the next ($r = 0.80$-1.00).
- Part B, basic mobility tests: Sit-and-reach, back scratch, and trunk rotation showed substantial or excellent correlations ($r = 0.72$-1.00). The tandem walk showed less consistent scoring ($r = 0.66$). Rikli and Jones (1999a) reported intrarater reliability of 0.95 for the chair sit-and-reach and 0.96 for the back scratch.
- Part C, performance mobility tests: The intrarater correlations were moderate to excellent; the interrater coefficients were slightly higher, with substantial to excellent correlations.

The tests are simple to administer but provide enough information (e.g., component weakness) to allow for valuable feedback from clients on their functional mobility, appropriate information to use as a stepping-stone to health and activity promotion, and effective design of interventions. The scoring system can identify progression in difficulty with the rubric-like numerical hierarchy of levels of efficiency of performance. Self-rating in conjunction with performance measures can reveal a pattern of recognition and may increase the sensitivity of questionnaires alone in which individuals misunderstand or overrate themselves.

All items of the functional mobility questionnaire (Griffin 2012) and all segments of the basic and performance mobility tests are associated with one or more of the following components.

- **Strength.** Muscle strength is the amount of force produced by a group of muscles to overcome a resistance or body weight and can involve short-ening or lengthening of the muscles. Repeated over time, this is called muscular endurance. Developing strength assists in moving the body and heavy objects.

- **Dynamic stability.** Dynamic stability is the ability to control or limit the movement of limbs during activities, to adapt or react to movement and regain balance or stabilize joints. Developing dynamic stability may decrease the risk of postural imbalances or injury and increase the feeling of steadiness.

- **Flexibility.** Flexibility is the range of motion around a joint or series of joints. Developing flexibility may enhance movement control and guard against injury.

- **Motor mechanics.** Motor mechanics refers to the performance of activities with normal and efficient movement patterns demonstrating coordination and agility. Developing motor mechanics may reduce unwanted compensation in activities, thereby reducing stress on the body.

The trainer needs to have a good understanding of these components, but it is important that the client does also. Assist your clients with good examples of movements, sport skills, or exercises that allow them to self-assess and discriminate between appropriate components. The following are examples:

- The strength of the hip in a squat versus the dynamic stability of the hip in getting into and out of a car
- The motor mechanics of a quick change of direction in a tennis game versus the strength of push-off to get to a ball
- The flexibility of the spine in bending sideways in a yoga class versus the spine's dynamic stability when one picks up a grocery bag from the floor

The evaluations consider efficiency in performing certain movements and identify potential compensatory movement patterns, therefore pinpointing fundamental movement deficits. The tests provide information on functional mobility, enabling feedback on status and design of a personalized exercise program. The evaluation assists with (1) targeting specific areas (domains) that present difficulty and (2) identifying physical components that may underlie mobility problems. These self-reported abilities or difficulties afford a simple process of evaluation within each activity domain.

Since the entire Functional Mobility Screening Tool can be self-administered, it can be done online at home. This provides a wider audience exposure, increases awareness, and encourages interest in seeking out more extensive functional mobility follow-up. Careful wording, clear photographs, and an organized layout for all test items are paramount to ensuring reliability, safety, and meaningful interpretation.

Fitness specialists working with seniors should be knowledgeable about the selection, administration, and interpretation of appropriate functional fitness assessments in order to have a basis for designing appropriate activity programs. Assessing functional mobility can help practitioners to

- identify people at risk of becoming functionally dependent,
- identify individuals who may need special services or treatment,

- obtain objective data to help determine client goals,
- identify component weaknesses,
- have a basis for the design of a personalized rehabilitative program,
- show specific areas of improvement during retest, and
- motivate clients with tangible goals.

A results report with interpretation outlines areas of difficulty for each test item (e.g., performance difficulty and component weakness). This type of interpretation facilitates future intervention programming. The following are sample explanations for the assessment report.

Part A: Questionnaire

The focus of the questionnaire items in each of the three domains was referenced back to a grouping of similar basic tasks or activities that were well documented in the gerontology research and were verified and expanded in our interviews and expert reflections on 50- to 70-year-olds (Griffin 2011b).

In responding to a series of eight questions for each domain, clients identify their degree of difficulty in completing the task (area of difficulty). For each task that presents difficulty, clients also identify their reason for the difficulty by selecting the critical underlying component(s), that is, strength, dynamic stability, flexibility, motor mechanics.

Part B: Basic Mobility Tests

The self-rating questionnaire and the basic mobility tests allow for both subjective and objective discovery. The basic mobility assessments are self-administered (i.e., at home) but may add an element of realism for those who tend to overrate themselves on questionnaires (figures 14.6-14.9). The scoring systems for the mobility assessments follow the same pattern as the questionnaire. Each domain has a possible total of 20 points, with 16 points from the questionnaire plus 4 points from the basic mobility assessment(s). The client identifies the critical underlying components for the questionnaire, and the underlying components for basic mobility are automatically assigned along with a score of 0, 1, or 2.

Sit-and-Reach

This test (figure 14.6) measures lower body flexibility including hamstrings and back muscles; lower body flexibility may also be restricted by tight calves. Difficulties with this test may be due to static or dynamic immobility in multiple or single joints.

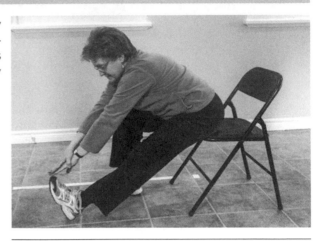

Figure 14.6 Sit-and-reach.

Tandem Walk

This test (figure 14.7) measures how well one moves and changes directions, as well as dynamic balance during moving. Difficulties with this test may relate to dynamic stability of the lower body or coordination and motor ability involving timing judgment.

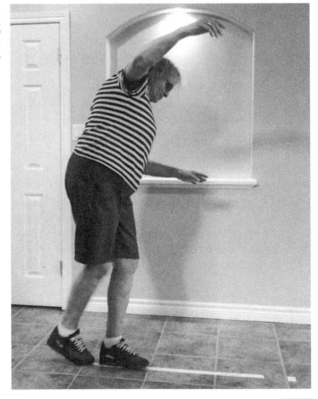

Figure 14.7 Tandem walk.

Back Scratch

This test (figure 14.8) requires shoulder mobility in a combination of motions including abduction–external rotation, flexion-extension, and adduction–internal rotation. It also requires shoulder girdle and thoracic spine mobility. Difficulties with this test beyond shoulder rotation immobility may be due to shortening of the pectoralis minor or latissimus dorsi muscles causing rounded shoulders.

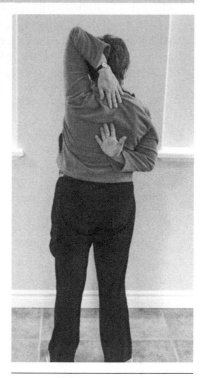

Figure 14.8   Back scratch.

Trunk Rotation

This test (figure 14.9) measures spinal flexibility. Difficulties with this test may be due to limited range of motion in the neck or tightness in the lumbar–thoracic musculature.

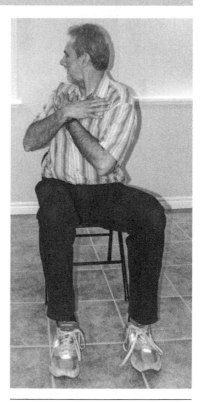

Figure 14.9   Trunk rotation.

Part C: Performance Mobility Tests

The performance mobility tests include level 1 tests that involve different physical components of the selected activity domain including strength, dynamic stability, flexibility, and motor mechanics (figures 14.10, 14.13, and 14.15). Performance level 2 tests involve more complex, multiple tasks, integrating and expanding on the physical components of the first level (figures 14.11, 14.12, 14.14, and 14.16). As the complexity of the tests increases, outcome measures involve a checklist approach to the evaluation, enabling the identification of specific areas of difficulty.

The performance mobility tests include a description for each test, its purpose, procedures, measurement, and interpretation. As the complexity of the tests increases and the multiple movement patterns are combined, outcome measures involve a rubric-type approach to the evaluation. A combined scoring system includes a measurement scale (0, 1, 2) in addition to detailed descriptors for each measurement point.

The following list represents score interpretation for the performance mobility section:

2: No difficulty; able to perform completely with good technique; minimal to no extraneous movement, loss of balance, or misalignment

1: Some difficulty; unwanted or discontinuous movement; loss of some alignment or balance

0: Cannot complete because of mobility difficulty, pain, or both

For example, a test score of 1 would be awarded for the timed up-and-go test if any of the following descriptors were checked:

- Some trouble getting up fast
- Some trouble with speed and/or controlling the movement
- Some trouble with moving the feet around the cone or felt unsteady at times
- Some trouble sitting down

The client receives his score (0, 1, or 2) for each test and for the left and right sides for the tests that involve two sides. Each box checked off in the performance mobility testing has been assigned corresponding underlying components inherent to that movement segment. These are accumulated throughout the performance mobility testing and combined with the results from the basic mobility testing and the questionnaire (part of the algorithm). For example, see table 14.2.

Table 14.2 Agility Course Test (C4) Algorithm

Rubrics	Specific mobility difficulty	Underlying components
Squat start and pick-up	(a) Somewhat unsteady with kneeling start; paused or had some trouble getting up fast	Domain 1, dynamic stability Domain 2, dynamic stability Domain 2, flexibility
	(b) Some trouble with a smooth and continuous bending of the hips and knees to go down and up for the juice box	Domain 1, strength Domain 1, flexibility Domain 2, strength Domain 2, dynamic stability
Straightaway and slalom	(a) Walking straight was slow to gain speed and was careful when turning around	Domain 2, dynamic stability Domain 2, motor mechanics
	(b) Walking speed was only moderate	Domain 2, motor mechanics
	(c) Moving around the markers did not flow well, moved feet slowly, or did not take the shortest distance	Domain 2, dynamic stability Domain 2, motor mechanics

Chair Stand

This test (figure 14.10) measures lower body strength and muscle endurance. Difficulties with this test may be due to limited range of motion or dynamic stability in the ankle, knee, or hip. Some clients may find the lowering or eccentric phase more difficult; others may change the motor mechanics by rocking to get up.

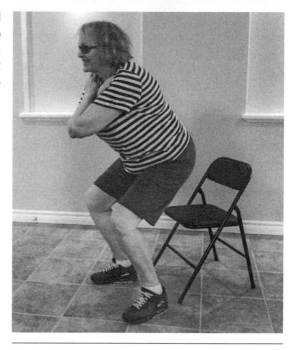

Figure 14.10   Chair stand.

In-Line Lunge

This test (figure 14.11) requires dynamic stability of the ankle, knee, and hip of the stance leg. It also requires mobility of the hip, ankle dorsiflexion, and rectus femoris flexibility of the step leg. The lateral stress can challenge the client's balance. Besides inadequate mobility or stability, an imbalance between relative adductor weakness and abductor tightness in one or both hips may cause poor test performance.

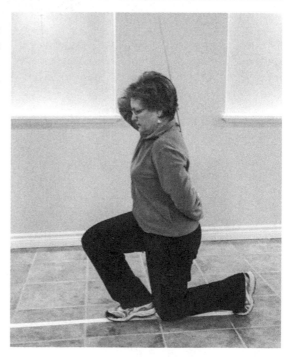

Figure 14.11   In-line lunge.

Hurdle Step

The hurdle step (figure 14.12) requires stance-leg stability of the ankle, knee, and hip as well as maximal closed kinetic chain extension of the hip. It also requires step-leg open kinetic chain dorsiflexion of the ankle and flexion of the knee and hip. There is a requirement for adequate balance and a need for dynamic stability to maintain alignments. Maximum hip flexion mobility of one leg during maintenance of a stable hip extension of the opposite leg requires bilateral, asymmetric hip mobility.

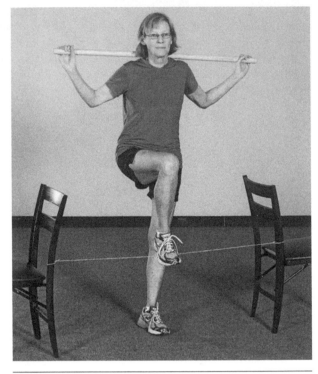

Figure 14.12   Hurdle step.

Timed Up-and-Go (TUG)

This test (figure 14.13) measures locomotor performance, more specifically motor ability, agility, speed, and dynamic balance. Difficulties with this test may be due to limited muscular power in the eccentric phases with rapid direction changes and sitting quickly.

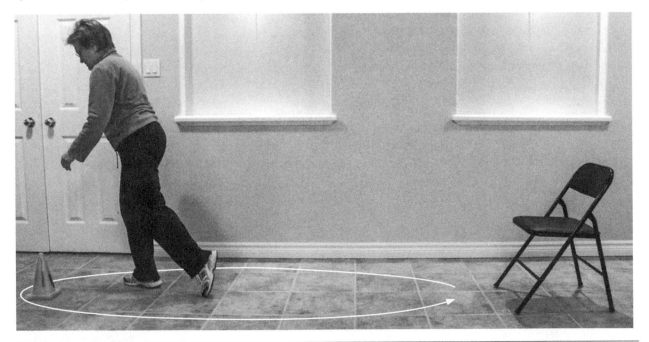

Figure 14.13   Timed up-and-go (TUG).

Agility Course

The agility course (figure 14.14) requires the ability to quickly change directions. Core stability is necessary to withstand shear forces on the spine. The agility course also calls for body coordination patterns involving a single-leg phase, as well as lower extremity movements demanding mobility of the lower extremities and stability of the upper body. Difficulties with this test may be due to multidirectional changes in speed and posture.

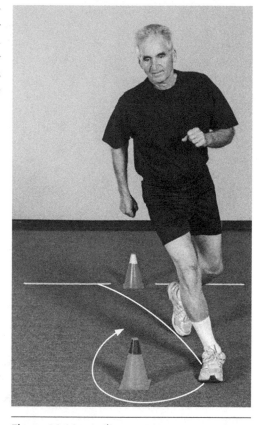

Figure 14.14   Agility course.

Side Bridge

The side bridge (figure 14.15) challenges the muscular endurance of the trunk musculature, especially lateral flexors like the quadratus lumborum and the core, to stabilize the trunk and shoulder in the coronal plane. In this test, the quadratus lumborum functions to stabilize flexion and extension and resist shearing force on the spine through activation of the core musculature. Difficulties with this test may be due to an inability to hold the position or difficulty with spine and hip alignment.

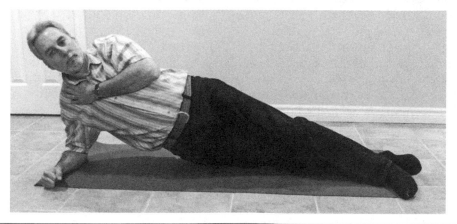

Figure 14.15   Side bridge.

Lift–Carry–Reach Course

This test (figure 14.16) measures upper body and trunk strength and dynamic stability, including the ability to withstand multidirectional forces, maneuver obstacles, and perform full ranges of motion under load. Difficulties with this test may be due to the motor mechanics involved in lifting and reaching, dynamic stability of the shoulder and spine in various movement tasks, and the range of motion of the shoulder during the reach.

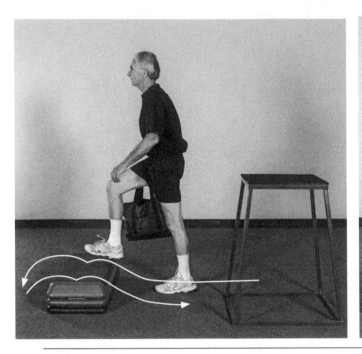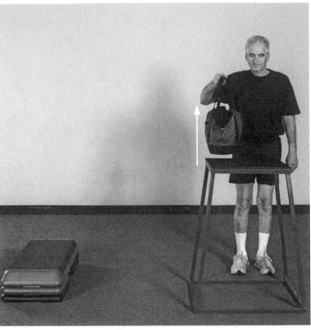

Figure 14.16 Lift–carry–reach course.

Assessment Interpretation and Activity Intervention

The series of tests that make up a functional mobility screening tool and the follow-up should involve a functional testing algorithm (FTA) (Reiman and Manske 2009). This is a systematic, objective procedure that uses quantitative and qualitative criteria to interpret test scores and direct the client to information or action, for example, prescribing remedial exercises to meet client needs at the appropriate level (see agility course rubric, table 14.2). The Functional Mobility Screening Tool can provide valuable direction and guidance toward a client's activity intervention whether self-administered at home or in a program administered by a health care practitioner from one of a number of different disciplines.

Within the functional mobility project, the exercises prescribed are based on the questionnaire and any mobility testing that was done. When a client achieves less than a perfect score,

the limiting factors (i.e., the essential components for that test) should be identified. For example, the timed up-and-go test is a performance level 1 test that requires agility with change of direction around the pylon, strength off the chair, dynamic balance with changes in posture and direction, and coordination (motor mechanics) in maneuvering on and off the chair as well as the footwork. The agility course test, performance level 2, is more advanced and complex, combining multiple movement patterns with more challenging underlying components of speed, agility, power, dynamic balance, coordination (mechanics), and range of motion. The tests differentiate the causes underlying a client's mobility problem, evaluating the phases of a given task and sensitizing the screening tool, indicating more specifically a problem in mobility. For example, in the timed up-and-go test, a slow or shuffling transition into or out of a turn may indicate sensorimotor or joint stability problems that would not be captured by a time or percentile score.

Client-Centered Functional Mobility Prescription

Each exercise is related to a domain, a component, and a level of difficulty. The body adapts to specific demands placed on it, so the exercises prescribed incorporate specific movements associated with results from the algorithm (e.g., table 14.2).

The Activity Domain

- Up-down, lower body
- Locomotor
- Carry–push–reach, upper body and trunk

The Key Component

- Strength
- Dynamic stability
- Flexibility
- Motor mechanics

As described in chapter 13, a functional progression is a series of basic movement patterns used in active daily living and recreation, graduated according to the difficulty of the exercise and the tolerance of the individual. In the sample functional mobility prescription presented here, exercises are marked as level 1, 2, or 3. In addition, at each level is a modification of the given exercise to make it easier and a second modification to make it more difficult. With these options, your client will be able to help fine-tune the degree of difficulty of their functional exercise program.

The Levels of Difficulty

- **Level 1** is for people who need the basics, are in poorer shape for the given component, or are at a therapeutic level. No equipment is needed in most cases. If this level is too difficult, advise your client to see a health care practitioner.

- **Level 2** is for the general public wanting to do a little bit but nothing too strenuous. Jarring movements are avoided.

- **Level 3** is for people who are currently active and need to make sure they are covering all areas. Tasks are at a "training" level. Your client may want to incorporate some or all of the functional mobility exercises as part of their regular exercise plan.

An exercise prescribed for your client will incorporate specific movements associated with results from the algorithm. In the following functional mobility exercise prescription, the algorithm selected the flexibility component of the first domain (lower body) at a level 3 difficulty score. The specific exercise was the scarf-assisted hamstring stretch.

Functional Mobility Prescription

Functional Mobility Assessment Interpretation:
Domain: 1—Up and Down (Lower Body)
Component: Flexibility
Level: 3

Scarf-Assisted Hamstring Stretch

The functional mobility benefits of this exercise help with

- putting on socks or pants;
- bending down or picking something up;
- tightness in the lower back or calves; and
- recreational activities such as gardening, picking up a golf ball, yoga, or exercise classes.

Loop a scarf around the arch of the right foot with a full circle, then lie on your back with your knees bent and feet on the floor. Hold the scarf on either side of the leg. Ensure that the scarf will not slip. Follow these instructions for 2 reps for each leg:

- Bend your right knee and pull on the scarf to bring your right thigh in close to your chest (position 1). Hold for 15 s, keeping the core stable.
- Keeping the upper thigh in position, extend the knee as far as you comfortably can. Gently pull with the scarf to assist the stretch (position 2). Hold for 30 s. Avoid holding your breath. Keep head and neck relaxed and keep looking upward.
- Repeat these steps on the left side (figure 14.17).
- **Hold:** as indicated above (position 1 for 15 s; position 2 for 30 s)
- **Reps:** 2 (each leg)

Modifications:

This exercise can be made easier by

- Lowering your thigh before straightening your knee
- Doing the exercise while seated on a chair.

This exercise can be made more difficult by

- Pulling your toes toward your shin in position 2 for an added stretch to the calf

Prescribed for: _____

Date: _____

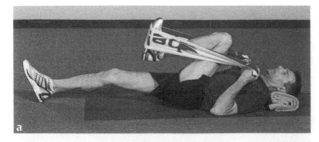

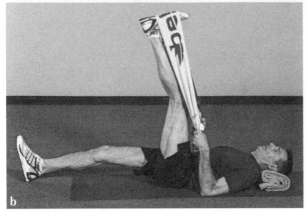

Figure 14.17 Scarf-assisted hamstring stretch: *(a)* position 1 and *(b)* position 2.

Summary

Functional mobility is the foundation of health and an aspect of everyday life, whether for the athlete, senior, student, or average adult. To be successful and safe in the skills of daily activities, everyone needs the essential abilities in one or more aspects of physical function.

Functional loss may be identified by difficulties in task (activity) performance. Typical of the natural history of disability, changes before its onset define a critical point when preventive measures would be most effective. Functional mobility reserve may be seen as the difference between a client's maximal capacity to perform a task successfully and the minimal capacity required to perform that task or to maintain a specific level of activity.

Alterations in functioning in terms of performance or capacity may be seen as impairments (e.g., altered mobility, altered muscle strength-power, altered gait pattern, pain). Impairment in function would affect the execution of an activity. Functional mobility is the ability to carry out activities one needs and wants to do (daily activities and recreation) efficiently for quality of life without undue fatigue or pain and to stay healthy, safe, and active. Lifestyle, inactivity, and aging can lead to these types of impairments even without pathology. Eventually, the accumulated impairments can lead to limitations in physical functioning (e.g., walking, stair climbing) and ultimately to disability.

Preclinical diminished functional mobility is an intermediate stage of early identifiable functional loss and may be identified by changes in task performance (impairment) in which the individual performs a task in an alternative manner (compensation). Compensation has the potential to lead to further mobility and stability imbalances; however, it is not necessarily a bad thing if it results in efficient movements that avoid normal pain patterns. Perhaps the exercise health practitioner not only should attempt to correct poor compensations but also may want to implement effective compensations with people who may benefit from them.

With the assistance of an effective screening tool, we can achieve early identification of changes in physical ability before overt limitations in functional behavior present themselves. Several assessment tools and data on mobility function are reviewed in the chapter.

Defining the domains as groupings of related tasks or activities with similar components allows some awareness of similar activities that may present difficulties in the future and identification of risks involved with that impairment. Evaluation must consider the client's efficiency in performing certain movements. Any functional movement (activity) difficulties in turn may reflect a deficit in one or more of the essential components of functional mobility, such as balance and proprioception, muscular strength (stability), muscular endurance, muscular power, flexibility, speed, coordination (mechanics), agility, and aerobic and anaerobic capacity.

Once the personal fitness trainer is aware of the client's functional mobility issue, perhaps through a screening process, the interventions that are planned need to recognize the limiting components and how they may affect each client individually. Exercises and tasks should be functional, that is, basic activities of daily living that are required and those that allow us to engage in recreational and meaningful activities related to work or leisure and to move effectively and efficiently in our environment. This may involve an exercise program to improve functional fitness consisting of aerobic training combined with resistance and balance training.

The Functional Mobility Screening Tool for Adults 50-70 Years of Age (Griffin 2011a, 2011b, 2012) identifies potential compensatory movement patterns, therefore identifying fundamental movement deficits. The tests provide the client information on functional mobility and serve as a guide for the design of a personalized preventive exercise program. The evaluation assists with (1) targeting specific areas (domains) that present difficulty and (2) identifying physical components that may underlie mobility problems.

FORM 14.1   Functional Mobility Self-Rating Questionnaire

Client name: _____   Trainer name: _____   Date: _____

Instructions: Examine the list of activities below. Circle the number to the left of the activity that corresponds to how you can or would be able to do the activity.

2: You can do the activity with **no trouble**.

1: You would have **some trouble** doing the activity.

0: You would have **lots of trouble** doing the activity, could not do the activity, would have pain, or would not do the activity.

If you circle a score of 1 or 0, then circle the letters in the column to the right of the activity that would most apply (choose no more than two).

S: Strength—you do not feel strong enough; it would be very hard.

D: Dynamic stability—your joints don't feel stable reacting to the movement, or you have trouble with balance (feel unsteady).

F: Flexibility—you lack enough flexibility or range of motion; you can't bend or reach far enough.

M: Motor mechanics—the coordination would be difficult, or you might have to change the movements to complete the activity.

Domain	Mobility score	Activity	Reason for the trouble			
Up and down activities: lower body focus	2 1 0	a. Getting in or out of a car	S	D	F	M
	2 1 0	b. Stepping on or off a bus	S	D	F	M
	2 1 0	c. Putting on socks from a seated position	S	D	F	M
	2 1 0	d. Taking the stairs	S	D	F	M
	2 1 0	e. Up and down activities (gardening, squatting down to pick something up)	S	D	F	M
	2 1 0	f. Getting up off of the floor	S	D	F	M
	2 1 0	g. Recreational activities involving changes in position and posture (golf, curling, dancing)	S	D	F	M
	2 1 0	h. Activities demanding lower body muscular work (lower body exercises with weights or resistance, more than 12 repetitions of a leg exercise)	S	D	F	M
Domain subtotal score:						

From J.C. Griffin, 2015, Client-centered exercise prescription, 3rd ed. (Champaign, IL: Human Kinetics).

Credits

Table 1.4: Source: *Canadian Physical Activity, Fitness & Lifestyle Approach: CSEP-Health & Fitness Program's Appraisal and Counselling Strategy,* 3rd edition, © 2003. Reprinted with permission from the Canadian Society for Exercise Physiology.

Figure 1.3: Source: *Canadian Physical Activity, Fitness & Lifestyle Approach: CSEP-Health & Fitness Program's Appraisal and Counselling Strategy,* 3rd edition, © 2003. Reprinted with permission from the Canadian Society for Exercise Physiology.

Figure 3.2: Adapted, by permission, from C. Bouchard, S. Blair, and W. Haskell, 2012, *Physical activity and health,* 2nd ed. (Champaign, IL: Human Kinetics), 18.

Figure 3.4: Source: *Canadian Physical Activity, Fitness & Lifestyle Approach: CSEP-Health & Fitness Program's Appraisal and Counselling Strategy,* 3rd edition, © 2003. Reprinted with permission from the Canadian Society for Exercise Physiology.

Figure 4.1: Source: *Canadian Physical Activity, Fitness & Lifestyle Approach: CSEP-Health & Fitness Program's Appraisal and Counselling Strategy,* 3rd edition, © 2003. Reprinted with permission from the Canadian Society for Exercise Physiology.

Table 4.5: Reprinted, by permission, from NSCA, 2008, Resistance training, T.R. Baechle, R.W. Earle, and D. Wathen. In *Essentials of strength training and conditioning,* 3rd ed., edited by T.R. Baechle and R. Earle (Champaign, IL; Human Kinetics), 394.

Table 5.2, illustrations: Adapted, by permission, from B.B. Cook and G.W. Stewart, 1996, *Strength basics: Your guide to resistance training for health and optimal performance* (Champaign, IL: Human Kinetics), 121.

Table 5.3, illustrations: Adapted, by permission, from B.B. Cook and G.W. Stewart, 1996, *Strength basics: Your guide to resistance training for health and optimal performance* (Champaign, IL: Human Kinetics), 91.

Table 5.5, illustrations: Adapted, by permission, from B.B. Cook and G.W. Stewart, 1996, *Strength basics: Your guide to resistance training for health and optimal performance* (Champaign, IL: Human Kinetics), 91.

Table 5.6, illustration: Reprinted, by permission, from E.T. Howley and B.D. Franks, 1997, *Health fitness instructors handbook,* 3rd ed. (Champaign, IL: Human Kinetics), 310.

Table 5.7, illustrations: Reprinted, by permission, from V. Heyward, 1998, *Advanced assessment and exercise prescription,* 3rd ed. (Champaign, IL: Human Kinetics), 272.

Table 6.3: Adapted from E. Fox and D. Mathews, 1974, *Interval training* (Columbus, OH: The Ohio State University), 60.

Table 6.5: From E. Fox and D. Mathews, 1974, *Interval training* (Philadelphia, PA: W.B. Saunders), 60. By permission of Donald Mathews.

Figure 8.9: Reprinted, by permission, from E.T. Howley and B.D. Franks, 1997, *Health fitness instructors handbook,* 3rd ed. (Champaign, IL: Human Kinetics), 259.

Figure 8.20, supine knees to chest: Illustration by Michael Richardson. Reprinted from M. Alter, 2004, *Science of flexibility,* 2nd ed. (Champaign, IL: Human Kinetics), 50. Used with permission of the author.

Figure 8.20, seated back stretch: Illustration by Michael Richardson. Reprinted from M. Alter, 2004, *Science of flexibility,* 2nd ed. (Champaign, IL: Human Kinetics), 38. Used with permission of the author.

Figure 8.20, one-joint hip flexor lunge: Illustration by Michael Richardson. Reprinted from M. Alter, 2004, *Science of flexibility,* 2nd ed. (Champaign, IL: Human Kinetics), 42. Used with permission of the author.

Figure 8.20, side-lying quad stretch: Illustration by Michael Richardson. Reprinted from M. Alter, 2004, *Science of flexibility,* 2nd ed. (Champaign, IL: Human Kinetics), 129. Used with permission of the author.

Figure 9.1: Reprinted, by permission, from N. Clark, 2014, *Nancy Clark's sports nutrition guidebook,* 5th ed. (Champaign, IL: Human Kinetics), 73.

Figure 10.1: Reprinted, by permission, from L. Jozsa and P. Kannus, 1997, *Human tendons* (Champaign, IL: Human Kinetics), 47.

Figure 10.2: Reprinted from *Clinics in Sports Medicine,* vol. 11(3), W.B. Leadbetter, "Cell-matrix response in tendon injury," pgs. 533-578, Copyright 1992, with permission of Elsevier.

Figure 13.1: Reprinted, by permission, from A.W. Taylor and M. Johnson, 2008, *Physiology of exercise and healthy aging* (Champaign, IL: Human Kinetics), xxviii.

Figure 13.2: Reprinted, by permission, from A.W. Taylor and M. Johnson, 2008, *Physiology of exercise and healthy aging* (Champaign, IL: Human Kinetics), 12.

Figure 13.3: Reprinted, by permission, from W. Spirduso, K. Francis, and P. MacRae, 2005, *Physical dimensions of aging,* 2nd ed. (Champaign, IL: Human Kinetics), 112.

Figure 13.4: Reprinted, by permission, from J. Signorile, 2007, *Power training for older adults* (Champaign, IL: Human Kinetics), 13.

Table 13.1: Adapted, by permission, from R.E. Rikli and C.J. Jones, 2013, *Senior fitness text manual,* 2nd ed. (Champaign, IL: Human Kinetics), 18, 19, 20, 21.

Figure 13.6: Adapted, by permission, from R.E. Rikli and C.J. Jones, 2013, *Senior fitness test manual,* 2nd ed. (Champaign, IL: Human Kinetics), 88.

Table 13.2: Source: *Canadian Physical Activity, Fitness & Lifestyle Approach: CSEP-Health & Fitness Program's Appraisal and Counselling Strategy,* 3rd edition, © 2003. Reprinted with permission from the Canadian Society for Exercise Physiology.

Figure 13.7: Adapted from B. Jam, 2010, *The pain truth . . . and nothing but!* (Thornhill, ON: Advanced Physical Therapy Education Institute), 8. By permission of Dr. Bahram Jam.

Table 13.5: Reprinted, by permission, from W. Spirduso, K. Francis, and P. MacRae, 2005, *Physical dimensions of aging,* 2nd ed. (Champaign, IL: Human Kinetics), 276.

Figure 14.6: © John C. Griffin.

Figure 14.7: © John C. Griffin.

Figure 14.8: © John C. Griffin.

Figure 14.9: © John C. Griffin.

Figure 14.10: © John C. Griffin.

Figure 14.11: © John C. Griffin.

Figure 14.13: © John C. Griffin.

Figure 14.15: © John C. Griffin.

Author photo: © John C. Griffin.

References

Chapter 1

Canadian Society for Exercise Physiology. 2003. *The Canadian Physical Activity, Fitness, and Lifestyle Approach*. 3rd ed. Ottawa: CSEP.

Clark, J., and S. Clark. 1993. *Prioritize, Organize, the Art of Getting It Done*. Shawnee Mission, KS: National Press.

DeBusk, R.F., U. Stenestrand, and M. Sheehan. 1990. Training effects of long versus short bouts of exercise. *American Journal of Cardiology* 65(15): 1010-1013.

Duffy, F.D., and L. Schnirring. 2000. How to counsel patients about exercise. *Physician and Sportsmedicine* 28(10): 53-58.

Egan, G. 1990. *The Skilled Helper*. Pacific Grove, CA: Brooks/Cole.

Fortier, M.S., et al. 2011. Impact of integrating a physical activity counsellor into the primary health care team: Physical activity and health outcomes of the Physical Activity Counselling randomized controlled trial. *Applied Physiology, Nutrition, and Metabolism* 36(4): 503-514.

Francis, L. 1990. Setting goals. *IDEA Today* (May): 8-10.

Jones, A.P. 1991. Communication and teaching techniques. In: *Program Design for Personal Trainers*. San Diego: IDEA.

Kolovou, T.A. 2011. Say what? The lost art of effective listening. *ACSM's Health & Fitness Journal* 15(4): 24-28.

Prochaska, J.O. 1994. Strong and weak principles for progressing from precontemplation to action on the basis of twelve problem behaviors. *Health Psychology* 13(1): 47-51.

Prochaska, J.O., C.C. DiClemente, and J.J. Norcross. 1992. In search of how people change: Applications to addictive behaviours. *American Psychologist* 47(9): 1102-1114.

Sotile, W.M. 1996. *Psychosocial Interventions for Cardiopulmonary Patients*. Champaign, IL: Human Kinetics.

Trottier, M. 1988. Client-driven programming. Keynote address: Fit Rendezvous, Edmonton, Canada, May.

Weylman, C.R. 1995. *Reaching the Potential Client*. Atlanta: The Achievement Group.

Wheeler, G.D. 2000. Counselling and behaviour change. Handout during PFLC training. Edmonton, Alberta, November.

Chapter 2

Alberta Centre for Active Living. 2011a. Alberta Survey on Physical Activity: A concise report. 1-3. http://centre4activeliving.ca/publications/surveys.html [accessed November 25, 2012].

Alberta Centre for Active Living. 2011b. Making a physical activity plan. B-1–B-4. http://centre4activeliving.ca/our-work/toolkit/about.html [accessed November 25, 2012].

Annesi, J. 2000. Retention crisis? Exercise dropouts and adherents. *Fitness Business Canada* (July-August): 6-8.

Ball, D.R. 2001. Cognitive strategies. *IDEA Personal Trainer* (November-December): 22-29.

Brehm, B.A. 2003. Cognitive restructuring supports behavior-change efforts. *Fitness Management* (April): 22.

Brooks, C.M. 2000. Marketing the active lifestyle. *Fitness Management* (July): 44-50.

Canadian Society for Exercise Physiology. 2003. *The Canadian Physical Activity, Fitness, and Lifestyle Approach*. 3rd ed. Ottawa: CSEP.

Cantwell, S. 2003. Lifestyle coaching. *Fitness Trainer Canada* (February-March): 10-15.

De Bourdeauhuij, I., and J. Sallis. 2002. Relative contribution of psychosocial variables to the explanation of physical activity in three population-based adult samples. *Preventive Medicine* 34: 279-288.

Dishman, R.K. 1990. Determinants of participation in physical activity. *Journal of Applied Sport Sciences* 8: 104-113.

Egan, G. 1990. *The Skilled Helper*. Pacific Grove, CA: Brooks/Cole.

Gabriele, J.M., D.L. Gill, and C.E. Adams. 2011. The roles of want to commitment and have to commitment in explaining physical activity behavior. *Journal of Physical Activity and Health* 8: 420-428.

Goldfine, H., A. Ward, P. Taylor, D. Carlucci, and J.M. Rippe. 1991. Exercising to health—What's really in it for your patients? *The Physician and Sports Medicine* 19(6): 81-93.

Jonas, S., and E. Phillips. 2009. *ACSM's Exercise Is Medicine. A Clinician's Guide to Exercise Prescription.* Philadelphia: Lippincott, Williams & Wilkins.

Kimiecik, J.C. 1998. The path of the intrinsic exerciser. *IDEA Health and Fitness Source* (March): 34-42.

Kimiecik, J.C. 2000. Bashing through the barriers. *IDEA Health and Fitness Source* (March): 42-46.

Kyllo, L.B., and D.M. Landers. 1995. Goal setting in sport and exercise: A research synthesis to resolve the controvercy. *Journal of Sport and Exercise Psychology* 17: 117-137.

Patrick, K., B. Long, W. Wooten, and M. Pratt. 1994. A new tool for encouraging activity. Project PACE. *Physician and Sportsmedicine* 22(11): 45-55.

Prochaska, J.O. 1992. Helping patients at every stage of change. *Behavioral Approaches to Addiction Journal* 1(1): 2-7.

Pronk, N.P., R.R. Wing, and R.W. Jeffery. 1994. Effects of increased stimulus control for exercise through use of a personal trainer. *Annals of Behavioral Medicine* 16: SO77.

Prukop, N. 1997. Selling with style. *IDEA Personal Trainer* (November/December): 41-47.

Temple, V., R. Rhodes, and J. Wharf Higgins. 2011. Unleashing physical activity: An observational study of park use, dog walking, and physical activity. *Journal of Physical Activity and Health* 8: 766-774.

Tod, D., and M. McGuigan. 2001. Maximizing strength training through goal setting. *Strength and Conditioning Journal* 23(4): 22-26.

Wheeler, G.D. 2000. Counselling and behavior change. Handout during PFLC training. Edmonton, Alberta, November.

Williams, E. 2011. Improve your member retention. *Fitness Business Canada* (November-December): 18-19.

Wilson, D.M.C., and D. Ciliska. 1984. Lifestyle assessment: Development and the use of the FANTASTIC Checklist. *Canadian Family Physician* 30: 1527-1531.

Chapter 3

Alberta Centre for Active Living. 2011. Benefits of physical activity. E-1–E-3. www.centre4activeliving. ca/media/filer_public/e-benefits.pdf: E2 [accessed November 25, 2012].

American College of Sports Medicine. 2006. *ACSM's Resource Manual for Guidelines for Exercise Testing and Prescription.* 5th ed. Baltimore: Lippincott, Williams & Wilkins.

American College of Sports Medicine. 2009. *Guidelines for Exercise Testing and Prescription.* 8th ed. Philadelphia: Lea & Febiger.

Åstrand, P.O., and K. Rodahl, eds. 2003. *Textbook of Work Physiology.* 6th ed. New York: McGraw-Hill.

Blair, S.N., H.W. Kohl III, R.S. Paffenbarger Jr., D.G. Clark, K.H. Cooper, and L.W. Gibbons. 1989. Physical fitness and all-cause mortality: A prospective study of healthy men and women. *Journal of the American Medical Association* 262(17): 2395-2401.

Bompa, T.O. 1999. *Periodization Theory and Methodology of Training.* 4th ed. Champaign, IL: Human Kinetics.

Bouchard, C., S. Blair, and W. Haskell, eds. 2007. *Physical activity and health.* Champaign, IL: Human Kinetics.

Burfoot, A. 1995. How much should you run? *Runner's World* (September): 66-67.

Canadian Society for Exercise Physiology. 2003. *The Canadian Physical Activity, Fitness, and Lifestyle Approach.* 3rd ed. Ottawa: CSEP.

Canadian Society for Exercise Physiology. 2011. Canadian Physical Activity Guidelines. www.csep.ca/guidelines.

DeBusk, R.F., U. Stenestrand, and M. Sheehan. 1990. Training effects of long versus short bouts of exercise. *American Journal of Cardiology* 65(15): 1010-1013.

Donnelly, J.E., et al. 2009. Appropriate physical activity intervention strategies for weight loss and prevention of weight regain for adults. *Medicine and Science in Sports and Exercise* 41(2): 459-471.

Ebisu, T. 1985. Splitting the distance of endurance running: On cardiovascular endurance and blood lipids. *Japanese Journal of Physical Education* 30(1): 37-43.

Edman, K.A.P. 1992. Contractile performance of skeletal muscle fibers. In: *Strength and Power in Sport.* Boston: Blackwell Scientific.

Feigenbaum, M.S., and M.L. Pollock. 1997. Strength training: Rationale for current guidelines for adult fitness programs. *Physician and Sportsmedicine* 25(2): 44-64.

Gledhill, N., and V. Jamnik. 1996. Figure 4-1. In: *The Canadian Physical Activity, Fitness, and Lifestyle Appraisal: CSEP's Plan for Healthy Active Living.* Ottawa: CSEP.

Goldfine, H., A. Ward, P. Taylor, D. Carlucci, and J.M. Rippe. 1991. Exercising to health—what's really in it for your patients? *Physician and Sportsmedicine* 19(6): 81-93.

Golshani, N.A. 2006. Exercise as medicine. *Fitness Business Canada* (November-December): 34-36.

Hagan, R.D. 1988. Benefits of aerobic conditioning and diet for overweight adults. *Sports Medicine* 5: 144-155.

Hamill, J., and K.M. Knutzen. 1995. *Biomechanical Basis of Human Movement.* Media, PA: Williams & Wilkins.

Haskell, W.H., et al. 2007. Physical activity and public health: Updated recommendations for adults from the American College of Sports Medicine and the American Heart association. *Circulation* 116(9): 1081-1093.

Hawley, C.J., and R.B. Schoene. 2003. Overtraining syndrome. A guide to diagnosis, treatment, and prevention. *Physician and Sportsmedicine* 31(6): 25-31.

Heyward, V.H. 2010. *Advanced Fitness Assessment and Exercise Prescription*. 6th ed. Champaign, IL: Human Kinetics.

Hoeger, W., and S. Hoeger. 1999. *Principles and Labs for Fitness and Wellness*. 5th ed. Englewood, CA: Morton.

International Federation of Sports Medicine position statement. 1990. Physical exercise: An important factor for health. *Physician and Sportsmedicine* 18(3): 155-156.

Jensen, K. 2010. *The Flexible Periodization Method*. Toronto: The Write Fit.

Jonas, S., and E. Phillips. 2009. *ACSM's Exercise Is Medicine. A Clinician's Guide to Exercise Prescription*. Philadelphia: Lippincott, Williams & Wilkins.

Katzmarzyk, P.T., and C.L. Craig. 2002. Musculoskeletal fitness and risk of mortality. *Medicine and Science in Sports and Exercise* 31(5): 740-744.

Kesaniemi, Y.I., et al. 2001. Dose-response issues concerning physical activity and health: An evidence-based symposium. *Medicine and Science in Sports and Exercise* 34(suppl): S351-S358.

Komi, P.V. 1992. Stretch-shortening cycle. In: *Strength and Power in Sport*. Boston: Blackwell Scientific.

Kuipers, H., and H.A. Keizer. 1988. Overtraining in elite athletes. *Sports Medicine* 5: 79-92.

La Forge, R. 2001. Exercise and health: Dose-response issues. *IDEA Health and Fitness Source* (September): 21-25.

Malkin, M. 2002. Exercise as preventive medicine. *Fitness Management* (February): 64-67.

Malkin, M. 2004. Warming up, cooling down and stretching. *Fitness Management* (January): 30-32.

Martin, C.K., et al. 2009. Exercise dose and quality of life: Results of a randomized controlled trial. *Archives of Internal Medicine* 169(3): 269-278.

Martin, C.K., B.D. Pence, and J.A. Woods. 2009. Exercise and respiratory tract viral infections. *Exercise and Sport Sciences Reviews* 37(4): 157-164.

Nieman, D.C. 2009. You asked for it. *ACSM's Health and Fitness Journal* 13(1): 5-6.

O'Brien, T. 1997. *The Personal Trainer's Handbook*. Champaign, IL: Human Kinetics.

Oliveira, N., and J. Oliveira. 2011. Excess post exercise oxygen consumption is unaffected by the resistance and aerobic exercise order in an exercise session. *Journal of Strength and Conditioning Research* 25(10): 2843-2850.

Paffenbarger, R.S. Jr., R.T. Hyde, A.L. Wing, and C. Hsieh. 1986. Physical activity, all-cause mortality, and longevity of college alumni. *New England Journal of Medicine* 314(10): 605-613.

Pate, R.R., M. Pratt, S.N. Blair, et al. 1995. Physical activity and public health: A recommendation from the Centers for Disease Control and Prevention and the American College of Sports Medicine. *Journal of the American Medical Association* 273(5): 402-407.

Payne, N., et al. 2000. Health implications of musculoskeletal fitness. *Canadian Journal of Applied Physiology* 25(2): 114-126.

Quinney, H.A., L. Gauvin, and A.E.T. Wall, eds. 1994. *Toward Active Living*. Champaign IL: Human Kinetics.

Ross, R., I. Janssen, and A. Tremblay. 2000. Obesity reduction through lifestyle modification. *Canadian Journal of Applied Physiology* 25(1): 1-18.

Skinner, J.S. 1987. General principles of exercise prescription. In: *Exercise Testing and Exercise Prescription for Special Cases,* ed. J.S. Skinner. Philadelphia: Lea & Febiger.

Stone, M.H., S.J. Fleck, N.T. Triplett, and W.J. Kraemer. 1991. Health- and performance-related potential of resistance training. *Sports Medicine* 11(4): 210-231.

Stone, M.H., R.E. Keith, J.T. Kearney, S.J. Fleck, G.T. Wilson, and N.T. Triplett. 1991. Overtraining: A review of the signs, symptoms and possible causes. *Journal of Applied Sports Science Research* 5(1): 35-50.

Warburton, D., N. Gledhill, and A. Quinney. 2001. The effects of changes in musculoskeletal fitness on health. *Canadian Journal of Applied Physiology* 26(2): 161-216.

Warburton, D.E.R., C.W. Nicol, and S.S.D. Bredin. 2006. Prescribing exercise as preventive therapy. *Canadian Medical Association Journal* 174(7): 961-973.

Wenger, H.A., and G.J. Bell. 1986. The interactions of intensity, frequency, and duration of exercise training in altering cardiorespiratory fitness. *Sports Medicine* 3: 346-356.

Westcott, W.L. 1989. When more isn't better. *IDEA Today* (February): 24.

Wilmore, J.H. 2003. Aerobic exercise and endurance: Improving fitness for health benefits. *Physician and Sportsmedicine* 31(5): 45-51.

Wilmore, J.H., and D.L. Costill. 2004. *Physiology of Sport and Exercise*. 3rd ed. Champaign, IL: Human Kinetics.

Chapter 4

Albert, W., J. Bonneau, J. Stevenson, and N. Gledhill. 2001. Back fitness and back health assessment considerations for the Canadian Physical Activity, Fitness, and Lifestyle Appraisal. *Canadian Journal of Applied Physiology* 26(3): 291-317.

Alter, M.J. 2004. *Science of Stretching*. 3rd ed. Champaign, IL: Human Kinetics.

American College of Sports Medicine. 2009. *Guidelines for Exercise Testing and Prescription*. 8th ed. Philadelphia: Lea & Febiger.

Anderson, G. 2003. Body composition: Weighing the options. Unpublished paper. University College Fraser Valley, British Columbia.

Baechle, T.R., and R.W. Earle. 2008. *Essentials of Strength Training and Conditioning.* 3rd ed. Champaign, IL: Human Kinetics.

Canadian Society for Exercise Physiology. 2003. *The Canadian Physical Activity, Fitness, and Lifestyle Approach.* 3rd ed. Ottawa: CSEP.

Canadian Society for Exercise Physiology. 2013. *Physical Activity Training for Health (CSEP-PATH).* Ottawa: CSEP.

Chen, W., C. Lin, C. Peng, C. Li, H. Wu, J. Chiang, J. Wu, and P. Huang. 2002. Approaching healthy body mass index norms for children and adolescents from health-related physical fitness. *Obesity Reviews* 3(3): 225-232.

Cook, G., L. Burton, and B. Hoogenboom. 2006a. Pre-participation screening: The use of fundamental movements as an assessment of function - part 1. *North American Journal of Sports Physical Therapy* 1(2): 62-72.

Cook, G., L. Burton, and B. Hoogenboom. 2006b. Pre-participation screening: The use of fundamental movements as an assessment of function - part 2. *North American Journal of Sports Physical Therapy* 1(3): 132-139.

DeLisa, J., ed. 1998. *Rehabilitation Medicine Principles and Practice.* Philadelphia: Lippincott.

Ellison, D. 1995. Beyond the sit-up. *IDEA Today* (September): 33-39.

Getchell, B., and W. Anderson. 1982. *Being Fit: A Personal Guide.* New York: Wiley.

Griffin, J.C. 1989. All the Right Moves. An unpublished manual. George Brown College, Ontario.

Griffin, J.C. 2006. *Client-Centered Exercise Prescription.* 2nd ed. Champaign, IL: Human Kinetics.

Heyward, V.H. 2010. *Advanced Fitness Assessment and Exercise Prescription.* 6th ed. Champaign, IL: Human Kinetics.

Heyward, V.H., and D.R. Wagner. 2004. *Applied Body Composition Assessment.* 2nd ed. Champaign, IL: Human Kinetics.

Hoeger, W., S. Hoeger, M. Locke, and L. Lauzon. 2009. *Principles & Labs for Fitness & Wellness.* Toronto: Nelson Education.

Hoffman, J. 2006. *Norms for Fitness, Performance, and Health.* Champaign, IL: Human Kinetics.

Imrie, D., and L. Barbuto. 1988. *The Back Power Program.* Toronto: Stoddard.

Janssen, I., S. Heymsfield, and R. Ross. 2002. Application of simple anthropometry in the assessment of health risk: Implications for the Canadian Physical Activity, Fitness, and Lifestyle Appraisal. *Canadian Journal of Applied Physiology* 27(4): 396-414.

Kaminsky, L.A., American College of Sports Medicine. 2010. *ACSM's Health-Related Physical Fitness Assessment Manual.* 3rd ed. Philadelphia: Wolters Kluwer/Lippincott, Williams and Wilkins.

Kendall, F.P., E.K. McCreary, and P.G. Provance. 2005. *Muscles, Testing and Function: With Posture and Pain.* 5th ed. Baltimore: Williams & Wilkins.

Kline, G.M., et al. 1987. Estimation of VO2 max from a one mile track walk, gender, age, and body weight. *Medicine and Science in Sports and Exercise* 19: 253-259.

Kravitz, L., and V. Heyward. 1997. The many aspects of fitness assessment body composition-skinfold technique. *IDEA Personal Trainer* (June): 19-23.

Michaelson, F., and P. Gagne. 2002. Upper limb evaluation. *Fitness Trainer Canada* (February): 30-33.

Morrison, C.A. 2001. Using the exercise test to create the exercise prescription. *Primary Care* 28(1): 137-158, vii.

National Institutes of Health, National Heart Blood and Lung Institute. 1998. *Clinical Guidelines on the Identification, Evaluation and Treatment of Overweight and Obesity in Adults.* NIH Publication No. 98-4083. www.nhlbi.nih.gov/guidelines/obesity/ob_home.htm.

Nieman, C. 2010. *Exercise Testing and Prescription: A Health-Related Approach.* 7th ed. Mountain View, CA: Mayfield.

Nieman, D.C. 1990. *Fitness and Sports Medicine: An Introduction.* Palo Alto: Bull.

Nordvall, M., and K. Sullivan. 2002. Pre-preparation health and fitness assessments. *Fitness Management* (February): 44-49.

Norkin, C., and D.J. White. 1995. *Measurement of Joint Motion: A Guide to Goniometry.* 2nd ed. Philadelphia: Davis.

Page, P., C. Frank, and R. Lardner. 2010. *Assessment and Treatment of Muscle Imbalance: The Janda Approach.* Champaign, IL: Human Kinetics.

Reiman, M.P., and R.C. Manske. 2009. *Functional Testing in Human Performance.* Champaign, IL: Human Kinetics.

Rockport Walking Institute. 1986. *Rockport Fitness Walking Test.* Marlboro, MA: Author.

Roskopf, G. 2001. When clients feel pain. *IDEA Personal Trainer* (February): 45-53.

Ross, R., J. Rissanen, and R. Hudson. 1996. Sensitivity associated with the identification of visceral adipose tissue levels using the waist circumference in men and women: Effects of weight loss. *International Journal of Obesity* 20: 533-538.

Sale, D., and J.D. MacDougall. 1981. Specificity in strength training: A review for the coach and athlete. *Canadian Journal of Applied Sport Science* 6: 87-92.

Shephard, R.J. 1988. PAR-Q, Canadian home fitness test and exercise screening alternatives. *Sports Medicine* 5: 185-195.

Shephard, R.J., and C. Bouchard. 1994. Population evaluations of health related fitness from perceptions of physical activity and fitness. *Canadian Journal of Applied Physiology* 19(2): 151-173.

Warburton, D.E., V.K. Jamnik, S.S. Bredin, and N. Gledhill. 2010. Enhancing the effectiveness of the PAR-Q and PARmed-X screening for physical activity participation. *Journal of Physical Activity and Health* 7: S338-S340.

Chapter 5

Baker, D. 2001. Science and practice of coaching a strength training program for novice and intermediate-level athletes. *Strength and Conditioning Journal* 23(2): 61-68.

Batman, P., and M. Van Capelle. 1992. *Exercise Analysis Made Simple.* 2nd ed. Arncliffe, NSW: F.I.A.

Cantwell, S. 1998. "On the floor" communication skills. *IDEA Personal Trainer* (February): 34-39.

Ellison, D. 1993. *Advanced Exercise Design for Lower Body.* San Diego: Movement That Matters.

Heyward, V. 1998. *Advanced Assessment and Exercise Prescription.* 3rd ed. Champaign, IL: Human Kinetics.

Howley, E.T., and B.D. Franks. 1997. *Health Fitness Instructors Handbook.* 3rd ed. Champaign, IL: Human Kinetics.

Tortora, G.J., and S.R. Grabowski. 2003. *Principles of Anatomy and Physiology.* 10th ed. New York: Wiley.

Westcott, W., et al. 2003. Using performance feedback in strength training. *Fitness Management* (September): 28-33.

Wilmore, J.H., and D.L. Costill. 2004. *Physiology of Sport and Exercise.* 3rd ed. Champaign, IL: Human Kinetics.

Chapter 6

Abel, M., et al. 2011. Determination of step rate thresholds corresponding to physical activity intensity classifications in adults. *Journal of Physical Activity and Health* 8: 45-51.

Allen, D., and L. Goldberg. 1986. Physiological comparison of two cross-country ski machines. Paper presented at the annual meeting of the American College of Sports Medicine, Indianapolis, May.

American College of Sports Medicine. 2009. *ACSM's Guidelines for Exercise Testing and Prescription.* 8th ed. Baltimore: Lippincott, Williams & Wilkins.

American College of Sports Medicine. 2010. *ACSM's Resource Manual for Guidelines for Exercise Testing and Prescription.* 4th ed. Baltimore: Lippincott, Williams & Wilkins.

Åstrand, P.-O., and K. Rodahl. 2003. *Textbook of Work Physiology.* 6th ed. New York: McGraw-Hill.

Baechle, T.R., and R.W. Earle. 2008. *Essentials of Strength Training and Conditioning.* 3rd ed. Champaign, IL: Human Kinetics.

Black, S.A. 2001. Heart rate training: A valuable exercise barometer. *Fitness Management* (August): 40-45.

Bouchard, C., S. Blair, and W. Haskell, eds. 2007. *Physical Activity and Health.* Champaign, IL: Human Kinetics.

Brooks, D. and C. Copeland-Brooks. 1991. Are you ready for the next step in circuit training? *IDEA Today* (November-December): 34-39.

Dishman, R.K. 1990. Determinants of participation in physical activity. *Journal of Applied Sports Science Research* 8: 104-113.

Fox, E.L. 1979. *Sports Physiology.* Philadelphia: Saunders.

Fox, E., and D. Mathews. 1974. *Interval training.* Philadelphia: W.B. Saunders.

Gaesser, G.A. 2003. On the move: Pedometer based walking initiative encourages physical activity. *Sports Medicine Digest* 25(8): 90, 92.

Gillen, J. 2012. Low-volume, high-intensity interval training: A practical fitness strategy. *WellSpring (ACAL)* 23(4): 1-4.

Golding, L.A., ed. 2000. *YMCA Fitness Testing and Assessment Manual.* 4th ed. Champaign, IL: Human Kinetics.

Graves, L., G. Stratton, N.D. Ridgers, and N.T. Cable. 2007. Comparison of energy expenditure in adolescents when playing new generation and sedentary computer games: Cross sectional study. *British Medical Journal* 335(7633): 1282-1284.

Haskell, W.L. 1995. Resolving the exercise debate: More vs. less. *IDEA Today* (October): 40-47.

Helgerud, J., et al. 2007. Aerobic high-intensity intervals improve VO2max more than moderate training. *Medicine and Science in Sports and Exercise* 39: 665-671.

Heyward, V.H. 2010. *Advanced Fitness Assessment and Exercise Prescription.* 6th ed. Champaign, IL: Human Kinetics.

Horswill, C.A., C.L. Kien, and W.B. Zipf. 1995. Energy expenditure in adolescents during low intensity, leisure activities. *Medicine and Science in Sports and Exercise* 27(9): 1311-1314.

Howard, M. 2003. Cardiovascular programming: Are we selling our clients short? A trainer's guide. *Fitness Trainer Canada* (February-March): 26-30.

Howley, E.T., and B.D. Franks. 1997. *Health and Fitness Instructor's Handbook.* 3rd ed. Champaign, IL: Human Kinetics.

Iknoian, T. 1992. 10 equipment trends that changed fitness. *IDEA Today* (July-August): 33-36.

Kaikkonen, H., et al. 2000. The effect of heart rate controlled low resistance circuit weight training and endurance training on maximal aerobic power in sedentary adults. *Scandinavian Journal of Medicine and Science in Sports* 10(4): 211-215.

Karp, J.R. 2000. Interval training. *Fitness Management* (August): 46-48.

Kesaniemi, Y.A., et al. 2001. Dose-response issues concerning physical activity and health: An evidence-based symposium. *Medicine and Science in Sports and Exercise* 34(suppl): S351-S358.

Marion, A., G. Kenny, and J. Thoden. 1994. Heart rate response as a means of quantifying training loads: Practical considerations for coaches. *Sports* 14(2): Part 1.

McArdle, W., F. Katch, and V. Katch. 1991. *Exercise Physiology: Energy, Nutrition, and Human Performance.* 3rd ed. Philadelphia: Lea & Febiger.

Nieman, D.C. 2010. *Exercise Testing and Prescription: A Health-Related Approach.* 7th ed. Mountain View, CA: Mayfield.

Pollock, M., L. Gettman, C. Milesis, M. Bah, L. Durstine, and R. Johnson. 1977. Effects of frequency and duration of training on attrition and incidence of injury. *Medicine and Science in Sports and Exercise* 9: 31-36.

Porcari, J., C. Foster, and P. Schneider. 2000. Exercise response to elliptical trainers. *Fitness Management* (August): 50-53.

Powers, S., and E. Howley. 2009. *Exercise Physiology: Theory and Application to Fitness and Performance.* 7th ed. New York: McGraw-Hill.

Rinne, M.B., S.I. Miilunpalo, and A.O. Heinonen. 2007. Evaluation of required motor abilities in commonly practiced exercise modes and potential training effects among adults. *Journal of Physical Activity and Health* 4: 203-214.

Schnirring, L. 2001. New formula estimates maximal heart rate. *Physician and Sportsmedicine* 29(7): 13-14.

Sharkey, B.J. 1984. *Physiology of Fitness.* 2nd ed. Champaign, IL: Human Kinetics.

Sillery, B. 1996. Essential technology guide to exercise and fitness. *Popular Science* (January): 65-68.

Stewart, G.W. 1995. *Active Living.* Champaign, IL: Human Kinetics.

Swain, D., and B. Leutholtz. 2007. *Exercise Prescription: A Case Study Approach to the ACSM Guidelines.* 2nd ed. Champaign, IL: Human Kinetics.

Tanaka, H., K.D. Monahan, and D.R. Seals. 2001. Age-predicted maximum heart rate revisited. *Journal of the American College of Cardiology* 37(1): 153-156.

Turki, O., et al. 2011. Ten minutes of dynamic stretching is sufficient to potentiate vertical jump performance characteristics. *Journal of Strength and Conditioning Research* 25(9): 2453-2463.

Wachner, P. 2012. Best Exercise and Fitness Apps for iPhone and iPod Touch. About.com Exercise. http://exercise.about.com/od/videosmusicsoftware/tp/fitnessapps.htm [accessed March 8, 2014].

Wilmore, J.H., and D.L. Costill. 2004. *Physiology of Sport and Exercise.* 3rd ed. Champaign, IL: Human Kinetics.

Yacenda, J. 1995. *Fitness Cross-Training.* Champaign, IL: Human Kinetics.

Chapter 7

Alcaraz, P.E., et al. 2011. Similarity in adaptations to high-resistance circuit vs traditional strength training in resistance-trained men. *Journal of Strength and Conditioning Research* 25(9): 2519-2527.

American College of Sports Medicine. 2002. Position stand: Progression models in resistance training for healthy adults. *Medicine and Science in Sports and Exercise* 34(2): 364-380.

American College of Sports Medicine. 2010. *ACSM's Guidelines for Exercise Testing and Prescription.* 8th ed. Baltimore: Lippincott, Williams & Wilkins.

Baechle, T.R., and R.W. Earle. 2008. *Essentials of Strength Training and Conditioning.* 3rd ed. Champaign, IL: Human Kinetics.

Benton, M.J., et al. 2011. Short-term effects of resistance training frequency on body composition and strength in middle-aged women. *Journal of Strength and Conditioning Research* 25(11): 3142-3149.

Bompa, T.O. 1999. *Periodization Theory and Methodology of Training.* 4th ed. Champaign, IL: Human Kinetics.

Burd, N.A., et al. 2012. Bigger weights may not beget bigger muscles: Evidence from acute muscle protein synthetic responses after resistance exercise. *Applied Physiology, Nutrition, and Metabolism* 37(3): 551-554.

Calder, A.W., P.D. Chilibeck, C.E. Webber, and D.G. Sale. 1994. Comparison of whole and split weight training routines in young women. *Canadian Journal of Applied Physiology* 19(2): 185-199.

Chu, D.A. 1992. *Jumping Into Plyometrics.* Champaign, IL: Leisure Press.

Escamilla, J., et al. 1998. Biomechanics of the knee during closed kinetic chain and open kinetic chain exercises. *Medicine and Science in Sports and Exercise* 24(4): 556-569.

Evangelista, R., et al. 2011. Rest interval between resistance exercise sets: Length affects volume but not creatine kinase activity or muscle soreness. *International Journal of Sports Physiology and Performance* 6: 118-127.

Farinatti, P., and A. Neto. 2011. The effect of between-set rest intervals on the oxygen uptake during and after resistance exercise sessions performed with large- and small-muscle mass. *Journal of Strength and Conditioning Research* 25(11): 3181-3190.

Fleck, S.J., and W.J. Kraemer. 2004. *Designing Resistance Training Programs.* 3rd ed. Champaign, IL: Human Kinetics.

Hagan, M. 2000. Training tips for today's fitness professionals. *Fitness Business Canada* (March-April): 38-39.

Heyward, V.H. 2010. *Advanced Fitness Assessment and Exercise Prescription.* 6th ed. Champaign, IL: Human Kinetics.

Jensen, K. 2010. *The Flexible Periodization Method.* Mississauga, ON: The Write Fit.

Kendall, F.P., E.K. McCreary, and P.G. Provance. 2005. *Muscles, Testing and Function: With Posture and Pain.* 5th ed. Baltimore: Williams & Wilkins.

Kraemer, W.J. 2003. Strength training basics: Designing workouts to meet patients' goals. *Physician and Sportsmedicine* 31(8): 39-45.

Lockwood, C.M. 1999. Troubleshooting: The most common training mistakes and how to fix them. Quads and glutes. *Muscle and Fitness* (October): 76-79.

Lyons, P.M., and J.F. Orwin. 1998. Rotator cuff tendinopathy and subacromial impingement syndrome. *Medicine and Science in Sports and Exercise* 30(4): S12-S17.

Marx, J.O., et al. 2001. Low-volume circuit versus high-volume periodized resistance training in women. *Medicine and Science in Sports and Exercise* 33(4): 635-643.

McGill, S.M., and L.W. Marshall. 2012. Kettlebell swing, snatch, and bottoms-up carry: Back and hip muscle activation, motion, and low back loads. *Journal of Strength and Conditioning Research* 26(1): 16-27.

Mohamad, N.I., J.B. Cronin, and K.K. Nosaka. 2012. Difference in kinematics and kinetics between high- and low-velocity resistance loading equated by volume: Implications for hypertrophic training. *Journal of Strength and Conditioning Research* 26(1): 269-275.

Norwood, J.T., et al. 2007. Electromyographic activity of the trunk stabilizers during stable and unstable bench press. *Journal of Strength and Conditioning Research* 21(2): 343-347.

O'Hagan, F.T., T.G. Sale, J.D. MacDougall, and S.H. Garner. 1995. Comparative effectiveness of accommodating and weight resistance training modes. *Medicine and Science in Sports and Exercise* 27(8): 1210-1219.

Pacheco, L., et al. 2011. The acute effects of different stretching exercises on jump performance. *Journal of Strength and Conditioning Research* 25(11): 2991-2998.

Robbins, D.W., et al. 2010. Agonist-antagonist paired set resistance training: A brief review. *Journal of Strength and Conditioning Research* 24(10): 2873-2882.

Signorile, J.F., et al. 2002. A comparative electromyographical investigation of muscle utilization patterns using various hand positions during the lat pull-down. *Journal of Strength and Conditioning Research* 16(4): 539-546.

Sorace, P., and T. LaFontaine. 2005. Resistance training muscle power: Design programs that work! *ACSM's Health and Fitness Journal* 9(2): 6-12.

Stone, M.H., et al. 1999. Periodization: Effects of manipulating volume and intensity. Part 1. *Strength and Conditioning Journal* 21(2): 56-62.

Thompson, W.R., ed. 2010. *ACSM's Resources for the Personal Trainer.* 3rd ed. Baltimore: Lippincott, Williams & Wilkins.

Turki, O., et al. 2011. Ten minutes of dynamic stretching is sufficient to potentiate vertical jump performance characteristics. *Journal of Strength and Conditioning Research* 25(9): 2453-2463.

Van Gelder, L., and S. Bartz. 2011. The effect of acute stretching on agility performance. *Journal of Strength and Conditioning Research* 25(11): 3014-3021.

Voight, M., and S. Tippett. 1994. Plyometric exercise in rehabilitation. In: *Rehabilitation Techniques in Sports Medicine.* 2nd ed., ed. W.E. Prentice. St. Louis: Mosby.

Chapter 8

Alter, M.J. 2004. *Science of Stretching.* 3rd ed. Champaign, IL: Human Kinetics.

Blievernicht, J. 2000. Round shoulder syndrome. *IDEA Health and Fitness Source* (September): 44-53.

Brooks, D. 1993. Where does PNF fit into a training program? In: *Program Design for Personal Trainers.* San Diego: IDEA.

Covert, C., et al. 2010. Comparison of ballistic and static stretching on hamstring muscle length using an equal stretching dose. *Journal of Strength and Conditioning Research* 24(11): 3008-3014.

Eitner, E. 1982. Loosening. In: *Physical Therapy for Sports,* ed. W. Kuprian. Philadelphia: Saunders.

Germann, W.J., and C.L. Stanfield. 2002. *Principles of Human Physiology.* San Francisco: Benjamin Cummings.

Hendrick, A. 2000. Dynamic flexibility training. *Strength and Conditioning Journal* 22(5): 33-38.

Heyward, V.H. 2010. *Advanced Fitness Assessment and Exercise Prescription.* 6th ed. Champaign, IL: Human Kinetics.

Holcomb, W.R. 2000. Improved stretching with proprioceptive neuromuscular facilitation. *Strength and Conditioning Journal* (February): 59-62.

Kendall, F.P., E.K. McCreary, and P.G. Provance. 2005. *Muscles, Testing and Function: With Posture and Pain.* 5th ed. Baltimore: Williams & Wilkins.

Kuprian, W., ed. 1982. *Physical Therapy for Sports.* Philadelphia: Saunders.

LaRoche, D., M. Lussier, and S. Roy. 2008. Chronic stretching and voluntary muscle force. *Journal of Strength and Conditioning Research* 22(2): 589-596.

McAtee, R., and J. Charland. 2007. *Facilitated Stretching.* 3rd ed. Champaign, IL: Human Kinetics.

Myers, T. 2009. *Anatomy Trains: Myofascial Meridians for Manual and Movement Therapists.* 2nd ed. Amsterdam: Elsevier.

National Strength and Conditioning Association. 1994. *Essentials of Strength Training and Conditioning.* Champaign, IL: Human Kinetics.

Ninos, J. 2001a. A chain reaction: The hip rotators. *Strength and Conditioning Journal* (April): 26-27.

Ninos, J. 2001b. Chain reaction: A tight gastroc-soleus group. *Strength and Conditioning Journal* (February): 60-61.

Nordin, M., and V. Frankel. 2001. *Basic Biomechanics of the Musculoskeletal System.* 3rd ed. Baltimore: Lippincott, Williams & Wilkins.

Norris, C.M. 2000. *Back Stability.* Champaign: Human Kinetics.

Osternig, L.R., R.N. Robertson, R.K. Troxel, and P. Hanson. 1990. Differential responses to PNF stretching techniques. *Medicine and Science in Sports and Exercise* 22: 106-111.

O'Sullivan, D., and S. Bird. 2011. Utilization of kinesio taping for fascia unloading. *International Journal of Athletic Therapy and Training* 16(4): 2127.

Page, P., C. Frank, and R. Lardner. 2010. *Assessment and Treatment of Muscle Imbalance: The Janda Approach.* Champaign, IL: Human Kinetics.

Roskopf, G. 2001. When clients feel pain. *IDEA Personal Trainer* (February): 45-53.

Sapega, A.A., T.C. Quendenfeld, R.A. Moyer, and R.A. Butler. 1991. Biophysical factors in range of motion exercise. *Physician and Sportsmedicine* 9(12): 57-65.

Shrier, I., and K. Gossal. 2000. Myths and truths of stretching: Individualized recommendations for healthy muscles. *Physician and Sportsmedicine* 28(8): 57-63.

Chapter 9

Ainsworth, B., et al. 2000. Compendium of physical activities: An update of activity codes and MET intensities. *Medicine and Science in Sports and Exercise* 32(suppl): S498-S516.

A lot on their plate. 2013. *YorkU* (Winter), 8.

American College of Sports Medicine. 2009. *ACSM's Guidelines for Exercise Testing and Prescription.* 8th ed. Baltimore: Lippincott, Williams & Wilkins.

American College of Sports Medicine, American Dietetic Association, Dietitians of Canada. 2009. Nutrition and athletic performance. *Medicine and Science in Sports and Exercise* 41: 709-731.

Andersen, R., and J. Jakicic. 2003. Physical activity and weight management. Building the case for exercise. *Physician and Sportsmedicine* 31(11): 39-45.

Bartlett, S. 2003. Motivating patients toward weight loss: Practical strategies for addressing overweight and obesity. *Physician and Sportsmedicine* 31(11): 29-36.

Bond Brill, J., A.C. Perry, L. Parker, A. Robinson, and K. Burnett. 2002. Dose-response effect of walking exercise on weight loss. How much is enough? *International Journal of Obesity* 26(11): 1484-1493.

Bushman, B. 2011. Wouldn't you like to know. *ACSM's Health & Fitness Journal* 15(5): 5-7.

Campbell, W.W., M.C. Crim, V.R. Young, and W.J. Evans. 1994. Increased energy requirements and changes in body composition with resistance training in older adults. *American Journal of Clinical Nutrition* 60: 167-175.

Clark, N. 2014. *Nancy Clark's Sports Nutrition Guidebook.* 5th ed. Champaign, IL: Human Kinetics.

Cullinen, K., and M. Caldwell. 1998. Weight training increases fat-free mass and strength in untrained young women. *Journal of the American Dietetic Association* 98(4): 414-418.

Dairy Farmers of Canada and CSEP. 2012a. Food Energy – A Current Reference for Fitness Professionals. www.csep.ca/CMFiles/publications/dfc/Energy_factsheet_e.pdf [accessed March 8, 2014].

Dairy Farmers of Canada and CSEP. 2012b. Fluid – A Current Reference for Fitness Professionals. dairy-nutrition.ca/fitness. www.csep.ca/CMFiles/publications/dfc/Hydration_factsheet_e.pdf [accessed March 30, 2014].

Dietary Guidelines for Americans 2010 [Internet]. 2011. http://www.health.gov/dietary guidelines/2010.asp. [accessed February 15, 2013].

Dietitians of Canada. 2005. Keep an Eye on Your Portion Size. www.bchu.org/pdf/Nutrition/Keep%20and%20Eye%20on%20Portions_lr.pdf [accessed March 8, 2014].

Donnelly, J.E., et al. 2009. American College of Sports Medicine position stand. Appropriate physical activity intervention strategies for weight loss and prevention of weight regain for adults. *Medicine and Science in Sports and Exercise* 41(2): 459-471.

Farinatti, P., and A. Neto. 2011. The effect of between-set rest intervals on the oxygen uptake during and after resistance exercise sessions performed with large- and small-muscle mass. *Journal of Strength and Conditioning Research* 25(11): 3181-3190.

Fleck, S.J., and W.J. Kraemer. 2004. *Designing Resistance Training Programs.* 3rd ed. Champaign, IL: Human Kinetics.

Garfinkel, P., and D. Coscina. 1990. Discussion: Exercise and obesity. In: *Exercise, Fitness and Health,* ed. C. Bouchard, R.J. Shephard, T. Stephens, J.R. Sutton, and B.D. McPherson. Champaign, IL: Human Kinetics.

Harvard Health Publications. The Healthy Eating Plate. 2014. www.hsph.harvard.edu/nutritionsource/pyramid.full.story/ [accessed March 8, 2014].

Heyward, V.H. 2002. *Advanced Fitness Assessment and Exercise Prescription.* 4th ed. Champaign, IL: Human Kinetics.

Heyward, V.H. 2010. *Advanced Fitness Assessment and Exercise Prescription.* 6th ed. Champaign, IL: Human Kinetics.

Hodgetts, V., et al. 1991. Factors controlling fat metabolism from human subcutaneous adipose tissue during exercise. *Journal of Applied Physiology* 71: 445-451.

Hoeger, W., S. Hoeger, M. Locke, and L. Lauzon. 2009. *Principles & Labs for Fitness & Wellness.* Toronto: Nelson Education.

Institute of Medicine. 2006. *Dietary Reference Intakes: The Essential Guide to Nutrient Requirements.* Washington, DC: National Academies Press.

Jakicic, K.M. 2009. The effect of physical activity on body weight. *Obesity (Silver Spring)* 17(suppl 3): S34-S38.

Klesges, R., et al. 1993. Effects of television on metabolic rate: Potential implications for childhood obesity. *Pediatrics* 91: 281-286.

Knab, A., et al. 2011. A 45-minute vigorous exercise bout increases metabolic rate for 14 hours. *Medicine and Science in Sports and Exercise* 43(9): 1643-1648.

Marks, B.L., A. Ward, D.H. Morris, J. Castellani, and J.M. Rippe. 1995. Fat-free mass is maintained in women following a moderate diet and exercise program. *Medicine and Science in Sports and Exercise* 27(9): 1243-1251.

McArdle, W., F. Katch, and V. Katch. 2010. *Exercise Physiology: Nutrition, Energy, and Human Performance.* 7th ed. Philadelphia: Lea & Febiger.

Miller, W.C. 1991. Diet composition, energy intake and nutritional status in relation to obesity in men and women. *Medicine and Science in Sports and Exercise* 23(3): 280-284.

National Heart Lung and Blood Institute. 2000, October. *Clinical Guidelines on the Identification, Evaluation, and Treatment of Overweight and Obesity in Adults: Executive Summary.* National Institutes of Health Publication No. 00-4084. Rockville, MD.

Nieman, D.C. 1990. *Fitness and Sports Medicine: An Introduction.* Palo Alto, CA: Bull.

Peterson, M.J., et al. 2004. Comparison of caloric expenditure in intermittent and continuous walking bouts. *Journal of Strength and Conditioning Research* 18(2): 373-376.

Powers, S., and E. Howley. 2009. *Exercise Physiology Theory and Application to Fitness and Performance.* 7th ed. New York: McGraw-Hill.

Romijn, J., et al. 1993. Regulation of endogenous fat and carbohydrate metabolism in relation to exercise intensity and duration. *American Journal of Physiology* 265: E380-E391.

Sass, C., et al. 2007. Crossing the line: Understanding the scope of practice between registered dietitians and health/fitness professionals. *ACSM's Health & Fitness Journal* 11(3): 12-19.

Shah, M., and A. James. 2013. Menu labels displaying amount of exercise needed to burn calories shows benefits. Paper presented at Experimental Biology 2013 Conference, Boston, April.

Spaccarotella, K., and W. Andzel. 2011. The effects of low fat chocolate milk on postexercise recovery in col-legiate athletes. *Journal of Strength and Conditioning Research* 25(12): 3456-3460.

Statistics Canada. 2006. Canadian Community Health Survey-Nutrition. www.hc-sc.gc.ca/fn-an/surveill/nutrition/commun/cchs_guide_escc-eng.php [accessed March 8, 2011].

Statistics Canada. 2011. Canadian Community Health Survey-Obesity. www.statcan.gc.ca/pub/82-003-x/2012003/article/11706-eng.htm [accessed November 18, 2013].

Thomas, J.G., et al. 2011. The National Weight Control Registry: A study of successful losers. *ACSM's Health & Fitness Journal* 15(2): 8-12.

Tremblay, A., et al. 1989. Impact of dietary fat content and fat oxidation on energy intake in humans. *American Journal of Clinical Nutrition* 47: 799-805.

U.S. Department of Agriculture. ChooseMyPlate.gov.

Vispute, S.S., et al. 2011. The effect of abdominal exercise on abdominal fat. *Journal of Strength and Conditioning Research* 25(9): 2559-2564.

Volpe, S.L. 2011. The 2010 USDA Dietary Guidelines for Americans and other tools to providing sound nutritional information. *ACSM's Health & Fitness Journal* 15(5): 37-39.

Walberg, J.L. 1989. Aerobic exercise and resistance weight training during weight reduction. *Sports Medicine* 47: 343-356.

Warburton, D.E.R., C.W. Nicol, and S.S.D. Bredin. 2006. Prescribing exercise as preventive therapy. *Canadian Medical Association Journal* 174(7): 961-973.

Williams, M.H. 1995. *Nutrition for Fitness and Sport.* 4th ed. Dubuque, IA: Brown and Benchmark.

Chapter 10

Anderson, M.K., and G.P. Parr. 2011. *Foundations of Sports Injury Management.* 3rd ed. Baltimore: Lippincott, Williams & Wilkins.

Andrish, J., and J.A. Work. 1990. How I manage shin splints. *Physician and Sportsmedicine* 18(12): 113-114.

Bahr, R., and S. Maehlum. 2004. *Clinical Guide to Sports Injuries.* Champaign, IL: Human Kinetics.

Chapman, D., et al. 2011. Effect of slow-velocity lengthening contractions on muscle damage induced by fast-velocity lengthening contractions. *National Strength and Conditioning Research* 25(1): 211-219.

Denegar, C., E. Saliba, and S. Saliba. 2010. *Therapeutic Modalities for Musculoskeletal Injuries.* 3rd ed. Champaign, IL: Human Kinetics.

Earle, R.W., and T.R. Baechle. 2004. *NSCA's Essentials of Personal Training.* Champaign, IL: Human Kinetics.

Frontera, W.R. 2003. Exercise and musculoskeletal rehabilitation. *Physician and Sportsmedicine* 31(12): 39-45.

Germann, W.J., and C.L. Stanfield. 2002. *Principles of Human Physiology.* San Francisco: Benjamin Cummings.

Gillespie, H. 2011. Nonsteroidal anti-inflammatory drugs. *ACSM's Health and Fitness Journal* (November-December): 46-47.

Griffin, J.C. 1987. Fitness injury survey: Fitness assessors and programmers. *Canadian Association for Health, Physical Education and Recreation Journal* 53(1): 15-17.

Hanson, R.W. 2009. Tendinopathy update. *Athletic Therapy Today* (March): 10-12.

Hess, G.P., W.L. Cappiello, R.M. Poole, and S.C. Hunter. 1989. Prevention and treatment of overuse tendon injuries. *Sports Medicine* 8(6): 371-384.

Houglum, P. 2001. *Therapeutic Exercise for Athletic Injuries.* Champaign, IL: Human Kinetics.

IDEA. 2001. Benefits of a working relationship between medical and allied health practitioners and personal fitness trainers. *IDEA Health and Fitness Source* (September): 48-54.

Jozsa, L., and P. Kannus. 1997. *Human Tendons.* Champaign, IL: Human Kinetics.

Kahn, K.M., et al. 2000. Overuse tendinosis, not tendinitis. *Physician and Sportsmedicine* 28(5): 38-48.

Kaul, M.P., and S.A. Herring. 1994. Superficial heat and cold. *Physician and Sportsmedicine* 22(12): 65-72.

Kraemer, W., et al. 2001. Influence of compression therapy on symptoms following soft tissue injury from maximal eccentric exercise. *Journal of Orthopaedic and Sports Physical Therapy* 31(6): 282-298.

Mayer, J.M., et al. 2006. Continuous low-level heat wrap therapy for the prevention and early phase treatment of delayed-onset muscle soreness of the low back. *Archives of Physical Medicine and Rehabilitation* 87: 1310-1317.

Molina, F., A. Rus, R. Lomas-Vega, and L. del Moral. 2011. The physiologic basis of tendinopathy development. *International Journal of Athletic Therapy and Training* (November): 5-8.

Nirschl, P.R. 1988. Prevention and treatment of elbow and shoulder injuries in the tennis player. *Clinical Sports Medicine* 7(2): 289-308.

O'Connor, F.G., J.R. Sobel, and R.P. Nirschl. 1992. Five-step treatment for overuse injuries. *Physician and Sportsmedicine* 20(10): 128-142.

Ralston, D.J. 2003. The RAMP System: A template for the progression of athletic-injury rehabilitation. *Journal of Sports Rehabilitation* 12: 280-290.

Ross, M. 1999. Delayed-onset muscle soreness. *Physician and Sportsmedicine* 27(1): 107-108.

Saidoff, D., and S. Apfel. 2005. *Healthy Body Handbook.* New York: Demos Medical.

Snyder, J., et al. 2011. Cryotherapy for treatment of delayed onset muscle soreness. *International Journal of Athletic Therapy and Training* (July): 28-31.

Stovitz, S.D., and R.J. Johnson. 2003. NSAIDs and musculoskeletal treatment. *Physician and Sportsmedicine* 31(1): 35-52.

Szymanski, D.J. 2001. Recommendations for the avoidance of delayed-onset muscle soreness. *Strength and Conditioning Journal* 23(4): 7-13.

Tokmakidis, S.P., E.A. Kokkinidid, I. Smilios, and H. Douda. 2003. The effects of ibuprofen on delayed muscle soreness and muscular performance after eccentric exercise. *Journal of Strength and Conditioning Research* 17(1): 53-59.

Chapter 11

Andrish, J., and J.A. Work. 1990. How I manage shin splints. *Physician and Sportsmedicine* 18(12): 113-114.

Bahr, R., and S. Maehlum. 2004. *Clinical Guide to Sports Injuries.* Champaign, IL: Human Kinetics.

Batt, M.E., and J.L. Tanji. 1995. Management options for plantar fasciitis. *Physician and Sportsmedicine* 23(6): 77-86.

Best, T.M., and W.E. Garrett. 1996. Hamstring strains. Expediting return to play. *Physician and Sportsmedicine* 24(8): 37-44.

Carter, J., et al. 2006. The effects of stability ball training on spinal stability in sedentary individuals. *Journal of Strength and Conditioning Research* 20(2): 429-435.

Cook, J.L., et al. 2000. Overuse tendinosis, not tendinitis. *Physician and Sportsmedicine* 28(6): 31-46.

Couture, C.J., and K.A. Karlson. 2002. Tibial stress injuries. *Physician and Sportsmedicine* 30(6): 29-36.

Craig, D. 2008. Medial tibial stress syndrome: Current etiological theories: part 1, background. *Athletic Therapy Today* (January): 17-20.

DeLisa, J.A. 1998. *Rehabilitation Medicine Principles and Practices.* Philadelphia: Lippincott-Raven.

De Palma, B. 1994. Rehabilitation of hip and thigh injuries. In: *Rehabilitation Techniques in Sports Medicine.* 2nd ed., ed. W.E. Prentice. St. Louis: Mosby.

DePalma, M.J., and E.W. Johnson. 2003. Detecting and treating shoulder impingement syndrome. *Physician and Sportsmedicine* 31(7): 25-32.

DePalma, M.J., and R.H. Perkins. 2004. Patellar tendinosis. *Physician and Sportsmedicine* 32(5): 41-45.

Doucette, S.A., and E.M. Goble. 1992. The effect of exercise on patellar tracking in lateral patellar compression syndrome. *American Journal of Sports Medicine* 20(4): 434-440.

Drezner, J.A., and S.A. Herring. 2001. Managing low-back pain. *Physician and Sportsmedicine* 29(8): 37-43.

Earle, R.W., and T.R. Baechle. 2004. *NSCA's Essentials of Personal Training.* Champaign, IL: Human Kinetics.

Faltus, J. 2009. Effective management of patellofemoral joint dysfunction. *Athletic Therapy Today* (November): 40-42.

Faltus, J. 2010. Optimal therapeutic management of chronic shoulder dysfunction. *Athletic Therapy Today* (November): 4-7.

Fick, D.S., J.P. Albright, and B.P. Murray. 1992. Relieving painful "shin splints." *Physician and Sportsmedicine* 20(12): 105-113.

Galea, A.M., and J.M. Albers. 1994. Patellofemoral pain. Beyond empirical diagnosis. *Physician and Sportsmedicine* 22(4): 48-58.

Hanney, W.J. 2000. Proprioceptive training for ankle instability. *Strength and Conditioning Journal* 22(5): 63-68.

Hanson, R.W. 2009. Tendinopathy update. *Athletic Therapy Today* (March): 10-12.

Houglum, P. 2010. *Therapeutic Exercise for Musculoskeletal Injuries.* 3rd ed. Champaign, IL: Human Kinetics.

Jackson, M.D. 1997. Evaluating and managing tennis elbow. *Your Patient & Fitness* 11(2): 104i-104l.

Jozsa, L., and P. Kannus. 1997. *Human Tendons.* Champaign, IL: Human Kinetics.

Korkola, M., and A. Amendola. 2001. Exercise-induced leg pain. *Physician and Sportsmedicine* 29(6): 35-50.

Liemohn, W. 2001. *Exercise Prescription and the Back.* New York: McGraw-Hill.

Martines-Silvestrini, J.A., et al. 2005. Chronic lateral epicondylitis: Comparative effectiveness of a home exercise program including stretching alone versus stretching supplemented with eccentric or concentric strengthening. *Journal of Hand Therapy* 18: 411-420.

McGill, S. 2007. *Low Back Disorders: Evidence-Based Prevention and Rehabilitation.* 2nd ed. Champaign, IL: Human Kinetics.

Myerson, M.S., and K. Biddinger. 1995. Achilles tendon disorders. Practical management strategies. *Physician and Sportsmedicine* 23(12): 47-54.

Page, P., C. Frank, and R. Lardner. 2010. *Assessment and Treatment of Muscle Imbalance: The Janda Approach.* Champaign, IL: Human Kinetics.

Post, W.R. 1998. Patellofemoral pain. *Physician and Sportsmedicine* 26(1): 68-78.

Prentice, W.E. 1994. *Rehabilitation Techniques in Sports Medicine.* 2nd ed. St. Louis: Mosby.

Reynolds, G. 2009. Phys ed: An easy fix for tennis elbow? *New York Times,* August 25.

Rizzo, T.D. 1991. Plantar fasciitis. Overcoming a nagging pain in the arch. *Physician and Sportsmedicine* 19(4): 129-130.

Sanders, M. 2007. Keep trekking with healthy happy feet. Understanding plantar fasciitis. *ACSM's Health & Fitness Journal* 4: 29-32.

Santana, J.C. 2000. Hamstrings of steel: Preventing the pull, part II – training the triple threat. *Strength and Conditioning Journal* 23(1): 18-20.

Schilling, J. 2008. Specific lumbar stabilization exercise: Theoretical underpinnings. *Athletic Therapy Today* (July): 34-36.

Sherry, M., and T. Best. 2004. A comparison of 2 rehabilitation programs in the treatment of acute hamstring strains. *Journal of Orthopaedic and Sports Physical Therapy* 34(3): 116-125.

Taunton, J.E., D.B. Clement, G.W. Smart, and K.L. McNicol. 1987. Non-surgical management of overuse knee injuries in runners. *Canadian Journal of Sports Science* 12(1): 11-18.

Tiidus, P.M. 2008. *Skeletal Muscle Damage and Repair.* Champaign, IL: Human Kinetics.

Toor, H. 2004. Calf pain. Common causes, treatment and preventive measures. *Fitness Trainer Canada* (February-March): 20-23.

Waddell, G. 1987. A new clinical model for the treatment of low back pain. *Spine* 12(7): 632-644.

Watkins, J. 1999. *The Structure and Function of the Musculoskeletal System.* Champaign, IL: Human Kinetics.

Whiting, W., and R. Zernicke. 2008. *Biomechanics of Musculoskeletal Injury.* 2nd ed. Champaign, IL: Human Kinetics.

Chapter 12

American College of Sports Medicine. 2010. *ACSM's Guidelines for Exercise Testing and Prescription.* 8th ed., 190-194. Philadelphia: Lippincott, Williams & Wilkins.

American Geriatrics Society Panel on Exercise and Osteoarthritis. 2001. Exercise prescription for older adults with osteoarthritis pain: Consensus practice recommendations. *Journal of the American Geriatrics Society* 49: 808-823.

Baker, B., and R. Cutlip. 2010. Skeletal muscle injury versus adaptation with aging: Novel insights on perplexing paradigms. *Exercise and Sport Sciences Reviews* 38(1): 10-16.

Brennan, F. 2002. Exercise prescriptions for active seniors. *Physician and Sportsmedicine* 30(2): 19-29.

Candow, D.G., et al. 2011. Short-term heavy resistance training eliminates age-related deficits in muscle mass and strength in healthy older males. *Journal of Strength and Conditioning Research* 25(2): 326-333.

Chakravarty, E.F., et al. 2008. Long distance running and knee osteoarthritis. A prospective study. *American Journal of Preventive Medicine* 35(2): 133-138.

Feland, J.B., et al. 2001. The effect of duration of stretching on the hamstring muscle group for increased range of motion in people aged 65 years or older. *Physical Therapy* 81(5): 1110-1117.

Janssen, I., S. Heymsfield, and R. Ross. 2002. Low relative skeletal legal muscle mass (sarcopenia) in older persons is associated with functional impairment and physical disability. *Journal of the American Geriatrics Society* 50: 889-896.

Jones, J., and D. Rose, eds. 2005. *Physical Activity Instruction of Older Adults.* Champaign, IL: Human Kinetics.

Kaplan, F.S. 1995. Prevention and management of osteoporosis. *Clinical Symposia* 47: 1-32.

Martin, M. 2010. *Exercise for Better Bones.* Ottawa, ON: Melioguide.

Matheson, G., et al. 1989. Musculoskeletal injuries associated with physical activity in older adults. *Medicine and Science in Sports and Exercise* 21(4): 379-385.

National Osteoporosis Foundation. 2008. Osteoporosis: Fast facts. http://med-docs.creighton.edu/images/Creighton_FIRST/Osteo_Spotlight/Fast_Facts.pdf [accessed October 21, 2012].

Pizzigalli, L., et al. 2011. Prevention of falling risk in elderly people: The relevance of muscular strength and symmetry of the lower limbs in postural stability. *Journal of Strength and Conditioning Research* 25(2): 567-574.

Porter, M. 2001. The effects of strength training on sarcopenia. *Canadian Journal of Applied Physiology* 26(1): 123-141.

Rose, D.J. 2010. *Fall Proof!* 2nd ed. Champaign, IL: Human Kinetics.

Roth, S.M., R.E. Ferrel, and B.F. Hurley. 2000. Strength training for the prevention and treatment of sarcopenia. *Journal of Nutrition, Health, and Aging* 4(3): 143-155.

Sayers, S.P. 2007. High-speed power training: A novel approach to resistance training in older men and women: A brief review and pilot study. *Journal of Strength and Conditioning Research* 21: 518-526.

Scott, W.A., and G.S. Couzens. 1996. Treating injuries in active seniors. *Physician and Sportsmedicine* 24(5): 63-68.

Seto, J.L., and C.E. Brewster. 1991. Musculoskeletal conditioning of the older athlete. *Clinics in Sports Medicine* 10(2): 401-429.

Signorile, J.K. 2011. *Bending the Aging Curve.* Champaign, IL: Human Kinetics.

Speers, K., ed. 2005. *Injury Prevention and Rehabilitation for Active Older Adults.* Champaign, IL: Human Kinetics.

Spirduso, W.W., K. Francis, and P. MacRae. 2005. *Physical Dimensions of Aging.* 2nd ed. Champaign, IL: Human Kinetics.

Taylor, A.W., and M.J. Johnson. 2008. *Physiology of Exercise and Healthy Aging.* Champaign, IL: Human Kinetics.

Vella, C.A., and L. Kravitz. 2002. Sarcopenia: The mystery of muscle loss. *IDEA Personal Trainer* 13(4): 30-35.

Warburton, D., C. Nicol, and S. Bredin. 2006. Health benefits of physical activity: The evidence. *Canadian Medical Association Journal* 174(6): 801-809.

Chapter 13

Aalbersa, T., M. Baarsa, and M. Olde-Rikkerta. 2011. Characteristics of effective Internet-mediated interventions to change lifestyle in people aged 50 and older: A systematic review. *Aging Research Review* 10(4): 487-497.

ALCOA. 2006. Health related quality of life in physical activity. *ALCOA NEWS* (September): 2-5.

American College of Sports Medicine. 2010. *ACSM's Guidelines for Exercise Testing and Prescription.* 8th ed., 190-194. Philadelphia: Lippincott, Williams & Wilkins.

American College of Sports Medicine. 2010. *ACSM's Resources for the Personal Trainer.* 3rd ed. Philadelphia: Lippincott, Williams & Wilkins.

Baker, B., and R. Cutlip. 2010. Skeletal muscle injury versus adaptation with aging: Novel insights on perplexing paradigms. *Exercise and Sport Sciences Reviews* 38(1): 10-16.

Barclay, L., and D. Lie. 2008. Regular exercise through middle age may delay biological aging. *British Journal of Sports Medicine.* Published online April 10.

Barke, C.R., and D.R. Nicholas. 1990. Physical activity in older adults: The stages of change. *Journal of Applied Gerontology* 9(2): 216-223.

Berg, K., S. Wood-Dauphinee, and J. Williams. 1995. The balance scale: Reliability assessment with elderly residents in patients with acute stroke. *Scandinavian Journal of Rehabilitation Medicine* 27: 27-36.

Blair, S.N., H. Kohl, D. Paffenbarger, D. Clark, K. Cooper, and L. Gibbons.1989. Health benefits of activity. *Exercise and Sport Science Reviews* 12: 205-244.

Brennan, F. 2002. Exercise prescriptions for active seniors. *The Physician & Sports Medicine,* 30(2): 19-29.

Bryant, C., and D. Green. 2005. *Exercise for Older Adults: ACE's Guide for Fitness Professionals.* 2nd ed. San Diego: American Council on Exercise.

Canadian Society for Exercise Physiology. 2003. *The Canadian Physical Activity, Fitness, and Lifestyle Approach.* 3rd ed. Ottawa: CSEP.

Canadian Society for Exercise Physiology. 2011. Canadian Physical Activity Guidelines. www.csep.ca/guidelines.

Candow, D.G., et al. 2011. Short-term heavy resistance training eliminates age-related deficits in muscle mass and strength in healthy older males. *Journal of Strength and Conditioning Research* 25(2): 326-333.

Cerny, F.J., and H.W. Burton. 2001. *Exercise Physiology for Health Care Professionals.* Champaign, IL: Human Kinetics.

Chodzko-Zajko, W.J., et al. 2009. Physical activity for older adults. *Medicine and Science in Sports and Exercise* 41(7): 1510-1530.

Conn, V., A. Hafdahl, and D. Mehr. 2011. Interventions to increase physical activity among healthy adults:

Meta-analysis of outcomes. *American Journal of Public Health* 101: 751-758.

Covinsky, K.E., et al. 2009. Pain, functional limitations, and aging. *Journal of the American Geriatrics Society* 57: 1556-1561.

Dartagan, G., et al. 2012. Quality of life and physical activity in a sample of Brazilian older adults. *Journal of Aging and Health* 24(2): 212-226.

Elble, R.J. 1997. Changes in gait with normal aging. In: *Gait Disorders of Aging: Falls and Therapeutic Strategies,* ed. J.C. Masdeu, et al., 93-106. Philadelphia: Lippincott-Raven.

Eurostat Press Office. 2012. At the age of 65, both women and men are expected to live a further nine years in a healthy condition. April 19. http://ec.europa.eu/eurostat. [accessed February 21, 2013]

Fatouras, K.G., et al. 2002. The effects of strength training, cardiovascular training and their combination on flexibility of inactive older adults. *International Journal of Sports Medicine* 23: 112-119.

Fern, A.K. 2009. Benefits of physical activity in older adults. *ACSM's Health & Fitness Journal* 13(5): 12-16.

Foldvari, M., et al. 2000. Association of muscle power with functional status in community dwelling elderly women. *Journal of Gerontology: Medical Sciences* 55A(4): M192-M199.

Freedman, V., L. Martin, and R. Schoeni. 2009. Recent trends in disability and functioning among older adults in the United States: A systematic review. *Journal of the American Medical Association* 288(24): 3137-3146.

Fries, J., et al. 2008. Running slows the aging clock. *Archives of Internal Medicine.* News release, August 11.

Frontera, W.R., et al. 1988. Strength conditioning in older men: Skeletal muscle hypertrophy and improved function. *Journal of Applied Physiology* 64: 1038-1044.

Gonzalez-Rave, J.M., et al. 2011. Changes in vertical jump height, anthropometric characteristics, and biochemical parameters after contrast training in master athletes and physically active older people. *Journal of Strength and Conditioning Research* 25(7): 1866-1878.

Griffin, J.C. 2011. Functional mobility screening in adults 50-70 years of age. Design principles and process. Unpublished paper. George Brown College, Ontario.

Griffin, J.C. 2012. Functional mobility screening in adults 50-70 years of age. *Journal of Active Aging* (January-February): 40-49.

Health Canada. 2001. *Canada's Physical Activity Guide to Healthy Active Living for Older Adults.* Ottawa: Health Canada.

Hernandez, D., D. Rose, and O. Theou. 2008. Can gait velocity predict which older adults will or will not fall? *Journal of Physical Activity and Aging* 16: S209.

Hoffman, J. 2006. *Norms for Fitness, Performance, and Health.* Champaign, IL: Human Kinetics.

Jam, B. 2010. *The Pain Truth . . . and Nothing But!* Thornhill, ON: APTEI.

Jones, J., and D. Rose. 2005. *Physical Activity Instruction of Older Adults.* Champaign, IL: Human Kinetics.

Jones, L., D. Waters, and M. Legge. 2009. Walking speed at self selected exercise pace is lower but energy cost higher in older versus younger women. *Journal of Physical Activity and Health* 6: 327-332.

Kalapotharakos, V., et al. 2005. Effects of a heavy and a moderate resistance training on functional performance in older adults. *Journal of Strength and Conditioning Research* 19(3): 652-657.

Kraemer, W.J., and F.S. Harman. 1998. Periodized training for older adults. *IDEA Personal Trainer* (July-August): 21-27.

Liffiton, J., S. Horton, J. Baker, and P. Weir. 2012. Successful aging: How does physical activity influence engagement with life? *European Review of Aging and Physical Activity* 9(2): 103-108.

Lusardi, M., G. Pellecchia, and M. Schulman. 2003. Functional performance in community living for adults. *Journal of Geriatric Physical Therapy* 26(3): 14-22.

Marcus, R. 2001. Role of exercise in preventing and treating osteoporosis. *Rheumatic Disease Clinics of North America* 27: 131-141.

Martyn-St. James, M., and S. Carroll. 2008. Meta-analysis of walking for preservation of bone mineral density in postmenopausal women. *Bone* 43(3): 521-531.

Moore, S.C., et al. 2012. Leisure time physical activity of moderate to vigorous intensity and mortality: A large pooled cohort analysis. *PLoS Medicine* 9(11): e1001335.

Morrison, C.A. 2001. Using the exercise test to create the exercise prescription. *Primary Care* 28(1): 137-158, vii.

Murias, J., et al. 2008. Time-course of adaptations in cardiorespiratory fitness with exercise training in older and younger subjects. *Applied Physiology, Nutrition, and Metabolism* 33(suppl 1): S69-S70.

Nashner, L.M. 2002. Maintaining safe balance and mobility: When is fitness enough and when is medical help needed? *Journal on Active Aging* (March-April): 31-34.

National Institute on Aging. 2009. Exercise & Physical Activity: Your Everyday Guide from the National Institute on Aging. www.nia.nih.gov/healthinformation/publications/exerciseguide [accessed March 8, 2014].

National Safety Council. 2009. www.nsc.org/safety_work/SafeCommunitiesAmerica/Documents/Networking Conference 2010/A Marr - Falls Prevention.ppt [accessed May 13, 2014].

Nelson, M.E., et al. 2007. Physical activity and public health in older adults: Recommendation from the American College of Sports Medicine and the American

Heart Association. *Medicine and Science in Sports and Exercise* 39(8): 1435-1445.

Nieman, D.C. 2009. You asked for it. *ACSM's Health and Fitness Journal* 13(1): 5-6.

Osness, W.H. 1996. *Functional Fitness for Assessment of Adults Over 60 Years.* Reston, VA: AAHPERD.

Parkatti, T., J. Perttunen, and P. Wacker. 2012. Improvements in functional capacity from Nordic walking: A randomized controlled trial among older adults. *Journal of Aging and Physical Activity* 20(1): 93-105.

Pizzigalli, L., et al. 2011. Prevention of falling risk in elderly people: The relevance of muscular strength and symmetry of the lower limbs in postural stability. *Journal of Strength and Conditioning Research* 25(2): 567-574.

Prochaska, J.O., and C.C. DiClemente. 1982. Transtheoretical therapy: Toward a more integrative model of change. *Psychotherapy: Theory, Research, and Practice* 20: 161-173.

Rejeski, W.J., and S.L. Mihalko. 2001. Physical activity and quality of life in older adults. *Journals of Gerontology. Series A, Biological Sciences and Medical Sciences* 56: 23-35.

Requa, R.K., and J.G. Garrick. 1996. Adult recreational fitness. In: *Epidemiology of Sports Injuries,* ed. D.J. Caine, et al. Champaign, IL: Human Kinetics.

Rikli, R.E., and J. Jones. 2001. *Senior Fitness Test Manual.* Champaign, IL: Human Kinetics.

Rose, D.J. 2010. *Fall Proof!* 2nd ed. Champaign, IL: Human Kinetics.

Rowe, J., and R. Kahn. 1987. Human aging: Usual and successful. *Science* 237: 143-149.

Sabia, S., et al. 2012. Influence of individual and combined healthy behaviors on successful aging. *Canadian Medical Association Journal* 184(18): 1985-1992.

Signorile, J.K. 2011. *Bending the Aging Curve.* Champaign, IL: Human Kinetics.

Sloan, K.S. 2001. Physical Activity and 50+. American Association of Retired Persons. http://lin.ca/resources/physical-activity-and-50-preliminary-findings-support-effective-communications-and [accessed November 25, 2012].

Speers, K., ed. 2005. *Injury Prevention and Rehabilitation for Active Older Adults.* Champaign, IL: Human Kinetics.

Spirduso, W.W., K. Francis, and P. MacRae. 2005. *Physical Dimensions of Aging.* 2nd ed. Champaign, IL: Human Kinetics.

Strawbridge, W.J., M.I. Wallhagen, and R.D. Cohen. 2002. Successful aging and well-being: Self-rated compared with Rowe and Kahn. *Gerontologist* 42(6): 727-733.

Tanaka, H., K.D. Monahan, and D.R. Seals. 2001. Age-predicted maximum heart rate revisited. *Journal of the American College of Cardiology* 37(1): 153-156.

Tannenbaum, C. 2012. Older Men's Hidden Health Concerns. www.alphagalileo.org/PrintView.aspx-?ItemId=118204&CultureCode=en [accessed March 8, 2012]

Taylor, A.W., and M.J. Johnson. 2008. *Physiology of Exercise and Healthy Aging.* Champaign, IL: Human Kinetics.

Tenetti, M.E. 1986. Performance oriented assessment of mobility problems in elderly patients. *Journal of the American Geriatrics Society* 34: 119-126.

Thielke, S.M., et al. 2012. Persistence and remission of musculoskeletal pain in community dwelling older adults: Results from the Cardiovascular Health Study. *Journal of the American Geriatrics Society* 60(8): 1393-1400.

Van Norman, K.A. 2010. *Exercise and Wellness for Older Adults.* Champaign, IL: Human Kinetics.

Vincent, K.R., and R.W. Braith. 2002. Resistance exercise and bone turnover in elderly men and women. *Medicine and Science in Sports and Exercise* 34: 17-23.

Vita, A., R. Terry, H. Hubert, and J. Fries. 1998. Aging, health risk, and cumulative disability. *New England Journal of Medicine* 338(15): 1035-1041.

Williamson, P. 2011. *Exercise for Special Populations.* Baltimore: Lippincott, Williams & Wilkins.

Woods, N.F., et al. 2012. Toward a positive aging phenotype for older women: Observations from the Women's Health Initiative. *Journals of Gerontology. Series A, Biological Sciences and Medical Sciences* 67(11): 1191-1196.

Zhu, W., and W. Chodzko-Zajko, eds. 2006. *Measurement Issues in Aging and Physical Activity.* Champaign, IL: Human Kinetics.

Chapter 14

Aronow, H., J. Hahn, and J. Branin. 2008. Use of a multi-dimensional health risk appraisal among adults aging with acquired disabilities. *Gerontologist* 48: 155.

Caldwell, C.A., S. Sahmann, and L. Van Dillen. 2007. Use of a movement system impairment diagnosis for physical therapy in the management of patient with shoulder pain. *Journal of Orthopaedic and Sports Physical Therapy* 37(9): 551-563.

Canadian Centre for Activity and Aging. 2004. *Functional Fitness for Older Adults Resource Manual.* Ch. 3, Fitness, Activity, Health, and Independence. London, ON: CCAA.

Chaves, P.H., E.S. Garrett, and L.P. Fried. 2000. Predicting the risk of mobility difficulty in older women with screening nomograms: The women's health and aging study II. *Archives of Internal Medicine* 160(16): 2525-2533.

Clemson, L., et al. 2012. Integration of balance and strength training into daily life activity to reduce the rate of falls in older people (the LIFE study): Randomized parallel trial. *British Medical Journal* 345: e4547.

Coalman, M. 2002. Functional fitness for older adults. *Journal on Active Aging* (January-February): 24-27.

Cook, G., L. Burton, and B. Hoogenboom. 2006a. Pre-participation screening: The use of fundamental movements as an assessment of function - part 1. *North American Journal of Sports Physical Therapy* 1(2): 62-72.

Cook, G., L. Burton, and B. Hoogenboom. 2006b. Pre-participation screening: The use of fundamental movements as an assessment of function - part 2. *North American Journal of Sports Physical Therapy* 1(3): 132-139.

Creel, G.L., K.E. Light, and M.T. Thigpen. 2001. Concurrent and construct validity of scores on the timed movement battery. *Physical Therapy* 81(2): 789-798.

Cunningham, D.A., et al. 1993. Determinants of independence in the elderly. *Applied Physiology, Nutrition, and Metabolism* 18(3): 243-254.

de Brito, L.B.B., et al. 2013. Ability to sit and rise from the floor as a predictor of all-cause mortality. *European Journal of Preventive Cardiology* (January) 9: 1-6.

DiPietro, L. 1996. The epidemiology of physical activity and physical function in older people. *Medicine and Science in Sports and Exercise* 28(5): 596-600.

DiStefano, L., M. Clark, and D. Padua. 2009. Evidence supporting balance training in healthy individuals: A systemic review. *Journal of Strength and Conditioning Research* 23(9): 2718-2731.

Ebrahim, S., et al. 2000. Locomotor disability in a cohort of British men: The impact of lifestyle and disease. *International Journal of Epidemiology* 29: 478-486.

Fatouros, I.G., et al. 2002. The effects of strength training, cardiovascular training and their combination on flexibility of inactive older adults. *International Journal of Sports Medicine* 23(2): 112-119.

Fisher, K.L., et al. 2007. 50+ and motion: Class vs. home-based exercise intervention for older adults – a longitudinal study. *Applied Physiology, Nutrition, and Metabolism* 32(S1): S30.

Foldvari, M., et al. 2000. Association of muscle power with functional status in community dwelling elderly women. *Journals of Gerontology. Series A, Biological Sciences and Medical Sciences* 55(4): M192-M199.

Fried, L.P., K. Bandeen-Roche, P. Chaves, and B. Johnson. 2000. Preclinical mobility disability predicts incident ability disability in older women. *Journals of Gerontology. Series A, Biological Sciences and Medical Sciences* 55(1): M43-M52.

Fried, L.P., S.J. Herdman, K.E. Kuhn, G. Rubin, and K. Turano. 1991. Preclinical disability: Hypotheses about the bottom of the iceberg. *Journal of Aging and Health* 3(2): 285-300.

Fries, J.F. 2005. Measuring and monitoring success in compressing morbidity. *Annals of Internal Medicine* 139(5 pt 2): 455-459.

Fujiwara, K., et al. 2011. Effects of regular heel-raise training aimed at the soleus muscle on dynamic balance associated with arm movement in elderly women. *Journal of Strength and Conditioning Research* 25(9): 2605-2615.

Gill, T.M., and E.A. Gahbauer. 2008. Evaluating disability over discrete periods of time. *Journals of Gerontology. Series A, Biological Sciences and Medical Sciences* 63(6): 588-594.

Gill, T.M., C.S. Williams, and M.E. Tinetti. 1995. Assessing risk for the onset of functional dependence among older adults: The role of physical performance. *Journal of the American Geriatrics Society* 43(6): 603-609.

Girouard, C.K., and B. Hurley. 1995. Does strength training inhibit gains in range of motion from flexibility training in older adults? *Medicine and Science in Sports and Exercise* 27(10): 1444-1449.

Griffin, J.C. 2011a. Functional mobility screening in adults 50-70 years of age. Design principles and process. Unpublished paper. George Brown College, Ontario.

Griffin, J.C. 2011b. Functional mobility screening in adults 50-70 years of age: Content validity and intra- and inter-rater reliability. Unpublished paper. George Brown College, Ontario.

Griffin, J.C. 2012. Functional mobility screening in adults 50-70 years of age. *Journal on Active Aging* (January-February): 40-49.

Groessi, E.J., et al. 2009. A cost analysis of a physical activity intervention for older adults. *Journal of Physical Activity and Health* 6: 767-774.

Guralnik, J.M., L. Ferrucci, E.M. Simonsick, M.E. Salive, and R.B. Wallace. 1995. Lower-extremity function in persons over the age of 70 years as a predictor of subsequent disability. *New England Journal of Medicine* 332(9): 556-561.

Hall, K.S., and E. McAuley. 2011. Examining indirect associations between physical activity, function, and disability independent and assisted-living residents. *Journal of Physical Activity and Health* 8: 716-723.

Hallage, T., et al. 2010. The effects of 12 weeks of step aerobics training on functional fitness of elderly women. *Journal of Strength and Conditioning Research* 24(8): 2261-2266.

Hanson, E., et al. 2009. Effects of strength training on physical function: Influence of power, strength, and body composition. *Journal of Strength and Conditioning Research* 23(9): 2627-2637.

Harris-Hayes, M., S. Sahmann, B. Norton, and G. Salsich. 2008. Diagnosis and management of the patient with knee pain using the movement system impairment classification system. *Journal of Orthopaedic and Sports Physical Therapy* 38(4): 203-213.

Holviala, J., et al. 2006. Effects of strength training on muscle strength characteristics, functional capabilities, and balance in middle-aged and older women.

Journal of Strength and Conditioning Research 20(2): 336-344.

Holviala, J., et al. 2010. Effects of combined strength and endurance training on treadmill load carrying walking performance in aging men. *Journal of Strength and Conditioning Research* 24(6): 1584-1595.

Janssen, W., H. Bussmann, and H. Stam. 2002. Determinants of the sit-to-reach movement: A review. *Physical Therapy* 82(9): 866-879.

Jette, A.M., and P.D. Cleary. 1987. Functional disability assessment. *Physical Therapy* 67(12): 1854-1859.

Jones, J., and D. Rose. 2005. *Physical Activity Instruction of Older Adults.* Champaign, IL: Human Kinetics.

Levelle, S., and L. Iezzoni. 2004. Trends in obesity, arthritis, and mobility difficulty among baby-boomers and their predecessors from 1971 to 2000. *Gerontologist* 44(1): 39.

Lindstrom, P.J., J. Suni, and C-H. Nygard. 2009. Associations of leisure-time physical activity with balance and lower extremity strength: A validation of the neuromuscular part of the physical activity pie. *Journal of Physical Activity and Health* 6: 493-502.

Lopopolo, R., et al. 2006. Effect of therapeutic exercise on gait speed in community-dwelling elderly people: A meta-analysis. *Physical Therapy* 86(4): 520-540.

McGill, S.M., A. Childs, and C. Liebenson. 1999. Endurance times for low back stabilization exercises: Clinical targets for testing and training from a normal database. *Archives of Physical Medicine and Rehabilitation* 80: 941-944.

Milner, C. 2001. Expanding horizons. *Fitness Business Canada* (November): 38-39.

Minick, K.I., K.B. Kiesel, L. Burton, A. Taylor, P. Plisky, and R.J. Butler. 2010. Interrater reliability of the Functional Movement Screen. *Journal of Strength and Conditioning Research* 24(2): 479-486.

Moxley, C. 2012. Floor freedom: How to get up from the floor. *Functional U (ICAA)* 10(5): 1-10.

Murtagh, K.N., and H.B. Hubert. 2004. Gender differences in physical disability among an elderly cohort. *American Journal of Public Health* 94(8): 1406-1411.

Nagi, S.Z. 1991. Disability concepts revisited: Implications for prevention. In: *Disability in America: Toward a National Agenda for Prevention,* ed. A.M. Pope and A.R. Tarlov, 309-327. Washington, DC: National Academy Press.

Nashner, L.M. 2002. Maintaining safe balance and mobility: When is fitness enough and when is medical help needed? *Journal on Active Aging* (March-April): 31-34.

Okada, T., K. Huxel, and T. Nesser. 2011. Relationship between core stability, functional movement, and performance. *Journal of Strength and Conditioning Research* 25(1): 252-261.

Ostchega, Y., T.B. Harris, R. Hirsch, V.L. Parsons, and R. Kington. 2000. The prevalence of functional limitations and disability in older persons in the US: Data from the national health and nutrition examination survey III. *Journal of the American Geriatrics Society* 48(9): 1132-1135.

Paterson, D., and D. Warburton. 2010. Physical activity function limitations older adults: A systematic review related to Canada's Physical Activity Guidelines. *International Journal of Behavioral Nutrition and Physical Activity* 7: 38.

PEI Health and Community Services Agency. 1996. FACTS: what is the circle of health? www.circleofhealth.net [accessed March 8, 2014].

Pizzigalli, L., et al. 2011. Prevention of falling risk in elderly people: The relevance of muscular strength and symmetry of the lower limbs in postural stability. *Journal of Strength and Conditioning Research* 25(2): 567-574.

Reiman, M.P., and R.C. Manske. 2009. *Functional Testing in Human Performance.* Champaign, IL: Human Kinetics.

Rikli, R.E., and C.J. Jones. 1999a. Development and validation of a functional fitness test for community-residing older adults. *Journal of Aging and Physical Activity* 7: 129-161.

Rikli, R.E., and C.J. Jones. 1999b. Functional fitness normative scores for community-residing older adults, ages 60-94. *Journal of Aging and Physical Activity* 7: 162-181.

Rikli, R.E., and J. Jones. 2001. *Senior Fitness Test Manual.* Champaign, IL: Human Kinetics.

Robinovitch, S., et al. 2012. Video capture of the circumstances of falls in elderly people residing in long-term care: An observational study. *Lancet* 381(9860): 47-54.

Rogers, H.L., R. Cromwell, and J. Grady. 2008. Adaptive changes in gait of older and younger adults as responses to challenges to dynamic balance. *Journal of Aging and Physical Activity* 16: 85-96.

Rogers, M. 2003. Balance and bands. *Journal on Active Aging* (September-October): 24-32.

Rogers, M., and P. Page. 2004. What is functional movement? *Changing the Way We Age (ICAA)*: 8-10. Adapted from the lecture "Functional Resistance Training for Older Adults" presented at ICAA Active Aging, Orlando, 2004.

Saliba, D., et al. 2000. Identifying a short functional disability screen for older persons. *Journals of Gerontology. Series A, Biological Sciences and Medical Sciences* 55(12): M750-M756.

Signorile, J.F. 2011. *Bending the Aging Curve.* 2nd ed. Champaign, IL: Human Kinetics.

Simonsick, E.M., et al. 1993. Risk due to inactivity in physically capable older adults. *American Journal of Public Health* 83: 1443-1450.

Siu, A.L., D.B. Reuben, and R.D. Hays. 1990. Hierarchical measures of physical function in ambulatory geriatrics. *Journal of the American Geriatrics Society* 38(10): 1113-1119.

Spirduso, W.W., K. Francis, and P. MacRae. 2005. *Physical Dimensions of Aging.* Champaign, IL: Human Kinetics.

Strawbridge, W.J., M.I. Wallhagen, and R.D. Cohen. 2002. Successful aging and well-being: Self-rated compared with Rowe and Kahn. *Gerontologist* 42(6): 727-733.

Taylor, A.W., and M.J. Johnson. 2008. *Physiology of Exercise and Healthy Aging.* Champaign, IL: Human Kinetics.

Trudelle-Jackson, E.J., A. Jackson, and J. Morrow. 2006. Muscle strength and postural stability in healthy, older women: Implications for fall prevention. *Journal of Physical Activity and Health* 3: 292-303.

Van Dillen, L., et al. 2001. Effect of active limb movements on symptoms in patients with low back pain. *Journal of Orthopaedic and Sports Physical Therapy* 31(8): 402-418.

Waltz, C.W., and R.B. Bausell. 1981. *Nursing Research: Design, Statistics and Computer Analysis.* Philadelphia: Davis.

Weiss, C.O., L.P. Fried, and K. Bandeen-Roche. 2007. Exploring the hierarchy of mobility performance in high-functioning older women. *Journals of Gerontology. Series A, Biological Sciences and Medical Sciences* 62(2): 167-173.

Whitehurst, M.A., et al. 2005. The benefits of a functional exercise circuit for older adults. *Journal of Strength and Conditioning Research* 19(3): 647-651.

Index